Innovations and Applications of Advanced Biomaterials in Healthcare and Engineering

Safaa Najah Saud Al-Humairi
Management and Science University, Malaysia

Erkan Koç
Karabuk University, Turkey

Amir Najah Saud Al-Humairi
Al-Mustaqabal University, Iraq

IGI Global
Scientific Publishing
Publishing Tomorrow's Research Today

Vice President of Editorial Melissa Wagner
Director of Acquisitions Mikaela Felty
Director of Book Development Jocelynn Hessler
Production Manager Mike Brehm
Cover Design Phillip Shickler

Published in the United States of America by
IGI Global Scientific Publishing
701 East Chocolate Avenue
Hershey, PA, 17033, USA
Tel: 717-533-8845
Fax: 717-533-7115
Website: https://www.igi-global.com E-mail: cust@igi-global.com

Library of Congress Cataloging-in-Publication Data

Names: Al-Humairi, Safaa, 1985- editor | Koç, Erkan, 1981- editor | Al-Humairi, Amir Najah Saud, 1993- editor
Title: Innovations and applications of advanced biomaterials in healthcare and engineering / edited by Safaa Al-Humairi, Erkan Koç, Amir Najah Al-Humairi.
Description: Hershey, PA : Engineering Science Reference, [2025] | Includes bibliographical references and index. | Summary: "The books' main objective is to provide comprehensive overview of the latest advancements and practical applications of biomaterials in these critical fields"-- Provided by publisher.
Identifiers: LCCN 2025004544 (print) | LCCN 2025004545 (ebook) | ISBN 9798337313054 hardback | ISBN 9798337313061 paperback | ISBN 9798337313078 ebook
Subjects: LCSH: Biomedical materials | Medical innovations | Biomedical engineering--Technological innovations
Classification: LCC R857.M3 I465 2025 (print) | LCC R857.M3 (ebook)
LC record available at https://lccn.loc.gov/2025004544
LC ebook record available at https://lccn.loc.gov/2025004545
British Cataloguing in Publication Data
A Cataloguing in Publication record for this book is available from the British Library.

This book is dedicated to the ones who inspire us daily with their unwavering love, encouragement, and support—our families, who have been the foundation of our strength and perseverance.

To my beloved wife, *Hanaa*, and my dear son, *Rayyan*, whose love, patience, and unwavering belief in me have been my guiding light throughout this journey. Your presence fills my life with joy and purpose, and I am forever grateful for your sacrifices and understanding. This work is as much yours as it is mine, and I dedicate it to you with all my love.

To my co-editor, Associate Professor Dr. *Erkan Koç*, whose dedication, expertise, and collaborative spirit have been instrumental in bringing this project to fruition. Your passion for advancing science and your tireless commitment to excellence continues to inspire us all.

To my co-editor, Dr. *Amir Najah Saud Al-Humairi*, whose vision, resilience, and scholarly contributions have enriched this book immeasurably. Your hard work and determination serve as a testament to the power of collaboration and shared goals.

We also dedicate this work to our parents, siblings, and extended families, whose constant encouragement and sacrifices have shaped us into who we are today. Your love has been the bedrock upon which we have built our careers and pursued our dreams.

Finally, to all those who believe in the transformative power of biomaterials to shape a healthier, more sustainable future—this book is for you. Together, may we continue to inspire innovation, foster collaboration, and leave a lasting impact on science and society.

This book is dedicated to you.

Table of Contents

Detailed Table of Contents

The impact of nanomaterials in healthcare has been transformative. In drug delivery, they enable targeted therapeutic delivery, improved drug solubility, and controlled release profiles, significantly enhancing treatment efficacy while reducing side effects. In tissue engineering, nanomaterial scaffolds provide ideal environments for cell growth and tissue regeneration, mimicking natural extracellular matrix structures. Diagnostic imaging has benefited from nanomaterial-based contrast agents that offer enhanced sensitivity and multimodal imaging capabilities. Their small size allows them to interact with cellular components, while their high surface area provides platforms for functionalization with targeting molecules, drugs, or imaging agents. The chapter discusses the ability to engineer these materials with specific surface properties for biomedical applications. It presents a comprehensive review of classification, properties, synthesis techniques, characterization techniques and applications of nanoparticles and nanofibers.

Biomaterials have attracted growing interest in the biomedical field thanks to their unique ability to interact with biological systems and make a significant contribution to advances in medicine, tissue engineering and sustainable technologies. Their importance lies in their dual potential: improving patients' quality of life while reducing their impact on the environment. This chapter first presents a detailed classification of biomaterials, distinguishing between natural, synthetic and hybrid categories. Next, the key properties of biomaterials are explored, showing their role in biocompatibility, durability and clinical performance. These fundamental characteristics directly influence the choice of biomaterials for a variety of applications. In addition, this chapter highlights the diversity of current biomaterial applications, while discussing the persistent challenges and limitations encountered in their design and use. Finally, future prospects are discussed, including the emergence of personalized biomaterials, which could revolutionize biomedical technologies.

Nanoparticle synthesis has gained significant interest over the years because of its unique characteristics and sustainable and productive applications in numerous fields. Metals exhibiting a friend-foe relationship with bacteria, possess the potential to inhibit their growth in specific forms and concentrations. The increase in antimicrobial resistance in recent years has drawn attention. Top-down and Bottom-up are the two approaches to metal nanoparticle synthesis. Gold, silver, copper, etc. have been used in medical fields from ancient times. Although these conventional methods of creating nanoparticles are effective and adaptable, they have very negative effects. On the other hand, green synthesis provides an economical and environmentally beneficial substitute by using natural resources. To address the current problem of antimicrobial resistance, this review highlights the antimicrobial activity of metal

regeneration, which makes them useful in regenerative medicine, drug delivery systems, and temporary medical implants. This chapter includes biodegradable engineering and dental care materials, representing new and sustainable options for temporary and permanent implants. Nanocomposites doped with nanoparticles such as hydroxyapatite and bioactive glasses can improve mechanical strength, biocompatibility, and bioactivity, proving more prominent in dental implants, as integration with the tissue is crucial here. Continued study is positioning such materials to dramatically change how sustainable and effective dental care is achieved, marrying the clinician's needs with the demands of environmental stewardship.

The intrinsic immune system activity awakens and trains the patient's immune system to destroy tumor cells. Immunotherapy has become a standard method for treating cancer since it is a more potent and secure option than conventional therapies like surgery, radiotherapy, and chemotherapy. Chimeric antigen receptor-modified T cells, immune checkpoint blockades, and cancer vaccines are the three primary forms of cancer immunotherapy that have been developed recently. Chemotherapy, radiation therapy, and surgery continue to be the mainstays of cancer treatment despite decades of advancements. Lung cancer, melanoma, advanced bladder, kidney, and other advanced tumors have all been successfully treated with immunotherapy. Immunotherapy is used to cure illnesses by regulating an overactive or underactive immune system. Biomaterials efficiency will be increased with the help of immune system engineering and targeted drug delivery. Chapter highlights the recent advancement in tailored biomaterials for cancer immunotherapy.

Tissue engineering, stem cells, and cloning are just a few of the technological fields that falls under regenerative medicine. Tissue engineering techniques utilize the cellular matrices, which rely on the body's inherent capacity for regeneration to ensure that new tissue growth is properly oriented and directed, and the use of matrices containing cells. Biomaterials give cells a three-dimensional environment in which to develop into new tissues with the right structure and function. They can also facilitate the distribution of cells and the right bioactive substances, such as growth factors and cell adhesion peptides, to the body's intended locations. Current regulations and ethical considerations advise that before a novel tissue engineering and regenerative medicine technique or instrument is implemented into standard clinical practice and used by numerous patients, controlled randomized clinical trials must be carried out. Clinical studies involving regeneration treatments have revealed some restrictions, difficulties, and unknowns.

Recently, Tissue engineering (TE) has been rapidly growing field in biomedical field, it provides the solutions to the problem such as immunological rejection and

chapter concludes with recommendations for optimizing biocomposite processes and informed material selection to improve their sustainability.

Girish Sharma, Amity University, Noida, India
Anusha Mittal, Amity University, Noida, India
Tejasvi Batra, Amity University, Noida, India
Jasmine Kaur, Amity University, Noida, India
Banashree Bandhopadhyay, Amity University, Noida, India

Despite the widespread use of traditional cancer therapies such as surgery, chemotherapy, and radiation, these approaches often suffer from significant drawbacks. Nanomaterials (NMs) are a promising alternative due to their distinct nanoscale properties which enable more precise drug delivery and reduced off-target effects. Recently, cuproptosis and ferroptosis have emerged as novel forms of programmed cell death regulated by metal ions, offering novel pathways for cancer therapy. Cuproptosis, caused by copper ion accumulation, leads to mitochondrial dysfunction, while ferroptosis, driven by iron-mediated lipid peroxidation, disrupts cellular integrity through oxidative stress. Here, we propose to explore how NMs can be harnessed to induce metalloptosis, for advanced cancer treatment strategies. Variations in NM size, morphology, and the synergistic effects of composite NMs complicate the identification of individual mechanisms. Use of NMs in cancer therapy, requires focusing on the precise design and regulation of metalloptosis pathways.

Imade Armadi, Cadi Ayyad University, Marrakech, Morocco
Abdessamad Abana, Cadi Ayyad University, Marrakech, Morocco
Youssef Ait Hamdan, Cadi Ayyad University, Marrakech, Morocco
Souad Loqman, Cadi Ayyad University, Marrakech, Morocco
Anass Belbachir, Cadi Ayyad University, Marrakech, Morocco

The application of biomaterials in the biomedical field represents a major advancement, offering effective and sustainable alternative solutions. These materials stand out for their unique properties, particularly their biocompatibility and biodegradability. However, the choice between animal or non-animal sources constitutes a primary challenge, directly influencing their use and effectiveness in various contexts. This chapter offers a comparative analysis of biomaterials of animal and non-animal origin, highlighting their distinct properties and adaptability to biomedical applications, while mentioning the limitations of each type of source. This multidimensional

Preface

INTRODUCTION

The field of biomaterials has witnessed unprecedented growth and innovation over the past few decades, revolutionizing healthcare, engineering, and technology. As we continue to push the boundaries of science and medicine, advanced biomaterials have emerged as a cornerstone of modern solutions, bridging the gap between fundamental research and practical applications. This book, *Advanced Biomaterials: Innovations and Applications in Healthcare and Engineering*, aims to provide a comprehensive exploration of the latest advancements in biomaterials, offering insights into their design, properties, and transformative applications across diverse domains.

Biomaterials are at the heart of numerous breakthroughs, from tissue engineering and regenerative medicine to drug delivery systems and medical implants. Their unique ability to interact with biological systems while maintaining biocompatibility and functionality has positioned them as critical tools in addressing some of the most pressing challenges in healthcare and engineering. This book delves into the intricate interplay between material science, biology, and engineering, highlighting how these disciplines converge to drive innovation.

Structured into thematic sections, this publication covers a wide spectrum of topics, ranging from biomaterials fundamentals to cutting-edge trends such as smart materials, additive manufacturing, and nanotechnology. Each chapter is meticulously crafted to provide foundational knowledge and advanced insights, ensuring that readers understand the subject holistically. Real-world case studies and practical examples are integrated throughout the text to bridge theoretical concepts with tangible outcomes, making it a valuable resource for researchers, engineers, educators, and clinicians.

The chapters included in this book span a variety of critical areas, including the role of nanomaterials in biomedical applications, sustainable and eco-friendly innovations, 3D-printed scaffolds for tissue regeneration, and strategies to overcome multidrug resistance in cancer therapy. Additionally, the book explores the environmental impacts of biomaterials through life cycle assessments and offers comparative insights into animal-based and non-animal sources of biomaterials. These diverse topics reflect the interdisciplinary nature of biomaterials research and underscore their potential to address global challenges in healthcare, sustainability, and technology.

This book is designed to cater to a broad audience, including academics, researchers, industry professionals, and students. For academics and researchers, it serves as a consolidated reference, offering both foundational principles and the latest advancements in biomaterials. Industry professionals will find practical guidance on integrating biomaterials into medical devices, implants, and other innovative solutions, aligning with current standards and emerging technologies. Educators and students will benefit from the systematic approach, which balances theory with real-world applications, making it an ideal teaching and learning resource. Clinicians and healthcare innovators will discover how biomaterials can enhance patient outcomes and advance treatment methodologies, fostering collaboration across academic, industrial, and clinical domains.

As editors, we are deeply grateful to the contributing authors whose expertise and dedication have made this publication possible. Their collective efforts have resulted in a work that reflects the current state of the art and inspires future directions in biomaterials research and application. This book will serve as a catalyst for innovation, encouraging readers to explore new possibilities and contribute to the ongoing evolution of this dynamic field.

It is our sincere belief that *Advanced Biomaterials: Innovations and Applications in Healthcare and Engineering* will inspire collaboration, spark creativity, and pave the way for transformative solutions in healthcare and beyond. We invite you to embark on this journey of discovery and innovation, as we collectively shape the future of biomaterials and their impact on society.

ORGANIZATION OF THE BOOK

In this volume, we delve into the frontier of biomedical innovation where nanomaterials, biomaterials, and regenerative medicine converge to redefine modern healthcare. **Chapter 1** lays the foundation by exploring the transformative role of nanomaterials—particularly nanoparticles and nanofibers—in biomedical applications. This chapter emphasizes their critical role in targeted drug delivery, tissue engineering, and diagnostic imaging, while also detailing the classification, synthesis, and characterization techniques pivotal to their application.

Expanding on the material-science perspective, **Chapter 2** offers a comprehensive overview of biomaterials, classifying them into natural, synthetic, and hybrid forms. It thoroughly examines their properties in relation to biocompatibility and durability, underscoring their significance in clinical applications and highlighting emerging trends such as personalized biomaterials that promise to reshape the future of medicine.

Addressing the urgent issue of antimicrobial resistance, **Chapter 3** focuses on the synthesis and antimicrobial applications of metal nanoparticles. It provides insight into both conventional and green synthesis methods, advocating for sustainable and safe practices while revealing the potent antibacterial properties of metals like silver and copper.

In **Chapter 4**, we shift to an interdisciplinary approach that integrates molecular science and environmental responsibility. This chapter champions sustainable nanomaterials for green healthcare, linking molecular mechanisms to pressing global issues such as climate change and waste management, and emphasizing a research-driven, educational model that fosters real-world problem-solving.

Turning to dentistry and engineering, **Chapter 5** explores biodegradable materials and their pivotal role in creating sustainable medical solutions. It discusses how nanocomposites and bioactive fillers are transforming dental implants and medical devices, promoting not only functional integration with biological tissues but also eco-conscious innovation.

Chapter 6 investigates the burgeoning field of cancer immunotherapy, highlighting the synergy between biomaterials and immune engineering. By enhancing targeted drug delivery and immunomodulation, biomaterials are instrumental in advancing therapies such as CAR-T cells, checkpoint inhibitors, and cancer vaccines.

The intersection of additive manufacturing and regenerative medicine is thoroughly examined in **Chapter 7**, which explores metallic 3D-printed scaffolds with functional coatings. These bioactive and antibacterial surfaces represent a breakthrough in tissue regeneration, offering customized, robust solutions for orthopedic and dental applications.

In **Chapter 8**, we turn our attention to chronic wound healing and tissue repair. This chapter surveys recent technological innovations—ranging from self-healing hydrogels to wearable sensors and gene therapies—that are revolutionizing wound management and improving patient outcomes through advanced biomaterials and devices.

Chapter 9 expands the discussion into the broader realm of regenerative medicine and tissue engineering. Highlighting the role of biomaterials in delivering bioactive substances and creating supportive cellular environments, this chapter also engages with the regulatory and ethical complexities surrounding clinical implementation.

Continuing the exploration of regenerative strategies, **Chapter 10** focuses on scaffold design for tissue engineering. Here, we examine how advances in nanotechnology and artificial intelligence are addressing key limitations such as vascularization and immune compatibility, setting the stage for highly functional, scalable therapeutic platforms.

In **Chapter 11**, the role of biomaterials in wound healing is revisited with greater depth. This chapter outlines how natural and synthetic polymers—enhanced with bioactive agents—create optimal environments for tissue regeneration while addressing challenges in scalability and biocompatibility.

Chapter 12 introduces a novel paradigm in cancer treatment through nano-engineered therapies designed to overcome multidrug resistance in breast cancer. By leveraging nanoparticles for precise drug delivery and genetic modulation, this chapter exemplifies how cutting-edge nanomedicine can disrupt traditional treatment limitations and pave the way for personalized oncology.

Chapter 13 delves into the growing emphasis on sustainability and the circular economy, illustrating how biocomposites are environmentally friendly alternatives to traditional materials. By applying Life Cycle Assessment (LCA), the chapter evaluates the environmental performance of biocomposites across various system boundaries, shedding light on their ecological footprints at different life cycle stages. It highlights the challenges and methodological considerations in conducting LCA while demonstrating its critical role in guiding sustainable material design and policymaking. The chapter compares biocomposites with conventional materials through case studies, showcasing their potential to reduce environmental impacts.

Chapter 14 delves into the limitations of traditional cancer therapies such as surgery, chemotherapy, and radiation, which often result in significant side effects. The chapter highlights the potential of nanomaterials (NMs) to revolutionize cancer treatment through precise drug delivery and reduced off-target impacts. It examines novel programmed cell death mechanisms, including cuproptosis, triggered by copper-induced mitochondrial dysfunction, and ferroptosis, driven by iron-mediated oxidative stress. The chapter provides insights into advanced cancer therapy strategies by exploring how NMs can be engineered to target these metalloptosis pathways. Challenges related to NM size, morphology, and composite synergies are discussed, emphasizing the need for precise design and regulation. Ultimately, this chapter underscores the transformative role of nanomaterials in advancing targeted and effective cancer treatments.

Finally, **Chapter 15** explores the pivotal role of biomaterials in advancing biomedical solutions, emphasizing their biocompatibility and biodegradability. The chapter addresses the critical challenge of selecting between animal-based and non-animal sources, significantly impacting the materials' suitability and performance in diverse applications. A comparative analysis examines the unique properties and adaptability of biomaterials derived from both sources while discussing their limitations. This multidimensional evaluation provides a framework for selecting biomaterials tailored to specific biomedical needs. Additionally, the chapter highlights opportunities for developing hybrid or alternative materials that can overcome existing constraints, paving the way for more effective and sustainable innovations in the field.

Together, these chapters illustrate a multidisciplinary journey through the evolving landscape of biomedical science—where sustainability, technology, and biology intersect to offer visionary solutions for global health challenges.

CONCLUSION

The exploration of advanced biomaterials has fundamentally transformed the landscape of healthcare, engineering, and technology. As we conclude this book, *Advanced Biomaterials: Innovations and Applications in Healthcare and Engineering*, it is evident that biomaterials are not merely tools or components but enablers of revolutionary solutions that address some of the most pressing challenges in modern science and society. From tissue engineering and regenerative medicine to drug delivery systems and sustainable innovations, biomaterials have demonstrated their unparalleled potential to bridge the gap between fundamental research and real-world applications.

Throughout this book, we have traversed a diverse array of topics, ranging from the fundamentals of biomaterial classification and properties to cutting-edge advancements in nanotechnology, 3D printing, and smart materials. The chapters collectively underscore the interdisciplinary nature of biomaterials research, highlighting how material science, biology, engineering, and clinical practice converge to drive innovation. By integrating theoretical insights with practical case studies, this publication has sought a comprehensive understanding of how biomaterials can be designed, optimized, and applied to improve human health, enhance sustainability, and advance technological frontiers.

One of the key takeaways from this book is the versatility of biomaterials. Whether derived from animal or non-animal sources, fabricated through additive manufacturing, or engineered at the nanoscale, biomaterials offer tailored solutions for specific biomedical and engineering challenges. Their ability to mimic natural tissues, deliver therapeutics precisely, and promote healing underscores their critical role in advancing patient care. Moreover, the growing emphasis on sustainability and eco-friendly innovations reflects the scientific community's responsibility to develop materials that not only benefit humanity but also minimize environmental impact.

However, as we celebrate these achievements, it is vital to acknowledge the remaining challenges. The complexity of designing biocompatible and biodegradable materials, ensuring scalability for industrial applications, and addressing regulatory hurdles are just a few of the obstacles that researchers and engineers must navigate. Furthermore, integrating emerging technologies such as artificial intelligence, machine learning, and advanced imaging into biomaterials development presents opportunities and challenges that warrant further investigation.

Looking ahead, the future of biomaterials lies in fostering collaboration across disciplines and industries. By bringing together material scientists, biomedical engineers, clinicians, and industry professionals, we can translate laboratory discoveries into clinical and commercial applications. Hybrid materials, bioinspired designs, and multifunctional platforms represent promising avenues for further exploration, offering the potential to overcome current limitations and unlock new possibilities.

In closing, *Advanced Biomaterials: Innovations and Applications in Healthcare and Engineering reflects* the progress made in this dynamic field and a call to action for continued innovation. As researchers, educators, clinicians, and industry leaders, we share a collective responsibility to push the boundaries of what is possible, ensuring that biomaterials play a pivotal role in shaping a healthier, more sustainable, and technologically advanced future. We hope this book inspires readers to contribute to this exciting journey, driving transformative change and leaving a lasting impact on science and society.

Acknowledgments

We are deeply grateful to all the contributors, researchers, and institutions whose dedication and expertise have made this book, *Innovations and Applications of Advanced Biomaterials in Healthcare and Engineering*, a reality. This compilation reflects the collective effort of numerous scholars and professionals who are at the forefront of advancing biomaterials research and its transformative applications in healthcare and engineering.

Our heartfelt thanks go to the authors of each chapter, whose insightful contributions have enriched the content of this book. Their commitment to sharing cutting-edge knowledge and innovative ideas has been instrumental in addressing the complex challenges faced in these dynamic fields. Special appreciation is extended to the universities, research centers, and organizations that supported the work of these esteemed contributors.

We would also like to acknowledge the editorial team and technical staff who worked tirelessly behind the scenes to ensure this publication's accuracy, coherence, and quality. Their meticulous efforts in organizing, reviewing, and refining the manuscript have been invaluable.

Finally, we extend our gratitude to the global scientific community for their continued pursuit of excellence and innovation. Through collaborative endeavors and shared knowledge, advancements in biomaterials are being realized, ultimately benefiting humanity and shaping the future of healthcare and engineering.

This book stands as a testament to what can be achieved when brilliant minds come together with a common purpose. Thank you to everyone who has played a role in bringing this vision to life.

The Editors

Introduction

In an era defined by rapid technological advancements and an ever-growing demand for sustainable, innovative solutions, the field of biomaterials stands at the forefront of transformative progress. Biomaterials have emerged as a cornerstone of modern science, bridging disciplines such as biology, engineering, medicine, and environmental sustainability to address some of the most pressing challenges of our time. From revolutionizing healthcare through regenerative medicine and drug delivery systems to fostering eco-friendly innovations in materials science, the potential applications of biomaterials are vast and far-reaching.

It is with great enthusiasm that I introduce *Advanced Biomaterials: Innovations and Applications in Healthcare and Engineering*, a comprehensive and timely contribution to this dynamic field. This book represents a remarkable synthesis of foundational principles and cutting-edge research, offering readers a deep dive into the design, properties, and applications of advanced biomaterials. Its carefully curated chapters span a wide array of topics, from nanotechnology and 3D printing to biocompatibility, tissue engineering, and sustainable materials, reflecting the interdisciplinary nature of biomaterials research.

What sets this book apart is its ability to seamlessly integrate theoretical insights with practical applications. Each chapter not only delves into the scientific underpinnings of biomaterials but also highlights real-world case studies and innovative solutions that demonstrate their transformative impact. The inclusion of emerging trends such as smart materials, additive manufacturing, and metalloptosis-targeted therapies underscores the forward-thinking approach of the editors and contributing authors. Moreover, the emphasis on sustainability and eco-friendly innovations aligns perfectly with the global imperative to develop technologies that benefit humanity while safeguarding our planet.

As we face unprecedented challenges in healthcare, environmental sustainability, and technological innovation, the role of biomaterials becomes increasingly critical. This book not only provides a comprehensive overview of current advancements but also inspires readers to envision new possibilities and contribute to the ongoing evolution of this vital discipline. It is my hope that *Advanced Biomaterials: Innovations and Applications in Healthcare and Engineering* will spark curiosity, foster collaboration, and catalyze groundbreaking discoveries that improve lives and shape a brighter future for generations to come.

I commend the editors and authors for their outstanding work and extend my gratitude to them for sharing their invaluable insights with the global scientific community. May this book serve as both a guide and an inspiration for all who seek to harness the power of biomaterials to transform healthcare, engineering, and society at large.

Chapter 1
Nanomaterials:
Nanoparticles, Nanofibers, and their Biomedical Applications

Himani Shukla
School of Basic and Applied Sciences, K.R. Mangalam University, Gurugram, India

Neeraj Kumari
School of Basic and Applied Sciences, K.R. Mangalam University, Gurugram, India

Rajni Gautam
https://orcid.org/0000-0003-0825-629X
School of Basic and Applied Sciences, K.R. Mangalam University, Gurugram, India

ABSTRACT

The impact of nanomaterials in healthcare has been transformative. In drug delivery, they enable targeted therapeutic delivery, improved drug solubility, and controlled release profiles, significantly enhancing treatment efficacy while reducing side effects. In tissue engineering, nanomaterial scaffolds provide ideal environments for cell growth and tissue regeneration, mimicking natural extracellular matrix structures. Diagnostic imaging has benefited from nanomaterial-based contrast agents that offer enhanced sensitivity and multimodal imaging capabilities. Their small size allows them to interact with cellular components, while their high surface area provides platforms for functionalization with targeting molecules, drugs, or imaging agents. The chapter discusses the ability to engineer these materials with specific surface properties for biomedical applications. It presents a comprehensive review of classification, properties, synthesis techniques, characterization techniques and applications of nanoparticles and nanofibers.

DOI: 10.4018/979-8-3373-1305-4.ch001

1. INTRODUCTION TO NANOMATERIALS

Nanomaterials have revolutionized modern science and technology through their unique properties at the nanoscale (1-100 nm). Because of their extremely high surface-to-volume ratio and properties of quantum effects, these nanoscale structures differ from bulk materials in their physical, chemical, and biological properties (Fu, 2024). Their capacity to be precisely manipulated in terms of composition, size, and shape has led to significant developments in a few domains, most notably biomedical applications. Advances in synthesis methods, better characterisation tools, and a better knowledge of how these materials interact with biological systems are all responsible for the exponential increase in nanomaterial research and development over the past few decades. Unprecedented control over the characteristics and behaviours of materials has been made possible by the capacity to change them at the molecular level. Because of this control over elements like tissue integration, drug release kinetics, and imaging contrast enhancement, nanomaterials are very useful in healthcare applications (Arif, 2024). Two basic types of nanomaterials that have demonstrated remarkable potential in biomedicine are nanoparticles and nanofibers. Applications requiring targeted administration and cellular penetration are well suited for nanoparticles, which are often spherical or almost spherical in shape. Nanofibers are extremely useful in tissue engineering and wound healing applications because of their high aspect ratio and linked structure. Numerous techniques, including as chemical, physical, and biological approaches, can be used to synthesize both groups; each has unique benefits and drawbacks (Goyal, 2016).

Nanomaterials have had a revolutionary effect on healthcare. They greatly increase treatment efficacy while lowering negative effects by enabling focused therapeutic delivery, enhanced drug solubility, and controlled release profiles in medication delivery. By simulating natural extracellular matrix architecture, nanomaterial scaffolds in tissue engineering offer optimal conditions for cell proliferation and tissue regeneration. Nanomaterial-based contrast agents, which provide improved sensitivity and multimodal imaging capabilities, have helped diagnostic imaging (Kurul, 2025). The molecular characteristics of nanomaterials have made it possible to manipulate biological interactions in a way that has never been possible before. They can interact with biological components due to their small size, and they can be functionalized with medicines, imaging agents, or targeting molecules thanks to their large surface area. The capacity to design these materials with certain surface characteristics guarantees that they are compatible with biological systems while preserving their functional capacities (Zhang, 2012). With new developments in smart nanomaterials that react to stimuli, enhanced targeting techniques, and the creation of theragnostic platforms that combine therapeutic and diagnostic capabilities, the area is still developing. Enhancing safety profiles, creating green synthesis techniques, and increasing scalability for commercial applications are the main goals of research. These developments point to an exciting future for nanomaterials in biomedicine, with potential uses that go beyond what is now possible (Sun, 2023).

Figure 1. Graph representing Number of publications of synthesized nanomaterial for biomedical application from year 2011 to 2024 (Machtakova, 2022) (Sanchez-Lopez., 2020)' (Hasan, 2018) (Niculescu & Grumezescu, 2022) (Nune, 2009)

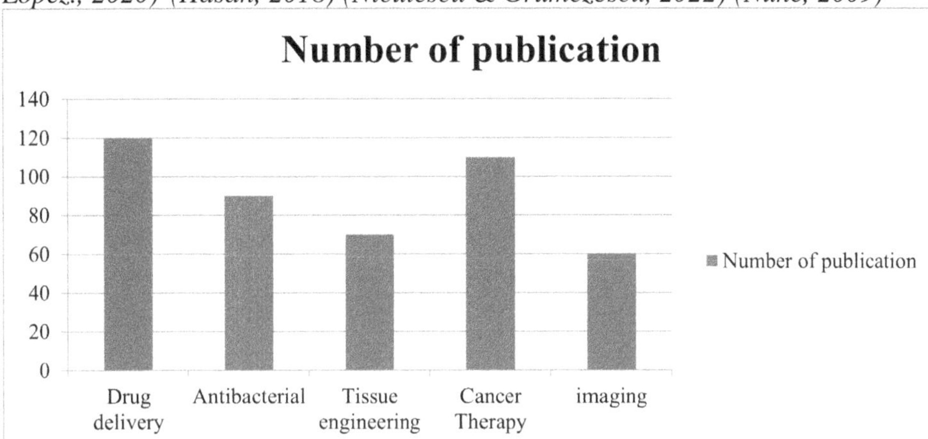

2. NANOPARTICLES: SYNTHESIS AND CLASSIFICATIONS

Nanoparticles are small and due to their incredibly small sizes from one to hundred nanometres in at least one-dimension nanoparticles found a special class of materials. When compared to bulk materials, their properties (physical and chemical) are fundamentally altered by this nanoscale dimension. Because a greater percentage of atoms are exposed on the surface, the sharply increased surface area to volume ratio of nanoparticles results in noticeably higher chemical reactivity and catalytic behaviour (Raut, 2024). These particles' interactions with light, electricity, and magnetic fields are drastically changed at the nanoscale by the dominance of quantum phenomena. These quantum events produce special optical characteristics that can be used for a variety of purposes, such as size-dependent colour changes in metallic nanoparticles and unique electronic behaviours. Superparamagnetic magnetic nanoparticles are those that get substantially magnetized in an external magnetic field but lose all their magnetism when the field is removed (Mimona, 2025). Nanoparticles' high surface energy and huge surface area contribute to their great chemical reactivity. Their increased reactivity makes them useful in a range of industrial and medicinal applications by facilitating more effective catalysis and chemical transformations. To avoid unintended aggregation or reactions, this same feature also necessitates careful surface modification and stabilization. The tiny size of nanoparticles in biological systems allows for special cellular and molecular interactions (Rathod, 2024). Through a variety of methods, they can enter cells, interact with cell membranes, and transcend biological barriers. They are very useful for drug administration, imaging, and therapeutic applications because of their altered biological interactions, but their biological safety and possible toxicity must also be carefully assessed.

Numerous applications in electronics, energy, health, and environmental cleanup have resulted from the combination of these unique qualities, which include improved reactivity, biological interactions, and quantum effects. As scientists create new techniques to create, describe, and work with nanoparticles, these uses (Figure 2) keep growing with ever-increasing control over their size, shape (Figure 3), and surface chemistry (Shelesh Krishna Saraswat, 2024).

Figure 2. Applications of nanomaterials

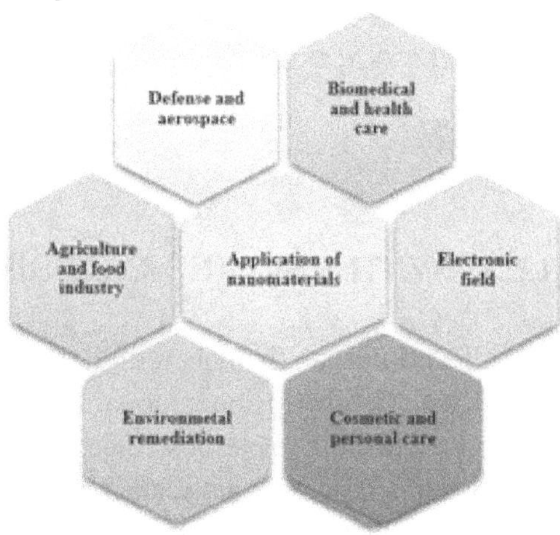

Figure 3. Different types of nanoparticles

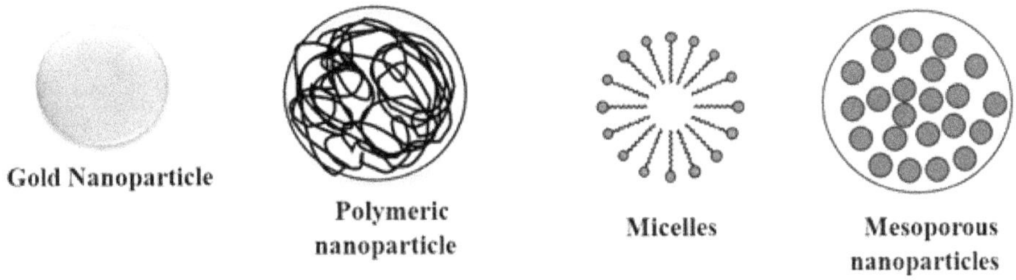

2.1 Classification of Nanoparticles

2.1.1 Organic Nanoparticles

Organic nanoparticles are tiny particles made only of organic compounds, usually with a size in nanometres. Lipids, polymers, and carbon-based materials are only a few examples of the variety of these molecules.

These nanoparticles are intriguing prospects for a variety of applications in medicine, cosmetics, and other sectors because of their special qualities, which include their small size, huge surface area, and capacity to be functionalized with certain molecules (Mirsasaani, 2019).

Classification of organic nanoparticles based on structure:

(a) **Liposomes:** Liposomes (Figure 4), which are spherical vesicles made of a phospholipid bilayer, are a good example. Liposomes are very biocompatible because of this bilayer, which resembles the structure of cell membranes. They may contain a range of substances at their core, such as drugs, genes, and imaging agents. This encapsulation allows for tailored distribution to tissues or cells while protecting the cargo from degradation. Liposomes, for example, can be engineered to selectively target cancer cells, delivering chemotherapeutic medications to the tumour with the least number of adverse effects on healthy organs (Nakhaei, 2021).

Figure 4. Liposomes (Liposomes, n.d.)

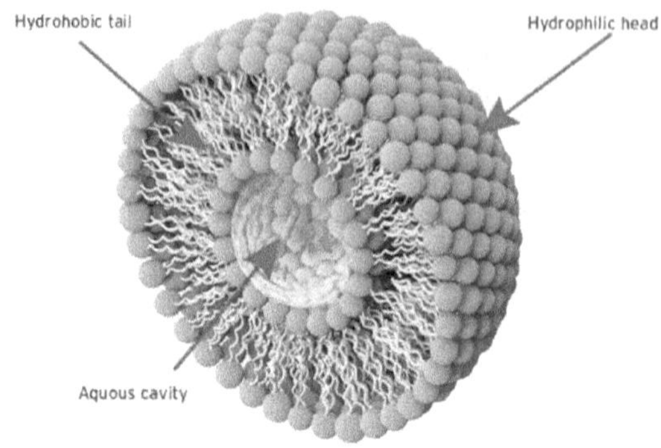

(b) **Micelles:** Micelles (Figure 5) that are created when amphiphilic molecules self-assemble frequently have diameters in the nanoscale range. Because of their small size, micelles have unique properties that set them apart from nanoparticles, such as a larger surface area-to-volume ratio and increased solubility. Like other nanoparticles, they are used in medication delivery applications where their small size enables more effective tissue penetration and tailored distribution (Ghezzi, 2021).

Figure 5. Micelles

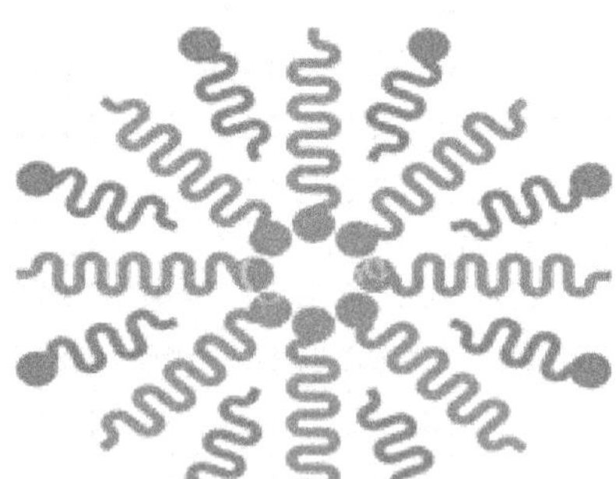

(c) **Dendrimers:** These are the kinds of nanoparticles that have a well-defined molecular weight and size and have extremely branching, tree-like architectures. Like other nanoparticles, dendrimers are employed in drug delivery because to their unique structure and small size, which allow for controlled release, targeted administration, and enhanced drug loading (Mittal, 2021).

(d) **Polymeric Nanoparticles:** One type of nanoparticle made completely of polymers is called a polymeric nanoparticle (Figure 6). These polymers may be manufactured or natural, biodegradable or not. In contrast to dendrimers, which have extremely branched, tree-like structures, or micelles, which self-assemble from amphiphilic molecules, polymeric nanoparticles are created via a variety of methods, including solvent evaporation, emulsion, and polymerization. Numerous polymers utilized in the creation of nanoparticles are biocompatible and biodegradable, reducing the possibility of toxicity (Han, 2023).

Figure 6. Polymeric nanoparticles

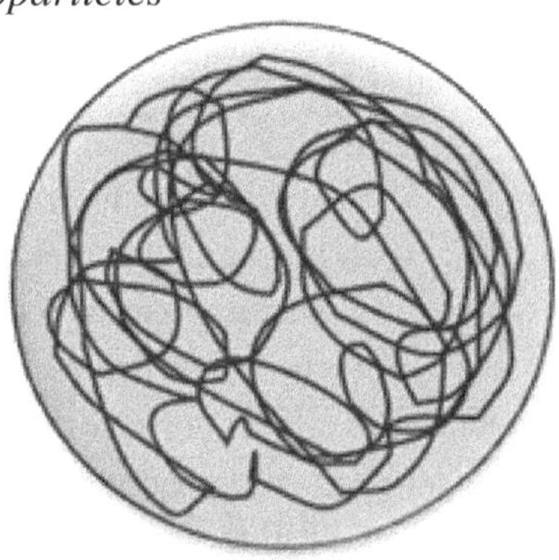

Classification of nanoparticles based on composition:

(a) **Lipid-based:** A class of organic nanoparticles known as "lipid-based nanoparticles" is made up mainly of lipids, including cholesterol, triglycerides, and phospholipids. Lipid-based nanoparticles take advantage of the biocompatibility and intrinsic qualities of lipids, in contrast to polymeric nanoparticles, which use natural or synthesized polymers as their main building element. Natural compounds found in biological systems, lipids frequently have strong biodegradability and low toxicity. Many lipid-based nanoparticles have a lipid bilayer shape that resembles biological membranes, improving their ability to interact with tissues and cells (Mehta, 2023).

(b) **Polymer-based:** One type of nanoparticle made completely of polymers is called a polymeric nanoparticle. These polymers may be manufactured or natural, biodegradable or not. Polymeric nanoparticles provide a greater variety of material options for customization than lipid-based nanoparticles, which mainly use lipids as their building components (Tivadar Feczkó, 2021).
(c) **Carbon-based:** A special class of nanoparticles made up only of carbon atoms are known as carbon-based nanoparticles. Because carbon bonding is so diverse, carbon-based nanoparticles have remarkable features in contrast to lipid-based or polymeric nanoparticles, which depend on organic molecules other than carbon. Incorporate fullerenes, graphene, and carbon nanotubes, which are renowned for their remarkable mechanical, electrical, and thermal characteristics (Rodoshi Khan & Bin Rashid, 2024).

2.1.2 Inorganic Nanoparticles

Inorganic nanoparticles are extremely small particles made of elements other than carbon, usually with a size range of one to hundred nanometres. Because of their nanoscale size, these materials have special and frequently better qualities than their bulk counterparts.

Gold nanoparticles, which have been well researched for their many uses, are a good example. They can absorb and scatter light at wavelengths because to their special optical characteristics, which are referred to as surface plasmon resonance. They are useful for biosensing, imaging, and photothermal treatment applications because of this characteristic. To target certain cancer cells, for example, gold nanoparticles can be coupled with antibodies. When the nanoparticles are exposed to near-infrared light, they absorb it, produce heat, and kill the targeted cells (Hassan, 2022).

Key characteristics of inorganic nanoparticles:

- **Size:** incredibly tiny; measured in billionths of a meter, or nanometres.
- **Composition:** composed of inorganic substances or elements, including semiconductors, metals, and metal oxides.
- **Structure:** can be spheres, rods, or more intricate structures, among other sizes and shapes.
- **Properties:** possess special qualities brought forth by their small size, such as improved optical, electrical, and magnetic qualities and a high surface area to volume ratio.

Classification of inorganic nanoparticles based on composition:

(a) **Metal Nanoparticles:** Made entirely of metallic materials, metal nanoparticles are incredibly small particles with at least one dimension in the nanoscale range, often one to one hundred nanometres. Gold, silver, platinum, iron, and other nanoparticles having unique optical, electrical, and magnetic properties (Zhou & Vijayavenkataraman, 2021).
(b) **Metal Oxide Nanoparticles:** Metal oxide nanoparticles, composed of metal atoms linked to oxygen atoms, have unique properties due to their nanoscale size. They are produced when a metal mixes with oxygen and are widely used in catalysis, sensing, and medicine. Examples of these are iron oxide, zinc oxide, and titanium dioxide (Patel & Munjal, 2022).
(c) **Semiconductor Nanoparticles:** Quantum dots are semiconductor nanoparticles, which are materials at the nanoscale with special size-dependent optical and electrical characteristics. The energy gap widens as their size shrinks, resulting in adjustable emission colors and improved uses in quantum computing, bio-imaging, and optoelectronics (S. Cathrin Lims, 2025).
(d) **Ceramic Nanoparticles:** Ceramic nanoparticles, including silica, zirconia, and alumina, are well known for their remarkable chemical resistance, hardness, and thermal stability. These characteristics make them perfect for use in coatings, biomedical implants, and catalysis (Kapil, 2023).

Classification of inorganic nanoparticles based on shape:

(a) **Spherical:** The most prevalent form of nanoparticles is spherical (Figure 7), which offers a high surface area-to-volume ratio. This increases their reactivity, which makes them perfect for sensing, catalysis, and drug delivery applications (Altammar, 2023).

Figure 7. Spherical nanoparticles

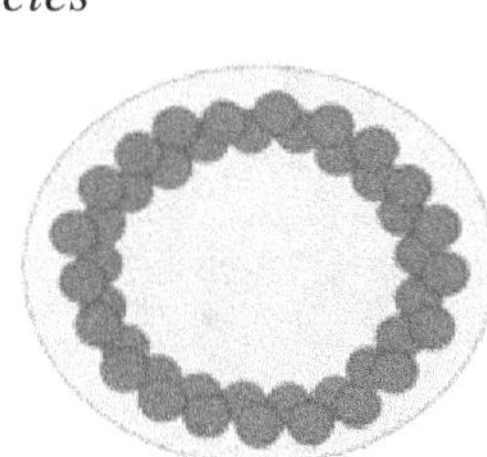

(b) **Rod-shaped:** Because of their anisotropic characteristics, rod-shaped nanoparticles (Figure 8) are ideal for use in photothermal therapy, electronics, and optics. Their longer design improves light absorption and directional conductivity (Huang & El-Sayed, 2010).

Figure 8. Rod-shaped nanoparticles

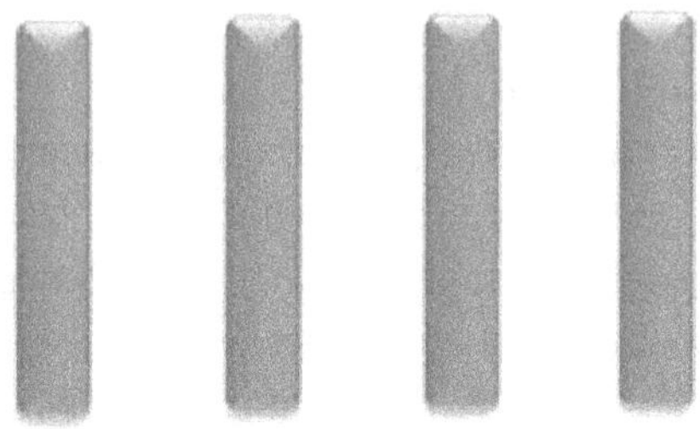

(c) **Platelet-shaped:** Because of their improved mechanical qualities, platelet-shaped (Figure 9) nanoparticles are perfect for strengthening composites and increasing material strength in coatings, polymers, and ceramic applications (Rashid, 2024).

Figure 9. Platelet shaped nanoparticles

(d) **Other shapes:** Because of their distinct geometries, nanoparticles of different shapes—like cubes, stars, and triangles—have special qualities. These forms allow for customized uses in advanced material creation, catalysis, and plasmonic (Jin, 2022).

2.2 Synthesis Methods

2.2.1 Top-Down Approaches

Top-down procedures (Figure 10) use mechanical or physical methods to break down bulk materials into nanoscale structures. Commonly employed methods include sputtering, lithography, laser ablation, and milling. Although these techniques are useful for creating distinct forms and structures, they may have drawbacks such as imperfections or uneven sizes. They are frequently used in the creation of thin films, semiconductors, and nanodevices. The method works well for producing large-scale nanostructured materials, but it usually requires a lot of energy (Kumari, 2023).

Figure 10. Top-down approach

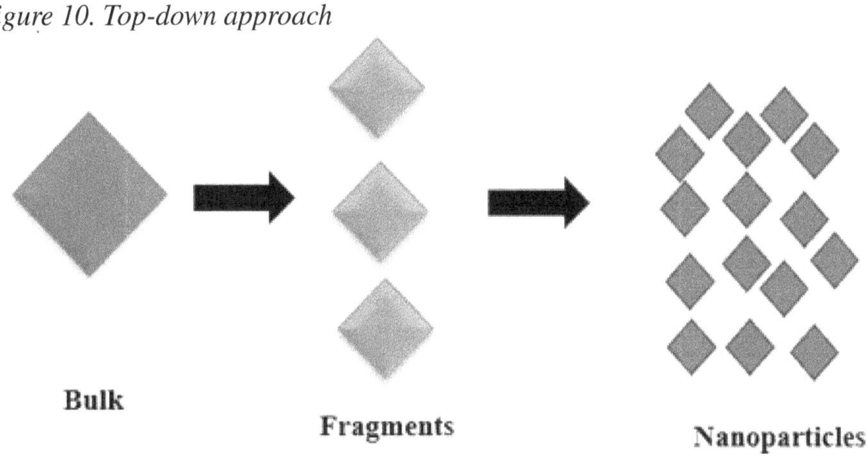

(a) Mechanical milling

A popular top-down method for creating nanostructured materials, such as nanoparticles, is mechanical milling (Figure 11). It involves high-energy ball milling, in which hard balls rotate inside a container and repeatedly collide, shatter, and cold weld bulk materials. The procedure results in structural and chemical alterations at the nanoscale as well as a reduction in particle size.

This process can create nanoparticles with precise sizes and shapes and is both economical and scalable. Its drawbacks include energy consumption, uneven forms, and contamination from milling medium. For the production of nanostructured alloys, ceramic nanoparticles, and composite materials for use in energy storage, electronics, and catalysis, mechanical milling is frequently used (Prasad Yadav, 2012).

Figure 11. Ball milling method

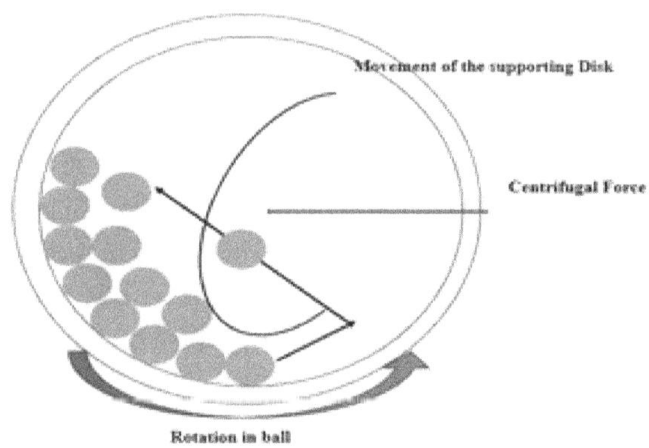

(b) Lithography

The manufacturing of electrical and photonic devices frequently uses lithography, a precise top-down method for producing nanoscale patterns on a substrate. Using a mask and a light source—usually ultraviolet (UV), electron, or ion beams—a pre-designed pattern is transferred onto a material.

This method makes it possible to produce complex and incredibly accurate structures with nanoscale resolution. Certain requirements in semiconductor production and nanotechnology are met by variations such as photolithography and electron beam lithography. Although lithography provides exceptional accuracy and consistency, it is limited by issues like as mask flaws and resolution limitations and necessitates costly equipment. It is essential for uses in integrated circuits, nanodevices, and microelectronics (Paras & Kumar, 2021).

(c) Laser ablation

A solid substance is exposed to a high-energy laser beam in a top-down process called laser ablation, which creates nanoparticles and nanostructures. Material is ejected by the laser's high intensity, creating tiny particles in a regulated setting, frequently in a liquid or gas medium.

This method allows to produce pure and contamination-free nanoparticles with adjustable size and composition by varying laser parameters. It is versatile, capable of processing a wide range of materials, including metals, ceramics, and semiconductors. However, laser ablation requires precise control of experimental conditions and is often limited by equipment cost and scalability. It finds applications in nanomaterial synthesis, thin-film deposition, and advanced material research (Balachandran, 2022).

(d) Thermal decomposition

A bottom-up synthesis technique called thermal decomposition breaks down a precursor material by heating it to high temperatures, which causes it to break down and generate nanoparticles. In order to regulate particle development and size distribution, the procedure is frequently conducted with a stabilizing agent or solvent present.

Benefits of this approach include ease of use, scalability, and the capacity to create nanoparticles with precise morphology and composition. It is frequently employed in the synthesis of carbon-based nanomaterials, semiconductor nanoparticles, and metal oxide nanoparticles. To prevent unwanted byproducts, however, exact control over temperature and reaction conditions is necessary. Energy storage systems, environmental cleanup applications, and catalyst preparation all make extensive use of thermal decomposition (Chiravoot Pechyen, 2024).

2.2.2 Bottom-up Approaches

Bottom-up methods (Figure 12) use chemical reactions or self-assembly to create nanoparticles from atomic or molecular constituents. Bottom-up approaches concentrate on assembling smaller units into nanoscale structures as opposed to top-down approaches, which disassemble large materials. Sol-gel, co-precipitation, hydrothermal synthesis, and chemical vapor deposition (CVD) are examples of common techniques.

By precisely controlling the nanoparticles' size, shape, and composition, these techniques produce materials of superior quality with consistent qualities. When creating nanoparticles with functions for a variety of uses, bottom-up methods are frequently more adaptable and economical. To guarantee reproducibility, they might necessitate meticulous control of reaction conditions and can be more time-consuming. They are widely employed in disciplines like materials science, electronics, nanomedicine, and catalysis (Kumar, 2017).

Figure 12. Bottom-up approach

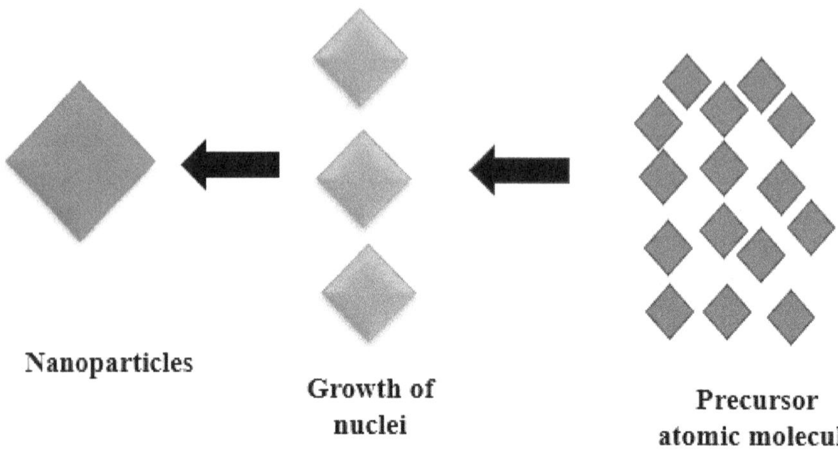

(a) Chemical synthesis

Chemical synthesis is a bottom-up method in which precursor materials, reducing agents, and stabilizing agents in solution undergo chemical reactions to generate nanoparticles. By modifying variables including concentration, temperature, and pH, this technique enables exact control over the nanoparticles' size, shape, and makeup.

Metal, metal oxide, and semiconductor nanoparticles are frequently produced using chemical synthesis methods such co-precipitation, sol-gel, and hydrothermal synthesis. Scalability, reproducibility, and the capacity to create complex materials with specific properties are some benefits of the technique. It may, however, require the use of hazardous chemicals or solvents, necessitating cautious handling and attention to the surroundings. Chemical synthesis is frequently used in energy storage, biomedical applications, and catalysis (Anesu Nyabadza, 2023).

(b) Sol-gel processing

A flexible bottom-up method for creating nanoparticles, sol-gel processing involves changing from a liquid (sol) to a solid (gel) phase. In order to create a gel network, the process starts with the manufacture of a precursor solution, usually metal alkoxides or salts, which then go through hydrolysis and condensation processes.

This process is appropriate for creating metal oxides, ceramics, and composite materials because it provides for the exact control of particle size, content, and morphology. Because sol-gel processing is so versatile, it can be used to create bulk materials, coatings, and thin films with special qualities. Although it provides superior uniformity and low-temperature processing, the procedure can be laborious and necessitates meticulous reaction parameter control. Applications for sol-gel processing are numerous and include optical coatings, sensors, and catalysis (Bokov, 2021).

(c) Chemical vapor deposition

A bottom-up method called chemical vapor deposition (CVD) creates thin films or nanoparticles by reacting gaseous precursors in a heated chamber, where they either break down or react to produce solid material that is deposited onto a substrate. High temperatures and a regulated environment are usually used in the procedure to promote the chemical processes that produce nanoparticles or films.

The thickness, structure, and composition of the deposited material can all be precisely controlled by CVD. High-purity semiconductors, metal films, and carbon-based nanomaterials like graphene and nanotubes are all produced using it extensively. Although CVD produces uniformly high-quality materials, it can be energy-intensive and requires specialized equipment. The process is frequently used in the production of semiconductors, coatings, and materials for energy storage, electronics, and optics (Bube, 2001).

(d) Biological synthesis

A bottom-up method called biological synthesis creates nanoparticles by using natural organisms like fungi, bacteria, or plants. This technique converts metal ions into nanoparticles by taking advantage of the metabolic activities of microorganisms or plant extracts. Because it frequently calls for mild reaction conditions and stays away from hazardous chemicals, the biological approach is regarded as environmentally beneficial.

Green chemistry, scalability, and the possibility to create biocompatible nanoparticles are just a few benefits of biological synthesis. Additionally, it can create nanoparticles with distinct sizes, shapes, and surface characteristics. However, the yield and particle size may vary, and the procedure might be slower than chemical approaches. The creation of nanoparticles for use in biocatalysis, environmental remediation, and medical applications frequently involves biological synthesis (Osman, 2024).

3. NANOFIBERS: STRUCTURE AND FABRICATION

Nanofibers are the fibres with diameters in the nanometre range which have unique mechanical, chemical, and physical properties due to their small size and large surface area. These fibres high degree of adaptability makes them useful in a variety of fields, such as biomedical engineering, electronics, energy storage, and filtration. The structure and production processes of nanofibers greatly influence their properties and applications (Kenry & Lim, 2017).

3.1 Structure of Nanofibers

Compared to bulk materials, nanofibers have special mechanical properties and are more reactive due to their high surface area-to-volume ratio. Depending on how they are made, nanofibers might have a smooth cylindrical shape or more intricate, branching, or porous architectures. Because of their small diameter, they have special optical, electrical, and thermal characteristics that set them apart from bulk materials or bigger fibres.

Nanofibers' surface-to-volume ratio makes them especially well-suited for uses where material-environment interactions are essential. For instance, because of their large surface area, which makes it possible for pharmacological substances to be loaded and released efficiently, nanofibers have been employed as drug delivery vehicles. Additionally, nanofibers have improved conductivity, strength, and flexibility, which make them perfect for structural uses in electronic devices and lightweight composites (Andre, 2021).

It is also possible to functionalize nanofibers (Figure 13), which entails attaching chemical or biological substances to their surfaces to give them certain properties or abilities. Because functionalized nanofibers may interact with target molecules or particles selectively, they are frequently utilized in sensors, filtration systems, and environmental clean-up procedures (Kulkarni, 2022).

Figure 13. Nanofibers

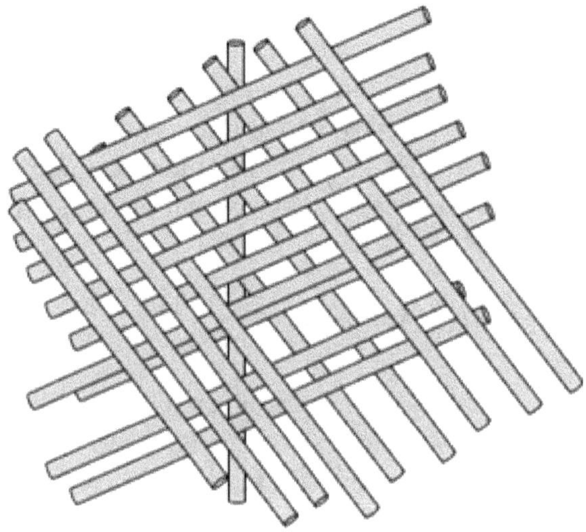

3.2 Fabrication Techniques

Several techniques are available for the fabrication of nanofibers, each with distinct advantages and challenges. The most widely used methods include electrospinning, solution blow spinning, and template-assisted methods (Thareja Rakhi, 2023).

3.2.1 Electrospinning

Electrospinning is the most widely used and studied method for producing nanofibers. A high-voltage electric field is applied to a polymer melt or solution, causing the material to produce a jet of liquid that stretches into a thin fiber when it is expelled from the needle. During the fiber's flight, the solvent evaporates, leaving behind a solid nanofiber. Electrospinning allows for the creation of fibers of controlled diameters, typically ranging from a few nanometers to several micrometres, and can be used with a wide range of natural and synthetic polymers. The electro spun fibers can also be orientated in a specific direction, which is useful for filtering and tissue engineering applications (Rand Abdulhussain, 2023).

3.2.2 Solution Blow Spinning

Solution blow spinning is a technique that creates nanofibers by blowing a polymer melt or solution onto a collector using a high-pressure air stream. Compared to electrospinning, this process is easier to use, more scalable, and capable of producing fibers in continuous lengths. Nanofiber mats are frequently made by solution blow spinning for uses like filtration, wound healing, and protective apparel (Daristotle, 2016).

3.2.3 Template-Assisted Methods

Template-assisted techniques direct the creation of nanofibers using a mold or template containing nanoscale pores. After the template is removed, continuous nanofibers are produced from components like metals, carbon-based compounds, or polymers that have been deposited into the pores. These techniques are frequently employed to create nanofibers with certain functions, such conductive or magnetic qualities, and they can provide exact control over the size and structure of the fiber (Pavlenko, 2022).

3.2.4 Other Fabrication Techniques

Chemical vapor deposition (CVD), self-assembly, and drawing are further techniques for creating nanofibers. While self-assembly uses the spontaneous arrangement of molecules or nanoparticles into nanofibers under specific conditions, drawing uses a micro-sized nozzle to pull a polymer melt or solution through to create fibers. Another method for creating carbon nanotubes and other nanofibers is chemical vapor deposition (CVD), in which gaseous precursors react and deposit onto a substrate to create nanofibers (Ganesan & Jaiganesh, 2022).

4. BIOMEDICAL APPLICATIONS OF NANOPARTICLES

Nanoparticles have garnered a lot of attention in the biomedical profession due to their unique properties, which include their small size, high surface area-to-volume ratio, and ability to be functionalized for specific needs. These features make nanoparticles suitable for a wide range of biomedical uses, such as drug transport, imaging, diagnosis, and treatment. By altering their size, shape, and surface chemistry, nanoparticles can be tailored for specific biological interactions, increasing their effectiveness as compared to traditional therapy methods (Meher, 2024).

4.1 Drug Delivery Systems

One of the most intriguing applications of nanoparticles in biomedicine is drug delivery. By employing nanoparticle engineering, medications can be administered to certain bodily areas, improving therapeutic efficacy and lowering side effects. For instance, drugs can be encapsulated in nanoparticles for controlled, progressive release. Nanoparticles can be designed to release their payload in response to certain stimuli, such as changes in pH, temperature, or the presence of specific enzymes. This feature minimizes systemic exposure and toxicity while guaranteeing that the medication is precisely delivered to the targeted spot, such as a tumour (Elumalai, 2024).

Liposomes, dendrimers, micelles, and polymeric nanoparticles are among the frequently utilized nanoparticle forms for drug delivery. Numerous medications, such as proteins, nucleic acids, and chemotherapeutic medicines, can be encapsulated in these carriers. Liposomes' capacity to transport both hydrophilic and hydrophobic medications has been extensively researched, making them extremely adaptable for a variety of therapeutic uses (Sultana, 2022).

4.2 Cancer Therapy

Nanoparticles are essential for improving the treatment of cancer. Nanoparticles can be targeted to tumor cells by functionalizing them with certain targeting ligands, which minimizes damage to healthy tissues and eliminates the need for large dosages of chemotherapeutic medications. In cancer treatment, when reducing the harmful side effects of traditional treatments is crucial, this type of focused drug administration is extremely beneficial (Ghazal, 2024).

The ability of nanoparticles to absorb energy (from magnetic fields or infrared radiation, for example) and transform it into heat makes them useful for hyperthermia treatment. Cancer cells may be destroyed by this localized heating, or it may increase their susceptibility to chemotherapy and radiation. By increasing the dose given to the tumor cells, gold nanoparticles have demonstrated potential in improving the effects of radiation therapy (Beik, 2016).

4.3 Advantages of Nanoparticle-based Drug Delivery

Drug delivery methods based on nanoparticles provide a number of benefits that increase the potency of medicinal substances. The improved drug solubility is one of the main advantages; this is especially important for hydrophobic medications with low water solubility. These medications' dispersion in biological fluids is improved by encapsulating them in nanoparticles, which enhances absorption and effectiveness. Another important benefit is controlled release kinetics, which allows nanoparticles to be designed to release medications at a triggered or sustained rate, minimizing the need for frequent administration and guaranteeing a long-lasting therapeutic impact (Patra, 2018).

Additionally, optimizing drug concentration at the desired site and reducing off-target effects depend heavily on focused delivery. Nanoparticles can selectively bind to sick cells, including malignant tissues, while avoiding healthy ones when they are functionalized with ligands or antibodies. Because it stops medications from building up in organs that are not the intended target, this focused strategy also helps to lessen side effects by reducing toxicity and unpleasant responses. Finally, a greater percentage of the prescribed medication will enter the systemic circulation in an active form thanks to enhanced bioavailability. Drug stability and therapeutic effect are increased by nanoparticles, which shield medications from early deterioration in the bloodstream or gastrointestinal system. When taken as a whole, these benefits make drug delivery via nanoparticles a viable approach to enhancing medication effectiveness and patient outcomes (Chehelgerdi, 2023).

4.4 Design Considerations

To maximize their effectiveness, a number of important criteria need to be taken into account while creating nanoparticles for biological purposes. The stability, cellular uptake, and biodistribution of nanoparticles are significantly influenced by their size and surface charge. While surface charge affects interactions with biological membranes and protein adsorption, smaller particles can readily pass through biological barriers. To increase the stability of nanoparticles, boost their biocompatibility, and accomplish targeted drug delivery, surface modification techniques are used. Reducing immunogenicity and increasing circulation time can be achieved through functionalization using polymers, ligands, or antibodies. Another important factor that influences the therapeutic potential of the nanoparticles is drug loading efficiency. High loading efficiency guarantees that an adequate dosage is administered while preserving the carrier's structural integrity (Waheed, 2022).

A prolonged and focused medication release also requires careful regulation of release mechanisms. In order to ensure accurate drug delivery at the site of action, these methods can be stimulus-responsive, such as pH-sensitive or enzyme-triggered systems. Finally, the safety of the nanoparticles and their removal from the body depend heavily on their biodegradation profiles. To avoid buildup and possible toxicity, nanoparticles should ideally break down into non-toxic components at a predictable rate. Researchers can create nanoparticles for biological purposes with improved efficacy and fewer adverse effects by carefully weighing these design factors (Karimi, 2016).

4.5 Diagnostic Imaging

(a) Magnetic Resonance Imaging (MRI)

Magnetic resonance imaging (MRI), a powerful non-invasive diagnostic method, uses contrast chemicals to enhance tissue differentiation and image quality. One of the often-used contrast agents, superparamagnetic iron oxide nanoparticles (SPIONs), has attracted a lot of attention due to its strong magnetic properties, biocompatibility, and ability to improve T2-weighted MRI contrast.

These nanoparticles produce local magnetic field disruptions that cause MRI scans to lose signal and allow for high-contrast tissue imaging, which is especially useful for identifying liver abnormalities, inflammation, and tumors (Busquets, 2015).

Another class of MRI contrast agents includes gadolinium-based contrast agents (GBCAs), which are commonly used to enhance T1-weighted imaging. Gadolinium ions (Gd^{3+}) possess unpaired electrons that shorten relaxation times, resulting in brighter signals in MRI scans. These agents are highly effective in imaging vascular structures, brain lesions, and tumors. However, concerns regarding gadolinium toxicity and its potential retention in the body have driven research into safer alternatives, such as nanoparticle-based gadolinium formulations that reduce free ion exposure while maintaining imaging efficiency (Nebal Iyad, 2023).

Multimodal imaging probes, which combine MRI with other imaging modalities such as computed tomography (CT), positron emission tomography (PET), or fluorescence, have been created to further increase diagnostic accuracy. By combining many imaging modalities, these hybrid nanoparticles enable the collection of complementary data from a single probe. For instance, SPIONs coated with fluorescent dyes can provide optical and MRI imaging, offering improved spatial resolution and real-time tracking. Precision medical applications, therapy monitoring, and disease identification are all improved by such multimodal techniques. Utilizing these cutting-edge contrast chemicals and imaging probes, MRI keeps developing as a vital instrument in contemporary medical diagnostics (Li, 2016).

(b) Optical Imaging

Because it provides high sensitivity and real-time observation of biological structures at the cellular and molecular levels, optical imaging is a commonly utilized tool in biomedical research and clinical diagnostics. Numerous nanomaterials have been created to improve optical imaging capabilities through increased brightness, photostability, and biocompatibility, including fluorescent nanoparticles, gold nanoparticles, and quantum dots (Evelien Hesemans, 2022).

Semiconductor nanocrystals known as quantum dots (QDs) have special optical characteristics such as size-tunable fluorescence emission, great photostability, and robust resistance to photobleaching. Because of these characteristics, QDs are ideal for multiplexed biomarker detection, molecular tracking, and long-term cellular imaging. Multiple targets can be detected simultaneously in a single sample thanks to QDs' shorter emission peaks and wider absorption spectra as compared to conventional organic fluorophores. However, current research into biocompatible coatings and substitute materials for safer biomedical uses has been prompted by worries about possible cytotoxicity due to heavy metal content (Kairdolf, 2013).

Because of their strong surface plasmon resonance (SPR), which improves light absorption and scattering, gold nanoparticles (AuNPs) have become useful instruments in optical imaging. AuNPs can be designed for a variety of uses, including surface-enhanced Raman scattering (SERS), dark-field imaging, and photoacoustic imaging, depending on their size and form. They are perfect for photothermal therapy, biosensing, and targeted imaging due to their biocompatibility and simplicity of functionalization. In the near-infrared (NIR) spectrum, gold nanorods show tunable SPR, enabling deeper tissue penetration for in vivo imaging (Wu, 2019).

Fluorescent nanoparticles provide a flexible platform for optical imaging, including fluorescent probes based on polymers and silica. By encasing fluorescent proteins or organic dyes, these nanoparticles reduce photobleaching and increase stability and brightness. Their surface can be altered with targeted ligands to detect certain biomolecules, opening up possibilities for cellular imaging, cancer diagnosis, and real-time biological process monitoring (Ruedas-Rama, 2012).

5. BIOMEDICAL APPLICATIONS OF NANOFIBERS

5.1 Tissue Engineering

Scaffold Design

Fluorescent nanoparticles provide a flexible platform for optical imaging, including fluorescent probes based on polymers and silica. By encasing fluorescent proteins or organic dyes, these nanoparticles reduce photobleaching and increase stability and brightness. Their surface can be altered with targeted ligands to detect certain biomolecules, opening up possibilities for cellular imaging, cancer diagnosis, and real-time biological process monitoring.

ECM mimicry is the process of creating scaffolds that closely resemble the extracellular matrix found in nature in order to create the best possible conditions for cell attachment, growth, and differentiation (Abdellah Aazmi, 2024).

(a) Scaffolds' mechanical qualities are crucial for preserving structural integrity and giving growing tissues mechanical support. Depending on the kind of tissue, the scaffold's stiffness, elasticity, and rate of disintegration must be adjusted (Chan & Leong, 2008).
(b) By enhancing cell adhesion, proliferation, and differentiation, surface modification improves scaffold biocompatibility and functionality. Scaffold surfaces can be altered using a variety of methods, including chemical grafting, plasma treatment, and coating with bioactive compounds(Teimouri, 2023).
(c) Because they dictate how cells adhere, proliferate, and communicate within the scaffold, cell-material interactions are essential to scaffold design. These interactions are strongly influenced by the scaffold's surface chemistry, topography, and porosity (Wang, 2023).

5.1.2. Tissue-Specific Applications

Strategies for scaffold-based tissue engineering are made to accommodate the distinct mechanical and biological needs of various tissues. The ability of a scaffold to promote cell proliferation, differentiation, and integration inside the targeted tissue determines how effective it is. Scaffolds are used in a variety of tissue-specific applications, such as bone, cartilage, skin, neural, and cardiovascular tissue engineering, each of which has distinct structural and biochemical requirements.

1. Scaffolds with high mechanical strength, osteoconductive properties, and biodegradability are essential for bone tissue engineering. Materials that replicate the natural bone matrix include composite polymers, bioactive glasses, and hydroxyapatite (Lee, 2022).
2. To enable chondrocyte function and extracellular matrix deposition, cartilage tissue engineering calls for scaffolds that are flexible, resilient, and highly hydrated. To mimic the characteristics of cartilage, hydrogels, collagen-based matrices, and synthetic polymers like polycaprolactone (PCL) are frequently utilized (Fariba Hashemi-Afzal, 2024).
3. The goal of skin tissue engineering is to create scaffolds that replicate the skin's layered structure and aid in the healing of wounds. Dermal scaffolds are often made of biodegradable polymers such as collagen, fibrin, and hyaluronic acid (Jorgensen, 2022).
4. Scaffolds that promote neuronal growth, direct axonal regeneration, and establish a favourable milieu for nerve repair is necessary for neural tissue engineering. Neuronal adhesion and electrical conductivity are enhanced by the introduction of biomaterials including fibrin, chitosan, and conductive polymers (Subramanian, 2009).

5. Scaffolds that support structural integrity and encourage the regeneration of heart tissue and blood vessels are used in cardiovascular tissue engineering. Vascular grafts and cardiac patches are created using biomaterials including decellularized extracellular matrix (dECM), scaffolds made of elastin, and biodegradable polymers like polylactic acid (PLA) (Hossein Rayat Pisheh, 2024).

5.2 Wound Healing

1. Controlling inflammation and maintaining hemostasis are essential during the early phases of wound healing. Cutting-edge biomaterials, including hemostatic dressings derived from gelatin, fibrin, or chitosan, aid in halting bleeding and establishing a stable wound environment (Kushwaha, 2022).
2. During the early phases of wound healing, hemostasis and inflammation management are essential. Haemostatic dressings consisting of gelatine, fibrin, or chitosan are examples of advanced biomaterials that assist control bleeding and establish a stable wound environment (B, 2024).
3. The formation of new tissue depends critically on cell proliferation and extracellular matrix remodeling. Biodegradable scaffolds, hydrogels, and nanofibrous dressings enhance fibroblast migration, collagen deposition, and keratinocyte proliferation by simulating the natural extracellular matrix (Komal Sindhi, 2025).
4. Additionally, silver and gold nanoparticles have antimicrobial qualities that help to promote angiogenesis and tissue healing while preventing wound infections (Jain, 2014).
5. 3D-printed bioactive scaffolds and electrospun nanofiber mats provide high surface area, moisture retention, and oxygen permeability, which further improve wound healing (Aliakbar Ahovan, 2022).

5.2.2 Drug-loaded Wound Dressings

1. Antimicrobial agents, growth factors, anti-inflammatory medications, and painkillers are all included in these dressings to address different facets of wound healing and enhance the rate and caliber of tissue regeneration (Saghazadeh, 2018).
2. Silver nanoparticles lower the chance of resistance development while maintaining antibacterial activity. By keeping the wound bed clean and avoiding issues like biofilm formation, which can slow healing, these substances not only stop microbiological growth but also aid in wound healing (Yousefian, 2023).
3. Growth factors that support tissue regeneration, cell migration, and angiogenesis include vascular endothelial growth factor, platelet-derived growth factor, and epidermal growth factor. Growth factor-releasing drug-loaded dressings promote

collagen deposition, epithelialization, and the development of new blood vessels, hastening wound healing and enhancing tissue regeneration (Steere, 2015).

4. To control the inflammatory stage of wound healing, anti-inflammatory medications are essential. Prolonged inflammation can cause problems like excessive scarring and delayed healing by impeding tissue repair (Huang, 2022).
5. Since pain can impede the healing process and patients' quality of life, pain management is another crucial component of wound care. Localized pain alleviation at the wound site can be achieved with drug-loaded dressings that contain analgesics such morphine, lidocaine, or local anaesthetics (Bechert & Abraham, 2019).

5.3 Drug Delivery Applications

(a) Mucoadhesive drug delivery, transdermal drug delivery, and implantable drug delivery devices are important examples of controlled release applications (Tobechukwu Christian Ezike, 2023).

(b) Mucoadhesive drug delivery provides controlled drug release by using polymers that stick to mucosal membranes, like those in the mouth, nose, or gastrointestinal system. When it comes to treating gastrointestinal disorders, nasal congestion, or oral infections, these systems are very helpful for localized drug delivery to mucosal tissues (Boddupalli, 2010).

(c) Transdermal patches are frequently used to administer nicotine to help people quit smoking, hormones like oestrogen, or painkillers like fentanyl. Drug penetration through the skin can be improved by using permeation enhancers and nanocarriers, including liposomes or nanoparticles, in transdermal patches. This enables continuous release over the course of hours or even days. This method provides continuous drug delivery and patient convenience, especially for managing chronic diseases (Won Fen Wong, 2023).

(d) Medical devices that are surgically or minimally invasively inserted into the body to deliver medications at a specific location over an extended period of time with regulated release are known as implantable drug delivery devices. These devices are perfect for controlling chronic disorders like cancer, diabetes, or infections because they may be made to dispense medications over a period of weeks to months (Huanbutta, 2024).

Table 1. Comparing about different types of nanoparticles have synthesized by using different method for biomedical application with advantages and limitations

S.N.	Name of NPs	Biomedical application	Synthesis method	Characterization	Advantages/ limitation	References
1.	AgNPs	Antibacterial	Chemical method	FTIR, DLS, XRD, TEM	Strong antimicrobial activity/ Expensive precursors; toxicity at higher doses	(Naganthran, 2022)
2.	Copper oxide nanoparticles	Antibacterial	Electrochemical reduction	UV, FTIR, XRD, SEM-EDS, TEM	Cost-effective, good stability/Less effective than Ag in some cases	(Jadhav, 2011)
3.	Copper oxide nanostructures	Drug delivery	Galvanic reaction	SEM-EDS, XRD, UV, TEM	Simple method, good control over morphology/Limited biomedical data	(Woźniak-Budych, 2016)
4.	Zinc oxide nanoparicles	Drug delivrey	Co-precipitation Method	XRD, SEM, TEM, UV, FTIR	Biocompatible, scalable method/Agglomeration issues	(Rasmussen, 2010)
5.	Zinc oxide nanoparticles	Antiviral	Microwave assisted	XRD, UV, FTIR, SEM-EDS	Rapid synthesis, uniform particles/Equipment dependency	(Salari, 2017)
6.	Nickel nanparticles	Anicancer, antibacterial, antiviral, antioxidant	Green method	XRD, FTIR, SEM	Eço-friendly multifunctional/Potential cytotoxicity	(Moulana Kareem, 2023)
7.	Nickel nanoparticles	Antioxidant	Plant mediated method	Uv, FTIR, DLA, TEM, TGA	Biocompatible synthesis/Plant extract standardization needed	(Hashem, 2021)
8.	Titanium oxide nanofiber	Removal from aqueous solution	Electrospinning	UV, FTIR, XRD, TEM	High surface area, efficient in adsorption/ Costly apparatus	(Abbasizadeh, 2013)
9.	Titanium oxide nanoparticles	Antibacterial and antioxidant activity	Plant mediated method	XRD, FTIR, FESEM, EDX	Environmentally friendly/Less crystallinity	(Santhoshkumar, 2014)
10.	Tin oxide nanoparitcles	Antibacterial actibity	Co-precipittaion method	XRD, BET, XPS, FTIR	Simple method, porous structure/Less explored for biomedical use	(Mahfooz-ur-Rehman, 2019)

6. CHARACTERIZATION TECHNIQUES

6.1 Physical Characterization

For the in-depth viewing and examination of biological, chemical, and material materials at the micro- and nanoscale, microscopy techniques are crucial instruments. These techniques enable high-resolution imaging and offer important information on the composition, characteristics, and structure of different materials. Atomic force microscopy, transmission electron microscopy, confocal microscopy, and scanning electron microscopy are a few of the most used microscopy method(Aziz, 2025).

(a) High-resolution, three-dimensional images of surfaces can be obtained using the potent imaging method known as scanning electron microscopy SEM detects secondary electrons released from a sample's surface by scanning it with a concentrated electron beam. The product is a comprehensive picture that offers details on the composition, morphology, and topography of the surface. SEM is frequently used to analyse biological samples, characterize materials, and examine the texture of thin films and nanoparticles. The method is appropriate for imaging large and complicated samples because it provides great resolution and outstanding depth of field (Yanet Rodríguez Herrero, 2023).
(b) The internal structure of thin samples can be studied at the atomic and molecular levels using Transmission Electron Microscopy (Figure 14), which has a better resolution than SEM. A TEM creates an image by passing an electron beam through a very thin sample and observing how the electrons and sample interact. TEM offers comprehensive details on the internal morphology of materials, including crystalline configurations, nanoparticles, and cellular structures. It is perfect for examining minute features such as flaws, surfaces, and delicate structural components of materials, including subcellular biological tissues (Darwesh, 2020).

Figure 14. Scanning electron microscope and transmission electron microscope

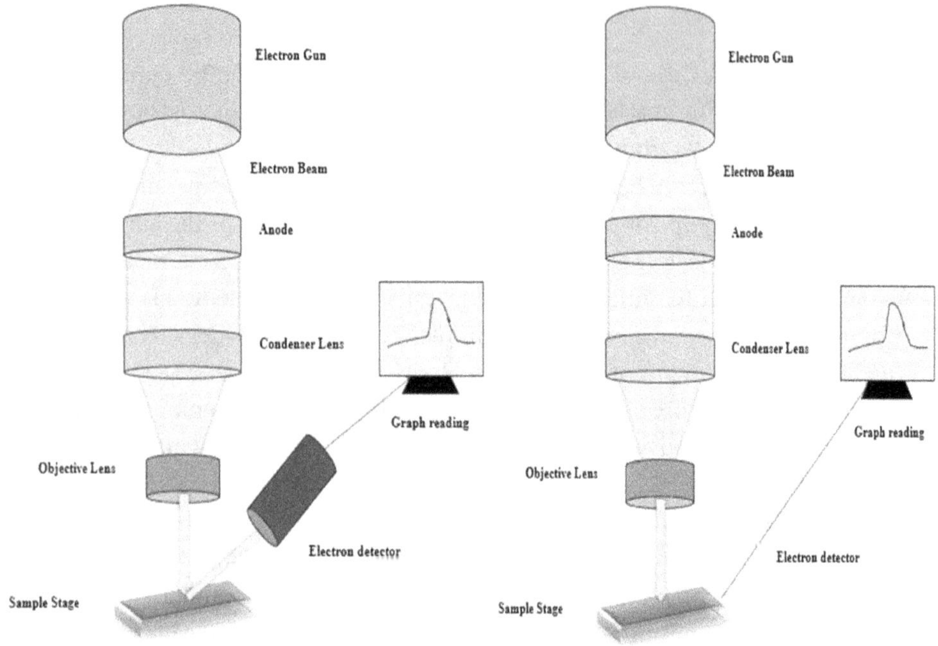

(c) Atomic Force Microscopy is a kind of scanning probe microscopy that scans a sample's surface at the nanoscale using a sharp point. High-resolution imaging of both soft and hard materials is made possible by AFM (Figure 15), which measures the contact forces between the tip and the surface. AFM can quantify surface roughness, create three-dimensional pictures of surfaces, and assess mechanical attributes like adhesion, stiffness, and elasticity. It provides topographic and mechanical property information in a single scan, making it particularly helpful for researching biomolecules, polymers, and nanomaterials (Sheppard, 2005).

(d) Confocal Microscopy is an optical imaging method that scans samples using laser light and creates high-resolution, three-dimensional images by concentrating light on a particular plane inside the sample. Compared to traditional fluorescence microscopy, confocal microscopy produces crisper and more detailed images by removing out-of-focus light. It is frequently used to image fluorescently labeled cells, tissues, and nanoparticles in the fields of material science, neuroscience, and cell biology. Optical sectioning and depth analysis of thick samples are made possible by confocal microscopy, which offers information on the distribution of molecules within cells and tissues (Stachowiak, 2004).

Figure 15. Atomic force microscopy

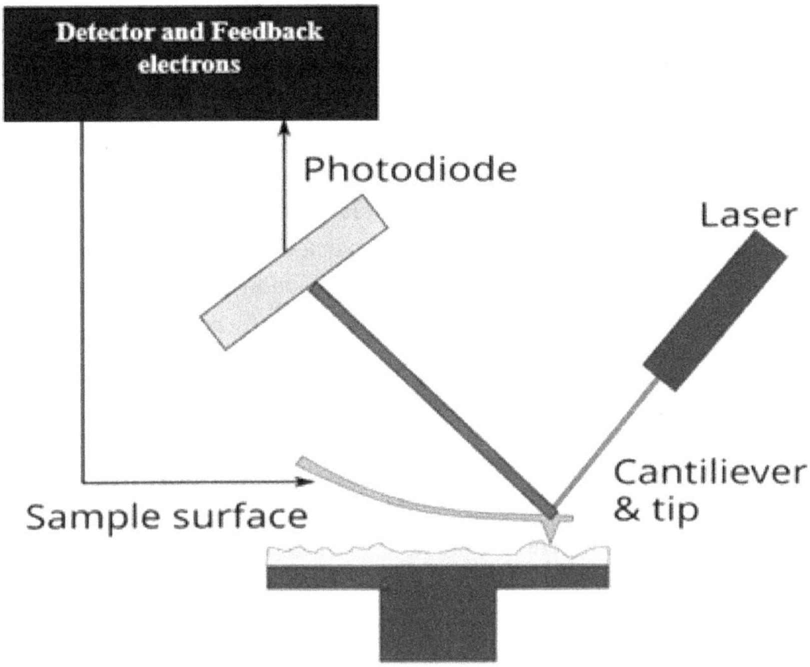

6.2 Particle Size and Distribution

For nanoparticles to be used in areas like drug delivery, diagnostics, and materials research, it is essential to comprehend their size and distribution. Consistent performance and efficacy are guaranteed by precise particle size and distribution measurements. The size, distribution, and surface charge of nanoparticles are analyzed using a variety of methods, including as zeta potential studies, dynamic light scattering (DLS), and nanoparticle tracking analysis (NTA).

(a) Dynamic Light Scattering is a popular technique for figuring out the size distribution of nanoparticles in solution. DLS quantifies the changes in scattered light intensity caused by the Brownian motion of particles. DLS is able to determine the hydrodynamic radius of nanoparticles since the rate of particle motion is inversely related to their size. The average size, size distribution, and polydispersity index (PDI) of the nanoparticles in a sample are all usefully revealed by this method. It is frequently used to describe proteins, polymers, and nanoparticles, especially in applications linked to drug delivery and nanomedicine (Caputo et al., 2021).

(b) Another method for determining the size and concentration of nanoparticles in a liquid suspension is Nanoparticle Tracking Analysis. NTA uses video microscopy to track the Brownian motion of particles illuminated by a laser beam. NTA can ascertain the size of individual particles and produce a comprehensive size distribution profile by examining their displacement over time. This method is very helpful for measuring nanoparticles between 10 nm and 1 μm in size, and it enables the measurement of both particle size and concentration. NTA is useful in fields like drug formulation and protein aggregation investigations since it also offers high-resolution data on particle size distribution, particularly for polydisperse materials (Rocca et al., 2013).

(c) Potential for Zeta The surface charge of suspended nanoparticles is measured because it affects their stability, aggregation behaviour, and interactions with biological systems. An electric field is applied to a suspension of nanoparticles, and the velocity of the particles as they approach the electrodes is measured to estimate the zeta potential. The zeta potential, which shows the strength of electrostatic repulsion between particles, is obtained from the resulting data. While low zeta potential values suggest the possibility of aggregation, a larger absolute zeta potential value indicates greater stability and less aggregation of nanoparticles. Understanding the behaviour of nanoparticles in biological systems, such as medication delivery systems or diagnostic agents, and evaluating the stability of colloidal suspensions depend on this measurement (Serrano-Lotina, 2022).

6.3 Chemical Characterization

Analysis of the structure, content, and chemical characteristics of materials—especially nanoparticles, polymers, and biomolecules—requires the use of chemical characterization techniques. By identifying a material's chemical identity, functional groups, crystal structures, and thermal stability, these methods aid in optimizing it for a certain use. X-ray diffraction, Fourier transform infrared spectroscopy, X-ray photoelectron spectroscopy and thermal analysis techniques are some of the primary techniques utilized for chemical characterization.

(a) One effective method for figuring out a material's crystalline structure is X-ray diffraction. When X-rays are directed at a sample, they interact with the crystal lattice and create a diffraction pattern, which is how XRD (Figure 16) operates. The material's crystal structure, phase composition, and lattice parameters are determined by the peaks' diffraction angles and intensities. With its ability to provide important details on crystallinity, phase transitions, and crystallite size, XRD is especially helpful for characterizing metals, ceramics, polymers, and nanomaterials. When it comes to nanoparticles, XRD can be used to verify their size, shape, and phase as well as to find any contaminants or structural alterations that might alter their characteristics (Adams, 2005).

Figure 16. X-ray diffractometer (Mahadeshwara, n.d.)

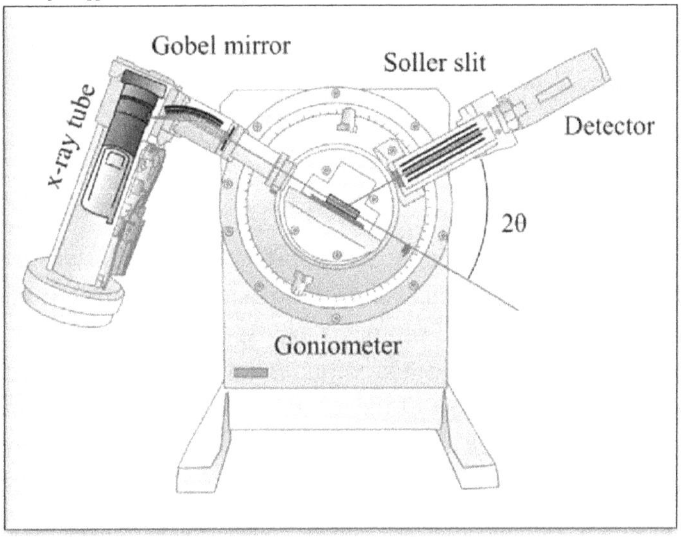

(b) A popular method for determining a material's functional groups and chemical bonds is Fourier Transform Infrared Spectroscopy (FTIR). FTIR (Figure 17) measures how much infrared light at different wavelengths is absorbed by the sample. Infrared light at frequencies is absorbed by each chemical link, creating a distinct spectrum that acts as a fingerprint for the chemical makeup of the material. FTIR is useful for studying surface functionalization, ligand binding, and chemical changes of nanoparticles. It is also useful for analysing organic chemicals, polymers, and coatings. It gives researchers information on the molecular structure, enabling them to pinpoint functional groups and confirm a material's chemical makeup (Kalra, 2023).

Figure 17. FTIR instrumentation (Infrared and FTIR Spectroscopy Instrument, n.d.)

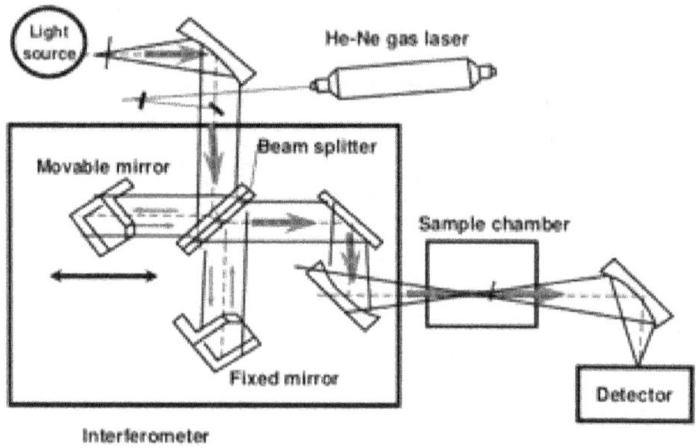

(c) X-ray A surface-sensitive method that offers comprehensive details on the elemental makeup and chemical states of a material's surface is photoelectron spectroscopy (XPS). When a sample is exposed to X-ray radiation, photoelectrons are released from the surface, which is how XPS (Figure 18) operates. By measuring the binding energy of the released electrons, the elements' identities and chemical states can be ascertained. Because it allows for the identification of surface functional groups, oxidation states, and elemental composition, XPS is very helpful for characterizing the surface chemistry of nanoparticles, thin films, and coatings. Because surface chemistry is essential to biological compatibility and reactivity, it is also useful for researching how nanoparticles interact with biological systems (Chakraborty, 2023).

Figure 18. X-ray photoelectron spectroscopy

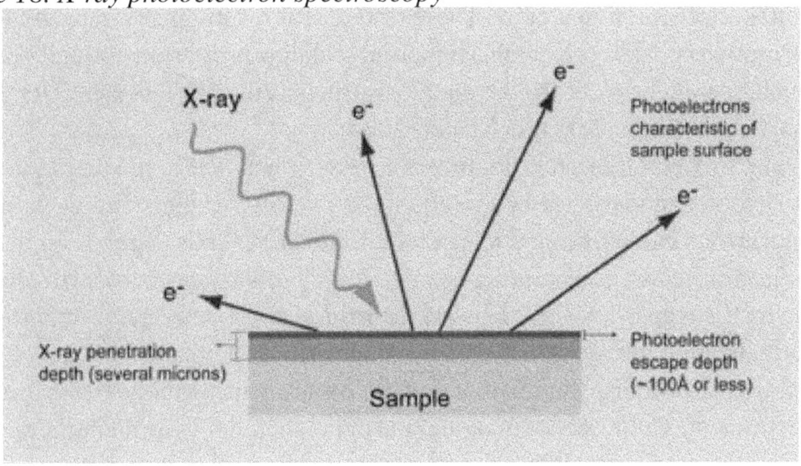

(d) Thermal analysis techniques include a variety of approaches to investigating the stability, phase transitions, and degradation behavior of materials' thermal characteristics. Common thermal analysis methods include Differential Scanning Calorimetry (DSC), which measures heat flow into or out of a material as it undergoes phase transitions, giving information about melting points, glass transition temperatures, and crystallization behavior; Thermogravimetric Analysis (TGA), which measures a material's weight loss as it is heated, providing information on its composition, moisture content, and thermal stability; and Differential Thermal Analysis (DTA), which tracks temperature differences between a sample and a reference material. The stability, breakdown, and processing behavior of nanoparticles and polymers can be better understood through thermal study, especially in the fields of medication delivery, material science, and food technology (Saadatkhah et al., 2019).

6.4 Biological Characterization

Particularly in biomedical applications like medication administration, tissue engineering, and diagnostic devices, biological characterisation is crucial for assessing the safety, efficacy, and biocompatibility of materials. By offering vital information on toxicity, cell contacts, distribution, and immunological responses, these methods aid in evaluating the interactions between materials (such as nanoparticles or biomaterials) and biological systems. Cytotoxicity assays, cell uptake investigations, biodistribution analysis, and immunogenicity testing are important biological characterization techniques.

(a) Cytotoxicity Assays are frequently used to evaluate a material's possible detrimental effects on living cells. These tests assess a substance's capacity to stop cell growth or cause cell death. Numerous techniques can measure cell viability, membrane integrity, or trigger apoptosis, such as the MTT assay, LDH release assay, and apoptosis assays (Khalef, 2024).
(b) Uptake of Cells Research is utilized to assess how well medication delivery devices or nanoparticles are internalized by cells. Understanding how well nanocarriers carry therapeutic medicines into target cells depends on these investigations. Fluorescence microscopy, flow cytometry, or confocal microscopy in which nanoparticles are labeled with fluorescent markers to monitor their internalization into cells can be used to quantify cell uptake (Behzadi, 2017).
(c) Nanoparticle biodistribution in vivo can be tracked using methods such as mass spectrometry, fluorescence imaging, and radiolabelling. To evaluate the targeting effectiveness of drug delivery systems and make sure that they minimize off-target effects while reaching the intended site of action, biodistribution analysis is essential (Kumar, 2023).
(d) In vitro or in vivo assessments of cytokine production, immune cell activation, and antibody response are frequently part of immunogenicity testing. Determining the safety of nanoparticles or biomaterials, especially in systemic or long-term applications, requires an understanding of their capacity to activate the immune system. For clinical usage, materials with low immunogenicity are desirable because they are less likely to result in negative consequences or immunological rejection (Kuriakose, 2016).

7. CONCLUSION

This chapter has explored the fundamental aspects of nanomaterials, with a particular focus on nanoparticles and nanofibers, covering their synthesis methods, characterization techniques, and diverse biomedical applications. The synthesis strategies discussed—ranging from top-down to bottom-up approaches—underscore the importance of controlled fabrication in achieving desired particle size, morphology, and surface functionality, which directly influence their performance in biomedical systems. Characterization tools such as XRD, SEM, TEM, FTIR, and UV-Vis spectroscopy play a pivotal role in confirming structural integrity, surface chemistry, and optical properties of these nanomaterials. A clear understanding of these characteristics is essential for optimizing their functionality in biological environments.

Nanoparticles and nanofibers have shown remarkable promise in various biomedical domains, including drug delivery, tissue engineering, diagnostics, and antimicrobial applications. Their ability to interact at the cellular level with high specificity and efficiency offers significant advantages over conventional therapeutic approaches. In conclusion, the convergence of precise synthesis techniques, thorough characterization, and innovative applications positions nanomaterials at the forefront of biomedical research. Continued interdisciplinary efforts and a focus on biocompatibility, toxicity assessment, and regulatory standards will be key to translating these materials from laboratory research to clinical realities.

8. FUTURE PERSPECTIVES AND CHALLENGES

Significant progress has been made in the subject of nanotechnology, especially in the creation of nanomaterials for industrial and biomedical uses. But even with the advancements, there are still a number of obstacles to overcome and chances for further research for example:

(a) A significant obstacle to the broad application of nanoparticles and nanomaterials in industry is scalability and manufacturing. Nanomaterial synthesis at the laboratory scale has been well researched, but transferring these techniques to large-scale manufacturing is still a challenging problem.

(b) One of the biggest obstacles in the field of nanomaterials is still safety and toxicity issues. The distinct characteristics of nanoparticles, namely their huge surface area and small size, can result in unexpected interactions with biological systems that could be harmful or have other negative impacts. The study of nanoparticles' long-term impacts on the environment and human health is still in its infancy. Comprehensive in vitro, in vivo, and human clinical studies are required to determine the safety of nanoparticles.

(c) It is anticipated that the capabilities of nanomaterials will be improved by integration with advanced technologies including artificial intelligence (AI), machine learning, and sophisticated imaging techniques. By forecasting the characteristics of nanomaterials and how they will interact with biological systems, artificial intelligence (AI) can aid in their design and optimization. Large experimental datasets can be analyzed using machine learning algorithms to find new links and patterns that could speed up the creation of novel materials. Furthermore, there is potential for bettering early illness identification and treatment monitoring through the integration of nanomaterials with cutting-edge diagnostic instruments like real-time imaging systems.

9. ETHICAL AND REGULATORY STANDARDS

Moral and Regulatory Problems are major obstacles to the clinical application and commercialization of nanomaterials. To ensure that goods based on nanomaterials are safe and effective for human use, regulatory bodies must create precise rules for their approval. However, it is challenging to create global standards due to the complexity and variety of nanomaterials. To address particular issues with the production, labeling, and disposal of nanomaterials, regulatory frameworks must change. It's also necessary to address ethical issues such possible harm to the environment, hazards to human health, and fair access to nanotechnology. To develop strong and clear regulatory norms, researchers, legislators, and industry must work together.

REFERENCES

Aazmi, A., Zhang, D., Mazzaglia, C., Yu, M., Wang, Z., Yang, H., Huang, Y. Y. S., & Ma, L. (2024). Biofabrication methods for reconstructing extracellular matrix mimetics. *Bioactive Materials, 31*, 475–496. DOI: 10.1016/j.bioactmat.2023.08.018 PMID: 37719085

Abbasizadeh, S., Keshtkar, A. R., & Mousavian, M. A. (2013). Preparation of a novel electrospun polyvinyl alcohol/titanium oxide nanofiber adsorbent modified with mercapto groups for uranium(VI) and thorium(IV) removal from aqueous solution. *Chemical Engineering Journal, 220*, 161–171. DOI: 10.1016/j.cej.2013.01.029

Abdulhussain, R., Adebisi, A., Conway, B. R., & Asare-Addo, K. (2023). Electrospun nanofibers: Exploring process parameters, polymer selection, and recent applications in pharmaceuticals and drug delivery. *Journal of Drug Delivery Science and Technology, 90*, 105156–105156. DOI: 10.1016/j.jddst.2023.105156

Adams, F. (2005). X-RAY ABSORPTION AND DIFFRACTION | Overview. *Encyclopedia of Analytical Science*, 365–377.

Aliakbar Ahovan, Z., Esmaeili, Z., Eftekhari, B. S., Khosravimelal, S., Alehosseini, M., Orive, G., Dolatshahi-Pirouz, A., Pal Singh Chauhan, N., Janmey, P. A., Hashemi, A., Kundu, S. C., & Gholipourmalekabadi, M. (2022). Antibacterial smart hydrogels: New hope for infectious wound management. *Materials Today. Bio, 17*, 100499. DOI: 10.1016/j.mtbio.2022.100499 PMID: 36466959

Altammar, K. A. (2023). A review on nanoparticles: Characteristics, synthesis, applications, and challenges. *Frontiers in Microbiology, 14*(1155622), 1155622. DOI: 10.3389/fmicb.2023.1155622 PMID: 37180257

Andre, R. S., Facure, M. H., Schneider, R., Migliorini, F. L., dos Santos, D. M., Mercante, L. A., & Correa, D. S. (2023). Sensing materials: Nanofibers produced by electrospinning and solution blow spinning.

Arif, M. D., Hoque, M. E., Rahman, M. Z., & Shafoyat, M. U. (2024). Emerging Directions in Green Nanomaterials: Synthesis, Physicochemical Properties and Applications. *Materials Today. Communications, 40*, 109335–109335. DOI: 10.1016/j.mtcomm.2024.109335

Aziz, A., Shaikh, H., Abbas, A., Zehra, K. E., & Javed, B. (2025). Microscopic Techniques for Nanomaterials Characterization: A Concise Review. *Microscopy Research and Technique, 88*(5), 1599–1614. DOI: 10.1002/jemt.24799 PMID: 39780429

Balachandran, A., Sreenilayam, S. P., Madanan, K., Thomas, S., & Brabazon, D. (2022). Nanoparticle production via laser ablation synthesis in solution method and printed electronic application-A brief review. *Results in Engineering*, *16*, 100646.

Bechert, K., & Abraham, S. E. (2019). Pain Management and Wound Care. *The Journal of the American College of Certified Wound Specialists*, *1*(2), 65–71. DOI: 10.1016/j.jcws.2008.12.001 PMID: 24527116

Behzadi, S., Serpooshan, V., Tao, W., Hamaly, M. A., Alkawareek, M. Y., Dreaden, E. C., Brown, D., Alkilany, A. M., Farokhzad, O. C., & Mahmoudi, M. (2017). Cellular uptake of nanoparticles: Journey inside the cell. *Chemical Society Reviews*, *46*(14), 4218–4244. DOI: 10.1039/C6CS00636A PMID: 28585944

Beik, J., Abed, Z., Ghoreishi, F. S., Hosseini-Nami, S., Mehrzadi, S., Shakeri-Zadeh, A., & Kamrava, S. K. (2016). Nanotechnology in hyperthermia cancer therapy: From fundamental principles to advanced applications. *Journal of Controlled Release*, *235*, 205–221. DOI: 10.1016/j.jconrel.2016.05.062 PMID: 27264551

Boddupalli, B. M., Mohammed, Z. N. K., Nath, R. A., & Banji, D. (2010). Mucoadhesive drug delivery system: An overview. *Journal of Advanced Pharmaceutical Technology & Research*, *1*(4), 381–387. DOI: 10.4103/0110-5558.76436 PMID: 22247877

Bokov, D., Turki Jalil, A., Chupradit, S., Suksatan, W., Javed Ansari, M., Shewael, I. H., Valiev, G. H., & Kianfar, E. (2021). Nanomaterial by Sol-Gel Method: Synthesis and Application. *Advances in Materials Science and Engineering*, *2021*(1), 1–21. DOI: 10.1155/2021/5102014

Bube, R. H. (2001). Cadmium Sulfide and Telluride. *Encyclopedia of Materials: Science and Technology*, 873–879.

Busquets, M. A., Estelrich, J., & Sánchez-Martín, M. J. (2015). Nanoparticles in magnetic resonance imaging: From simple to dual contrast agents. *International Journal of Nanomedicine*, *10*, 1727. DOI: 10.2147/IJN.S76501 PMID: 25834422

Caputo, F., Vogel, R., Savage, J., Vella, G., Law, A., Della Camera, G., Hannon, G., Peacock, B., Mehn, D., Ponti, J., Geiss, O., Aubert, D., Prina-Mello, A., & Calzolai, L. (2021). Measuring particle size distribution and mass concentration of nanoplastics and microplastics: Addressing some analytical challenges in the sub-micron size range. *Journal of Colloid and Interface Science*, *588*, 401–417. DOI: 10.1016/j.jcis.2020.12.039 PMID: 33422789

Cathrin Lims, S., Tran, N. A., Dao, V.-D., & Pham, P. V. (2025). The world of quantum dot-shaped nanoparticles: Nobel prize in chemistry 2023: Advancements and prospectives. *Coordination Chemistry Reviews*, *528*, 216423–216423. DOI: 10.1016/j.ccr.2024.216423

Chakraborty, R., Asthana, A., Singh, A. K., Adhikari, R., & Susan, M. A. B. H. (2023). Collagen-a highly developed and abundant fibrous protein: synthesis and characterization. In *Handbook of Natural Polymers* (Vol. 1, pp. 489–508). Elsevier.

Chan, B. P., & Leong, K. W. (2008). Scaffolding in tissue engineering: General approaches and tissue-specific considerations. *European Spine Journal : Official Publication of the European Spine Society, the European Spinal Deformity Society, and the European Section of the Cervical Spine Research Society*, *17*(S4), 467–479. DOI: 10.1007/s00586-008-0745-3 PMID: 19005702

Chehelgerdi, M., Chehelgerdi, M., Allela, O. Q. B., Pecho, R. D. C., Jayasankar, N., Rao, D. P., Thamaraikani, T., Vasanthan, M., Viktor, P., Lakshmaiya, N., Saadh, M. J., Amajd, A., Abo-Zaid, M. A., Castillo-Acobo, R. Y., Ismail, A. H., Amin, A. H., & Akhavan-Sigari, R. (2023). Progressing nanotechnology to improve targeted cancer treatment: Overcoming hurdles in its clinical implementation. *Molecular Cancer*, *22*(1), 169. DOI: 10.1186/s12943-023-01865-0 PMID: 37814270

Daristotle, J. L., Behrens, A. M., Sandler, A. D., & Kofinas, P. (2016). A Review of the Fundamental Principles and Applications of Solution Blow Spinning. *ACS Applied Materials & Interfaces*, *8*(51), 34951–34963. DOI: 10.1021/acsami.6b12994 PMID: 27966857

Darwesh, O. M., Ali, S. S., Matter, I. A., Elsamahy, T., & Mahmoud, Y. A. (2020). Enzymes immobilization onto magnetic nanoparticles to improve industrial and environmental applications. *Methods in Enzymology*, *630*, 481–502. DOI: 10.1016/bs.mie.2019.11.006 PMID: 31931999

Elumalai, K., Srinivasan, S., & Shanmugam, A. (2024). Review of the efficacy of nanoparticle-based drug delivery systems for cancer treatment. *Biomedical Technology*, *5*, 109–122. DOI: 10.1016/j.bmt.2023.09.001

Ezike, T. C., Okpala, U. S., Onoja, U. L., Nwike, C. P., Ezeako, E. C., Okpara, O. J., Okoroafor, C. C., Eze, S. C., Kalu, O. L., Odoh, E. C., Nwadike, U. G., Ogbodo, J. O., Umeh, B. U., Ossai, E. C., & Nwanguma, B. C.Tobechukwu Christian Ezike. (2023). Advances in drug delivery systems, challenges and future directions. *Heliyon*, *9*(6), e17488–e17488. DOI: 10.1016/j.heliyon.2023.e17488 PMID: 37416680

Feczkó, T. (2021). Polymeric nanotherapeutics acting at special regions of body. *Journal of Drug Delivery Science and Technology*, *64*, 102597–102597. DOI: 10.1016/j.jddst.2021.102597

Fu, Y., Liu, T., Wang, H., Wang, Z., Hou, L., Jiang, J., & Xu, T. (2024). Applications of nanomaterial technology in biosensing. *Journal of Science. Advanced Materials and Devices*, *9*(2), 100694–100694. DOI: 10.1016/j.jsamd.2024.100694

Ganesan, A., & Jaiganesh, R. (2022). A review on fabrication methods of nanofibers and a special focus on application of cellulose nanofibers. *Carbohydrate Polymer Technologies and Applications*, •••, 100262.

Ghazal, H., Waqar, A., Yaseen, F., Shahid, M., Sultana, M., Tariq, M., Bashir, M. K., Tahseen, H., Raza, T., & Ahmad, F. (2024). Role of nanoparticles in enhancing chemotherapy efficacy for cancer treatment. *Next Materials*, *2*, 100128–100128. DOI: 10.1016/j.nxmate.2024.100128

Ghezzi, M., Pescina, S., Padula, C., Santi, P., Del Favero, E., Cantù, L., & Nicoli, S. (2021). Polymeric micelles in drug delivery: An insight of the techniques for their characterization and assessment in biorelevant conditions. *Journal of Controlled Release*, *332*, 312–336. DOI: 10.1016/j.jconrel.2021.02.031 PMID: 33652113

Goyal, R., Macri, L. K., Kaplan, H. M., & Kohn, J. (2016). Nanoparticles and nanofibers for topical drug delivery. *Journal of Controlled Release*, *240*, 77–92. DOI: 10.1016/j.jconrel.2015.10.049 PMID: 26518723

Han, H., Li, S., Xu, M., Zhong, Y., Fan, W., Xu, J., Zhou, T., Ji, J., Ye, J., & Yao, K. (2023). Polymer- and lipid-based nanocarriers for ocular drug delivery: Current status and future perspectives. *Advanced Drug Delivery Reviews*, *196*, 114770. DOI: 10.1016/j.addr.2023.114770 PMID: 36894134

Hasan, A., Morshed, M., Memic, A., Hassan, S., Webster, T., & Marei, H. (2018). Nanoparticles in tissue engineering: Applications, challenges and prospects. *International Journal of Nanomedicine*, *13*, 5637–5655. DOI: 10.2147/IJN.S153758 PMID: 30288038

Hashem, A. H., Al, M. A., Alawlaqi, M. M., Abdelghany, T. M., & Hasanin, M. (2021). Synthesis of Nanocapsules Based on Biosynthesized Nickel Nanoparticles and Potato Starch: Antimicrobial, Antioxidant, and Anticancer Activity. *Stärke*, *74*(1-2), 2100165. DOI: 10.1002/star.202100165

Hassan, H., Sharma, P., Hasan, M. R., Singh, S., Thakur, D., & Narang, J. (2022). Gold nanomaterials – The golden approach from synthesis to applications. *Materials Science for Energy Technologies*, *5*, 375–390. DOI: 10.1016/j.mset.2022.09.004

Hashemi-Afzal, F., Fallahi, H., Bagheri, F., Collins, M. N., Eslaminejad, M. B., & Seitz, H. (2025). Advancements in hydrogel design for articular cartilage regeneration: A comprehensive review. *Bioactive Materials*, *43*, 1–31.

Herrero, Y. R., Camas, K. L., & Ullah, A. (2023). Characterization of biobased materials. In *Advanced Applications of Biobased Materials* (pp. 111–143). Elsevier.

Hesemans, E., Buttiens, K., Manshian, B., & Soenen, S. (2022). The Role of Optical Imaging in Translational Nanomedicine. *Journal of Functional Biomaterials*, *13*(3), 137–137. DOI: 10.3390/jfb13030137 PMID: 36135572

Rayat Pisheh, H., Nojabaei, F. S., Darvishi, A., Rayat Pisheh, A., & Sani, M. (2024). Cardiac tissue engineering: An emerging approach to the treatment of heart failure. *Frontiers in Bioengineering and Biotechnology*, *12*, 1441933.

Huanbutta, K., Puri, V., Sharma, A., Singh, I., Sriamornsak, P., & Sangnim, T. (2024). Rise of implantable drugs: A chronicle of breakthroughs in drug delivery systems. *Saudi Pharmaceutical Journal : SPJ : the Official Publication of the Saudi Pharmaceutical Society*, *32*(12), 102193. DOI: 10.1016/j.jsps.2024.102193 PMID: 39564378

Huang, C., Dong, L., Zhao, B., Lu, Y., Huang, S., Yuan, Z., Luo, G., Xu, Y., & Qian, W. (2022). Anti-inflammatory hydrogel dressings and skin wound healing. *Clinical and Translational Medicine*, *12*(11), e1094. DOI: 10.1002/ctm2.1094 PMID: 36354147

Huang, X., & El-Sayed, M. A. (2010). Gold nanoparticles: Optical properties and implementations in cancer diagnosis and photothermal therapy. *Journal of Advanced Research*, *1*(1), 13–28. DOI: 10.1016/j.jare.2010.02.002

Delloyd. (n.d.). Infrared and FTIR spectroscopy Instrument. Delloyd.50megs.com. http://delloyd.50megs.com/MOBILE/infrared_spectroscopy.html

Iyad, N., Ahmad, M. S., Alkhatib, S. G., & Hjouj, M. (2023). Gadolinium contrast agents-challenges and opportunities of a multidisciplinary approach: Literature review. *European Journal of Radiology Open*, *11*, 100503.

Jadhav, S., Gaikwad, S., Nimse, M., & Rajbhoj, A. (2011). Copper Oxide Nanoparticles: Synthesis, Characterization and Their Antibacterial Activity. *Journal of Cluster Science*, *22*(2), 121–129. DOI: 10.1007/s10876-011-0349-7

Jain, R. K., D. Fukumura, & Duda, D. G. (2014). Modes of Neovascularization in Tumors and Clinical Translation of Antiangiogenic Therapy. *Elsevier EBooks*, 2926–2957.

Jin, C., Wu, Z., Molinski, J. H., Zhou, J., Ren, Y., & Zhang, J. H. (2022). Plasmonic nanosensors for point-of-care biomarker detection. *Materials Today. Bio*, *14*, 100263–100263. DOI: 10.1016/j.mtbio.2022.100263 PMID: 35514435

Jorgensen, A., Mahajan, N., Atala, A., & Murphy, S. V. (2022).. . *Advances in Skin Tissue Engineering and Regenerative Medicine.*, *44*(Supplement_1), S33–S41.

Kairdolf, B. A., Smith, A. M., Stokes, T. H., Wang, M. D., Young, A. N., & Nie, S. (2013). Semiconductor Quantum Dots for Bioimaging and Biodiagnostic Applications. *Annual Review of Analytical Chemistry (Palo Alto, Calif.)*, *6*(1), 143–162. DOI: 10.1146/annurev-anchem-060908-155136 PMID: 23527547

Kalra, A., Nag, A., Khandelwal, A., & Singh, R. (2023). Nanoparticles: Characters, applications, and synthesis by endophytes. *Elsevier EBooks*, 237–276.

Kapil, N., Mayani, S. V., & Gopal Bhattacharyya, K. (2023). Environmental implications of nanoceramic applications. *Results in Chemistry*, *5*, 100724. DOI: 10.1016/j.rechem.2022.100724

Karimı, M., Eslami, M., Sahandi-Zangabad, P., Mirab, F., Farajisafiloo, N., Shafaei, Z., Ghosh, D., Bozorgomid, M., Dashkhaneh, F., & Hamblin, M. R. (2016). pH-Sensitive stimulus-responsive nanocarriers for targeted delivery of therapeutic agents. *Wiley Interdisciplinary Reviews. Nanomedicine and Nanobiotechnology*, *8*(5), 696–716. DOI: 10.1002/wnan.1389 PMID: 26762467

Khalef, L., Lydia, R., Filicia, K., & Moussa, B. (2024). Cell viability and cytotoxicity assays: Biochemical elements and cellular compartments. *Cell Biochemistry and Function*, *42*(3), e4007. DOI: 10.1002/cbf.4007 PMID: 38593323

Kulkarni, D., Musale, S., Panzade, P., Paiva-Santos, A. C., Sonwane, P., Madibone, M., Choundhe, P., Giram, P., & Cavalu, S. (2022). Surface Functionalization of Nanofibers: The Multifaceted Approach for Advanced Biomedical Applications. *Nanomaterials (Basel, Switzerland)*, *12*(21), 3899. DOI: 10.3390/nano12213899 PMID: 36364675

Kumar, M., Kulkarni, P., Liu, S., Chemuturi, N., & Shah, D. K. (2023). Nanoparticle biodistribution coefficients: A quantitative approach for understanding the tissue distribution of nanoparticles. *Advanced Drug Delivery Reviews*, *194*, 114708. DOI: 10.1016/j.addr.2023.114708 PMID: 36682420

Kumar, S., Bhushan, P., & Bhattacharya, S. (2017). Fabrication of Nanostructures with Bottom-up Approach and Their Utility in Diagnostics, Therapeutics, and Others. *Energy. Environmental Sustainability*, •••, 167–198.

Kumari, S., Raturi, S., Kulshrestha, S., Chauhan, K., Dhingra, S., András, K., Thu, K., Khargotra, R., & Singh, T. (2023). A comprehensive review on various techniques used for synthesizing nanoparticles. *Journal of Materials Research and Technology*, *27*, 27. DOI: 10.1016/j.jmrt.2023.09.291

Kuriakose, A., Chirmule, N., & Nair, P. (2016). Immunogenicity of Biotherapeutics: Causes and Association with Posttranslational Modifications. *Journal of Immunology Research*, *2016*, 1–18. DOI: 10.1155/2016/1298473 PMID: 27437405

Kurul, F., Turkmen, H., Cetin, A. E., & Topkaya, S. N. (2025). Nanomedicine: How nanomaterials are transforming drug delivery, bio-imaging, and diagnosis. *Next Nanotechnology*, *7*, 100129. DOI: 10.1016/j.nxnano.2024.100129

Kushwaha, A., Goswami, L., & Kim, B. S. (2022). Nanomaterial-Based Therapy for Wound Healing. *Nanomaterials (Basel, Switzerland)*, *12*(4), 618. DOI: 10.3390/nano12040618 PMID: 35214947

Lee, S. S., Du, X., Kim, I., & Ferguson, S. J. (2022). Scaffolds for bone-tissue engineering. *Matter*, *5*(9), 2722–2759. DOI: 10.1016/j.matt.2022.06.003 PMID: 35673575

Li, X., Li, X., Zhang, X.-N., Li, X.-D., Chang, J., Zhang, X.-N., Li, X.-D., & Chang, J. (2016). Multimodality imaging in nanomedicine and nanotheranostics. *Cancer Biology & Medicine*, *13*(3), 339–348. DOI: 10.20892/j.issn.2095-3941.2016.0055 PMID: 27807501

Liposomes. (n.d.). InProcess-LSP. https://www.inprocess-lsp.com/liposomes/

Machtakova, M., Thérien-Aubin, H., & Landfester, K. (2022). Polymer nano-systems for the encapsulation and delivery of active biomacromolecular therapeutic agents. *Chemical Society Reviews*, *51*(1), 128–152. DOI: 10.1039/D1CS00686J PMID: 34762084

Mahadeshwara, M. R. (n.d.). *XRD – X-ray diffraction - About Tribology*. https://www.tribonet.org/wiki/xrd-x-ray-diffraction/

Mahfooz-ur-Rehman, , Rehman, W., Waseem, M., Shah, B. A., Shakeel, M., Haq, S., Zaman, U., Bibi, I., & Khan, H. D.Mahfooz-ur-Rehman. (2019). Fabrication of Titanium–Tin Oxide Nanocomposite with Enhanced Adsorption and Antimicrobial Applications. *Journal of Chemical & Engineering Data*, *64*(6), 2436–2444. DOI: 10.1021/acs.jced.8b01243

Meher, A., Tandi, A., Moharana, S., Chakroborty, S., Mohapatra, S. S., Mondal, A., ... & Chandra, P. (2024). Silver nanoparticle for biomedical applications: A review. Hybrid Advances, 100184.

Mehta, M., Bui, T. A., Yang, X., Aksoy, Y. A., Goldys, E. M., & Deng, W. (2023). Lipid-Based Nanoparticles for Drug/Gene Delivery: An Overview of the Production Techniques and Difficulties Encountered in Their Industrial Development. *ACS Materials Science Au, 3*(6).

Mimona, M. A., & Hossain, I. (2025). Quantum Dot Nanomaterials: Empowering Advances in Optoelectronic Devices. *Chemical Engineering Journal Advances*, *21*, 100704–100704. DOI: 10.1016/j.ceja.2025.100704

Mirsasaani, S. S., Hemati, M., Dehkord, E. S., Yazdi, G. T., & Poshtiri, D. A. (2019). Nanotechnology and nanobiomaterials in dentistry. *Nanobiomaterials in Clinical Dentistry*, 19–37.

Mittal, P., Saharan, A., Verma, R., Altalbawy, F. M. A., Alfaidi, M. A., Batiha, G. E.-S., Akter, W., Gautam, R. K., Uddin, M. S., & Rahman, M. S. (2021). Dendrimers: A New Race of Pharmaceutical Nanocarriers. *BioMed Research International*, *2021*(1), e8844030. DOI: 10.1155/2021/8844030 PMID: 33644232

Moulana Kareem, M., & Babu, H. (2023). Anticancer, antibacterial, antioxidant, and photo-catalytic activities of eco-friendly synthesized Ni nanoparticles. *Inorganic Chemistry Communications*, *148*, 110274. DOI: 10.1016/j.inoche.2022.110274

Naganthran, A., Verasoundarapandian, G., Khalid, F. E., Masarudin, M. J., Zulkharnain, A., Nawawi, N. M., Karim, M., Che Abdullah, C. A., & Ahmad, S. A. (2022). Synthesis, Characterization and Biomedical Application of Silver Nanoparticles. *Materials (Basel)*, *15*(2), 427. DOI: 10.3390/ma15020427 PMID: 35057145

Nakhaei, P., Margiana, R., Bokov, D. O., Abdelbasset, W. K., Jadidi Kouhbanani, M. A., Varma, R. S., Marofi, F., Jarahian, M., & Beheshtkhoo, N. (2021). Liposomes: Structure, Biomedical Applications, and Stability Parameters With Emphasis on Cholesterol. *Frontiers in Bioengineering and Biotechnology*, *9*, 705886. DOI: 10.3389/fbioe.2021.705886 PMID: 34568298

Niculescu, A.-G., & Grumezescu, A. M. (2022). Novel Tumor-Targeting Nanoparticles for Cancer Treatment—A Review. *International Journal of Molecular Sciences*, *23*(9), 5253. DOI: 10.3390/ijms23095253 PMID: 35563645

Nune, S. K., Gunda, P., Thallapally, P. K., Lin, Y.-Y., Laird Forrest, M., & Berkland, C. J. (2009). Nanoparticles for biomedical imaging. *Expert Opinion on Drug Delivery*, *6*(11), 1175–1194. DOI: 10.1517/17425240903229031 PMID: 19743894

Nyabadza, A., McCarthy, É., Makhesana, M., Heidarinassab, S., Plouze, A., Vazquez, M., & Brabazon, D. (2023). A review of physical, chemical and biological synthesis methods of bimetallic nanoparticles and applications in sensing, water treatment, biomedicine, catalysis and hydrogen storage. *Advances in Colloid and Interface Science, 321*, 103010–103010. DOI: 10.1016/j.cis.2023.103010 PMID: 37804661

Osman, A. I., Zhang, Y., Farghali, M., Rashwan, A. K., Eltaweil, A. S., Abd El-Monaem, E. M., Mohamed, I. M. A., Badr, M. M., Ihara, I., Rooney, D. W., & Yap, P.-S. (2024). Synthesis of green nanoparticles for energy, biomedical, environmental, agricultural, and food applications: A review. *Environmental Chemistry Letters, 22*(2), 841–887. DOI: 10.1007/s10311-023-01682-3

Patel, N., & Munjal, S. (2022). *Metal Oxide Nanoparticles and Their Applications: A Report. ArXiv*. Cornell University.

Patra, J. K., Das, G., Fraceto, L. F., Campos, E. V. R., Rodriguez-Torres, M. del P., Acosta-Torres, L. S., Diaz-Torres, L. A., Grillo, R., Swamy, M. K., Sharma, S., Habtemariam, S., & Shin, H.-S. (2018). Nano Based Drug Delivery systems: Recent Developments and Future Prospects. *Journal of Nanobiotechnology, 16*(1), 71. DOI: 10.1186/s12951-018-0392-8 PMID: 30231877

Pavlenko, V., Khosravi, H. S., Żółtowska, S., Haruna, A. B., Zahid, M., Mansurov, Z., Supiyeva, Z., Galal, A., Ozoemena, K. I., Abbas, Q., & Jesionowski, T. (2022). A comprehensive review of template-assisted porous carbons: Modern preparation methods and advanced applications. *Materials Science and Engineering R Reports, 149*, 100682. DOI: 10.1016/j.mser.2022.100682

Pechyen, C., Tangnorawich, B., Toommee, S., Marks, R., & Parcharoen, Y. (2024). Green synthesis of metal nanoparticles, characterization, and biosensing applications. *Sensors International, 5*, 100287–100287. DOI: 10.1016/j.sintl.2024.100287

Prasad Yadav, T., Manohar Yadav, R., & Pratap Singh, D. (2012). Mechanical Milling: A Top Down Approach for the Synthesis of Nanomaterials and Nanocomposites. *Nanoscience and Nanotechnology, 2*(3), 22–48. DOI: 10.5923/j.nn.20120203.01

Rakhi, T., Pragati, M., Prerna, B., & Jyoti, S. (2023). Multifaceted approach for nanofiber fabrication. In *Fiber and Textile Engineering in Drug Delivery Systems* (pp. 253–283). Woodhead Publishing.

Rashid, A. B., Haque, M., Islam, S. M. M., & Uddin Labib, K. M. R. (2024). Nanotechnology-enhanced fiber-reinforced polymer composites: Recent advancements on processing techniques and applications. *Heliyon, 10*(2), e24692. DOI: 10.1016/j.heliyon.2024.e24692 PMID: 38298690

Rasmussen, J. W., Martinez, E., Louka, P., & Wingett, D. G. (2010). Zinc oxide nanoparticles for selective destruction of tumor cells and potential for drug delivery applications. *Expert Opinion on Drug Delivery*, *7*(9), 1063–1077. DOI: 10.1517/17425247.2010.502560 PMID: 20716019

Rathod, S., Preetam, S., Pandey, C., & Bera, S. P. (2024). Exploring Synthesis and Applications of Green Nanoparticles and the Role of Nanotechnology in Wastewater Treatment. *Biotechnology Reports (Amsterdam, Netherlands)*, *41*, 00830. DOI: 10.1016/j.btre.2024.e00830 PMID: 38332899

Raut, S. S., Singh, R., & Lekhak, U. M. (2024). Naturally occurring nanoparticles (NONPs): A review. *Next Sustainability*, *3*, 100037–100037. DOI: 10.1016/j.nxsust.2024.100037

Rocca, A. L., Liberto, G. D., Shayler, P. J., Parmenter, C. D. J., & Fay, M. W. (2013). Application of nanoparticle tracking analysis platform for the measurement of soot-in-oil agglomerates from automotive engines. *Tribology International*, *70*, 142–147. DOI: 10.1016/j.triboint.2013.09.018

Khan, N. R., & Rashid, A. B. (2024). Carbon-based nanomaterials: A paradigm shift in biofuel synthesis and processing for a sustainable energy future. *Energy Conversion and Management*, *X*, 100590.

Ruedas-Rama, M. J., Walters, J. D., Orte, A., & Hall, E. A. H. (2012). Fluorescent nanoparticles for intracellular sensing: A review. *Analytica Chimica Acta*, *751*, 1–23. DOI: 10.1016/j.aca.2012.09.025 PMID: 23084048

Saadatkhah, N., Carillo Garcia, A., Ackermann, S., Leclerc, P., Latifi, M., Samih, S., Patience, G. S., & Chaouki, J. (2019). Experimental methods in chemical engineering: Thermogravimetric analysis—TGA. *Canadian Journal of Chemical Engineering*, *98*(1), 34–43. DOI: 10.1002/cjce.23673

Saghazadeh, S., Rinoldi, C., Schot, M., Kashaf, S. S., Sharifi, F., Jalilian, E., Nuutila, K., Giatsidis, G., Mostafalu, P., Derakhshandeh, H., Yue, K., Swieszkowski, W., Memic, A., Tamayol, A., & Khademhosseini, A. (2018). Drug delivery systems and materials for wound healing applications. *Advanced Drug Delivery Reviews*, *127*, 138–166. DOI: 10.1016/j.addr.2018.04.008 PMID: 29626550

Salari, Z., Ameri, A., Forootanfar, H., Adeli-Sardou, M., Jafari, M., Mehrabani, M., & Shakibaie, M. (2017). Microwave-assisted biosynthesis of zinc nanoparticles and their cytotoxic and antioxidant activity. *Journal of Trace Elements in Medicine and Biology*, *39*, 116–123. DOI: 10.1016/j.jtemb.2016.09.001 PMID: 27908402

Sánchez-López, E., Gomes, D., Esteruelas, G., Bonilla, L., Lopez-Machado, A. L., Galindo, R., Cano, A., Espina, M., Ettcheto, M., Camins, A., Silva, A. M., Durazzo, A., Santini, A., Garcia, M. L., & Souto, E. B. (2020). Metal-Based Nanoparticles as Antimicrobial Agents: An Overview. *Nanomaterials (Basel, Switzerland)*, *10*(2), 292. DOI: 10.3390/nano10020292 PMID: 32050443

Santhoshkumar, T., Rahuman, A. A., Jayaseelan, C., Rajakumar, G., Marimuthu, S., Kirthi, A. V., Velayutham, K., Thomas, J., Venkatesan, J., & Kim, S.-K. (2014). Green synthesis of titanium dioxide nanoparticles using Psidium guajava extract and its antibacterial and antioxidant properties. *Asian Pacific Journal of Tropical Medicine*, *7*(12), 968–976. DOI: 10.1016/S1995-7645(14)60171-1 PMID: 25479626

Saraswat, S. K., Mustafa, M. A., Ghadir, G. K., Kaur, M., Lozada, D. F. G., & Al-Ani, A. M. & huseen Redhee, A. (2024). Carbon quantum dots: A comprehensive review of green Synthesis, characterization and investigation their applications in bioimaging. *Inorganic Chemistry Communications*, •••, 112279.

Serrano-Lotina, A., Portela, R., Baeza, P., Alcolea-Rodriguez, V., Villarroel, M., & Avila, P. (2022). Zeta potential as a tool for functional materials development. *Catalysis Today*.

Sheppard, C. J. R. (2005). MICROSCOPY I Overview. *Encyclopedia of Modern Optics*, 61–69.

Sindhi, K., Pingili, R. B., Beldar, V., Bhattacharya, S., Rahaman, J., & Mukherjee, D. (2025). The role of biomaterials-based scaffolds in advancing skin tissue construct. *Journal ofTissue Viability*, *34*(2), 100858–100858. DOI: 10.1016/j.jtv.2025.100858 PMID: 39827732

Stachowiak, G. W., Batchelor, A. W., & Stachowiak, G. B. (2004). Characterization of Test Specimens. *Tribology Series*, 115–150.

Steere, A. C., Strle, K., & Drouin, E. E. (2015). Infection and Autoimmunity in Antibiotic-Refractory Lyme Arthritis. In Infection and Autoimmunity (pp. 519-534). Academic Press.

Subramanian, A., Krishnan, U., & Sethuraman, S. (2009). Development of biomaterial scaffold for nerve tissue engineering: Biomaterial mediated neural regeneration. *Journal of Biomedical Science*, *16*(1), 108. DOI: 10.1186/1423-0127-16-108 PMID: 19939265

Sultana, A., Zare, M., Thomas, V., Kumar, T. S. S., & Ramakrishna, S. (2022). Nano-based drug delivery systems: Conventional drug delivery routes, recent developments and future prospects. *Medicine in Drug Discovery*, *15*, 100134. DOI: 10.1016/j.medidd.2022.100134

Sun, L., Li, H., Ye, Y., Yang, L., Islam, R., Tan, S., Tong, R., Miao, Y., & Cai, L. (2023). Smart nanoparticles for cancer therapy. *Signal Transduction and Targeted Therapy*, *8*(1), 418. DOI: 10.1038/s41392-023-01642-x PMID: 37919282

Teimouri, R., Abnous, K., Taghdisi, S. M., Ramezani, M., & Alibolandi, M. (2023). Surface modifications of scaffolds for bone regeneration. *Journal of Materials Research and Technology*, *24*, 7938–7973. DOI: 10.1016/j.jmrt.2023.05.076

Waheed, S., Li, Z., Zhang, F., Chiarini, A., Armato, U., & Wu, J. (2022). Engineering nano-drug biointerface to overcome biological barriers toward precision drug delivery. *Journal of Nanobiotechnology*, *20*(1), 395. DOI: 10.1186/s12951-022-01605-4 PMID: 36045386

Wang, F., Cai, X., Shen, Y., & Meng, L. (2023). Cell–scaffold interactions in tissue engineering for oral and craniofacial reconstruction. *Bioactive Materials*, *23*, 16–44. DOI: 10.1016/j.bioactmat.2022.10.029 PMID: 36406245

Wong, W. F., Ang, K. P., Sethi, G., & Looi, C. Y. (2023). Recent advancement of medical patch for transdermal drug delivery. *Medicina*, *59*(4), 778.

Woźniak-Budych, M. J., Langer, K., Peplińska, B., Przysiecka, Ł., Jarek, M., Jarzębski, M., & Jurga, S. (2016). Copper-gold nanoparticles: Fabrication, characteristic and application as drug carriers. *Materials Chemistry and Physics*, *179*, 242–253. DOI: 10.1016/j.matchemphys.2016.05.036

Wu, Y., Ali, M. R. K., Chen, K., Fang, N., & El-Sayed, M. A. (2019). Gold nanoparticles in biological optical imaging. *Nano Today*, *24*, 120–140. DOI: 10.1016/j.nantod.2018.12.006

Yousefian, F., Hesari, R., Jensen, T., Obagi, S., Rgeai, A., Damiani, G., Bunick, C. G., & Grada, A. (2023). Antimicrobial Wound Dressings: A Concise Review for Clinicians. *Antibiotics (Basel, Switzerland)*, *12*(9), 1434. DOI: 10.3390/antibiotics12091434 PMID: 37760730

Zhang, X.-Q., Xu, X., Bertrand, N., Pridgen, E., Swami, A., & Farokhzad, O. C. (2012). Interactions of nanomaterials and biological systems: Implications to personalized nanomedicine. *Advanced Drug Delivery Reviews*, *64*(13), 1363–1384. DOI: 10.1016/j.addr.2012.08.005 PMID: 22917779

Zhou, J., & Vijayavenkataraman, S. (2021). 3D-printable conductive materials for tissue engineering and biomedical applications. *Bioprinting (Amsterdam, Netherlands)*, *24*, e00166. DOI: 10.1016/j.bprint.2021.e00166

Chapter 2
Overview of Biomaterials Classification, Properties, and Biomedical Applications

Imade Armadi
https://orcid.org/0009-0003-3063-5058
Cadi Ayyad University, Marrakech, Morocco

Adil El Housseini
https://orcid.org/0009-0007-9294-2685
Ibn Zohr University, Marrakech, Morocco

Samia Elouali
Cadi Ayyad University; University of Mons, Marrakech, Morocco

Souad Loqman
Cadi Ayyad University, Marrakech, Morocco

Abdessamad Abana
Cadi Ayyad University, Marrakech, Morocco

Anass Belbachir
https://orcid.org/0009-0002-4828-0251
Cadi Ayyad University, Marrakech, Morocco

ABSTRACT

Biomaterials have attracted growing interest in the biomedical field thanks to their unique ability to interact with biological systems and make a significant contribution to advances in medicine, tissue engineering and sustainable technologies. Their importance lies in their dual potential: improving patients' quality of life while reducing their impact on the environment. This chapter first presents a detailed classification of biomaterials, distinguishing between natural, synthetic and hybrid categories. Next, the key properties of biomaterials are explored, showing their role in biocompatibility, durability and clinical performance. These fundamental characteristics directly influence the choice of biomaterials for a variety of applications.

DOI: 10.4018/979-8-3373-1305-4.ch002

In addition, this chapter highlights the diversity of current biomaterial applications, while discussing the persistent challenges and limitations encountered in their design and use. Finally, future prospects are discussed, including the emergence of personalized biomaterials, which could revolutionize biomedical technologies.

INTRODUCTION

From prehistoric times to the mid-19th century, the era of modern medicine, the word biomaterials has attracted the interest of scientific researchers, evolving over time in line with technological advances and scientific knowledge. (Cohen, 1967), was one of the first to propose a definition of biomaterials. For him, they are defined as any material used as an implant. This concept, though elementary, laid the foundations for a line of thinking that was to become progressively more refined. In 1974, the first approach was enriched by integrating the word inert substance, so that the definition of biomaterials is a systematically and pharmacologically inert substance designed to be implanted or incorporated into a living system (Marin et al., 2020). A few years later, the definition was redefined, this time emphasizing the importance of biomedical function. It therefore refers to a substance of synthetic or natural origin, which can be used for a given period of time, as a whole or as part of a system that treats, augments or replaces a tissue, organ or function of the body (Nitesh R. Patel & Piyush P. Gohil, 2012). In 1987, Professor David Franklyn Williams proposed a more systematic approach, incorporating the notion of non-viability into the definition, for what takes the form of a non-viable material used in a medical device, intended to interact with biological systems (Williams DF, 1987). It took until 1991, at the "Consensus Conference", to get the most complete definition, accepted today by the scientific community. Biomaterials are therefore any substance or combination of substances, other than drugs, of synthetic or natural origin, which can be used for a given period of time, which partially or totally augment or replace a tissue, organ or function of the body, in order to maintain or improve the individual's quality of life. This definition takes into account the concept of improving quality of life (Marin et al., 2020). Thus, the progressive evolution of the definition of biomaterials reflects their growing role in scientific research and their multiple applications. Today, biomaterials are no longer considered simply as biological substitutes, but as key elements of biomedical innovation. The evolution of their definition has been accompanied at the same time by a diversification of their classification, notably according to their origin (natural or synthetic), their structure (polymers, metals, ceramics, composites) and their function (mechanical support, biological interface, tissue regeneration, etc.) (Agrawal et al., 2023). This multifactorial approach enables us to better adapt to the specific requirements of each clinical application. In addition, their physico-chemical and biological properties - such as biocompatibility, biodegradability and non-toxicity, in plus bioactivity, thermal, chemical and mechanical stability, not forgetting hydrophilic/hydrophobic properties - are rigorously studied to guarantee their efficacy and safety in vivo. Thanks to these qualities, biomaterials have a wide range of applications: orthopedic implants, cardiovascular devices, tissue engineering, drug delivery systems, and many others. Against a dynamic backdrop of rapid technological progress, current trends are moving towards intelligent, bio-inspired materials that can be customized via 3D printing or nanotechnology. However, major challenges remain, notably in terms of immune response, long-term durability, and large-scale manufacturing. This chapter explores these aspects to better understand the impact and future prospects of biomaterials in the biomedical field (Chong et al., 2023).

I. CLASSIFICATION OF BIOMATERIALS

Biomaterials are materials designed to interact with biological systems for medical purposes, such as replacing or repairing tissues and organs. The classification of biomaterials is essential for understanding their properties and optimizing their use in various applications, various criteria are based to classification of biomaterials, including chemical composition, structure, and biological properties, mean classification methods are chemical, functional, source-based, and structural properties (Mahdi et al., 2024). Common categories comprise bioceramic, polymeric, and metallic biomaterials, each with specific advantages and disadvantages (Chong et al., 2023). Crucial considerations for biomaterial selection include biocompatibility, bioinertness, bioactivity, biodegradability, sterilizability, mechanical properties, manufacturability, weight, and cost (Barutça et al., 2018). High speeds evolution of biomaterials has guided to multifunctional, customizable, and biologically active materials, necessitating more sophisticated classification systems (Arjunan et al., 2022). These classification methods are essential for understanding biomaterial properties, guarantying optimal use in medical devices and implants, and facilitating regulatory processes (Chong et al., 2023).

1. Classification of Biomaterials by Origin

Biomaterials can be classified by origin into two primary categories: natural and synthetic materials. Natural biomaterials, such as collagen, chitosan, and silk, are obtained from biological sources and demonstrate inherent biocompatibility and bioactivity, making them suitable for applications in tissue engineering and regenerative medicine. In opposition, synthetic biomaterials, including polymers like polypropylene and metals, take into account the precise control over material properties, enabling customization for specific medical applications. Besides, hybrid biomaterials, which are a combine of natural and synthetic components made to leverage the advantages of both. They are designed to enhance properties like biocompatibility, mechanical strength, and functionality, making them suitable for advanced biomedical applications (Datta et al., 2020). Natural biomaterials are often more biocompatible resulting from their origin, which makes them fit for purpose for applications in direct contact with biological tissues, such as implants and tissue scaffolds, in other hands synthetic biomaterials yield in precise control over their properties, which is beneficial for applications requiring specific mechanical or chemical characteristics, for instance in drug delivery systems and orthopedic devices. While hybrid biomaterials are utilized in cutting-edge applications like smart drug delivery systems and bioimaging, where the integration of natural and synthetic elements can provide enhanced functionality and performance (Chelu & Musuc, 2023). Additionally, biomaterials can be further categorized based on their processing methods, such as unmodified, extracted, or derived materials, which influence their final properties and applications (Chakraborty & Prasad, 2024).

- **Biomaterials From Natural Origin**

Biomaterials that originate from natural sources consist of broad variety of materials from plants, animals, and even microorganisms that are being used more often in medical applications because they're bio-compatible and can be broken down. From polysaccharides such as cellulose, alginate, chitosan and agarose, to collagens, elastins, fibronectins, silk proteins and minerals such as hydroxyapatite and calcium carbonate mimic the structures of human tissues which makes them useful tissue engineering and regenerative medicine (P. Mishra et al., 2024). Natural biomaterials have been used since ancient times for wound healing, bone grafting and tissue formation. However, great progress has been made towards their uses for long term implants and scaffolds (Alamgir & Haider, 2023). Innovations made recently include bioactive scaffold development and injectable biomaterials enhancement for better drug delivery and tissue regeneration. The emergence of advanced technologies, such as 3D printing and biofabrication, now makes it possible to design customized three-dimensional scaffolds, promoting better cellular integration and architecture adapted to targeted tissues (Bhatti & Singh, 2023; H. Zhang & Wu, 2023). These efforts address challenges like immune rejection and infection (Jasni et al., 2023). Research being made for these materials is to stamp out issues faced and broaden the potential to be used in more biomedical improvements (Chouhan et al., 2023).

Due to their resemblance with the extracellular matrix, natural biomaterials are highly used in tissue engineering because they allow cells to adhere, proliferate and differentiate as well as stimulate tissue regeneration. They also used in the formulation of drug delivery systems, and their biocompatibility and biodegradability are very important for controlled release of drugs and in synergy with biological tissues (Troy et al., 2021). Another unique bioactive potential of natural biomaterials is that their particular chemistries can be used to actively improve therapeutic outcomes. The processing preservation of bioactivity, however, is difficult to meet. These properties can be retained and optimized with techniques such as cross-linking as well as decellularization, in the perspective of realizing a material that could be used as drug delivery systems or tissue engineered constructs (Joyce et al., 2021).

- **Biomaterials From Synthetic Origin**

Customizable in their properties, such biomaterials represent the spearhead of modern biomedical practice with contents specific to improved functionality and biological compatibility of synthetic materials. Polymeric materials, such as polypropylene, polyurethanes, polymethyl methacrylate (PMMA) and polyethylene terephthalate (PET), can be used to produce scaffolds, offer a higher degree of specificity for mechanical as well as chemical properties are useful in a variety of applications from tissue engineering or drug delivery (Aldana et al., 2023). Mean type of synthetic biomaterials comprise metabolically derived synthons that can be made up from metabolism-derived building blocks, e.g. lactic acid and glycerol which provides them with a myriad of possible structural features as well functions. For example they are widely used in drug delivery and tissue engineering due to their bio-deliverable properties (Chelu & Musuc, 2023). Polymers that are sequence-controlled other synthetic biomaterials have been developed via advanced synthetic methods to replicate the linear sequence of biopolymers. Used mostly for the fabrication of tailorable biomaterials (Austin & Rosales, 2019). With in drug delivery medical implants and tissue engineering scaffolds, synthetic biomaterials have accurate properties, at times these lacks the time and space complexity of the natural ECM. However, future studies are needed to further extrapolate these natural principles in order to achieve viable tissue and organ-specific applications (Todros et al., 2021). A promising artificial integration of additive manufacturing with synthetic biomaterials is needed to design patient specific medical device. However, there are still challenges in terms of material selection and processing technologies to upscale this technology (Satchanska et al., 2024). The advancements in synthetic biomaterials have facilitated the development of innovative solutions, comprehending bioactive scaffolds that support cell growth and tissue regeneration, as well as, injectable systems for targeted therapeutic delivery (Alamgir & Haider,

2023). Despite their advantages, challenges such as bioactivity and resorption remain critical areas of research. However convergence of synthetic biology and biomaterials research had lead in creation of hierarchically structured and 'living' materials that can sense and respond to their environment, with potential applications in medicine and biotechnology (A. P. Liu et al., 2022). Mostly, the integration of synthetic biomaterials into medical practice continues to evolve, driven by ongoing innovations and the need for improved biocompatibility and functionality (Tsouknidas, 2024).

- **Biomaterials From Hybrid Origin**

Hybrid biomaterials were all intended as a combination of natural and synthetic sources, which are seeing increasing interest for both biomedical applications like tissue engineering, and regenerative medicine in particular. These materials are designed to combine the desirable features of both kinds: biocompatibility/bioactivity of natural materials and mechanical robustness/service-life properties of synthetic polymers; Hybrid biomaterials are generally polymeric materials, natural polymers for example: collagen, chitosan, elastin, keratin,silk etc. with synthetic polymers mixed to generate blends with improved properties (Rana & De la Hoz Siegler, 2024). Polyhydroxyalkanoates (PHAs), for instance are biodegradable and biocompatible polyesters which can be incorporated into other materials to modulate their mechanical as well as functional properties for tissue engineered applications (Pryadko et al., 2021). Further, Hybrid biomaterials are used widely in tissue engineering because they provide characteristics similar to natural tissues. They are used in bone, cartilage, nerve tissues engineering, and skin. They also allow for the tuning of properties towards specific tissue requirements, so as to orientate the cell transmigration and support extracellular matrix formation when fabricated with organic-inorganic hybrid material composites (Pryadko et al., 2021). They can also be used in a functional way by e.g. adding drug delivery systems (Abalymov et al., 2020). For example, hybrid constructs have been shown to promote cell growth and differentiation as observed in biohybrids made up of lipid vesicles with phytosynthesized NP; the antioxidant and antimicrobial properties of which were examined with considerable values (Barbinta-Patrascu et al., 2024). Moreover, hybrid materials have been taken as a promising approach to overcoming the constraints of synthetic or natural materials with special attention such as infection risks and mechanical issues in cardiovascular and urological applications (Casarin et al., 2023). Moreover, several natural hybrid biomaterials was approved in clinical trials as osteogenic differentiation promoting and analgesic compounds showing their therapeutic potentials (Izadyari Aghmiuni et al., 2024). Although some important applications of hybrid biomaterials have been demonstrated, all still need optimization for the particular biomedical usage. The modular and orthogonal synthesis of hybrid polymers intends for materials with tunable and distinct properties (Ana, 2022). However, an appropriate equilibrium between structure,bio-compatibilityand stability is also necessary. Ongoing studies are expected to yield further refinements of these materials that will underpin their potential for regenerative medicine and subsequent biomedical applications.

2. Classification of Biomaterials by Structure

Drugs delivery by different molecular structures i.e bioceramics, polymers and metals are possible and each have certain advantages & applications (controlled drug delivery, cancer studies, etc), which in turn show individual properties and applyments with Biomaterials by Structural Classification or topologically functional organization of molecular building block, like covalent interactions in case of proteins (Chong et al., 2023), which are integrally linked and functionalised; Dendritic glucans are one example of a novel molecular architecture featuring highly branched structures that enhance versatility in diverse application fields e.g. biomedical (Chen et al., 2023). On the other hand, structural polymeric biomaterials such as polyesters and polyurethanes are crucial because they exhibit high mechanical strength combined with excellent biocompatibility (Rohani Shirvan et al., 2021). Moreover, the structure some decides of proprieties biomaterials including molecular structure; as matter such as polysaccharide carbohydrates are biocompatible support and applied in drug delivery or tissue engineering; carbohydrates as information such glycans mediate cell-cell and cell-matrix interations (Su et al., 2021). Subsequently, molecular organization, handedness, and configuration are important in designing synthetic biomaterials in order to improve their interactions with biomolecules, cells, and tissues. Synthetic biomaterials that mimic the ordered structures found in nature, such as helical peptides, nucleic acids, and polysaccharides, can greater cell adhesion, proliferation, and differentiation. By means of biomaterial design that can increase ligand accessibility and reciprocal interactions with proteins, cells, and tissues, conducting to better performance in biomedical applications (Hendrikse et al., 2022).

- **Polymeric**

Positioning of polymers molecular structure in defining the properties and function for biomaterial applications. Biomedical devices with macromolecular architectures (random/block/star/cross-linked) determining biocompatibility and biodegradability i.e. polymers (Patil & Misra, 2018). Concretely, the polymeric biomaterials like polyesters, polyethylenes and polyurethanes are intended to support systemic mechanical loads so they can be used for orthopedic implants and scaffolds within tissue engineering (Rohani Shirvan et al., 2021). Molecularly imprinted polymers (MIPs) are tailored into a specific ligand capture with higher stability and selectivity which would make them widely used in diagnostics as well as drug delivery (Göktürk et al., 2024). Furthermore, non-covalent-interactions based supramolecular polymers exhibit properties like self-healing and environmental responsiveness which are capable for biomedical applications like regenerative medicine or 3D bioprinting (H. Zhang & Wu, 2023). Hence polymers can be shaped to become more like the ECM and induce cell responses comparable to natural physiological systems. The Basis, Assembly Structure, Chemical composition and Physical properties of polymer-made biomaterials are set to direct their capability to producing unique stimuli, replicating biological cell functions. Laurence With a comprehensive knowledge of structure-property-function relationships provides the essential underpinning for constructing improved biomedical polymers that will be able to tackle current and emerging healthcare demands (Donati et al., 2024).

- **Ceramic**

Properties and applications of ceramic biomaterials differ in molecular scheme, which leads to the applications in medicine, particularly in the dentistry and orthopaedics. Calcium phosphate such as hydroxyapatite HAp and β-tricalcium phosphate β-TCP), main components of these materials can be combined with silica and alumina to increase their mechanical properties and biocompatibility (Dash et al., 2022). For this reason, as ceramics are characterized by porosity or glassy features they can be regarded as effective fillers, scaffolds and coatings that allow tissue adhesion and regeneration (Dash et al., 2022). Hence, development in syntheses, such as sol-gel and additive manufacturing due to the resulting of well-controlled porosity with ideal surface area, together with corrosion resistance (Punj et al., 2021). And besides that in-vitro computational techniques (e.g. molecular dynamics and finite element analysis) that enables the design optimisation and prediction of these biomaterials under physiological conditions (Dash et al., 2022). As a result silicon nitride has been identified as a promising ceramic to enable medical applications offering the unique properties required for spinal/orthopedic/dental implants, antibacterial coatings and biosensors. Well, the new surface modification of ceramic materials is focused in fostering the biointegration of these materials with further implications on efficiency for therapeutic applications (Fernández-Lahore et al., 2023).

- **Metallic**

Metals Biomaterials featured widely in feasible medical therapies:orthopedic implants, dental implants and cardiovascular devices (Sharma et al., 2021). Particular metals such as stainless steel and titanium alloys, cobalt-based alloys are the most commonly used for their apparent mechanical properties, biocompatibility and corrosion resistant behaviour suggested in (Nagay et al., 2020) study. Metallic alloy nanoparticles comprising at the nanoscale have more plasmonic catalytic and/or magnetic properties than monometallic nanoparticles (Huynh et al., 2020). For example, the formation of polynuclear complexes Nd(III)-Cu(II) shows that metal ions can be coupled to form complex structures through ionic/covalent bonding to organic ligands markedly improving their biocompatibility and coordination properties introducing Europium, osteoinduction to host tissue (Katkova et al., 2023). Metal nanoparticles (e.g., AgNPs, AuNPs) are characterized by their nanoscale surface with distinctive features that are essential for applications in biosensing and drug delivery because the surface of nanoparticles can be easily functionalised for enhanced biomolecular interactions (Proniewicz, 2023). Biodegradable metals are another emerging trend to minimize the long-term sequel as well as the need for multiple treatments. Some metal ion-mediated assembly of peptides due to their collagen and generally coiled-coil structure illustrates that metal-binding ligands which allows to vary the morphologies and properties of biomaterials thereby providing en route guidance for new supramolecular architectures (Curtis & Chmielewski, 2021). While, development of bio-metal-organic frameworks (bio-MOFs) which is exemplifies the integration of biomolecules with metallic components, leading to materials with exceptional physicochemical properties and multifunctionality for therapeutic and diagnostic applications (Pathak et al., 2024).

- **Composite Materials**

Due to its attributes and capability to contain two to more constituent materials in it, composite materials are broadly used in biomedical with many applications (Egbo, 2021).These materials afford engineering materials that can fulfill specific demands, so they are also good enough to use in tissue engineering and regenerative medicine (Nagabushanam et al., 2023). Compared to traditional biomaterials (metals ceramics and polymers) composites offer advantages in that they can be engineered so that they mimic the mechanical properties of the surrounding tissues. Therefore, the molecular structures of composites components are involved with regulatory their own property and applications (Kostag et al., 2021). For example synthetic collagen and proteins of spider silk both form hydrogen bonds, so their self-assembly behavior which is essential for scaffolding applications is crucial (Rawal et al., 2020). The characteristics of collagen-chitosan (from food industry byproducts) foams appear to be good for regenerative medicine (Kervran et al., 2022). Apart from that, another composite is formed by cellulose and silk fibroin with multi-functional, biocompatible and biodegradable properties for tissue engineering applications (Kostag et al., 2021). Despite extensive research, the commercial production and distribution of composite-based medical devices have only recently been realized, emphasizing the need for a thorough understanding of their limitations and intended goals (Nagabushanam et al., 2023).

3. Classification of Biomaterials by Function

Functional classification emphasizes the specific applications of biomaterials, in the range of implants, biosensors, and scaffolds, which are designed to interact with biological systems for therapeutic purposes (S. Atheena et al., 2024). Additionally, biomaterials are evaluated base on their biocompatibility, mechanical properties, and ability to promote tissue integration, which are essential for their effectiveness in applications, such as orthopedic and dental surgeries (Nasiri et al., 2024). Moreover, functional classification considers safety, performance, and application, facilitating material selection (Arjunan et al., 2022). These materials can guide cell migration, alignment, and stem cell differentiation. The classification of biomaterials is decisive for selecting safer, biocompatible materials for medical devices and implants, such as heart valves, bone plates, and cardiac pacemakers (Chong et al., 2023).

- **Biomaterials for Repair**

Biomaterials effects the repair and replacement of damaged tissues through implant, leading to beneficial biological responses making its selection essential so as to achieve adequate functionality, despite the fact that titanium alloys are the most preferred material for orthopedic (e.g., hip, knee) and dental implant applications due to its strength and there high biocompatibility, there are often hampered by ion leaching to inflammation. Another are the implant materials like stainless steel and many ceramic fillers polymers by going from metals in some orthopedics devices try to solve metal-on-metal related complications (Al-Shalawi et al., 2023). Such materials have to be biocompatible, osteoconductive and mechanically stable thereby providing a substrate for cellular hom lodging and tissue remodelling (Garg et al., 2003). Advances are aimed towards the fabrication of biomaterials with features mimicking natural tissues and containing anti-infective agents to reduce implant-related infections (Agrawal et al., 2023). However, the key aspects for biomaterial selection remain biocompatibility, mechanical property and corrosion resistance and osseointegration (Abraham & Venkatesan, 2023). The field evolves with continued efforts reporting in vitro to improve implant performance and solve problems that are inherent to this type of procedure like infection, fracture, oversized loading etc. As the demand for effective biomaterials grows, particularly with an aging population, research aims to enhance their performance and application in medical devices (Drevet & Benhayoune, 2024).

- **Regeneration Biomaterials**

Tissue engineering and regenerative medicine mints to replace the damaged tissues with biomaterials, which are needed in the repair and reconstruction of damaged tissues. The optimization of scaffolds for such cellular integration and long-term functionality must provide scaffolds with a set of essential characteristics including good biocompatibility, sensibility and specific mechanical properties for effective cellular incorporation in vivo (Sultana et al., 2024). Hence, a variety of biomaterials (combination of natural and synthetic polymers, bioceramics with decellularized tissues) are used to make scaffolds customized for the improved structure, mechanical properties, and biological function (Farag, 2023). From scaffold fabrication methods, mainly two: 3D printing and hydrogel manufacturing, are never still regular to satisfy tissue-specifc demands (Farag, 2023). Subsequently, these approaches were directed on biocomposite hydrogels by intertwining natural and artificial polymers with inorganic components, implying increased mechanical strength together with biochemical for tissues regeneration (Farag, 2023). This leads to a suite of multiphase scaffolds by incorporating functionally modified biomaterials (bioresorbable and hybrid) that not only provides for cell encapsulation but also offer opportunity to controlled release bioactive drugs (Yadav et al., 2024). Additionally, emerging fabrication techniques (3D printing) are shaping scaffold design for specimen-specific microstructural control on cell-adhesion and functional tissue. Thereby, the field is progressing towards creating more complex, multi-cellular in vitro models that better mimic native tissues (Yadav et al., 2024). Overall, the evolution of scaffold technology continues to address the complex challenges in regenerative medicine (Todros et al., 2021).

- **Biomaterials for Diagnostics**

In diagnostics, bioimaging and biosensors, biomaterials (especially nanomaterials) had remarkable advancement for the improved sensitivity, specificity and also overall diagnostic capacity in different field [a placed underscore indicates an excellent in that category. Nanomaterials used in medical imaging as contrast agents i.e. based on metal nanoparticles, carbon nanodynamic as well quantum dots are used to improve tissue distinguish ability from MRI and CT scans (Gade et al., 2024). In biosensing these materials are capable to detect a low concentration level biomarkers (microRNAs/pathogens etc.) essential for early disease detection and monitoring (Jasni et al., 2023). Also, metal sulfide nanostructures are promising for different imaging modalities as fluorescence, magnetic resonance, acoustic imaging with comparator on fluorescent, calorimetric and electrochemical biosensors (Joicy & Thangadurai, 2021). More recently, biorecognition nanomaterials are receiving considerable attention due to their diagnostic benefit of responding to specific bio-relevant stimuli through shape or rate of chemical reaction modification (Jiang et al., 2022). Graphene-based materials including 2D films, 3D architectures and grapheme hybrids are also envisaged as universal platforms for cancer diagnosis in biosensing and bioimaging. This unique characteristic by virtue of high selectivity, sensitivity and biocompatibility make this ideal target for early detection of cancer biomarkers (Göktürk et al., 2025). Accordingly, the application of nanomaterials in rapid diagnostics, particularly for COVID-19, showcases their potential for real-time detection and response to health crises (Turab et al., 2024). All-inclusive, the integration of nanotechnology in diagnostics promises to revolutionize healthcare by facilitating personalized medicine and improving patient outcomes (Chouhan et al., 2023).

II. PROPERTIES OF BIOMATERIALS

1. Physicochemical Properties

- **Thermal, Chemical and Mechanical Stability**

Several biobased materials exhibit adequate thermal, mechanical and chemical stability to function effectively in physiological environment (Chang et al., 2020) . These properties are essential for maintaining the integrity and performance of medical devices and implants over time. Thermal stability ensures that biomaterials can withstand temperature fluctuations within the body without degrading or losing their functional properties. Most biomaterials are designed to remain stable at 37°C and during sterilization processes (up to 100°C), which may involve higher temperatures. Polylactic acid (PLA), chitin, chitosan and alginate exhibit good thermal stability up to 180°C (Ablouh et al., 2019; Elouali et al., 2025; Kervran et al., 2022), making them suitable for various biomedical applications due to their thermal stability, such as wound healing and drug delivery systems. However, collagen denatures at low temperature around 40°C, which limits its use in high-temperature applications (Lin et al., 2023).

Chemical stability is also considered a key factor to prevent degradation of the biomaterial when exposed to bodily fluids and tissues. This property ensures that the material maintains its structure and function over time, avoiding the release of potentially harmful degradation products (Bunzen, 2021). According to (Aristizábal et al., 2020) the PEEK material demonstrates an excellent chemical stability in physiological environments, making it suitable for long-term implants. Conversely, as reported by (Tatu et al., 2022), biodegradable polymers such as polycaprolactone

(PCL) undergo hydrolytic degradation, which can be advantageous for temporary implants but unsuitable for long-term applications (Dias et al., 2022). Additionally, carrageenan exhibits chemical stability in aqueous environments, making it useful for drug delivery and wound healing applications (Neamtu et al., 2022).

For load bearing applications, the study of mechanical properties of the biomaterial is necessary, especially for orthopedic implants (Szczęsny et al., 2022). In general, the mechanical properties of biomaterials should ideally match those of the surrounding tissues to prevent stress shielding and ensure proper integration (Hu et al., 2020; Moltasov et al., 2023). For instance, titanium alloys, which is widely used in orthopedic implants, have excellent mechanical properties, with a tensile strength up to 1000 MPa and an elastic modulus vary from 110 to 114 GPa (J. Liu et al., 2023). However, even hydrogels are biocompatible, often lack the mechanical strength required for load-bearing applications (Fuchs et al., 2020; Petelinšek & Mommer, 2024). However, for alginate, it provides structural support in tissue engineering but requires reinforcement for high-load applications.

- **Hydrophilic/Hydrophobic Properties and Their Role in Biomedical Applications**

The hydrophilic or hydrophobic nature of a biomaterial significantly influences its interaction with biological systems and its suitability for specific biomedical applications. For instance, hydrogels, such as those based on polyethylene glycol (PEG), are highly hydrophilic and can absorb large amounts of water, making them useful for wound dressings and drug delivery systems (Díaz-Marín et al., 2024). Similarly, alginate and carrageenan are highly hydrophilic polysaccharides, allowing them to form gels that mimic extracellular matrices.

2. Biological Properties

- **Biocompatibility**

To be considered biocompatible for clinical use by regulatory agencies, biomaterials must satisfy several key criteria, as defined by the International Organization for Standardization (ISO 10993) (Huzum et al., 2021). They must be non-toxic, non-thrombogenic, non-carcinogenic, non-antigenic and non-mutagenic, in order to present an appropriate biological response (Huzum et al., 2021). Biocompatibility is therefore a fundamental requirement for biomaterials. This property guarantees their efficacy in the body without undesirable effects. Biocompatibility does not depend solely on the absence of toxicity, but results from a harmonious interaction between the biomaterial and the biological environment in which it is implanted

(Karakullukcu et al., 2023). This property is influenced by several key factors, including chemical composition, mechanical and structural properties, and the biological environment in which the material is used. Other critical parameters include surface texture, degree of crystallinity, wettability, surface chemistry, degradation products, stiffness and the type of application envisaged (Hakim et al., 2024). Several biomaterials exemplify these properties: titanium and its alloys are distinguished by their corrosion resistance, high biocompatibility and long-term stability, making them the materials of choice in orthopedics (prostheses, plates) and dentistry. Chitosan, a natural polymer, offers controlled degradability, non-toxicity and excellent biological compatibility (Wang, 2023). It is particularly used as a carrier for drugs in the oral cavity. Magnesium alloys (such as Mg-Ca and Mg-Zn) are promising for biodegradable orthopedic implants, thanks to their good osteoconductivity and ability to promote osteogenesis. As for synthetic polymers, PLA, PGA, polyethylene and polyesters offer adjustable properties. Their biocompatibility depends on molecular structure, molecular weight and surface morphology. Metallic nanoparticles, such as those based on gold or silver, are used as drug delivery systems. Silver, in particular, is renowned for its antibacterial properties, while gold has good biological tolerance. Finally, natural polymers such as gelatin, alginate, hyaluronic acid and calcium phosphates are widely used in dentistry and for controlled drug delivery, thanks to their compatibility with living tissue.(Ansari & Darvishi, 2024; Yang et al., 2023).

- **Degradability and Biodegradability**

Degradability and biodegradability are critical properties for biomaterials used in temporary implants or drug delivery systems. For example, polylactic-co-glycolic acid (PLGA) is a biodegradable polymer widely used in drug delivery systems and tissue engineering scaffolds due to its controlled degradation profile. Similarly, chitin and chitosan degrade enzymatically in vivo, making them suitable for biodegradable medical applications (Ait Hamdan et al., 2024; Boulila et al., 2017; Santhosh et al., 2019). Alginate also undergoes biodegradation, allowing for controlled release in drug delivery systems (Abdollahi et al., 2024). Conversely, ceramics like alumina and zirconia are non-biodegradable and are used in applications requiring long-term stability, such as joint replacements.

- **Potential Toxicity and Assessment Criteria**

The evaluation of biomaterial toxicity is a fundamental aspect of ensuring their safety for clinical applications. Biocompatibility assessments constitute a critical requirement in the development and regulatory approval of orthopedic materials (Huzum et al., 2021). Hydroxyapatite, a calcium phosphate-based ceramic, is well-documented for its superior biocompatibility and minimal cytotoxicity (Balu et al., 2020; Venkatesan et al., 2018), rendering it highly suitable for bone tissue engineering. In contrast, metal ions released from certain alloys, such as cobalt-chromium, have been associated with adverse tissue reactions, necessitating thorough evaluation for long-term biomedical use. Polysaccharide-based biomaterials, including chitin, chitosan, alginate, and carrageenan, are widely regarded as non-toxic, as their degradation products are biocompatible, metabolizable and non-detrimental to biological tissues (Ait Hamdan et al., 2023, 2024).

3. Specific Functional Properties

Electrical and thermal conductivity are fundamental properties of biomaterials utilized in neural interfaces, biosensors and tissue engineering (Majumdar et al., 2021; Nasiri et al., 2024). Conductive polymers, such as polyaniline, have attracted significant interest in neural tissue engineering due to their capacity to facilitate electrical signal transmission (Yi et al., 2023). In contrast, the majority of ceramics employed in biomedical applications, including alumina, function as electrical insulators (Licciardello et al., 2024).

Antimicrobial properties are critical for medical devices, particularly those intended for implantation or prolonged contact with biological tissues (Yang & Xiao, 2020), as they play a key role in preventing infections and biofilm formation factors that can compromise device functionality and lead to severe health complications. Silver nanoparticles exhibit potent antimicrobial activity and are frequently incorporated into biomaterials for use in wound dressings and catheter coatings (Sam et al., 2023). Conversely, many conventional polymers, such as polyethylene, inherently lack antimicrobial properties and often require surface modifications or the integration of antimicrobial agents to mitigate bacterial colonization. Chitosan, owing to its intrinsic antimicrobial activity, is extensively utilized in wound healing applications, as a coating for medical devices and in drug delivery systems (Ait Hamdan et al., 2024; El-Mansoury et al., 2023).

III. BIOMATERIALS APPLICATIONS

Thanks to their unique properties, as described above, biomaterials have made their mark in many fields. Their development over time has led to significant advances in tissue engineering, where they serve as a support for cell regeneration and the regeneration of damaged tissue (Dhavalikar et al., 2020). In the field of drug delivery, biomaterials enable controlled and targeted release, thus increasing the efficacy of treatments taken, while reducing the adverse effects caused (Pires et al.,

2023). In addition to biomedical applications, they also have their part to play in the industrial and technological sectors, where they are exploited for their mechanical performance, biodegradability and green engineering potential (Amandine Magnaudeix & et Julie Usseglio-Grosso, 2020).

- **Tissue Engineering**

We first recall that tissue engineering in general is a concept that combines the principles of engineering and biology, thus aiming to replace damaged tissue (H. M. Khan et al., 2022). Biomaterials, on the other hand, are any substance, other than drugs, of synthetic or natural origin, which can be used for a given period of time, that partially or totally augments or replaces a tissue, organ or body function, in order to maintain or improve the individual's quality of life (Marin et al., 2020). The biomaterials used can therefore be of either synthetic or natural origin. The choice of biomaterial remains a very important step, and depends mainly on the specific tissue to be developed, as well as the desired properties and clinical application envisaged (Trucillo, 2024). However, these biomaterials must undoubtedly support the attachment, maintenance, proliferation and sometimes differentiation of selected cell populations. Not to mention that the biomaterial, must be a structural support adequate to the target site (H. M. Khan et al., 2022).

More clearly, in the skin, the literature shows that biomaterials (generally chitosan and collagen) are used to provide epidermal coating, dermal replacement or epidermal/dermal replacement(Gray et al., 2022). For bone, biomaterials such as Spongostan (gelatin) and scaffolds composed of collagen and hydroxyapatite, in combination with bone marrow stem cells, are used to repair bone defects (Biswal, 2021; M. U. A. Khan et al., 2023; Ressler, 2022). And of course in the trachea we find allogeneic decellularized tracheae saturated with bone marrow stem cells, have been used for tracheal replacement, according to the work of (M. U. A. Khan et al., 2023). In addition, for blood vessels, vascular grafts based on autologous bone marrow mononuclear cells seeded onto a degradable tubular scaffold have been used in the treatment of patients with unique ventricular physiology (Biswal, 2021).

Synthetic biomaterials, such as polyethylene glycol (PEG), poly(lactic-co-glycolic acid) (PLGA), polyethylene terephthalate and polyglycolic acid, previously described in the biomaterial classifications section, can be manufactured in a more customized way, since strength, structure and degradation rate can be more controlled (Ul-Islam et al., 2024). Natural materials include natural polymers, such as silk and chitosan, the latter being widely used and discussed, in the biomedical field, not least because of their natural origins, which is part of a waste recovery framework, and extracted recently using eco-responsible methods (Elouali et al., 2025).

Figure 1. Global classification of biomaterials and key biomedical applications

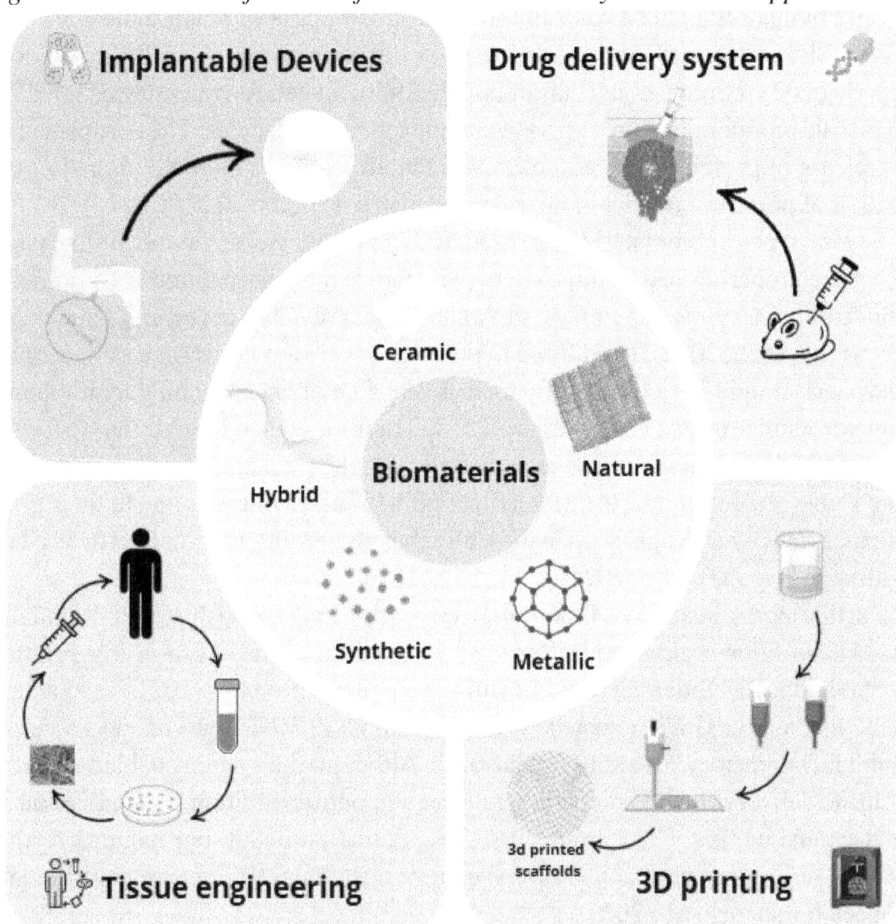

- **Drug Delivery**

Moving on to drug delivery, where biomaterials have attracted the interest of several scientific researchers, mainly in the biomedical field, offering innovative and alternative solutions for more efficient and targeted administration (Trucillo, 2024). According to, (Wan et al., 2021), the various biomaterials, each with its own properties, not only make it possible to control the release of therapeutic agents, but also to minimize the problem of adverse effects as much as possible. The first studies on the incorporation of biomaterials, particularly polymers, were developed as far back as the 1960s and 1970s, when the need forced researchers to turn to alternative solutions (Fenton et al., 2018).

In the same work by (Fenton et al., 2018), silicone rubber is depicted as one of the first biomaterials to be used in the controlled release of small molecules, due to its ability to tolerate hydrophobic dyes to diffuse through its wall. In addition, (Trucillo, 2024) demonstrated that around the 1970s, genetic engineering enabled the large-scale production of proteins and complex macromolecules. The encapsulation and release of proteins from polymers was therefore only brought to light after the creation of porous networks in the polymer matrix (Sood et al., 2021).

Several types of biomaterials are used: firstly, polymers, both synthetic and natural, whose properties can be adjusted to personalize delivery parameters. Examples include polyesters such as PLGA, PLA and PGA, polyanhydrides, PEG and many others (Han et al., 2022). In addition to polymers, there are lipids such as liposomes and spherical lipid vesicles, all of which are capable of encapsulating hydrophobic and hydrophilic drugs (Fenton et al., 2018; Trucillo, 2024). In addition, there are nanomaterials such as, dendrimers, polymeric micelles and inorganic nanoparticles, which have revolutionized the biomedical field in recent decades due to their great potential to deliver drugs at the nanoscale, thus increasing treatment efficacy in a significant way (Trucillo, 2024).

Furthermore, scaffolds functionalized with CRISPR (Clustered Regularly Interspaced Short Palindromic Repeats) biomaterials offer a promising solution for stable, localized delivery and in situ gene editing. Ho et al (2021) used an extracellular matrix (ECM)-coated hydrogel with Cas9 RNP-lipid nanoparticles to inhibit inflammatory pathways in leukemia. Although the system enabled efficient CRISPR delivery, it lacked spatial and kinetic control, limiting its application to precise gene editing. This approach suggests great potential, but requires further research to refine spatial and temporal control techniques to improve gene therapy efficacy (Graham et al., 2023).

And finally, we highlight the importance of natural materials, such as chitosan, alginate, hyaluronic acid (HA), pectin and collagen, which are used primarily for their biocompatibility and biodegradability (Insuasti-Cruz et al., 2022). We would point out here that several of these biomaterials have been used in clinical and commercial applications, the most relevant of which are grouped in Table 1.

Table 1. Biomaterials used in both clinical and commercial sectors

Trade name	Description	References
Lupron Depot	Formulation of PLGA microspheres encapsulating the hormone leuprolide, approved for the treatment of advanced prostate cancer and endometriosis.	(Anselmo & Mitragotri, 2014)
Doxil	Liposomal formulation of doxorubicin, improves circulation half-life and tumor absorption while reducing toxicity.	(Barenholz, 2012)
Abraxane	Formulation of albumin-bound paclitaxel nanoparticles for the treatment of breast cancer.	(Fenton et al., 2018)

There are four essential steps in drug delivery:

- **Encapsulation:** Drugs are enclosed in a carrier system, such as nanoparticles, liposomes or microspheres, to protect them and control their release (Abdul Hameed et al., 2023).
- **Entrapment:** Drugs are entrapped in a polymer matrix (Trucillo, 2024).
- **Attachment:** Drugs are attached to the surface of a carrier (Trucillo, 2024).
- **Controlled release:** Biomaterials release locked-in drugs at a specific rate, constant or variable, over a given period, depending on customization (Abdul Hameed et al., 2023; Trucillo, 2024).
- **Implantable Devices**

Over the last few decades, researchers have been focusing on the development and research of implantable medical devices, be they orthopedic implants, cardiovascular, dental, neurological devices or even for tissue healing and regeneration. However, this need is accompanied by requirements, such as being biocompatible, biodegradable, controllable etc. It is at this point that biomaterials endowed with these qualities represent the most suitable candidates for this need. In this sense, titanium alloy, a strong and resistant biomaterial, is widely used in particular applications, and for bone plate replacement (Chatterjee et al., 2019). Even stronger cobalt-chromium alloys are targeted for use in heart valves and as joint prostheses (D. Zhang et al., 2021). For temporary implants, researchers have chosen to study polylactic acid (PLA) as a synthetic biomaterial thanks to its ability to degrade naturally and, above all, provoke no rejection reaction from the application site (Pidhatika et al., 2022). Polyetheretherketone (PEEK), meanwhile, has been described as a biocompatible thermoplastic polymer, applied mainly in spinal implants, and dental devices (D. Zhang et al., 2021).

- **Biomaterials for 3D Printing**

Thanks to technological, industrial and scientific advances, the 3D printer has come into its own, so researchers have taken advantage of this technique to use it in a variety of medical applications, in particular craniofacial implants (Park et al., 2021), dental molds, crowns and implants, (S. Liu et al., 2022) prosthetic parts, (de León et al., 2023) medical equipment on demand, (A. Mishra & Srivastava, 2021) surgical models, (Pugliese et al., 2021) scaffolds for the regeneration of tissues such as skin and bone, (Fu et al., 2022) and many others...The major reason for this use is to meet the specific needs of patients by tailoring more, biomaterials, by controlling porosity and combining several materials (Chae & Cho, 2023). In other words, this technology has reenergized the biomedical field in particular. To be used as 3D printer inks, biomaterials must certainly satisfy a number of basic criteria: biodegradability, biocompatibility, printability, good degradation kinetics and appropriate mechanical properties (Chae & Cho, 2023).

Polymers in this sense are the most suitable candidates to be printed, on the one hand because they are cheaper, and on the other hand they present key properties such as biocompatibility, mechanical degradation. Examples of polymers include Poly(lactic acid) (PLA), Poly(D,L-lactide) (PDLLA), Poly(caprolactone) (PCL), Poly(propylene fumarate) (PPF), Polyetheretherketone (PEEK), Poly(butylene terephthalate) (PBT) and Acrylonitrile Butadiene Styrene (ABS) (de León et al., 2023; S. Liu et al., 2022). In addition to these types of biomaterials, we can even find hydrogels, which are used as bioinks when they carry cells and/or biochemical molecules (Pina et al., 2019). Not forgetting, of course, ceramics, such as Hydroxy-apatite (HA) and Tricalcium Phosphates (TCP) (Chae & Cho, 2023).

IV. CHALLENGES AND PERSPECTIVES

- **Challenges**

Due to their multiple beneficial properties, previously discussed different bio-materials are developed to interact with biological systems, their biodegradability, bioactivity as well as their compatibility with different tissues make biomaterials particularly interesting in different applications. For example, in the ecological field, biomaterials could provide a sustainable alternative to the traditional materials usually used, by exploiting environmentally-friendly green technologies, thus considerably reducing their impact on the environment.

This notion of biomaterials constitutes a complementary path to that of sustainable resources, which elucidates the integration of an interdisciplinary approach in any study that deals with biomaterials, in particular the valorization of high biomass waste as well as the use of green technologies (Mabrouk et al., 2021).

However, biomaterials, and despite their multiple advantages, their use triggers several challenges to overcome (Table 2), essentially, the reproducibility of these biomaterials, as well as their high porosity, the control of their properties and the stability of the products. These challenges remain major obstacles in any use (Biswal et al., 2020). This requires optimal handling and precise control of their characteristics during the synthesis of these biomaterials, this synthesis which is recognized by its complexity as well as by the presence of impurities that could alter the performance of these biomaterials (Mabrouk et al., 2021). Thus, it would be very essential to evaluate the types of biomaterials before their use in order to curb the adverse effects that may appear during handling in the different fields of application. This assessment is based on various essential criteria, including the biodegradability of biomaterials, their biological activities, their surface reactivity, biological inertia, sterilization capacity, their mechanical and chemical properties and finally, the manufacturing cost, which is a fundamental factor in their large-scale exploitation (Siraparapu et al., 2014).

Table 2. Advantages and disadvantages of different biomaterials

Biomaterials	Advantages	Disadvantages
Polymer	Easy to produce Low density	Low mechanical strength Easily degradable
Metal	Ductility High resistance to wear and impact	Low biocompatibility Susceptible to corrosion in physiological environments Mechanical properties different from biological tissues
Ceramic	High biocompatibility Corrosion resistance Inert Low thermal and electrical conductivity	Low impact strength Difficult to reproduce properties Complex manufacturing and processing
Composite	High biocompatibility Corrosion resistance Inert	Variable properties Difficult to replicate

(Festas et al., 2020)

- **Regulatory Challenges and Approval Routes for Biomaterials**

Another key issue is regulatory and ethical considerations. Indeed, the development of biomaterials for medical devices is subject to strict processes governed by international standards (Schuh & Funk, 2019). Jurczak et al (2025) indicate that recent developments in the Medical Device Regulation (MDR) and the In Vitro Diagnostic Devices Regulation (IVDR) in the EU, while essential for patient safety, may be holding back innovation (Jurczak et al., 2025). Bayon et al's (2024) approach highlights the need to integrate regulatory strategies tailored to clinical needs to facilitate the adoption of new biomaterials. Moreover, translating biomaterials into clinical products remains complex, as they are integrated into final devices approved by regulators (Song et al., 2022). In addition, shortcomings in the design of animal studies, as well as specific challenges related to plant-based materials, further complicate their standardization and clinical integration (Cheng et al., 2022). Close collaboration between researchers, clinicians, industry and regulatory authorities is therefore essential to ensure early integration of safety criteria and accelerate the commercialization of these innovations.

- **Perspectives**

Biomaterials play a vital role in many fields. Whether based on polymers, metals, ceramics or composites, these materials offer promising prospects for the development of humanity (UludaÄŸ, 2014). However, this development is now closely linked to environmental issues, a major concern for political and economic decision-makers.

The use of biomaterials thus represents an opportunity both to valorize biomass waste and to exploit their varied properties in diversified applications. However, a thorough understanding of these materials remains necessary. The development of environmentally friendly production methods is essential in order to overcome challenges such as reproducibility, stability and control of properties.

According to the use of biomaterials in different application fields, the prospects of use vary, for example, in the medical field, the use of biomaterials in tissue engineering and regenerative medicine requires in-depth studies of hydrogels and matrices derived from the extracellular matrix (ECM) that could improve the biocompatibility of biomaterials. As well as in pharmacology, especially in the process of drug release, the use of biomaterials could be a good choice, especially with the advancement of nanotechnology, which can facilitate the diffusion of active ingredients in a precise and prolonged manner, thus optimizing therapeutic efficacy.

In addition, in the use of biomaterials in implants, the durability or degradability of these compounds remains a major challenge. This is why it would be essential to optimize the mechanical and chemical properties of these products to improve their resistance and solve the problems related to their degradation in the human body. In another aspect, the use of biomaterials in environmental applications could be a promising prospect, particularly in water treatment and in carbon dioxide (CO_2) capture. Studies in this context could constitute a highly valuable research axis.

To conclude, and by exploiting advances in the fields of nanoscience, biotechnology and artificial intelligence, the use of biomaterials could be an innovative and high-caliber research avenue, first in the optimization of their properties, and then in the development of new applications of these biomaterials.

CONCLUSION

Since biomaterials first appeared on the scene, they have continued to evolve, in line with technological, industrial and scientific advances. Their development is ushering in a new era of medicine. Indeed, in a world where the need for urgent medical solutions is growing, biomaterials, thanks to their key properties such as biocompatibility and biofunctionality, are making their mark. Today, these materials represent the perfect candidates for various applications, mainly in tissue engineering, skin regeneration, orthopedics, cardiology, drug delivery and even nanomedicine (Marin et al., 2020; Trucillo, 2024).

Thanks to the various studies carried out over the last few decades, which affirm and confirm that these biomaterials remain effective and safe, increasing their adoption in clinical practice. Their influence is not limited to the repair or replacement of damaged tissues/organs, but extends to improving patients' quality of life (Keane & Badylak, 2014; Trucillo, 2024).

Innovations and creations continue today, with new techniques such as 3D bioprinting, smart polymer engineering and nanotechnology integration adding value to various fields. However, challenges remain, in particular biodegradability, immunocompatibility and large-scale industrialization (Chae & Cho, 2023)

As a result, our biomaterials represent not only scientific and technological advances, but also revolutionary alternative therapies, pushing back the boundaries of modern medicine. Their potential, still far from fully exploited, opens up fascinating prospects for the future of science and healthcare.

REFERENCES

Abalymov, A., Parakhonskiy, B., & Skirtach, A. (2020). Polymer- and Hybrid-Based Biomaterials for Interstitial, Connective, Vascular, Nerve, Visceral and Musculoskeletal Tissue Engineering. *Polymers*, *12*(3), 620. DOI: 10.3390/polym12030620 PMID: 32182751

Abdollahi, H., Amiri, S., Amiri, F., Moradi, S., & Zarrintaj, P. (2024). Antibacterial Biocomposite Based on Chitosan/Pluronic/Agarose Noncovalent Hydrogel: Controlled Drug Delivery by Alginate/Tetracycline Beads System. *Journal of Functional Biomaterials*, *15*(10), 286. DOI: 10.3390/jfb15100286 PMID: 39452585

Abdul Hameed, M. M., Mohamed Khan, S. A. P., Thamer, B. M., Rajkumar, N., El-Hamshary, H., & El-Newehy, M. (2023). Electrospun nanofibers for drug delivery applications: Methods and mechanism. *Polymers for Advanced Technologies*, *34*(1), 6–23. DOI: 10.1002/pat.5884

Ablouh, E., Essaghraoui, A., Eladlani, N., Rhazi, M., & Taourirte, M. (2019). Uptake of Pb(<scp>II</scp>) onto nanochitosan/sodium alginate hybrid beads: Mechanism and kinetics study. *Water Environment Research*, *91*(3), 239–249. DOI: 10.1002/wer.1050 PMID: 30624837

Abraham, A. M., & Venkatesan, S. (2023). A review on application of biomaterials for medical and dental implants. *Proceedings of the Institution of Mechanical Engineers, Part L: Journal of Materials: Design and Applications, 237*(2), 249–273. DOI: 10.1177/14644207221121981

Agrawal, R., Kumar, A., Mohammed, M. K. A., & Singh, S. (2023). Biomaterial types, properties, medical applications, and other factors: A recent review. *Journal of Zhejiang University. Science A*, *24*(11), 1027–1042. DOI: 10.1631/jzus.A2200403

Ait Hamdan, Y., El Amerany, F., Desbrières, J., Aghrinane, A., Oudadesse, H., & Rhazi, M. (2023). The evolution of the global COVID-19 epidemic in Morocco and understanding the different therapeutic approaches of chitosan in the control of the pandemic. *Polymer Bulletin*, *80*(10), 10633–10659. DOI: 10.1007/s00289-022-04579-3 PMID: 36466080

Ait Hamdan, Y., El-Mansoury, B., Elouali, S., Rachmoune, K., Belbachir, A., Oudadesse, H., & Rhazi, M. (2024). A review of chitosan polysaccharides: Neuropharmacological implications and tissue regeneration. *International Journal of Biological Macromolecules*, *279*, 135356. DOI: 10.1016/j.ijbiomac.2024.135356 PMID: 39244136

Al-Shalawi, F. D., Mohamed Ariff, A. H., Jung, D.-W., Mohd Ariffin, M. K. A., Seng Kim, C. L., Brabazon, D., & Al-Osaimi, M. O. (2023). Biomaterials as Implants in the Orthopedic Field for Regenerative Medicine: Metal versus Synthetic Polymers. *Polymers, 15*(12), 2601. DOI: 10.3390/polym15122601 PMID: 37376247

Alamgir, W., & Haider, A. (2023). The Past, Present and Future of Biomaterials. *Life Sciences*, *4*(4), 2. DOI: 10.37185/LnS.1.1.500

Aldana, A. A., Bauer, J., & Baker, M. B. (2023). *Synthetic biomaterials* (3rd ed.). Tissue Engineering., DOI: 10.1016/B978-0-12-824459-3.00006-8

Ana, I. D. (2022). Hybrid Biomaterials in Drug Delivery and Biomedical Applications. In *Functional Biomaterials* (pp. 409–434). Springer Singapore., DOI: 10.1007/978-981-16-7152-4_15

Ansari, M., & Darvishi, A. (2024). A review of the current state of natural biomaterials in wound healing applications. *Frontiers in Bioengineering and Biotechnology*, *12*, 1309541. Advance online publication. DOI: 10.3389/fbioe.2024.1309541 PMID: 38600945

Anselmo, A. C., & Mitragotri, S. (2014). An overview of clinical and commercial impact of drug delivery systems. *Journal of Controlled Release*, *190*, 15–28. DOI: 10.1016/j.jconrel.2014.03.053 PMID: 24747160

Aristizábal, S. L., Chisca, S., Pulido, B. A., & Nunes, S. P. (2020). Preparation of PEEK Membranes with Excellent Stability Using Common Organic Solvents. *Industrial & Engineering Chemistry Research*, *59*(12), 5218–5226. DOI: 10.1021/acs.iecr.9b04281

Arjunan, A., Baroutaji, A., Praveen, A. S., Robinson, J., & Wang, C. (2022). Classification of Biomaterial Functionality. In *Encyclopedia of Smart Materials* (pp. 86–102). Elsevier., DOI: 10.1016/B978-0-12-815732-9.00027-9

Atheena, S., M. P., Rashika, M., N. Sri, M. K., Sudherson, M., & M. Kriya, S. (. (2024). Exploring the role of biomaterials in organ implants. *I-Manager's. Journal of Materials Science*, *11*(4), 15. DOI: 10.26634/jms.11.4.20622

Austin, M. J., & Rosales, A. M. (2019). Tunable biomaterials from synthetic, sequence-controlled polymers. *Biomaterials Science*, *7*(2), 490–505. DOI: 10.1039/C8BM01215F PMID: 30628589

Balu, S., Sundaradoss, M. V., Andra, S., & Jeevanandam, J. (2020). Facile biogenic fabrication of hydroxyapatite nanorods using cuttlefish bone and their bactericidal and biocompatibility study. *Beilstein Journal of Nanotechnology*, *11*, 285–295. DOI: 10.3762/bjnano.11.21 PMID: 32117667

Barbinta-Patrascu, M.-E., Nichita, C., Enculescu, M., Maraloiu, V.-A., Bacalum, M., Ungureanu, C., Negrila, C. C., & Zgura, I. (2024). Bioactive Hybrids Containing Artificial Cell Membranes and Phyto-Gold–Silver Chloride Bio-Nanoparticles. *International Journal of Molecular Sciences*, *25*(22), 11929. DOI: 10.3390/ijms252211929 PMID: 39596000

Barenholz, Y. (2012). Doxil® — The first FDA-approved nano-drug: Lessons learned. *Journal of Controlled Release*, *160*(2), 117–134. DOI: 10.1016/j.jconrel.2012.03.020 PMID: 22484195

Barutça, B., Köroğlu, L., Ayas, E., & Koparal, A. T. (2018). In vitro cytotoxicity of monticellite based bioactive ceramic powder synthesized from boron derivative waste. *Ceramics International*, *44*(7), 8094–8099. DOI: 10.1016/j.ceramint.2018.01.252

Bhatti, S. S., & Singh, J. (2023). 3D printing of biomaterials for biomedical applications: A review. [IJIDeM]. *International Journal on Interactive Design and Manufacturing*. Advance online publication. DOI: 10.1007/s12008-023-01525-z

Biswal, T. (2021). Biopolymers for tissue engineering applications: A review. *Materials Today: Proceedings*, *41*, 397–402. DOI: 10.1016/j.matpr.2020.09.628

Biswal, T., BadJena, S. K., & Pradhan, D. (2020). Sustainable biomaterials and their applications: A short review. *Materials Today: Proceedings*, *30*, 274–282. DOI: 10.1016/j.matpr.2020.01.437

Boulila, S., Oudadesse, H., Kallel, R., Lefeuvre, B., Mabrouk, M., Chaabouni, K., Makni-Ayedi, F., Boudawara, T., Elfeki, A., & Elfeki, H. (2017). In vivo study of hybrid biomaterial scaffold bioactive glass–chitosan after incorporation of Ciprofloxacin. *Polymer Bulletin*, *74*(10), 4153–4173. DOI: 10.1007/s00289-017-1936-z

Bunzen, H. (2021). Chemical Stability of Metal-organic Frameworks for Applications in Drug Delivery. *ChemNanoMat : Chemistry of Nanomaterials for Energy, Biology and More*, *7*(9), 998–1007. DOI: 10.1002/cnma.202100226

Casarin, M., Todesco, M., Fontanella, C. G., Morlacco, A., Dal Moro, F., & Bagno, A. (2023). Hybrid Materials for Tissue Repair and Replacement: Another Frontier in Biomaterial Exploitation Focusing on Cardiovascular and Urological Fields. *Processes (Basel, Switzerland)*, *11*(7), 2013. DOI: 10.3390/pr11072013

Chae, S., & Cho, D.-W. (2023). Biomaterial-based 3D bioprinting strategy for orthopedic tissue engineering. *Acta Biomaterialia*, *156*, 4–20. DOI: 10.1016/j.actbio.2022.08.004 PMID: 35963520

Chakraborty, G., & Prasad, A. (2024). 1 Bio-based materials: origin, synthesis, and properties. In *Sustainable Bio-Based Composites* (pp. 1–24). De Gruyter., DOI: 10.1515/9783111321530-001

Chang, B. P., Mohanty, A. K., & Misra, M. (2020). Studies on durability of sustainable biobased composites: A review. *RSC Advances*, *10*(31), 17955–17999. DOI: 10.1039/C9RA09554C PMID: 35517220

Chatterjee, S., Saxena, M., Padmanabhan, D., Jayachandra, M., & Pandya, H. J. (2019). Futuristic medical implants using bioresorbable materials and devices. *Biosensors & Bioelectronics*, *142*, 111489. DOI: 10.1016/j.bios.2019.111489 PMID: 31295710

Chelu, M., & Musuc, A. M. (2023). Advanced Biomedical Applications of Multifunctional Natural and Synthetic Biomaterials. *Processes (Basel, Switzerland)*, *11*(9), 2696. DOI: 10.3390/pr11092696

Chen, L., Zhao, N., McClements, D. J., Hamaker, B. R., & Miao, M. (2023). Advanced dendritic glucan-derived biomaterials: From molecular structure to versatile applications. *Comprehensive Reviews in Food Science and Food Safety*, *22*(5), 4107–4146. DOI: 10.1111/1541-4337.13201 PMID: 37350042

Cheng, M., Liu, W., Zhang, J., Zhang, S., Guo, Z., Liu, L., Tian, J., Zhang, X., Cheng, J., Liu, Y., Deng, G., Gao, G., & Sun, L. (2022). Regulatory considerations for animal studies of biomaterial products. *Bioactive Materials*, *11*, 52–56. DOI: 10.1016/j.bioactmat.2021.09.031 PMID: 34938912

Chong, E. T. J., Ng, J. W., & Lee, P.-C. (2023). Classification and Medical Applications of Biomaterials–A Mini Review. *BIO Integration*, *4*(2). Advance online publication. DOI: 10.15212/bioi-2022-0009

Chouhan, A. P. S., Verma, A., & Singh, V. (2023). *The Significance of Nanomaterials in Medical Imaging and Diagnostics*., DOI: 10.4018/979-8-3693-0448-8.ch012

Cohen, J. (1967). Biomaterials in orthopedic surgery. *American Journal of Surgery*, *114*(1), 31–41. DOI: 10.1016/0002-9610(67)90037-2 PMID: 5338210

Curtis, R. W., & Chmielewski, J. (2021). A comparison of the collagen triple helix and <scp>coiled-coil</scp> peptide building blocks on metal <scp>ion-mediated</scp> supramolecular assembly. *Peptide Science (Hoboken, N.J.)*, *113*(2), e24190. Advance online publication. DOI: 10.1002/pep2.24190

Dash, R., Rajak, A. K., Kumar, R. P., Kommu, P., Sharma, S., Gurjar, M., & Bhattacharyya, A. (2022). *Bioceramics for medical applications: a computational view*. DOI: 10.26434/chemrxiv-2022-n3tjf

Datta, L. P., Manchineella, S., & Govindaraju, T. (2020). Biomolecules-derived biomaterials. *Biomaterials*, *230*, 119633. DOI: 10.1016/j.biomaterials.2019.119633 PMID: 31831221

de León, E. H.-P., Valle-Pérez, A. U., Khan, Z. N., & Hauser, C. A. E. (2023). Intelligent and smart biomaterials for sustainable 3D printing applications. *Current Opinion in Biomedical Engineering*, *26*, 100450. DOI: 10.1016/j.cobme.2023.100450

Dhavalikar, P., Robinson, A., Lan, Z., Jenkins, D., Chwatko, M., Salhadar, K., Jose, A., Kar, R., Shoga, E., Kannapiran, A., & Cosgriff-Hernandez, E. (2020). Review of Integrin-Targeting Biomaterials in Tissue Engineering. *Advanced Healthcare Materials*, *9*(23), 2000795. Advance online publication. DOI: 10.1002/adhm.202000795 PMID: 32940020

Dias, J. R., Sousa, A., Augusto, A., Bártolo, P. J., & Granja, P. L. (2022). Electrospun Polycaprolactone (PCL) Degradation: An In Vitro and In Vivo Study. *Polymers*, *14*(16), 3397. DOI: 10.3390/polym14163397 PMID: 36015652

Díaz-Marín, C. D., Masetti, L., Roper, M. A., Hector, K. E., Zhong, Y., Lu, Z., Caylan, O. R., Graeber, G., & Grossman, J. C. (2024). Physics-based prediction of moisture-capture properties of hydrogels. *Nature Communications*, *15*(1), 8948. DOI: 10.1038/s41467-024-53291-5 PMID: 39419983

Donati, L., Valicenti, M. L., Giannoni, S., Morena, F., & Martino, S. (2024). Biomaterials Mimicking Mechanobiology: A Specific Design for a Specific Biological Application. *International Journal of Molecular Sciences*, *25*(19), 10386. DOI: 10.3390/ijms251910386 PMID: 39408716

Drevet, R., & Benhayoune, H. (2024). Biomaterials Design for Human Body Repair. *Designs*, *8*(4), 65. DOI: 10.3390/designs8040065

Egbo, M. K. (2021). A fundamental review on composite materials and some of their applications in biomedical engineering. *Journal of King Saud University. Engineering Sciences*, *33*(8), 557–568. DOI: 10.1016/j.jksues.2020.07.007

El-Mansoury, B., Smimih, K., Hamdan, Y. A., El Khiat, A., Elouali, S., El Fatimi, H., Draoui, A., El Hiba, O., & Jayakumar, A. R. (2023). *The Interplay Between Environmental Pollutants*. Gut Microbiota, and Infections., DOI: 10.4018/978-1-7998-9414-8.ch008

Elouali, S., Ait Hamdan, Y., Benali, S., Lhomme, P., Gosselin, M., Raquez, J. M., & Rhazi, M. (2025). Extraction of chitin and chitosan from Hermetia illucens breeding waste: A greener approach for industrial application. *International Journal of Biological Macromolecules, 285*, 138302. DOI: 10.1016/j.ijbiomac.2024.138302 PMID: 39638207

Farag, M. M. (2023). Recent trends on biomaterials for tissue regeneration applications [review]. *Journal of Materials Science, 58*(2), 527–558. DOI: 10.1007/s10853-022-08102-x

Fenton, O. S., Olafson, K. N., Pillai, P. S., Mitchell, M. J., & Langer, R. (2018). Advances in Biomaterials for Drug Delivery. *Advanced Materials, 30*(29), 1705328. Advance online publication. DOI: 10.1002/adma.201705328 PMID: 29736981

Fernández-Lahore, M., Yelemane, V., Islam, T., & Carbajal, M. L. (2023). Ceramic-Based Adsorbents in Bioproduct Recovery and Purification. In *Surface-Functionalized Ceramics* (pp. 407–437). Wiley., DOI: 10.1002/9783527698042.ch11

Festas, A., Ramos, A., & Davim, J. (2020). Medical devices biomaterials <scp>– A</scp> review. *Proceedings of the Institution of Mechanical Engineers, Part L: Journal of Materials: Design and Applications, 234*(1), 218–228. DOI: 10.1177/1464420719882458

Fu, Z., Ouyang, L., Xu, R., Yang, Y., & Sun, W. (2022). Responsive biomaterials for 3D bioprinting: A review. *Materials Today, 52*, 112–132. DOI: 10.1016/j.mattod.2022.01.001

Fuchs, S., Shariati, K., & Ma, M. (2020). Specialty Tough Hydrogels and Their Biomedical Applications. *Advanced Healthcare Materials, 9*(2), 1901396. Advance online publication. DOI: 10.1002/adhm.201901396 PMID: 31846228

Gade, R. (2024). *M., L. P., Dwarampudi, L. P., Yamuna, K., Maraba, N., & Fufa, G.* Advanced Nanomaterials in Imaging and Diagnostics., DOI: 10.4018/979-8-3693-6326-3.ch004

Garg, G., Ramanujachary, K. V., Lofland, S. E., Lobanov, M. V., Greenblatt, M., Maddanimath, T., Vijayamohanan, K., & Ganguli, A. K. (2003). Crystal structure, magnetic and electrochemical properties of a quaternary thiospinel: Ag2MnSn3S8. *Journal of Solid State Chemistry, 174*(1), 229–232. DOI: 10.1016/S0022-4596(03)00240-8

Göktürk, I., Güler, K. Ç., Yılmaz, F., Oktar, C., Yılmaz, G. E., & Denizli, A. (2024). Molecularly Imprinted Polymeric Biomaterials in Diagnosis and Medical Practice. *Biomedical Materials & Devices*. Advance online publication. DOI: 10.1007/s44174-024-00192-2

Göktürk, I., Güler, K. Ç., Yılmaz, F., Oktar, C., Yılmaz, G. E., & Denizli, A. (2025). Molecularly Imprinted Polymeric Biomaterials in Diagnosis and Medical Practice. *Biomedical Materials & Devices*, *3*(1), 299–316. DOI: 10.1007/s44174-024-00192-2

Graham, J., Werba, L., Federico, I., & Gonzalez-Fernandez, T. (2023). Crispr strategies for stem cell engineering: A new frontier in musculoskeletal regeneration. *European Cells & Materials*, *46*, 91–118. DOI: 10.22203/eCM.v046a05

Gray, V. P., Amelung, C. D., Duti, I. J., Laudermilch, E. G., Letteri, R. A., & Lampe, K. J. (2022). Biomaterials via peptide assembly: Design, characterization, and application in tissue engineering. *Acta Biomaterialia*, *140*, 43–75. DOI: 10.1016/j.actbio.2021.10.030 PMID: 34710626

Guvendiren, M., Molde, J., Soares, R. M. D., & Kohn, J. (2016). Designing Biomaterials for 3D Printing. *ACS Biomaterials Science & Engineering*, *2*(10), 1679–1693. DOI: 10.1021/acsbiomaterials.6b00121 PMID: 28025653

Hakim, L. K., Yari, A., Nikparto, N., Mehraban, S. H., Cheperli, S., Asadi, A., Darehdor, A. A., Nezaminia, S., Dortaj, D., Nazari, Y., Dehghan, M., Hojjat, P., Mohajeri, M., & Hasani Jebelli, M. S. (2024). The current applications of nano and biomaterials in drug delivery of dental implant. *BMC Oral Health*, *24*(1), 126. DOI: 10.1186/s12903-024-03911-9 PMID: 38267933

Han, X., Alu, A., Liu, H., Shi, Y., Wei, X., Cai, L., & Wei, Y. (2022). Biomaterial-assisted biotherapy: A brief review of biomaterials used in drug delivery, vaccine development, gene therapy, and stem cell therapy. *Bioactive Materials*, *17*, 29–48. DOI: 10.1016/j.bioactmat.2022.01.011 PMID: 35386442

Hendrikse, S. I. S., Contreras-Montoya, R., Ellis, A. V., Thordarson, P., & Steed, J. W. (2022). Biofunctionality with a twist: The importance of molecular organisation, handedness and configuration in synthetic biomaterial design. *Chemical Society Reviews*, *51*(1), 28–42. DOI: 10.1039/D1CS00896J PMID: 34846055

Hu, H., Qi, Q., Dong, Z., Yu, X., Mo, Y., Luo, J., Wang, Y., Du, S., & Lu, Y. (2020). Albumin coated trimethyl chitosan-based targeting delivery platform for photothermal/chemo-synergistic cancer therapy. *Carbohydrate Polymers*, *241*, 116335. DOI: 10.1016/j.carbpol.2020.116335 PMID: 32507205

Huynh, K.-H., Pham, X.-H., Kim, J., Lee, S. H., Chang, H., Rho, W.-Y., & Jun, B.-H. (2020). Synthesis, Properties, and Biological Applications of Metallic Alloy Nanoparticles. *International Journal of Molecular Sciences*, *21*(14), 5174. DOI: 10.3390/ijms21145174 PMID: 32708351

Huzum, B., Puha, B., Necoara, R., Gheorghevici, S., Puha, G., Filip, A., Sirbu, P., & Alexa, O. (2021). Biocompatibility assessment of biomaterials used in orthopedic devices: An overview [Review]. *Experimental and Therapeutic Medicine*, *22*(5), 1315. DOI: 10.3892/etm.2021.10750 PMID: 34630669

Insuasti-Cruz, E., Suárez-Jaramillo, V., Mena Urresta, K. A., Pila-Varela, K. O., Fiallos-Ayala, X., Dahoumane, S. A., & Alexis, F. (2022). Natural Biomaterials from Biodiversity for Healthcare Applications. *Advanced Healthcare Materials*, *11*(1), 2101389. Advance online publication. DOI: 10.1002/adhm.202101389 PMID: 34643331

Izadyari Aghmiuni, A., Heidari keshel, S., Aghababai, A., Zahraei, M., & Rezaei-tavirani, M. (2024). The design of natural hybrid biomaterial to promote osteogenic differentiation, collagen i and II expression and relief of musculoskeletal pains: Bone tissue-engineering applications (in-vitro and clinical studies). *Arabian Journal of Chemistry*, *17*(6), 105766. DOI: 10.1016/j.arabjc.2024.105766

Jasni, A. H., Azmi, A. S., Puad, N. I. M., Ali, F., & Nor, Y. A. (2023). *Naturally Derived Biomaterials: Advances and Opportunities* (pp. 3–41). DOI: 10.1007/978-981-99-6698-1_1

Jiang, Z., Han, X., Zhao, C., Wang, S., & Tang, X. (2022). Recent Advance in Biological Responsive Nanomaterials for Biosensing and Molecular Imaging Application. *International Journal of Molecular Sciences*, *23*(3), 1923. DOI: 10.3390/ijms23031923 PMID: 35163845

Joicy, S., & Thangadurai, P. (2021). *Metal Sulfide Nanostructures for Bioimaging and Biosensing Applications*., DOI: 10.1007/978-3-030-56413-1_1

Joyce, K., Fabra, G. T., Bozkurt, Y., & Pandit, A. (2021). Bioactive potential of natural biomaterials: Identification, retention and assessment of biological properties. *Signal Transduction and Targeted Therapy*, *6*(1), 122. DOI: 10.1038/s41392-021-00512-8 PMID: 33737507

Jurczak, K. M., van der Boon, T. A. B., Devia-Rodriguez, R., Schuurmann, R. C. L., Sjollema, J., van Huizen, L., De Vries, J. P. M., & van Rijn, P. (2025). Recent regulatory developments in <scp>EU Medical Device Regulation</scp> and their impact on biomaterials translation. *Bioengineering & Translational Medicine*, *10*(2), e10721. Advance online publication. DOI: 10.1002/btm2.10721 PMID: 40060767

Karakullukcu, A. B., Taban, E., & Ojo, O. O. (2023). Biocompatibility of biomaterials and test methods: A review. *Materialprüfung (Munchen), 65*(4), 545–559. DOI: 10.1515/mt-2022-0195

Katkova, M. A., Zhigulin, G. Y., Baranov, E. V., Zabrodina, G. S., Muravyeva, M. S., Ketkov, S. Y., Fomina, I. G., & Eremenko, I. L. (2023). Specific Features of Binding Bioactive Organic Molecules with the Metallic Matrix of Heteronuclear 3d-4f Structures Containing Soft and Hard Metallocenters Using the Nd(III)–Cu(II) Complex as an Example. *Координационная химия, 49*(9), 590–600. DOI: 10.31857/S0132344X23600157

Keane, T. J., & Badylak, S. F. (2014). Biomaterials for tissue engineering applications. *Seminars in Pediatric Surgery, 23*(3), 112–118. DOI: 10.1053/j.sempedsurg.2014.06.010 PMID: 24994524

Kervran, M., Vagner, C., Cochez, M., Ponçot, M., Saeb, M. R., & Vahabi, H. (2022). Thermal degradation of polylactic acid (PLA)/polyhydroxybutyrate (PHB) blends: A systematic review. *Polymer Degradation & Stability, 201*, 109995. DOI: 10.1016/j.polymdegradstab.2022.109995

Khan, H. M., Liao, X., Sheikh, B. A., Wang, Y., Su, Z., Guo, C., Li, Z., Zhou, C., Cen, Y., & Kong, Q. (2022). Smart biomaterials and their potential applications in tissue engineering. *Journal of Materials Chemistry. B, 10*(36), 6859–6895. DOI: 10.1039/D2TB01106A PMID: 36069198

Khan, M. U. A., Aslam, M. A., Bin Abdullah, M. F., Hasan, A., Shah, S. A., & Stojanović, G. M. (2023). Recent perspective of polymeric biomaterial in tissue engineering– a review. *Materials Today. Chemistry, 34*, 101818. DOI: 10.1016/j.mtchem.2023.101818

Kostag, M., Jedvert, K., & El Seoud, O. A. (2021). Engineering of sustainable biomaterial composites from cellulose and silk fibroin: Fundamentals and applications. *International Journal of Biological Macromolecules, 167*, 687–718. DOI: 10.1016/j.ijbiomac.2020.11.151 PMID: 33249159

Licciardello, M., Traldi, C., Bortolameazzi, M., Testore, D., Ciardelli, G., & Tonda-Turo, C. (2024). Aligned polycaprolactone/polyaniline electrospun nanofibers for directing neural stem cell differentiation and neuron arrangement. *Frontiers in Biomaterials Science, 3*, 1362599. Advance online publication. DOI: 10.3389/fbiom.2024.1362599

Lin, A. H., Slater, C. A., Martinez, C.-J., Eppell, S. J., Yu, S. M., & Weiss, J. A. (2023). Collagen fibrils from both positional and energy-storing tendons exhibit increased amounts of denatured collagen when stretched beyond the yield point. *Acta Biomaterialia, 155*, 461–470. DOI: 10.1016/j.actbio.2022.11.018 PMID: 36400348

Liu, A. P., Appel, E. A., Ashby, P. D., Baker, B. M., Franco, E., Gu, L., Haynes, K., Joshi, N. S., Kloxin, A. M., Kouwer, P. H. J., Mittal, J., Morsut, L., Noireaux, V., Parekh, S., Schulman, R., Tang, S. K. Y., Valentine, M. T., Vega, S. L., Weber, W., & Chaudhuri, O. (2022). The living interface between synthetic biology and biomaterial design. *Nature Materials, 21*(4), 390–397. DOI: 10.1038/s41563-022-01231-3 PMID: 35361951

Liu, J., Wang, K., Li, X., Zhang, X., Gong, X., Zhu, Y., Ren, Z., Zhang, B., & Cheng, J. (2023). Biocompatibility and osseointegration properties of a novel high strength and low modulus β- Ti10Mo6Zr4Sn3Nb alloy. *Frontiers in Bioengineering and Biotechnology, 11*, 1127929. Advance online publication. DOI: 10.3389/fbioe.2023.1127929 PMID: 36865033

Liu, S., Wang, T., Li, S., & Wang, X. (2022). Application Status of Sacrificial Biomaterials in 3D Bioprinting. *Polymers, 14*(11), 2182. DOI: 10.3390/polym14112182 PMID: 35683853

Mabrouk, M., Das, D. B., Salem, Z. A., & Beherei, H. H. (2021). Nanomaterials for Biomedical Applications: Production, Characterisations, Recent Trends and Difficulties. *Molecules (Basel, Switzerland), 26*(4), 1077. DOI: 10.3390/molecules26041077 PMID: 33670668

Amandine Magnaudeix, & et Julie Usseglio-Grosso. (2020). 9. Biomatériaux métalliques. In *La métallurgie* (pp. 69–70). EDP Sciences. DOI: 10.1051/978-2-7598-0906-6.c026

Mahdi, N. M. S., Hassan, A. K., Al-Hasani, F. J., & Al-Jawher, W. A. M. (2024). Classification Of Biomaterials and Their Applications. *Journal Port Science Research, 7*(3), 281–299. DOI: 10.36371/port.2024.3.7

Majumdar, S., Gupta, S., & Krishnamurthy, S. (2021). Multifarious applications of bioactive glasses in soft tissue engineering. *Biomaterials Science, 9*(24), 8111–8147. DOI: 10.1039/D1BM01104A PMID: 34766608

Marin, E., Boschetto, F., & Pezzotti, G. (2020). Biomaterials and biocompatibility: An historical overview. *Journal of Biomedical Materials Research. Part A, 108*(8), 1617–1633. DOI: 10.1002/jbm.a.36930 PMID: 32196949

Mishra, A., & Srivastava, V. (2021). Biomaterials and 3D printing techniques used in the medical field. *Journal of Medical Engineering & Technology*, *45*(4), 290–302. DOI: 10.1080/03091902.2021.1893845 PMID: 33929285

Mishra, P., Kumar, S., Kumar Maurya, A., Tiwari, P., Tirkey, S., & Sharma, S. (2024). 5 Bio-based materials in drug delivery. In *Sustainable Bio-Based Composites* (pp. 79–106). De Gruyter., DOI: 10.1515/9783111321530-005

Moltasov, A. V., Voinaroych, S. G., Dyman, M. M., Kalyuzhnyi, S. M., & Burburska, S. V. (2023). Methods to prevent the stress shielding effect in implant-body system [Review]. *The Paton Welding Journal*, *2023*(1), 31–38. DOI: 10.37434/tpwj2023.01.05

Nagabushanam, M., Devade, K., Aravind Reddy, G., Nagaraj Goud, B., Sayed, R. M., Sood, S., & Sonia, P. (2023). Advance biomedical engineering – A fundamental review of composite materials and its applications. *Materials Today: Proceedings*. Advance online publication. DOI: 10.1016/j.matpr.2023.08.216

Nagay, B. E., Cordeiro, J. M., & Barão, V. A. R. (2020). Alloy Materials for Biomedical Applications. In *Alloy Materials and Their Allied Applications* (pp. 159–189). Wiley., DOI: 10.1002/9781119654919.ch9

Nasiri, H., Abbasian, K., Salahandish, M., & Elyasi, S. N. (2024). Sensitive surface plasmon resonance biosensor by optimized carboxylate functionalized carbon nanotubes/chitosan for amlodipine detecting. *Talanta*, *276*, 126249. DOI: 10.1016/j.talanta.2024.126249 PMID: 38743970

Neamtu, B., Barbu, A., Negrea, M. O., Berghea-Neam u, C., Popescu, D., Zăhan, M., & Mire an, V. (2022). Carrageenan-Based Compounds as Wound Healing Materials. *International Journal of Molecular Sciences*, *23*(16), 9117. DOI: 10.3390/ijms23169117 PMID: 36012381

Park, Y., Huh, K. M., & Kang, S.-W. (2021). Applications of Biomaterials in 3D Cell Culture and Contributions of 3D Cell Culture to Drug Development and Basic Biomedical Research. *International Journal of Molecular Sciences*, *22*(5), 2491. DOI: 10.3390/ijms22052491 PMID: 33801273

Patel, N. R., & Gohil, P. P. (2012). A Review on Biomaterials: Scope, Applications & Human Anatomy Significance. *International Journal of Emerging Technology and Advanced Engineering*, *2*(4).

Pathak, S., Sahu, P., Begum, J. P. S., Kashaw, S. K., Pandey, A., Semwal, P., & Sharma, R. (2024). Formulation and assessment of penetration potential of Risedronate chitosan nanoparticles loaded transdermal gel in the management of osteoporosis: In vitro and ex vivo screening. *Carbohydrate Polymer Technologies and Applications*, *7*, 100440. DOI: 10.1016/j.carpta.2024.100440

Patil, S. S., & Misra, R. D. K. (2018). The significance of macromolecular architecture in governing structure-property relationship for biomaterial applications: An overview. *Materials Technology*, *33*(5), 364–386. DOI: 10.1080/10667857.2018.1447266

Petelinšek, N., & Mommer, S. (2024). Tough Hydrogels for Load-Bearing Applications. *Advancement of Science*, *11*(12), 2307404. Advance online publication. DOI: 10.1002/advs.202307404 PMID: 38225751

Pidhatika, B., Widyaya, V. T., Nalam, P. C., Swasono, Y. A., & Ardhani, R. (2022). Surface Modifications of High-Performance Polymer Polyetheretherketone (PEEK) to Improve Its Biological Performance in Dentistry. *Polymers*, *14*(24), 5526. DOI: 10.3390/polym14245526 PMID: 36559893

Pina, S., Ribeiro, V. P., Marques, C. F., Maia, F. R., Silva, T. H., Reis, R. L., & Oliveira, J. M. (2019). Scaffolding Strategies for Tissue Engineering and Regenerative Medicine Applications. *Materials (Basel)*, *12*(11), 1824. DOI: 10.3390/ma12111824 PMID: 31195642

Pires, P. C., Mascarenhas-Melo, F., Pedrosa, K., Lopes, D., Lopes, J., Macário-Soares, A., Peixoto, D., Giram, P. S., Veiga, F., & Paiva-Santos, A. C. (2023). Polymer-based biomaterials for pharmaceutical and biomedical applications: A focus on topical drug administration. *European Polymer Journal*, *187*, 111868. DOI: 10.1016/j.eurpolymj.2023.111868

Proniewicz, E. (2023). Metallic nanoparticles as effective sensors of bio-molecules. *Spectrochimica Acta. Part A: Molecular and Biomolecular Spectroscopy*, *288*, 122207. DOI: 10.1016/j.saa.2022.122207 PMID: 36502763

Pryadko, A., Surmeneva, M. A., & Surmenev, R. A. (2021). Review of Hybrid Materials Based on Polyhydroxyalkanoates for Tissue Engineering Applications. *Polymers*, *13*(11), 1738. DOI: 10.3390/polym13111738 PMID: 34073335

Pugliese, R., Beltrami, B., Regondi, S., & Lunetta, C. (2021). Polymeric biomaterials for 3D printing in medicine: An overview. *Annals of 3D Printed Medicine, 2*, 100011. DOI: 10.1016/j.stlm.2021.100011

Punj, S., Singh, J., & Singh, K. (2021). Ceramic biomaterials: Properties, state of the art and future prospectives. *Ceramics International*, *47*(20), 28059–28074. DOI: 10.1016/j.ceramint.2021.06.238

Rana, M. M., & De la Hoz Siegler, H. (2024). Evolution of Hybrid Hydrogels: Next-Generation Biomaterials for Drug Delivery and Tissue Engineering. *Gels (Basel, Switzerland)*, *10*(4), 216. DOI: 10.3390/gels10040216 PMID: 38667635

Rawal, A., Rhinehardt, K. L., & Mohan, R. V. (2020). Molecular Dynamics Investigation of Self- Association of Synthetic Collagen and Spider Silk Composite System for Biomaterial Applications. *MRS Advances*, *5*(16), 797–804. DOI: 10.1557/adv.2019.490

Ressler, A. (2022). Chitosan-Based Biomaterials for Bone Tissue Engineering Applications: A Short Review. *Polymers*, *14*(16), 3430. DOI: 10.3390/polym14163430 PMID: 36015686

Rohani Shirvan, A., Nouri, A., & Wen, C. (2021). Structural polymer biomaterials. In *Structural Biomaterials* (pp. 395–439). Elsevier., DOI: 10.1016/B978-0-12-818831-6.00010-0

Sam, S., Joseph, B., & Thomas, S. (2023). Exploring the antimicrobial features of biomaterials for biomedical applications. *Results in Engineering*, *17*, 100979. DOI: 10.1016/j.rineng.2023.100979

Santhosh, S., Mukherjee, D., Anbu, J., Murahari, M., & Teja, B. V. (2019). Improved treatment efficacy of risedronate functionalized chitosan nanoparticles in osteoporosis: Formulation development, in vivo, and molecular modelling studies. *Journal of Microencapsulation*, *36*(4), 338–355. DOI: 10.1080/02652048.2019.1631401 PMID: 31190594

Satchanska, G., Davidova, S., & Petrov, P. D. (2024). Natural and Synthetic Polymers for Biomedical and Environmental Applications. *Polymers*, *16*(8), 1159. DOI: 10.3390/polym16081159 PMID: 38675078

Schuh, J. C. L., & Funk, K. A. (2019). Compilation of International Standards and Regulatory Guidance Documents for Evaluation of Biomaterials, Medical Devices, and 3-D Printed and Regenerative Medicine Products. *Toxicologic Pathology*, *47*(3), 344–357. DOI: 10.1177/0192623318804121 PMID: 30392453

Sharma, N., Modak, C., Singh, P. K., Kumar, R., Khatri, D., & Singh, S. B. (2021). Underscoring the immense potential of chitosan in fighting a wide spectrum of viruses: A plausible molecule against SARS-CoV-2? *International Journal of Biological Macromolecules*, *179*, 33–44. DOI: 10.1016/j.ijbiomac.2021.02.090 PMID: 33607132

Siraparapu, Y. D., Bassa, S., & Sanasi, P. D. (2014). *A Review on Recent Applications of Biomaterials*. https://api.semanticscholar.org/CorpusID:30296635

Song, X., Tang, Z., Liu, W., Chen, K., Liang, J., Yuan, B., Lin, H., Zhu, X., Fan, Y., Shi, X., Zhao, P., Yang, L., Zhang, K., Mikos, A. G., & Zhang, X. (2022). Biomaterials and regulatory science. *Journal of Materials Science and Technology*, *128*, 221–227. DOI: 10.1016/j.jmst.2022.04.018

Sood, A., Gupta, A., & Agrawal, G. (2021). Recent advances in polysaccharides based biomaterials for drug delivery and tissue engineering applications. *Carbohydrate Polymer Technologies and Applications*, *2*, 100067. DOI: 10.1016/j.carpta.2021.100067

Su, H., Fujiwara, T., Anderson, K. M., Karydis, A., Ghadri, M. N., & Bumgardner, J. D. (2021). A comparison of two types of electrospun chitosan membranes and a collagen membrane in vivo. *Dental Materials*, *37*(1), 60–70. DOI: 10.1016/j.dental.2020.10.011 PMID: 33208266

Sultana, N., Cole, A., & Strachan, F. (2024). Biocomposite Scaffolds for Tissue Engineering: Materials, Fabrication Techniques and Future Directions. *Materials (Basel)*, *17*(22), 5577. DOI: 10.3390/ma17225577 PMID: 39597399

Szczęsny, G., Kopec, M., Politis, D. J., Kowalewski, Z. L., Łazarski, A., & Szolc, T. (2022). A Review on Biomaterials for Orthopaedic Surgery and Traumatology: From Past to Present. *Materials (Basel)*, *15*(10), 3622. DOI: 10.3390/ma15103622 PMID: 35629649

Tatu, R. R., Oria, M., Rao, M. B., Peiro, J. L., & Lin, C.-Y. (2022). Biodegradation of poly(l-lactic acid) and poly(ε-caprolactone) patches by human amniotic fluid in an in-vitro simulated fetal environment. *Scientific Reports*, *12*(1), 3950. DOI: 10.1038/s41598-022-07681-8 PMID: 35273223

Todros, S., Todesco, M., & Bagno, A. (2021). Biomaterials and Their Biomedical Applications: From Replacement to Regeneration. *Processes (Basel, Switzerland)*, *9*(11), 1949. DOI: 10.3390/pr9111949

Troy, E., Tilbury, M. A., Power, A. M., & Wall, J. G. (2021). Nature-Based Biomaterials and Their Application in Biomedicine. *Polymers*, *13*(19), 3321. DOI: 10.3390/polym13193321 PMID: 34641137

Trucillo, P. (2024). Biomaterials for Drug Delivery and Human Applications. *Materials (Basel)*, *17*(2), 456. DOI: 10.3390/ma17020456 PMID: 38255624

Tsouknidas, A. (2024). Advancements in Biomaterials for Bioengineering and Biotechnology. *International Journal of Molecular Sciences*, *25*(14), 7840. DOI: 10.3390/ijms25147840 PMID: 39063082

Turab, N. M., Abu Owida, H., Al-Nabulsi, J. I., & Alnaimat, F. (2024). Applications of nanostructured materials for severe acute respiratory syndrome-CoV-2 diagnostic. *Bulletin of Electrical Engineering and Informatics*, *13*(4), 2913–2921. DOI: 10.11591/eei.v13i4.7325

Ul-Islam, M., Alabbosh, K. F., Manan, S., Khan, S., Ahmad, F., & Ullah, M. W. (2024). Chitosan-based nanostructured biomaterials: Synthesis, properties, and biomedical applications. *Advanced Industrial and Engineering Polymer Research*, *7*(1), 79–99. DOI: 10.1016/j.aiepr.2023.07.002

Uluda, Ä. Ÿ. (2014). Grand Challenges in Biomaterials. *Frontiers in Bioengineering and Biotechnology*, *2*. Advance online publication. DOI: 10.3389/fbioe.2014.00043 PMID: 25368868

Venkatesan, J., Rekha, P. D., Anil, S., Bhatnagar, I., Sudha, P. N., Dechsakulwatana, C., Kim, S.-K., & Shim, M. S. (2018). Hydroxyapatite from Cuttlefish Bone: Isolation, Characterizations, and Applications. *Biotechnology and Bioprocess Engineering; BBE*, *23*(4), 383–393. DOI: 10.1007/s12257-018-0169-9

Wan, M., Qin, W., Lei, C., Li, Q., Meng, M., Fang, M., Song, W., Chen, J., Tay, F., & Niu, L. (2021). Biomaterials from the sea: Future building blocks for biomedical applications. *Bioactive Materials*, *6*(12), 4255–4285. DOI: 10.1016/j.bioactmat.2021.04.028 PMID: 33997505

Wang, H. (2023). Biomaterials in Medical Applications. *Polymers*, *15*(4), 847. DOI: 10.3390/polym15040847 PMID: 36850130

Williams, D. F. (1987). Definitions in biomaterials. *Proceedings of a consensus conference of the european society for biomaterials*. Amsterdam; New York : Elsevier, 4.

Yadav, S., Khan, J., & Yadav, A. (2024). Applications of Scaffolds in Tissue Engineering: Current Utilization and Future Prospective. *Current Gene Therapy*, *24*(2), 94–109. DOI: 10.2174/0115665232262167231012102837 PMID: 37921144

Yang, Y., Li, B., Wang, M., Pan, S., Wang, Y., & Gu, J. (2023). Effect of natural polymer materials on skin healing based on internal wound microenvironment: A review. *Frontiers in Chemistry*, *11*, 1257915. Advance online publication. DOI: 10.3389/fchem.2023.1257915 PMID: 37731458

Yang, Y., & Xiao, Y. (2020). Biomaterials Regulating Bone Hematoma for Osteogenesis. *Advanced Healthcare Materials*, *9*(23), 2000726. Advance online publication. DOI: 10.1002/adhm.202000726 PMID: 32691989

Yi, H., Patel, R., Patel, K. D., Bouchard, L.-S., Jha, A., Perriman, A. W., & Patel, M. (2023). Conducting polymer-based scaffolds for neuronal tissue engineering. *Journal of Materials Chemistry. B*, *11*(46), 11006–11023. DOI: 10.1039/D3TB01838E PMID: 37953707

Zhang, D., Chen, Q., Shi, C., Chen, M., Ma, K., Wan, J., & Liu, R. (2021). Dealing with the Foreign-Body Response to Implanted Biomaterials: Strategies and Applications of New Materials. *Advanced Functional Materials*, *31*(6), 2007226. Advance online publication. DOI: 10.1002/adfm.202007226

Zhang, H., & Wu, C. (2023). 3D printing of biomaterials for vascularized and innervated tissue regeneration. *International Journal of Bioprinting*, *9*(3), 706. DOI: 10.18063/ijb.706 PMID: 37273994

Chapter 3
The Nano Revolution, Metal Nanoparticles in Antibiotic-Resistant Era: Synthesis, Properties, and Antimicrobial Applications

Shilpa Rudra
https://orcid.org/0000-0003-0291-2225
Vellore Institute of Technology, Vellore, India

Danie Kingsley
https://orcid.org/0000-0001-7838-5017
Vellore Institute of Technology University, Vellore, India

ABSTRACT

Nanoparticle synthesis has gained significant interest over the years because of its unique characteristics and sustainable and productive applications in numerous fields. Metals exhibiting a friend-foe relationship with bacteria, possess the potential to inhibit their growth in specific forms and concentrations. The increase in antimicrobial resistance in recent years has drawn attention. Top-down and Bottom-up are the two approaches to metal nanoparticle synthesis. Gold, silver, copper, etc. have been used in medical fields from ancient times. Although these conventional methods of creating nanoparticles are effective and adaptable, they have very negative effects. On the other hand, green synthesis provides an economical and environmentally beneficial substitute by using natural resources. To address the current problem of antimicrobial resistance, this review highlights the antimicrobial activity of metal nanoparticles and highlights their contributions to sustainability, safety and efficiency in nanoparticle production as well as their synthesis process,

DOI: 10.4018/979-8-3373-1305-4.ch003

benefits, and drawbacks.

1. INTRODUCTION

Nanotechnology is currently regarded as an intriguing field for research and is gaining continuous, vast, and enormous attention worldwide, (Lee, Jeong, & Kanmani, 2019). Professor Norio Taniguchi first used the term "nanotechnology" in 1974 in his thesis, but it achieved popularity from a book named Engines of Creation – The Coming Era of Nanotechnology written by Eric Dexter, (K.M.A et al., 2008). Nanotechnology includes synthesis techniques, structure, and size modification of nano-sized particles and is featured as a strong platform for metal nanoparticle synthesis, (Kadam et al., 2019). The word "nanoparticle" comes from the Greek word "nano," meaning "small or dwarf," (Ealia & Saravanakumar, 2017). Nanoparticles (NPs) are the particulate matters with at least 1-dimensional particles size ranging from 1-100 nm concerning 1nm equals 10^{-9} or one billionth of 1 meter and demonstrate potential biological activities such as antimicrobial, antifungal, etc. The decreased particle size of nanoparticles to nano-level particle size exhibits improved particle size distribution and morphology and shows a high surface-to-volume ratio. A nanoparticle's surface-to-volume ratio is 35–45% greater than a large molecule. The distinct surface area of NPs contributes to size-dependent strong surface reactivity. The unique and multifunctional characteristics of nanoparticles such as specific size, shape, different compositions, flexibility, ductility, rigidity, quantum size, hardness, and rigidity lead to the great expansion of the application of nanoparticles into various fields including agriculture, food, medical, material sciences, environmental aspects, space technology, magnetism, optoelectronics and electronics, cosmetics, catalytic, and energy use, (Lee, Jeong, & Kanmani, 2019).

Antibiotic resistance, a worldwide health emergency, poses a danger to decades of medical progress. traditional antibiotics are losing their effectiveness against multidrug-resistant (MDR) pathogens, necessitating alternative approaches. Different types of bacteria i.e. *Streptococcus pneumoniae*, Methicillin-resistant *Staphylococcus aureus* (MRSA), beta-lactamase (ESBL) producing *Escherichia coli* are developing as prevalent community spread multidrug-resistant bacteria due to overuse and unrequired overconsumption of antibiotics. NPs synthesized from gold, silver, zinc etc. open promising opportunities as efficient alternatives to antibacterial agents due to their diverse antimicrobial mechanisms such as membrane disruption, destabilization, production of Reactive oxygen species (ROS), and inhibition of cellular process and biofilm formation, diminishing the currently raised global concerns of an antibiotic-resistant era. Three categories of nanoparticles can be distinguished: (a) organic, (b) inorganic, and (c) carbon-based. Ferritin, dendrimers, liposomes, and micelles are examples of the organic ones. Metals and metal oxide nanoparticles are two types of inorganic nanoparticles, which are based on metals. Silver, gold, copper, iron, manganese, selenium, and zinc can all be used to create metal-based nanoparticles. Fullerenes, graphene, carbon nanotubes, carbon nanofibers, and carbon black are the several types of carbon-based nanoparticles, (Ealia & Saravanakumar, 2017). The synthesis of nanoparticles, nanostructures, and nanomaterials has received a lot of attention lately because of its numerous applications in sensor technology, composite-like polymer creation, illness diagnostics, and treatment. As Nanotechnology is effective and environmentally beneficial, it can provide cleaner air and water as well as clean renewable energy, which is essential for a sustainable and clean future. Silver, copper, and gold are examples of metal nanomaterials that have been shown to have antibacterial activity against strains of bacteria and fungi, both Gram-positive and Gram-negative, with a unique mode of action and a variety of target properties (Regiel-Futyra et al., 2017) and heat stability, (Shankar & Rhim, 2015). Gold and silver NPs are widely applied in numerous technologies like medicine, chemistry, electronics, and other biotechnological approaches. Silver nanoparticles possess antibacterial, antifungal, and antiviral properties. The crystalline feature of silver nanoparticles confers their applications in the fields of therapeutics, diagnostics, antimicrobials, catalysis, and high-sensitivity biomolecular detection. Metal nanoparticles are found in cosmetics like moisturizers, sunscreen, body wash, wash detergents, medicine, and other pharmaceutical products. Researchers are enormously focusing on implementing its use in drug development, targeted drug delivery, and disease diagnosis. As a result, the research work on nanoparticle synthesis has grown exponentially over the last three to four decades. Nanoparticles are created employing a variety of physical and chemical techniques. The conventional extensively used methods are top-down (such as mechanical milling, laser ablation, ion sputtering, and thermal decomposition) and bottom-up (such as solid-state procedures, liquid-state synthesis methods, and gas-phase methods). Although these traditional physical and chemical methods of creating nanoparticles are effective and adaptable, they involve elements like high pressure and temperature, poisonous chemicals, and the generation of dangerous byproducts. Green synthesis, also known as biosynthesis, provides an environmentally friendly substitute by using natural resources and methods to produce nanoparticles with minimal harm to the environment. Metal nanoparticles have emerged as versatile agents in pharmaceutical research, facilitating targeted drug delivery, enhanced imaging, and elevated crop protection.

Correct choice and use of specific NPs synthesis techniques play a crucial role as the kinetics of the interaction of metals and metal ion-reducing agents and the use of the stabilizing agent impact the properties of NPs like morphology and stability. Alternative safe and environmentally acceptable technologies are needed to produce metallic nanoparticles because chemical and physical procedures are costly and extremely harmful to living things. Consequently, the usage of biological resources, including bacteria, fungi, plant extract, algae, yeasts, actinomycetes, oils, and natural biopolymers is prioritized, (Lee, Jeong, & Kanmani, 2019). The present review provides a comprehensive overview of various kinds of metal nanoparticles, and methods employed in the synthesis of metallic nanoparticles, along with a critical analysis of their advantages, disadvantages, and antibacterial applications, (Rudra & D.K.J., 2024).

Figure 1. Number of papers published in different databases across the last few years indicating the exponential increase and emerging interest in nanoparticle synthesis and its application. 1A: PubMed; 1B: Google Scholar; 1C: Science Direct

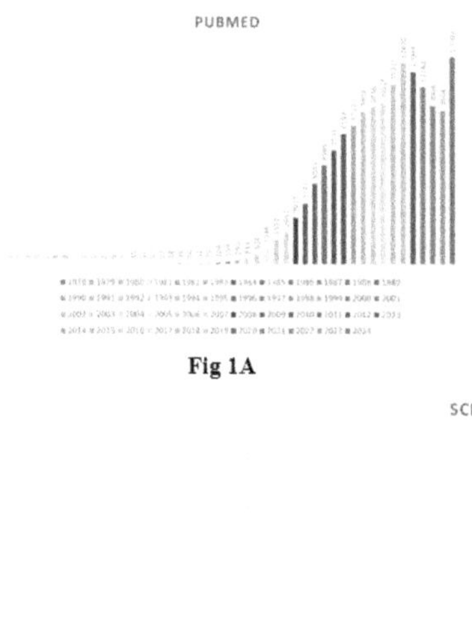

Fig 1A

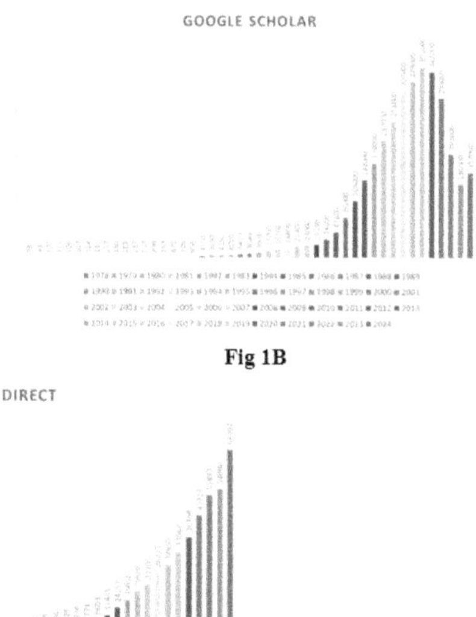

Fig 1B

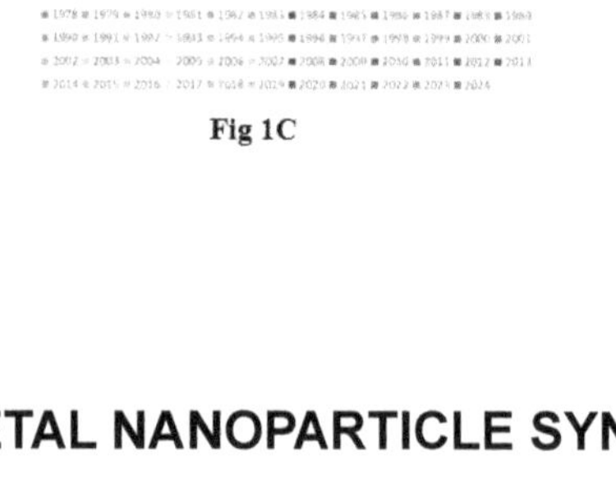

Fig 1C

2. METHODS OF METAL NANOPARTICLE SYNTHESIS

Nanoparticles can be synthesized using a variety of techniques, mostly top-down and bottom-up approaches. The initial substance utilized for the creation of the nanoparticles is the main difference between the two methods. While the top-down approach, sometimes referred to as a destructive approach, reduces bulk material to nanometric scale particles, the bottom-up approach, also known as a constructive approach, builds material from atoms to clusters to nanoparticles. This process reduces particle size to nanoparticles. Nanolithography, mechanical milling, laser ablation, thermal decomposition, sputtering, synthesis from biological resources are some of the methods most widely used for synthesizing nanoparticles, (Chauhan, 2024).

Table 1. Overview of historical evolution nanoparticle synthesis techniques

Name of Synthesis Techniques	Historical Evolution of Nanoparticle Synthesis Techniques
Mechanical Milling	**1961** – Introduced as **mechanical alloying** by John Benjamin. **1970** – Applied to nanoparticle synthesis, especially for metals and ceramics. **1990** – Used in materials processing industries. **Present** – Extensively employed for top-down nanoparticle synthesis.
Laser Ablation	**1987** – Initial studies on **laser ablation in liquid (LAL)**. **1990** – **Pulsed laser ablation (PLA)** refined for precise nanoparticle generation. **2000** – Improved for biomedical and optoelectronic applications. **Present** – Key method for producing high-purity nanoparticles.
Physical Vapor Deposition (PVD)	**1970** – Developed as an alternative to electroplating. **1980** – Applied in **magnetron sputtering** and **electron beam evaporation**. **1990** – **Atomic Layer Deposition (ALD)** introduced for nanoscale control. **Present** – Used in nano-coatings, optics, and microelectronics.
Chemical Vapor Deposition (CVD)	**1960** – First used for thin film deposition. **1980** – Applied for **carbon nanotube (CNT) growth** (Sumio Iijima). **1990** – Adapted for **graphene and nanowire fabrication**. **Present** – Core technique for 1D and 2D nanostructures.
Sol-Gel Method	**1968** – First studies on **silica gel nanoparticles**. **1970** – Applied for metal oxide nanoparticle synthesis. **1990** – Adapted for hybrid organic-inorganic nanomaterials. **Present** – Used in coatings, catalysts, and biomedical fields.
Chemical Reduction Method	**1900** – Used in colloidal gold synthesis (Faraday). **1950** – Applied for metal nanoparticle synthesis. **1980** – **Turkevich method** for citrate-reduced gold nanoparticles. **Present** – A widely used wet-chemical NP synthesis method.
Hydrothermal Method	**1960** – Developed for controlled nanoparticle synthesis under high pressure. **1980** – Used for oxide nanoparticles and zeolites. **2000** – Applied in **green chemistry** for eco-friendly synthesis. **Present** – Used for high-crystalline nanoparticles and quantum dots.
Solvothermal Method	**1980** – First introduced for organic solvent-assisted nanoparticle synthesis. **1990** – Used for oxide and sulfide nanoparticle growth. **Present** – Extensively used for controlled morphology in nanomaterials.
Spray Pyrolysis	**1960** – Developed for thin film deposition and ceramics. **1980** – Used in catalyst and energy storage applications. **2000** – Adapted for drug delivery systems. **Present** – Applied in coatings, electronics, and environmental catalysis.

continued on following page

Table 1. Continued

Name of Synthesis Techniques	Historical Evolution of Nanoparticle Synthesis Techniques
Laser Pyrolysis	**1990** – Developed for rapid synthesis of oxide and carbide nanoparticles. **2000** – Applied for high-purity nanoparticle production. **Present** – Used in **nanoceramics, nanocomposites,** and fuel research.
Flame Pyrolysis	**1940** – First used for **industrial-scale silica production**. **1980** – Applied to metal oxides and advanced ceramics. **2000** – Optimized for **large-scale nanoparticle synthesis**. **Present**– Key method in pharmaceuticals, pigments, and catalysts.
Spinning	**1934** – **Electrospinning** concept first patented. **1990 –** Applied to nanofiber and nanoparticle synthesis. **2000**– Advanced for biomedical, filtration, and textile applications. **Present** – Used in **biopolymers, energy storage**, and advanced textiles.

2.1. Top-Down Method

The bulk substance is broken down into little, nanoscale particles. The process of synthesizing nanoparticles begins with reducing the size of the starting substance with the help of various physical as well as chemical processes, (Abid et al., 2022). Despite being an easy and convenient technique for nanoparticle synthesis, this approach is not considered an appropriate method for preparing extremely tiny and irregularly shaped particles. The modification of nanoparticles' surface chemistry and physicochemical characteristics continues to be the fundamental obstacle to this approach, (Nadagouda, Speth, & Varma, 2011).

2.1.1. Mechanical Milling

It is one of the first methods implemented before the 2000s and is considered the most immensely used technique to produce different kinds of nanoparticles. In the case of large-scale production, mechanical millings are referred to as economical processes. In the mechanical milling process, several components are ground in an inert atmosphere to mill and post-anneal nanoparticles, (Ealia & Saravanakumar, 2017). A variety of ball milling techniques are often employed for the synthesis of nanomaterials where involved balls make the powder charge. The balls either fall freely and thrash the balls and powder underneath them or roll down. For the synthesis of nanomaterials, several ball milling techniques are often employed, in which balls strike the powder charge. The balls either fall freely and thrash the balls and powder underneath them, or they roll down the chamber's surface in a succession of parallel layers, (Yadav, Yadav, & Singh, 2012). ZnO NPs are produced in a steel cell by milling the ZnO powder with the help of hardened steel balls, (Salah et al.,

2011). The requirement of high energy and long duration of milling are the disadvantages of this process. Another process known as the mechanochemical synthesis process is the mixture of reactants' repetitive deformation, welding, and fracture. The initial components (e.g., sodium carbonate and chloride hexahydrate used in Fe_3O_2 nanoparticles synthesis) are ground using the mechanochemical synthesis method and mixed stoichiometrically. Reactions requiring high temperatures will occur at low temperatures without needing external heat application due to several chemical reactions that take place between surface interface between the reagent and substrate, (Chauhan, 2024). The main drawbacks of this approach are the extreme sensitivity of the produced nanoparticles to grinding circumstances and the possibility of undesired contamination owing to milling media and environment. $CuAlS_2$ nanoparticles have been synthesized by using Cu, Al, and S powder, (Shojaei, Shokuhfar, & Zolriasatein, 2021). Copper Oxide nanoparticles have been synthesised by this technique and reported with antibacterial activity against *Vibrio eltor*, *Bacillus subtilis*, *Staphylococcus aureus*, *Candida tropicalis*, and *Saccharomycetes cerevisiae*. Variable sizes and surface defects limit their effectiveness, (Amal *et al.,* 2019).

2.1.2. Laser Ablation

Laser Ablation Synthesis in Solution (LASiS) is a known nanoparticle synthesis method where NPs are produced from several solvents. A laser beam irradiates metal immersed in a liquid solution, causing it to condense a plasma plume that triggers the formation of nanoparticles. No stabilizing agent or chemicals are required here as it can provide continuous production of nanoparticles in organic solvents, (Dell'Aglio et al., 2024). Gold nanoparticles are one of the nanoparticles that could be synthesized under helium gas at the pressure of 3 to 90 kPa by the laser ablation method, (Kvítek et al., 2014). The period of time and energy of the laser pulse determine the overall number of particles and ablated atoms produced. When a large concentration of nanoparticles is generated in the colloidal solution by prolonged laser ablation, the laser's path is obstructed, absorbing laser energy into the already-formed nanoparticles rather than the target surface, (Ghorbani, 2014). According to the study, silver nanoparticles synthesized by laser liquid ablation have been conjugated with hydroxychloroquine, which could demonstrate various antimicrobial applications in biofilm disruption and wound healing effectively, (Mwenze et al., 2023). Mohammed et al. produced some nanoparticles that exhibit potential antibacterial activity against Sphingomonas paucimobilis, Serratia plymuthica, and Staphylococcus hyicus, isolated from people with dental caries, (Mohammed et al., 2022).

2.1.3. Ion Sputtering

A chemical is vaporized by sputtering an inert gas ion beam by using this method. It involves ejecting particles off a surface by colliding with ions, which results in the deposition of nanoparticles on that surface, (Shah & Gavrin, 2006). It includes annealing after a thin layer of nanoparticles is deposited. The nanoparticles' size and shape are affected by many things, such as the material type, temperature, annealing time, and the thickness of the layer. The process is executed in an evacuated vacuum chamber at very low pressure. The surface morphology, composition, texture, and optical properties of nanocrystalline metal oxide coatings can be affected by natural sputtering gases as He, Ne, Ar, Kr, and Xe. Silver nanoparticles can also be produced in this way using argon as the sputtering gas, (Asanithi, Chaiyakun, & Limsuwan, 2012). Au-Ag bimetallic nanostructures with sucrose sensing abilities have been formed based on former research, (Devi et al., 2024).

2.1.4. Thermal Decomposition

This endothermic chemical breakdown process involves heat where heat breaks the compound's chemical bonds. At particular temperatures, the metal's breakdown produces nanoparticles through a chemical reaction that also produces secondary compounds, (Görke et al., 2024).

The thermal decomposition method for synthesizing magnetic nanoparticles involves heating precursors in a non-aqueous environment, leading to well-defined products. In the case of ZnO nanoparticles, varying the decomposition temperature from 400°C to 700°C alters the morphology and structural properties, which is crucial for applications like photocatalysis, (Gritsenko, 2023). Co3O4 nanoparticles have been synthesized by thermal decomposition and revealed as a potent antibacterial agent, (Kavitha et al., 2017).

2.2. Bottom-Up Method

The bottom-up techniques of NPs synthesis rely on combining atoms, molecules, or tiny particles to produce nanoparticles from smaller molecules. It produces the final nanoparticle by first forming nanostructured building components, which are subsequently assembled, (Abid *et al.*, 2022).

2.2.1. Solid State Methods

The solid-state synthesis of metal NPs is a flexible, versatile, and efficient nanoparticle synthesis technique that can produce metal nanoparticles of regulated size and form, less agglomeration, and increased stability. This synthesis method is very helpful for producing nanoparticles with special qualities, such as UV-plasmonic responses, which are beneficial for several uses, such as photocatalysis and bioimaging, (Darwish et al., 2022). Karen L. Rincón-Granados et al. (2021) constructed NiO and NiFe2O4 nanoparticles which are found to be effective against *Pseudomonas aeruginosa* (ATCC 43,636) and *Staphylococcus aureus* (ATCC 23,235).

2.2.1.1. Physical Vapor Deposition (PVD) Method

PVD is a bottom-up approach that provides high-quality thin films and nanoparticles with controlled morphology and stability. Thermal evaporation and sputtered deposition techniques, considered as highly controlled vacuum techniques, are involved in the vaporization of solid material which then condenses on substrate resulting in the formation of thin films or nanoparticles. It can be regulated to stop particles from growing larger than desired as demonstrated by the production of nano-sized metal particles on substrates such as Al_2O_3 powder, (Koh et al., 2016). A type of PVD is frequently used to create a thin layer of lanthanum strontium cobalt by using laser ablation on a solid target to create a plasma of ablated species. These ablated species are placed on a substrate to make a film. The main drawback of this approach is the high cost of materials with very little production volume, (Jamkhande et al., 2019). Rodianah Alias et al. (2020) designed a silver–tantalum-oxide-based nanostructure that showed a prominent zone of inhibition against *S. aureus* and *E. coli*.

2.2.1.2. Chemical Vapour Deposition (CVD) Method

In this method, a thin coating of gaseous reactants is applied to the substrate, where substrate temperature acts as the influencing factor. During the chemical reaction, a heated substrate comes in touch with the combined gas, which contributes to the formation of a thin layer of product on the surface of substrate that is recovered and utilized further. The target material acts as a precursor and appears like a volatile molecule, (Pedersen & Elliot, 2014). The precursor fragment and substrate surface then undergo a series of chemical reactions to form a thin layer. This method usually uses a surface chemical reaction to create atomic layer deposition (ALD) thin films, (Miikkulainen et al., 2013). Since it can work at very minimal temperatures, it is suitable for the production of graphene nanostructures and nanotubes as well as large-scale industrial synthesis, (Bhuyan et al., 2016). The carbon nanofibers are synthesized by CVD. The disadvantages of this technique are the production of toxic gaseous by-products, chemical hazards due to corrosive and explosive precursor gases, and the need for special equipment. The deposition of multicomponent materials is challenging, (H.R.I.H. et al., 2007). Ponja et al. (2015) stated deposition of silver thin film on fluorine-doped tin-oxide (FTO) glass, regular glass coated with a SiO_2 barrier, Activ glass, and TiO_2 coated glass could potentially results in higher *E. coli* and *Staphylococcus aureus* inhibiting properties. *S. aureus* was eliminated by FTO/Ag in 15 minutes, while *E. coli* was totally eradicated in 60 minutes. 66.6% and 99.9% of S. aureus were destroyed by Activ/Ag and TiO_2/Ag respectively in 60 minutes.

2.2.2. Liquid State Synthesis Methods

2.2.2.1. Sol-Gel

This process is one of the most preferred and frequently used bottom-up nanoparticles synthesizing methods where the sol, a colloidal solution of particles floating in a liquid phase, and the gel, a solid macromolecule submerged in a solvent, are used. In this wet-chemical process, a chemical solution serves as a precursor for an integrated system of distinct particles, (Ramesh, 2013). The precursor is then sonicated, shaken, or stirred to spread it throughout the host liquid. The resulting system has a liquid phase, a solid phase, and a phase separation that aids in the recovery of the nanoparticles by a variety of techniques, including filtration, centrifugation, and sedimentation. The drying process also eliminates moisture, (Mahmoudi et al., 2024). Perveen et al. (2020) synthesised ZnO nanoparticles having antimicrobial activity against *Bacillus subtilis*, *Salmonella typhimurium*, *Staphylococcus aureus*.

2.2.2.2. Chemical Reduction Method

The synthesis of nanoparticles takes place by the reduction of ionic salt in a specific medium with the help of surfactant in the presence of several reducing agents like ethylene glycol, glucose, citrate of sodium, sodium borohydride, hydrazine hydrate, ethanol, etc. Stabilizing agent as well as reducing agents is used in many cases. There are numerous drawbacks, including toxicity, high expenses, inadequate reduction ability, and impurities, (Zhang et al., 2010). Gudikandula and Maringanti (2016) compared two kinds of silver nanoparticles synthesized by chemical reduction methods with the help of a chemical solution and biogenic methods through nitrate, demonstrating their comparative inhibiting activity of *S. aureus* and *E.coli*.

2.2.2.3. *Hydrothermal Method*

Small particles are deposited via the hydrothermal process, which is based on the interaction of solid solids at high temperatures and pressures with vapors from aqueous solutions. The high temperatures and pressures involved enhance the dehydration and kinetics of the process, leading to the formation of nanoparticles with desired properties. This has led to the development of semiconducting nanoparticles and nanostructured arrays, (Tripathi, 2021). Cations are precipitated as polymeric hydroxides that accelerate the production of the metal oxide crystal structure by dehydrating the material. The difficulty of controlling the process and the limitation of reliability and reproducibility are considered the biggest challenges for this technique, (Modabberasl et al., 2024). AgNPs synthesized through this process reported in Zhang et al. (2019), possesses excellent bactericidal activity. CuNPs with bacterial cellulose produced through this method demonstrated higher antimicrobial efficacy against *Salmonella, E. coli,* and *S. aureus*, suggesting its use in bactericidal films, (Araújo et al., 2018). The hydrothermal method-produced TiO2 nanoparticles have been reported to form significant zones of inhibition against *K. aerogenes, E. coli, P. desmolyticum* (Gram-ve), and *S. aureus* (Gram+ve), (Huang et al., 2022).

2.2.2.4. *Solvothermal Method*

This process involves heating the solvents (water and alcohol) over their boiling temperatures in a pressure vessel. This approach is applied to the creation of nanophases when water and solvents such as methanol, ethanol, and polyol are present, (Majerič, Friedrich, & Rudolf, 2015). The solvothermal method obtained ZnO nanoparticles demonstrated antimicrobial properties, highlighting scopes of being used in biomedical fields, (Wang & Gao, 2019).

2.2.3. Gas-Phase Methods

Pyrolysis is one of the most used gas-phase methods that is commonly implemented in industrial processes for large-scale production of nanoparticles. In this case, flame is used to burn a liquid or vapor precursor. The precursor must enter the furnace at high pressure through a small orifice in order to burn. Some contemporary furnaces generate high temperatures that promote evaporation by using lasers and plasma instead of flames. Despite being a straightforward, efficient, economical, and continuous process with an enhanced yield, it releases a number of hazardous gasses as a byproduct, (Ealia & Saravanakumar, 2017) (yadav, Yadav, & Singh, 2012).

2.2.3.1. Spray Pyrolysis

When tiny droplets start to form inside the heated reactor, a nebulizer is used to introduce the precursors of the nanoparticles into the reactor in vapor form. Spray pyrolysis is composed of three setups i.e. a) a fluid nebulizer, b) a thermostatic; temperature ranging from 200 °C to 1200 °C in a controlled reactor which is vertically tubular c) a nanoparticle collecting precipitator. An improved method called ultrasonic spray pyrolysis produces atomized droplets from precursor solution with the help of ultrasound, (Rashdan *et al.,* 2013).

2.2.3.2. Laser Pyrolysis (LP)

LP is the interaction of a sensitizer, a gaseous reactant species, and laser photons. This technique utilizes laser energy mostly from infrared CO_2 laser for the nanoparticle synthesis, (Prabakaran & Rajan, 2021). The nucleation reaction is initiated after the absorption of laser energy by the precursor. The powerful laser beam is one of the main disadvantages of laser pyrolysis. This results in a small portion of the polymer sample having local temperatures above 10,000 °C. At those temperatures, atoms, electrons, ions, and radicals are produced as plasma, (Tai et al., 2007).

2.2.3.3. Flame Pyrolysis

Liquid precursor is sprayed into the flame to form nanostructures. Precursors with vapor pressures that are not high enough can be delivered using this method. Other than liquid, gas is also used for spraying into flame for the production of nanoparticles, (Iravani et al., 2014). Scaling up the process and managing safety concerns can be expensive and challenging.

2.2.4. Spinning

Nanoparticles are produced by spinning in a spinning disc reactor. It consists of a rotating disk that may control physical parameters like temperature inside a reactor or chamber. For removing oxygen and stop chemical reactions, nitrogen or other inert gases are usually fed into the reactor, (Al-Badaii et al., 2024). The atoms or molecules fuse as a result of the spinning, causing precipitation, product accumulation, and finally drying. The properties of the SDR-made nanoparticles are influenced by several variables, such as feed position, disc surface, liquid/precursor ratio, liquid flow rate, and disc rotation speed, among other operating parameters, (Dheyab et al., 2023).

Figure 2. Nanoparticle synthesis procedures with top-down and bottom-up methods

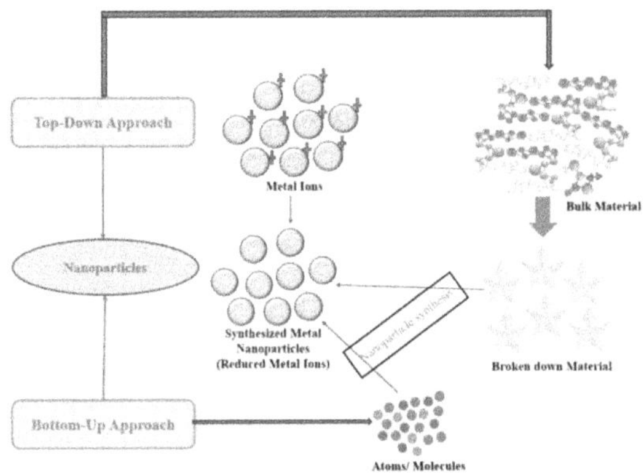

Table 2. Overview of different types of metal nanoparticle synthesis processes along with their advantages and disadvantages

Name of synthesis technique	Types	Advantages	Disadvantages
Mechanical milling	Ball milling	a) Standardised for Large scale production. b) Cost-effective. c) No temperature and pressure should be controlled. d) Solid and liquid raw materials could be used.	a) Required high energy b) Possibility of contamination c) Long time duration
	Mechanochemical synthesis	a) Simple b) Efficient	a) The produced nanoparticles are extremely sensitive to grinding circumstances. b) The possibility of undesired contamination owing to milling media and environment.
Laser ablation	--	a) Comparatively Simple and efficient	a) Nanoparticles formed in colloidal solution blocks further laser path inhibiting the production rate. b) It prevents the absorption of laser energy as well. c) High energy consumption and low yield.

continued on following page

Table 2. Continued

Name of synthesis technique	Types	Advantages	Disadvantages
Ion Sputtering	--	a) Comparatively economical b) Easy and versatile technique	a) Surface morphology, composition, texture, and the optical properties of the nanostructured films could be impacted by noble gases.
Thermal Decomposition	--	a) Versatile b) Easy to handle	a) Difficult to adjust particle size
Solid state methods	Physical Vapor Deposition (PVD) method	a) Simple method	a) Expensive b) A low volume of material is produced.
	Chemical Vapour Deposition (CVD) method	a) Characteristics such as surface morphology and crystal structure could be under control. b) This type of coating provides higher durability.	a) Toxic b) Chemical hazards c) Use of corrosive and explosive gas
Liquid state synthesis methods	Sol-gel	a) Simple method b) Particle size and morphology could be controlled.	a) Reliability b) Reproducibility
	Chemical reduction method	a) Easy and convenient method	a) Expensive b) Toxic c) Low reducing power d) Presence of impurities
	Hydrothermal method	a) Size and morphology could be controlled. b) High crystalline nanocrystals could be produced.	a) Factors are difficult to be controlled. b) Not reliable process c) Hard to reproduce the same results.
	Solvothermal method	a) Nanocrystals could be produced with high crystallinity. b) Rapid synthesis technique	a) Long time duration of process b) Inhomogeneity of the heating.

continued on following page

Table 2. Continued

Name of synthesis technique	Types	Advantages	Disadvantages
Gas-phase methods	Spray pyrolysis	a) Simple b) Reproducible	a) High-temperature use b) Environmental hazards
	Laser pyrolysis	a) Forms Nanoparticles with uniform and controllable size distribution.	a) Use of intense laser beam b) Use of high-temperature
	Flame pyrolysis	a) Most effective b) Use of liquid precursor is advantageous to dissolve less volatile raw materials	a) Pure coating quality
	Spinning	a) Efficient	a) Complicated technique b) Several factors should be under control
Green Synthesis	By Bacteria	a) Abundant in nature b) Can adapt to different environmental conditions	a) Growth optimization
	By Fungi	a) Scalable downstream process b) Economical c) Efficient due to the activity of mycelia	a) Different sizes of nanoparticles are produced. b) Safety issues due to overgrowth.
	By Algae	a) Versatile b) Sustainable c) Environment friendly d) Biocompatible e) Cost-effective	a) Different sizes of nanoparticles produced.
	By Plant and Plant Products	a) Scalable b) Safe c) No pathogenicity d) Homogeneous nanoparticle production e) Renewable	a) Sometimes costly due to sample availability
	By Polymer	a) Biocompatible b) Biodegradable, c) Non-immunogenicity, d) Non-toxic e) High tensile strength f) Low antigenicity	a) Nanoparticles produced are hydrophobic, but proteins, peptides, and nucleic acids are hydrophilic.

3. GREEN SYNTHESIS METHOD (GS)

The synthesis of nanoparticle processes with the help of natural resources such as microorganisms, their enzymes, and plant products is gaining attention worldwide because they are ecologically safe, abundant in nature, and possess the potential to overcome issues including reaction conditions and high expenses. The requirement for high pressure, temperature, energy, aseptic handling, and toxic substances could be opted out of in biosynthesis methods. Bioreduction and biosorption are the two kinds of biological synthesis methods.

Figure 3. Overview of Intracellular and Extracellular green synthesis of nanoparticles

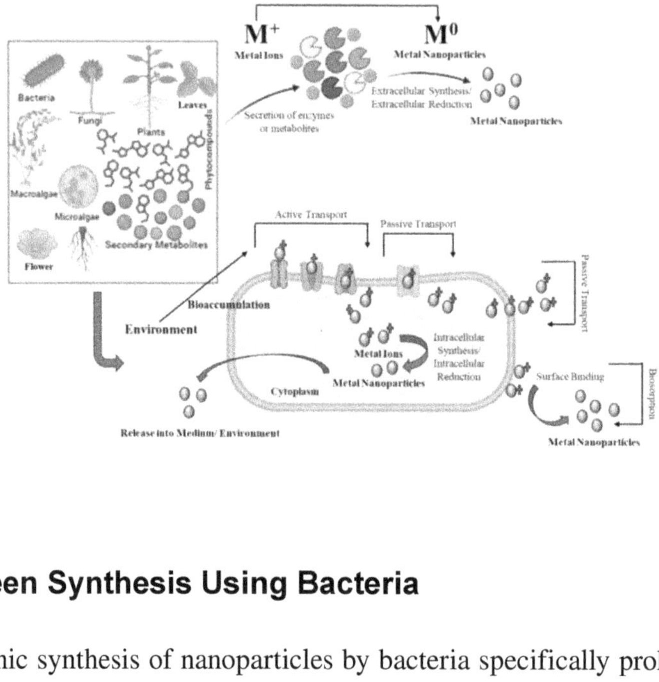

3.1. Green Synthesis Using Bacteria

Biogenic synthesis of nanoparticles by bacteria specifically prokaryotes is increasingly drawing attention as bacteria can adapt to extreme conditions and grow rapidly and easily. Various sizes and shapes of nanoparticles could be formed, and this approach could be industrially scalable due to convenient controlling factors such as temperature, pressure, pH, oxygenation, and incubation time. Psychrophilic bacteria such as *Pseudomonas meridiana, Pseudomonas antarctica, Arthrobacter gangotriensis, Bacillus indicus,* and *Bacillus cecembensis* have been reported to be able to synthesize AgNPs, (Andrade et al., 2024).

3.2. Green Synthesis Using Fungi

Metal nanoparticles are synthesized in the presence of enzymes and proteins secreted by fungi. Various fungi including *Fusarium oxysporum, Aspergillus fumigates*, and *Trichoderma reesei* produce enzymes as reducing agents, (Kaabo et al., 2024). The silver nanoparticles synthesized from endophytic fungi like *Phyllosticta capitalensis* and *Annona muricata* have been reported with significant therapeutic potential including antibacterial, anti-inflammatory, antidiabetic, and antioxidant activities, (Acay *et al.,* 2024). *Penicillium oxalicum* has been employed to produce silica nanoparticles, that exhibit excellent photocatalytic activity and heavy metal bioremediation capabilities effectively degrading dyes and removing heavy metals from the environment, (Rakamanikkam *et al.,* 2024) (Govindaraju et al., 2009). One study discusses the green synthesis of a novel nanomaterial, Pleurotus eryngii-Lecithin-Chitosan Nanomaterial (PEELCN), derived from the extract of the fungus *Pleurotus eryngii,* (Govindaraju et al., 2009).

3.3. Green Synthesis Using Algae

The extract of algae works as a reducing agent in the conversion of metal salt into metal nanoparticles. This extract is further used for various metal nanoparticle synthesis viz., gold, silver, iron, copper, and zinc are synthesized. Algae are most favoured for green synthesis due to their easy and rapid growth. Several types of algae such as red algae, brown algae, green algae, and blue-green algae are utilized. Several brown algae like *Turbinaria conoides*, *Cystophora moniliformis, Padina pavonica*, and *Sargassum sp.* are used in silver nanoparticle synthesis. Raja Rajamanikkam et al emphasised the copper nanoparticles synthesized from brown algae *Turbinaria* sp, (Singaravelu et al., 2007). It has been found that *Sargassum myriocystum, Sargassum wightii, Fucus vesiculosus,* and *Dictyota bartayresianna* are capable of green synthesis of AuNPs. AuNPs and AgNPs are synthesised by marine algae, *Sargassum wightii,* (Sharma et al., 2014) (Bishovi, Sahoo, & Padhy, 2023). The use of red algae named *Lemanea fluviatilis* for gold nanoparticles, (Nawak *et al.,* 2021). Blue-green algae including *Oscillatoria willei*, and *Cylindrospermum stagnale* for silver nanoparticles, (Jalali, Ghanavati, & Osfouri, 2024). *Chlamydomonas reinhardtii* for cadmium sulfide nanoparticles, green algae like *Pithophora oedogonia*, *Chlorella vulgaris*, and *Enteromorpha flexuosa* for gold nanoparticles have been recorded in previous studies, (Singh et al., 2016). Green algae like *Spirogyra hyalina* and marine brown algae *Cystoseira* are utilized for synthesizing ZnO nanoparticles. The bioactive molecules in the algae extract aid in the bio reduction and capping of nanoparticles and are characterized by their crystalline structure and antibacterial efficacy, (Awwad & Salem, 2012).

3.4. Green Synthesis by Plant and Plant Products

Plant and phytocompounds play a crucial role in nanoparticle synthesis. This approach uses several plant parts such as leaves, flowers, roots, stems, seeds, fruits, and fruit waste. Compounds such as phenolic acid, flavonoids, alkaloids, and terpenoids are abundant in the plant extracts. The environmentally benign production of nanoparticles results from the reduction of metal ions brought on by plant metabolites, (Rama et al., 2023). These nanoparticles could be employed in medical imaging, bioremediating heavy metals, wastes, and plastics, drug discovery, and delivery. The method could be applied in industries in bulk production because of convenient handling, availability, and safe by-products. Leaves of various plants such as *Aegle marmelos*, *Vernonia amygdalina*, Mulberry plant, *Cinnamomum tamala*, *Oxalis griffithii*, and radish seeds are used in studies for metal nanoparticle synthesis, (Shende et al., 2015) (Jadoun et al., 2021). Fruit juice of *Citrus medica,* (Das & Kingsley, 2023*)*, waste residues produced from bilberry juices and pineapple leaves have also been reported in green synthesis, (Hazarika & Borah, 2024). Vishnu et.al synthesized AgNPs nanotubes of size 79 nm from *Asparagus racemosus* that exhibit antibacterial activity against *Staphylococcus aureus* and *Salmonella typhimurium.* The study explains the efficacy of nanotubes in antibacterial activity due to their unique shape for penetrating the cell wall and cell membrane, (Vardar, Mehmetoğlu, & Yıldırım, 2024).

3.5. Green Synthesis Using Biopolymers

Biogenic nanoparticle synthesis by using biopolymers is a potential area of research due to the biodegradability, biocompatibility, and lower immunogenicity of biopolymers. These characteristics make those appropriate for their uses in magnetic hyperthermia, drug delivery, and other biomedical domains, (Banik & Kaur, 2024). Various methods and materials such as Ionic Gelation Method, Aqueous Solution Synthesis, and Sonochemical Assisted Method are employed to optimize the synthesis and functionality of biopolymer-based nanoparticles, (Atabaki, 2024). These properties allow for controlled release and targeted delivery of therapeutic agents, (Rhim, Wang, & Hong, 2013). Biopolymer nanoparticles synthesized through green methods are used in environmental treatment and smart packaging while reducing environmental impact, (Jafarzadeh et al., 2023). Spraying antimicrobial chemicals on the food surface helps prevent food contamination or spoiling, which is one of the deadliest problems in the world. Packaging materials generated from synthetic plastic leads to abrupt disposal and accumulation of plastic polymers because of their weak sustainability and degradability resulting in serious and emerging environmental problems. The biopolymer has several qualities such as environmental-friendliness, biodegradability, biocompatibility, and even edibility. It has outstanding mechanical and physical qualities that may serve as a barrier to lipids, carbon dioxide, oxygen, and scent. They can even be applied as suitable carrier systems for a variety of active ingredients such as antibacterial, antioxidant, antifungal, and coloring properties, (Kadam et al., 2019). Proteins like gelatin, gluten, casein, whey protein, soy, lipids like beeswax, and polysaccharides like agar, chitosan, carrageenan, pectin, alginate, cellulose, starch, and its derivatives are examples of biopolymers that are vividly used in the food industry to create eco-friendly and biodegradable packaging films, (El-Sherbiny & Sedki, 2019).

Table 3. Various kinds of metal nanoparticles with biomedical applications

Type of Metal Nanoparticles	Source of nanoparticles	Characteristics	Applications
Gold Nanoparticles (AuNP)	i. Gold(III) chloride	a) It shows strong absorption. b) High biocompatibility and stability.	a) Diagnostics tests b) Targeted drug delivery c) Imaging d) Therapeutic applications
Silver Nanoparticles (AgNP)	i. Silver Nitrate ($AgNO_3$)	a) Shows optical properties like gold b) Shows strong antimicrobial properties due to the release of silver ions, that have the potential to disrupt microbial cell walls and DNA.	a) Antimicrobial coatings, b) Wound dressings c) Water purification d) Electronics.
Copper Nanoparticles (CuNP)	i. Copper Sulphate ($CuSO_4$) ii. Copper chloride ($CuCl_2.2H_2O$) iii. Copper nitrate ($Cu(NO_3)_2$)	a) Possesses antimicrobial activities b) Shows electrical conductivity.	a) Catalyst b) Antimicrobial coatings c) Electronics d) Conductive materials.
Iron Nanoparticles (FeNP)	i. Ferrous sulfate ($FeSO_4$) ii. Ferrous chloride ($FeCl_2$) iii. Ferric Chloride ($FeCl_3$)	a) Exhibits superparamagnetic properties b) Environmentally safe	a) Magnetic resonance imaging (MRI) contrast agents, b) Targeted drug delivery c) Magnetic separation d) Bioremediation
Platinum Nanoparticles (PtNP)	i. Platinum (II) acetate ($Pt(CH_3COO)_2$) ii. Platinum (IV) chloride ($PtCl_4$) iii. Platinum (II) chloride ($PtCl_2$)	a) Catalytic properties like hydrogenation and oxidation b) Highly stable c) Resistant to poisoning	a) Catalysts b) Electrocatalysts c) Fuel cells

continued on following page

Table 3. Continued

Type of Metal Nanoparticles	Source of nanoparticles	Characteristics	Applications
Cobalt Nanoparticles (CoNP)	i. cobalt nitrate ii. cobalt sulfate iii. cobalt acetate	a) Magnetic properties b) Catalytic activity	a) Magnetic materials b) Catalysis reaction c) Storage technologies
Nickel Nanoparticles (NiNP)	i. Nickel (II) Chloride (NiCl2) ii. Nickel (II) Sulfate (NiSO4) iii. Nickel (II) Nitrate (Ni(NO3)2) iv. Nickel Acetate (Ni(CH3COO)2)	a) Magnetic properties b) Used in hydrogenation	a) Magnetic materials b) Catalysis reaction c) Energy Storage technologies
Tungsten Nanoparticles (WNP)	i. Tungsten (VI) Chloride (WCl6) ii. Tungsten (IV) Chloride (WCl4) iii. Tungsten (VI) Sulfide (WS3)	a) High melting point b) Density c) Strength d) Highly stable and durable	a) Used in electronics b) Radiation shielding
Palladium Nanoparticles (PdNP)	i. Palladium (II) Chloride (PdCl2) ii. Palladium (II) Nitrate (Pd(NO3)2) iii. Palladium (II) Acetate (Pd(CH3COO)2) iv. Palladium (II) Sulfate (PdSO4) v. Palladium (II) Carbonate (PdCO3)	a) Catalysts in carbon-carbon coupling reactions b) Can interact with gases	a) Sensors b) Hydrogen storage
Rhodium Nanoparticles (RhNP)	i. Rhodium (III) Chloride (RhCl3) ii. Rhodium (III) Nitrate (Rh(NO3)3) iii. Rhodium (III) Acetate (Rh(CH3COO)3) iv. Rhodium (III) Sulfate (Rh2(SO4)3)	a) Resistant to temperature b) Resistant to corrosion	a) Catalysis b) Chemical manufacturing
Ruthenium Nanoparticles (RuNP)	i. Ruthenium(III) chloride (RuCl3) ii. Ruthenium(III) acetate (Ru(CO2CH3)3)	a) Catalytic activity b) Hydrogenation and oxidation	a) Sensors b) Fuel cells c) Catalysis reactions
Silver Gold Alloy Nanoparticles (Ag-Au NP)	Salts of Gold and Silver	a) Combination of silver and gold b) Electronic properties	a) Sensors b) Imaging c) Therapeutic approaches

4.1. Advantages of the Green Synthesis Method

Green synthesis techniques for metal nanoparticles are shown to be less costly, safe, biocompatible, scalable, reproducible, and relatively toxic-free. They also do not require the use of hazardous chemicals and have a little detrimental impact on the environment and biological systems, (Medarametla *et al.,* 2024). Therefore, it can be regarded as an environmentally beneficial approach in which physical and chemical approaches have an impact on ecological systems. It represents environmental sustainability, and functional diversity as well. Conventional methods include requirements of toxic and harmful substances posing health risks and environmental hazards. The green synthesis of nanoparticles utilizes inexpensive and abundant natural materials and involves mild conditions like room temperature and atmospheric pressure. The production cost is reduced due to the low cost of materials and reasonable conditioning factors. The formation of safe end products minimizes the potential damage risks to human health. These attributes are crucial for applications such as drug delivery, imaging, and diagnostics. Several kinds of disadvantages such as the difficulties of scaling up and conserving cell cultures, are faced while synthesizing nanoparticles in collaboration with the use of microorganisms, (Hamilton & Kingston, 2024). Nanoparticles could be produced with the help of plant compounds and biopolymers that have the potential to mitigate the scaling-up issue. Researchers as well as companies may advance the science of nanotechnology and contribute to the development of sustainable and environmentally friendly technologies by adopting green synthesis processes.

Figure 4. FESEM results indicating the presence of nanotubes synthesized from Asparagus racemosus

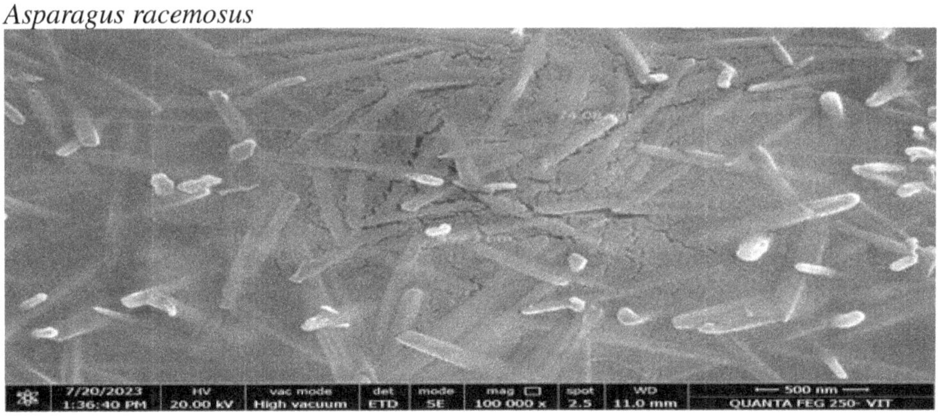

4.2. Role of Computational Modelling and Artificial Intelligence (AI) in NP Design

Computational modeling and artificial intelligence (AI) have transformed the design optimization of nanoparticles, reducing the need for expensive and time-consuming experimental trials by allowing researchers to forecast the characteristics and behaviour of nanoparticles, (Pater et al., 2010). In order to optimize the selection of the optimal nanoparticle carrier, computational methods can be employed to assist the design of nanomedicine formulations, evaluate interactions between nanoparticles and biological systems with potential toxicity, and generate models using high-throughput screening methods, (Singh et al., 2020). Understanding the physicochemical characteristics of metal nanoparticles has been made possible by computational methods such as density functional theory (DFT), finite element modeling (FEM), and molecular dynamics (MD) simulations. The rational construction of more potent antimicrobial medicines is aided by MD simulations, which anticipate NP stability, shape, and size-dependent interactions with bacterial membranes, (Tian, Liu, & Chen, 2021). DFT simulations offer valuable information about their electronic structure and reactivity in order to maximize metal nanoparticles' antibacterial activity while reducing their toxicity. Additionally, by helping to comprehend how NPs disperse and aggregate in various biological settings, computational fluid dynamics (CFD) models guarantee improved control over their behaviour in therapeutic applications. Computational modelling and machine learning highly contribute to the screening of large datasets on compounds by physiologically based pharmacokinetic (PBPK) modeling and absorption, distribution, metabolism, and excretion (ADME)-based in silico methods, (Mohammadjani et al., 2023). According to the study, silica nanoparticles have been designed and docked against bacterial cell wall synthesis (β-lactamase) and fatty acid biosynthesis (FabI and FabH), indicating adherence to the surface of E. coli and S. aureus by hydrogen bonds formation with amino acid residue, (Karthik et al., 2021). Mohammadjani et al. performed a comparative study on metal oxide nanoparticle docking against antibacterial targets and reported MgO and Fe_2O_3 NPs as better than standard drugs, (Serov & Vinogradov, 2022). Karthik et al. (2021) constructed chitosan silver nanoparticle decorated with benzodioxane-coupled piperazine as an effective antibacterial and anti-biofilm agent against methicillin-resistant Staphylococcus aureus (MRSA) validated by molecular docking approach. Machine learning (ML) and artificial intelligence (AI) have become effective techniques for speeding up NP design. Large datasets can be analyzed by ML algorithms to determine the best NP compositions, forecast their antibacterial effectiveness, and evaluate any possible cytotoxic consequences, (Fu & Chen, 2025). Researchers are able to develop prediction frameworks that simplify NP synthesis and formulation by training AI models on theoretical and experimental data. This eliminates the need for a great deal of trial-and-error experimentation. In an attempt to quickly identify NP candidates with exceptional antibacterial qualities, deep learning methods have been used to assess high-throughput screening findings. Through the prediction of structure-function correlations and the recommendation of creative design approaches, AI generative models also aid in the discovery of unique NP formulations. Le et. al. (2016) exhibited the generation of different models of ZnO nanoparticle synthesis, making it feasible for commercial availability and safety to humans and the environment. Translating lab-developed NPs into real-world applications involves integrating computational modeling and artificial intelligence with experimental and clinical studies. Though interpretability is a vital factor in this case, AI-assisted optimization of NP synthesis ensures reproducibility and scalability, enhanced antimicrobial efficacy, stability, and biocompatibility, paving the way for their clinical and commercial deployment in combating antibiotic-resistant infections and addressing key challenges in industrial and pharmaceutical production, (Mohammadjani et al., 2023). Furthermore, safety evaluations are improved by computational toxicity prediction models, which reduce possible future hazards prior to in vivo and clinical studies, (Fernández et al., 2021).

Table 4. Detailed comparision of traditional approach and computer modelling and AI-based nanoresearch

Aspect	Traditional Approach	Computational Modelling	Artificial Intelligence (AI)
Nanoparticle Formulation	It includes conventional physical and chemical synthesis methods such as milling, sol gel, etc.	• It enhances understanding of drug self-assembly, molecular interactions, and biological functions. • Quantum and molecular dynamics methods predict structure, binding energies, and surface interactions. • Mechanic pharmacokinetic/ pharmacodynamic (PK/PD) and physiologically based pharmacokinetic models (PBPK) assist to monitor nanoparticle distribution and elimination in biological systems.	• It helps in the optimization of manufacturing NPs. • Accelerates the processes such as selection of materials, optimization process, accessing real-time monitoring, forecasting properties of NPs.
Drug Delivery	Traditional drug delivery techniques have some drawbacks, such as poor targeting, poor drug release kinetics, and potential toxicity. These challenges are addressed by nanoparticles, which provide controlled drug release, improved targeting, and fewer side effects.	• Understanding drug self-assembly, molecular interactions, and the biological function of nanoparticles is improved by computational modeling. • From excipient screening to drug-excipient combination optimization, it is essential at every stage of formulation. • This simplifies and speeds up the creation of nanoparticles.	• By enabling precision targeting using patient-specific data and improving treatment efficacy, AI has completely changed the way drugs are distributed. • On the basis of drug kinetics and solubility, machine learning forecasts the best nanoparticle formulations. • AI-powered devices can also modify medication release in real time, guaranteeing individualized and successful treatment.
Cost	High (lab experiments)	Low (in silico prediction)	
Time	Time-consuming	Rapid screening and optimization	
Scale	Limited samples	Massive data and high-throughput screening	
Accuracy	Empirical	Predictive and tunable accuracy	
Customization	Trial-and-error	Rational design with specific targets	

5. MECHANISM OF ANTIBACTERIAL ACTION OF NANOPARTICLES

Pathogenic bacteria play a role of major contributor to the infectious disease burden due to the significant elevation of single and multidrug-resistant bacteria leading to health threats, (Huang et al., 2024). NPs have emerged as a viable remedy by interfering with bacterial pathways, interacting with cell walls and cell membranes, hampering internal structure, removing bacterial toxins from the body, and targeted delivery of conventional antibiotics, (Wang et al., 2023). Nanovaccine development is highlighting efficient and long-lasting antimicrobial vaccines. Recent prospects of NPs include the detection, prevention, and treatment of bacterial infections, (Yang et al., 2020).

5.1. Generation of Damaging Cellular Components and ROS

One of the greatest strategies to inhibit microbial growth is by hampering their cellular component maturation. Nanomedicine promotes the ROS production pathway in bacteria leading to increased ROS concentration at the infection sites. Ang reported the hike in ROS level by gold-silver carbon QDs presenting antibacterial activity, (Gao et al., 2021). Xu et al. found that CeO_2 NPs after administration to *Escherichia coli*, could prevent the expression of genes linked to DNA intake by decreasing ROS levels and cell membrane permeability with the help of directly binding to eDNA. This antibacterial approach can stop germs from growing and reproducing right at their source. As pathogenic infection induces inflammatory responses resulting in ROS generation, nanoenzymes, artificial enzymes, are being used lately to activate ROS formation, (Sasaninia et al., 2023). These nanoenzymes mimic enzyme activity and bacterial binding capability in a single medication attaching to the surface of the bacteria and specifically destructing them in mammalian cells, (Dey et al., 2022). GSH-cyclodextrin NP has been reported to reduce the presence of Mycobacterium avium in whole blood from patients and has progressed to clinical trials. A study by Fresneda shows SeNPs to impart antibacterial therapeutic effects with increased ROS levels causing 80% of DNA damage, (Kim et al., 2018).

5.2. Cell Wall and Membrane Disruption

One of the important parts of bacteria in pathogenicity is their cell wall (CW) and membrane (CM) that serve as primary targets for developing antimicrobial agents. As a result, NPs direct the breakdown of CW and CM interrupting the CM's efflux pumps and alteration of transmembrane electron transport by targeting proteins particularly, (Khare et al., 2021). Metallic nanoparticles are vividly used here due to their charges, the contradiction of NPs carried charge and charge of CW surface led to the rupture of the structure. The potential antibacterial mechanisms of NPs are prevention of adhesion of bacteria, biofilm development, maturation of CW and CM, and finally proceeding to deformation of cells. Domyoung Kim (2018) designed CBD-EGFP-B-based silver NPs to target specific cells. Khare et al. (2021) emphasized that multi-combined gold nanoparticles can suppress efflux pumps of MDR bacteria cell membrane. ZnO NPs increase their efficacy against resistant strains of bacteria by disrupting their membranes and preventing the formation of biofilms, (Mocan et al., 2017). The antibacterial activity of CuNPs is size-dependent, with smaller particles (20 nm) demonstrating higher potency. They contribute to the death of bacterial cells by causing membrane disruption and producing reactive oxygen species (ROS), (Huang et al., 2022). Nanorods can easily penetrate cells due to their unique size and structure. Nanorods are also able to increase permeability of CW and CM and leakage of intracellular contents, (Hu et al., 2013).

5.3. Removal of Bacterial Toxins

During bacterial infection, harmful toxin secretion is facilitated that helps in penetration of bacteria into deeper tissues damaging host tissues, (Luo et al., 2024). Nanoparticles (NPs) have demonstrated the ability to mitigate bacterial toxins by inhibiting their secretion, binding to, and eliminating them. Metal NPs can capture lipopolysaccharides or peptidoglycans. Han et al. explored a toxin-responsive NP that elucidates the absorption and degradation of bacterial toxins upon encountering bacteria within the body. In addition, nanosponge coated with red blood cell (RBC) membranes neutralizes multiple pore-forming toxins, providing an effective treatment for bacterial sepsis, (Duncan et al., 2017). GLA-loaded NPs signal the downregulation of cytotoxic toxins which are also pore-forming, resulting in minimizing damage to the macrophage, also promoting wound healing. Zinc and copper nanoparticles ranging from 25nm to 50nm in size emphasize increased effectiveness in impeding the formation of biofilms, with zinc oxide nanoparticles showing better antibacterial action than copper, (Zhao et al., 2017). Metal-containing nanorods can release metals to damage enzyme functions and interfere with cellular respiration.

Figure 5. Mechanism of action of metal nanoparticles on inhibiting growth of bacteria

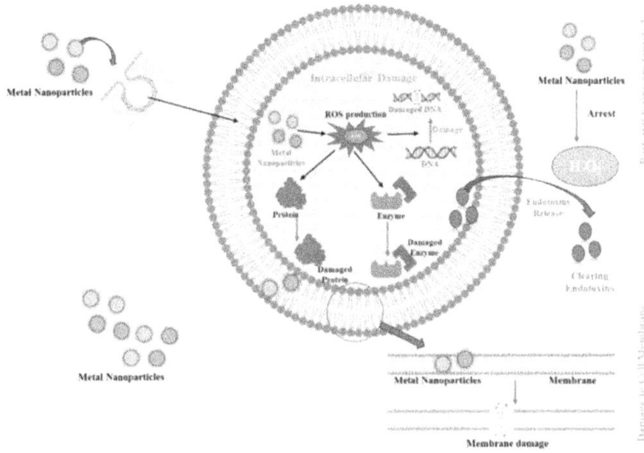

Figure 6. Metal nanoparticles used in the prevention of bacterial spread

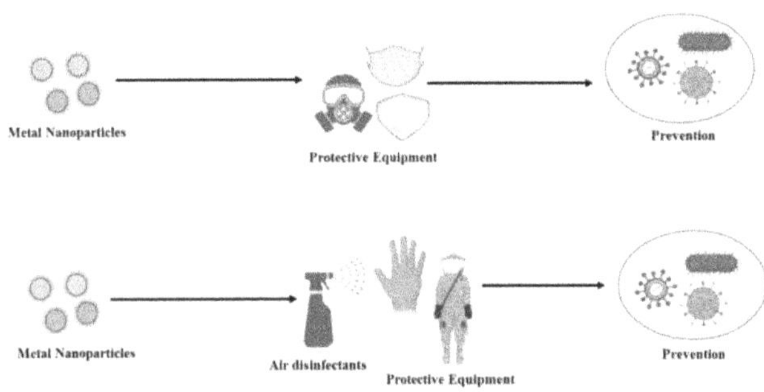

5.4. Nanotechnology Developed and Utilized in the Detection of Pathogenic Bacteria

Recent research focuses on pathogen detection based on nanotechnology detectors rendering a crucial tool for the present antibiotic-resistant, (Huang et al., 2017). Modified NPs are usually found using spectroscopy, electrochemical detection, or optical imaging to identify bacterial ligands. Based on the theory of NPs binding and preventing lipase, the highly sensitive sensors convert odorless molecules to odored molecules restoring the lipase activity representing swift sensing. Material design plays a key role in the detection and diagnosis of intricate and microscopic materials, such as metabolites. Phage-based, olfactory system-based, and antibody or aptamer-based tests are the three categories of pathogen detection-based nanotechnology. D-amino acid-AuNPs, developed by Yang et al., can potentially distinguish between Staphylococcus aureus and Methicillin-resistant Staphylococcus aureus (MRSA) by the change of colors. Nanoprobe in treating MRSA infection is currently under development that instigates NIRF imaging and continuous monitoring of MRSA infections, (Zhang et al., 2023). Nanodisk sensors containing silica NPs with labeled antibodies have been observed to detect extrapulmonary tuberculosis and culture-positive pulmonary tuberculosis with high sensitivity and specificity. AuNPs transfer the colour from purple to gray in the presence of Salmonella typhimurium DT104 facilitating the selective detection of the pathogen. Huang et al. (2017) designed and developed SiO_2-Ag for identifying metabolites and biomarkers in humans suffering from brain infection after surgery, this is in a clinical trial at present, (Bruna et al., 2021).

5.5. Nanotechnology in the Eradication and Prevention of Transmission of Pathogenic Bacteria

In addition to detection, prevention is also explored by nanotechnology. A substance's bactericidal activity enables it to be utilized as an antibacterial agent. Besides, anti-biofilm and antiadhesive properties act as beneficial characteristics for an antibacterial material. Nanotechnology has the vast scope to attenuate pathogenic bacterial infections reducing the burden of treatment of drug-resistant bacteria. The size and shape of AgNPs help them to enter bacteria cells destructing the cells by degrading cellular components like CW and CM. Also, it has the potential to ROS formation that directs cell-to-cell death by damaging cellular contents, (Ali et al., 2021). NPs aim and concentrate on the infection site halting transmission routes effectively. Common applications of NPs include wound dressing and wound healing. A variety of metallic nanoparticles such as AgNPs, (Román et al., 2020) AuNPS, (López-Ruiz et al., 2022) CuNPs, CeO-NPs, carbon-modified NPs, and Polymeric NPs are included as antimicrobial agents in disinfectants and protective gear. The presence of CuO NPs in protective equipment like masks, and gloves exhibits antibacterial impacts, (Webster, Wang, & Larese-Casanova, 2015). Silica NPs coated L-arginine can prevent dental caries, (dos Santos, Ingle, & Rai, 2020). Webster et al. (2015) emphasized that Se-NPs coated tissues potentially halt gram-positive and gram-negative bacterial growth. A wide range of sanitizers, disinfectants, and soaps contains AgNPs killing a broad spectrum of bacteria, (Chlumsky et al., 2021). Food-borne pathogens are considered one of the prime targets for nanomaterials as it is found effective in stopping the infection entry through the mouth resulting in the elimination of pathogens, (Franck et al., 2021), total NPs are employed in food packaging as well. Chlumsky et al. (2021) mentioned that PdNPs, and PtNPs are found to be utilized in packaging bags to inhibit the growth of bacteria such as *E.coli*, *Staphylococcus aureus*, *Salmonella*, *Listeria monocytogenes*, etc. AgNPs and FeNPs can alter the surface of implants for post-implant infection in surgery, (Wang et al., 2021).

5.6. Nanotechnology-Based Antimicrobial Vaccines

Nanolevel vaccine development including DNA vaccine, (Muhammad et al., 2012) mRNA vaccine, (Micoli & MacLennan, 2020) protein vaccine, (Meza-Segura et al., 2021) OMV, (Mellbye & Schuster, 2011) (Lee et al., 2018) and nanotoxoids (Simmons et al., 2018) is interestingly gaining attention due to their wide range of use and minimal side effects. DNA vaccine stimulates cellular and antibody-mediated immunity for arresting foreign particles, (Chatzikleanthous, O'Hagan, & Adamo, 2021). Incorporation of nanotechnology addresses the low immunogenicity-related issues in DNA vaccine development, (Li, Yu, & Cai, 2008). Numerous NPs formations with polymers, liposomes, (Mikušová & Mikuš, 2021) virus-like proteins, or specific proteins are involved in DNA vaccine delivery, (Crane, 2020). PGLA-combined DNA vaccines with standard biocompatibility can be used against tuberculosis infection, (Schwendener et al., 2010). Metal NPs have the potential to act as vaccine adjuvants. Metal NPs can emigrate to the site of action from the administration site instigating host immune defenses though the toxicity should be carefully regulated, (Lorenzi et al., 2010). Compared to bare plasmid-DNA vaccines, delivery with liposomal NPs increases the effectiveness of plasmid DNA transfection by effectively preventing extracellular nucleic acid endonucleases from degrading DNA through contact with the cell membrane, (Mayer et al., 2022). Developed liposomes with accurate target compounds trigger PRRs-based signaling pathways forming matured APCs at last, (Mikušová & Mikuš, 2021), mRNA vaccine, which swiftly evolved in COVID pandemic, is playing an important role in treating bacterial infections along with viral infections. The limitation of advancing research on mRNA vaccines to combat bacterial infection is to find accurate proteins from large numbers of bacterial proteins involved, (Fan & Lowrie, 2021). Despite these, mRNA vaccine could positively deal with antimicrobial resistance (AMR). Mayer et al. (2022) presented immune peptides of *Listeria monocytogenes* and combined them in mRNA vaccines that led to the considerable reduction of bacterial concentration from the spleen and liver, (Tan et al., 2018). The self-amplified mRNA has been reported to exert protective impacts against group A and Group B streptococcus inducing antigen-specific lgG2a (Th1) responses, (Camacho et al., 2013). OMV can be produced in 20-250nm by genetic engineering or when bacterial cell membrane vesiculates. OMVs consist of various membrane proteins that demonstrate enhanced binding of PRR to PAMP on the APCs leading to the activation of immune systems, (Gao et al., 2015). OMV can penetrate lymph nodes accelerating APCs uptake due to having a small size and shape in nm. OMV, derived from *Streptococcus meningitidis* and *Staphylococcus aureus*. are under clinical trial now. NP delivery system containing OMV results in increased vaccine efficiency. Poly(anhydride) NPs combined with Shigella release OMVs that improve bioadhesive interactions stimulating TLR2 and TLR4 mediated innate immunity, (Angsantikul, Fang, & Zhang, 2018). Gao et al. (2015) reported that the efficiency level of OMVs encapsulated with NPs is enhanced. The AuNPs encapsulated with OMVs exploit the multivalent antigenic qualities of OMVs in addition to increasing the stability of AuNPs, (Chen et al., 2018). Harmful toxins are secreted in presence of bacterial infections that damage the cell, and immune system causing haemolysis and sepsis. The detrimental consequences of infections could be obviated with the help of toxoid vaccine lowering the host stress, (Chen et al., 2016). NP-designed nanotoxins strengthen vaccine efficacy. In contrast to traditional inactivated toxin vaccines, nanotoxins produce antibody-boosting protective immunity in mice after vaccination with less cytotoxicity. Bacterial toxins such as alpha toxin, bee toxin, haemolysin O, etc. could be neutralized in presence of nano toxins developed with erythrocytes, (Thamphiwatana et al., 2017). They block toxins from binding to cell membranes as membrane of NPs mimics the cell membrane. It results in an increase of versatility, (Agreles, Cavalcanti, & Cavalcanti, 2022). Macrophage membrane mimicking nanoparticles designed by Thamphiwatana S et al. can capture endotoxins like lipopolysaccharides. It can additionally bind to cytokines resulting downstream of inflammation and inhibition of cytokine storm, (Alavi & Rai, 2019). The development of a nanotoxin as a vaccination against a variety of dangerous bacteria, including both Gram-positive and Gram-negative strains, is because of the adaptability of the cell membrane coating and the diversity of the different toxins.

5.7. Antibacterial Therapy and Delivery Vehicles

A series of inflammatory responses are initiated due to bacterial infection damaging tissues. Drugs developed by NPs are gaining importance for treating this disease, (Pelgrift & Friedman, 2013) (Osman et al., 2022). The size and shape of NPs could be maintained by several factors that render them suitable for delivering antibacterial compounds. The shortcomings of conventional antibiotic medicine including inappropriate targeting, and low bioavailability could be overcome by NP-based drugs. Antimicrobial drug delivery by NPs improves the antibiotic's bioavailability while also minimizing side effects and toxicity of the drug overcoming drug tolerance and enhancing intracellular infection resistance. Encapsulating multiple antibacterial compounds in one NPs decreases the scope of resistance development killing bacteria, (Nguyen & Pieters, 2005). Research on NPs surface modification for carrying antimicrobial compounds has progressed now, (Zou et al., 2023). Nps acts as a potent agent in treating intracellular infection of bacteria and preventing the recurrence of bacterial infection. When a drug is loaded with NPs, it is identified as a foreign particle undergoing phagocytosis by macrophages that release the drug inside it removing the bacteria, (Paredes da Rocha et al., 2023). Cinnamaldehyde-dextran combined NPs composed by Zou et al. (2023) target MRSA-infected macrophages by killing intracellular MRSA decreasing the possibility of macrophage injury. This also lowers the scope of drug resistance, (Hatamie et al., 2012). The nanocrystal formation with antibiotics could also be a way out of overcoming low bioavailability. Nataly et al. constructed a dapsone nanocrystal that is small and comparatively more soluble and stable than conventional drugs, (Gounani et al., 2019). Hatamie et al. (2012) synthesized cobalt nanoparticles showing the strong antibacterial activity of cobalt nanoparticles when subjected to E. coli, (Cinteza et al., 2018). The drawbacks of antibiotics are their adverse effects including GI irritation, and alterations of natural human microbiota causing severe toxicity to human organs such as kidneys and liver. Formulations of multiple drugs packed in one nanocarrier could also be used to overcome the adverse side effects elevating efficacy. NPs loaded with polymyxin B and vancomycin as designed by Gounani et al. (2019) have been used for the local delivery of antibiotics that require reduced dosages against gram-positive and gram-negative bacteria. Ludmila et al. prepared AgNPs from chitosan that is found to be non-toxic to fibroblasts at increased concentrations, (Hartmann, Rode, & Kramer, 2016). Self-assembled NPs composed of chitosan solve the issues of poor water solubility, instability, and low bioavailability, (Kuo et al., 2017). Carbon nanotube conjugated drug delivery elevates the efficiency of antibacterial medication due to its photothermal therapeutic properties, (Hu et al., 2013).

6. REAL-WORLD APPLICATIONS OF NANOPARTICLES AS ANTIBACTERIAL AGENTS

Nanoparticles have emerged as powerful tools in the fight against bacterial infections due to their unique properties such as small size, large surface area, and ability to interact at the cellular and molecular levels. They span across several sectors including biomedical fields, healthcare, cosmetics, food industries, textiles and environmental sections. They are widely applied in medical fields such as Wound Healing & Dressings, Coatings for Medical Devices, Drug Delivery Systems etc. The antibacterial potential of silver nanoparticles to act upon open wounds, burns and surgical rates make them eligible to be used in bandages and wound dressings.

Acticoat™ dressings coated with nanosilver, (Davies, McCarthy, & Hamberg, 2017) Aquacel® Ag for surgical dressing Girija, Balasubramanian, & Cowin, 2022), Mepilex Ag, a silver-impregnated foam dressing (Kang et al., 2017), CuraFoam AG Silver Foam (Ip et al., 2006), KoCarbonAg (Nguyen et al., 2024) have been reported to contain silver nanoparticles with antibacterial efficacy. Ip et al. (2006) evaluated the antimicrobial efficacy of numerous Ag dressings including Aquacel® Ag, Acticoat™, Urgotol® SSD, PolyMem® Silver, and Contreet® that reported their effectiveness against gram negative bacteria mostly whereas Acticoat and Contreet have also been found to exhibit antimicrobial efficacy against S. aureus, (Sathiyaseelan et al., 2023). Silver coated urinary catheters contribute to the control of urinary tract infections (UTI). According to the reports lipid-based nanoparticles, polymeric nanoparticles could be used as nanocarriers of medicine to the infection sites. Chitosan nanoparticles have the potential to carry ampicillin for targeted drug delivery and treating bacterial infections like S. aureus, (Deus et al., 2017). Chitosan-based ampicillin PEGylated zinc oxide nanoparticles (CS-AMP-P-ZnO NPs) demonstrates distinct antimicrobial potential against E. coli, (Shraouba & Makkia, 2022). In the food industry, nanoparticles of chitosan and zinc oxide (ZnO) prolong the shelf life of food by preventing bacterial growth on its surfaces. Meat packaging uses NanoAg+ and Nano-silver spray coatings to prevent microorganisms from spoiling. Chitosan/ZnO NPs extend shelf life of poultry meat, (Joseph, Nair, & Arya, 2025), beef meat (Abedi, Ghasemi, & Nemati, 2024) in food packaging due to their antibacterial potency. NanoSeptic® is utilised in surface cleaning on different sections like elevators, (Labille et al., 2020). Toothpaste and cosmetics like cream, sunscreen contains zinc oxide nanocrystals.

7. CHALLENGES AND FUTURE PERSPECTIVES

Metal nanoparticles could be signified antimicrobial agents due to their unique physicochemical properties, however, challenges such as toxicity, stability, and scalability hinder their widespread applications.

7.1. Challenges

Biocompatibility and Toxicity: Biocompatibility remains as the biggest hurdle in pharmaceutical sciences for development and use of metal NPs due to several sizes, shapes, and coating materials. NPs display potential cytotoxic effects on human cells at higher concentrations limiting their therapeutic impacts. This cytotoxic impact warrants thorough evaluation and regulatory frameworks.

Standardization of Synthesis Methods: Reproducibility is impacted by variations in nanoparticle characteristics caused by inconsistent production methods differing in size, shape, and purity of nanomedicine.
Batch to Batch Variability: Small changes in synthesis conditions lead to alterations of nanoparticles behaviour.
Scalability and Cost: Large-scale industrial-level synthesis with maintained control over their characteristics is expensive and technically challenging. Preparation of a budget for cost-effective production while maintaining efficacy is yet to be focused on by industrialists.
Nanoparticle Resistance: There is a high chance of the development of adaptive resistance in bacteria as noticed with antibiotics, dragging the importance of continuous evaluation of resistance patterns. Emerging evidence of nanoparticle resistance in some microbes demands the need for combination therapies and periodic monitoring.
Unclear Regulatory Classification: The scope of consideration of nanoparticle based antibacterial agents as drugs or medication are still ambiguous.
Lack of Nanoparticle-Specific Guidelines: Most regulatory frameworks (by FDA, EMA) were developed for traditional drugs, lacking for nanomaterials.

7.2. Future Perspectives

Green synthesis: Scalable processes of eco-friendly synthesis techniques with the help of plant extracts, microorganisms, biopolymers, etc. should be focused on for industrial applications to minimize environmental concerns.
Design of target delivery system:
Nanoparticles can be incorporated into ingenious delivery systems through nanocarriers or nanocomposites for site-specific antibacterial action improving therapeutic outcomes.
Synergistic Therapies of Metal Nanoparticles:
Incorporating metal nanoparticles with natural antibacterial agents, peptides, or antibiotics can enhance efficacy delaying resistance.
Artificial Intelligence and Computational Tools:
Applying AI and machine learning to optimize synthesis, anticipate nanoparticle behaviour, assess antibacterial activity, and use computer technologies to speed up the process of finding new formulations for nanoparticles could direct toward the alleviation of antibiotic resistance era.
Policy:
Policy and initiatives on commercializing nano-based antimicrobials would promote more research and their forefront use in medications.

8. CONCLUSION

In summary, the diverse methodologies for nanoparticle synthesis ranging from chemical and physical techniques to biological and green synthesis, present unique benefits and limitations tailored to specific applications and material properties. Particle size and composition can be precisely controlled using chemical techniques like sol-gel and hydrothermal synthesis, although these approaches can involve complex processes and higher costs. Physical techniques, including laser ablation, and ball milling enable the production of nanoparticles with varied sizes and shapes but often face challenges related to efficiency and uniformity. Biological synthesis methods leverage natural processes to create nanoparticles with potential advantages like biocompatibility and environmental sustainability, albeit with consistency issues. Green synthesis approaches emphasize eco-friendly practices and can align with sustainable development goals, yet they often require further refinement to achieve the precision and scalability of conventional methods. The optimal choice of synthesis technique is contingent upon the type of application, encompassing factors such as cost, environmental impact, scalability, and the desired physicochemical properties of the nanoparticles. The overuse of antibiotics gave rise to antibiotic-resistant bacteria. Antibiotic-resistant era is evolving drastically which could be resolved with the help of nanotechnology. The application of metal nanoparticles in detection, and prevention of wildtype and resistant bacteria and treatment of bacterial infection is through nanoparticle-based drug and drug delivery. AuNPs could distinguishably detect SA and MRSA, the presence of *Salmonella typhimurium*. Metal nanoparticle including AgNPs, AuNPS, CuNPs, and CeO-NPs enhances the effectivity of antimicrobial agents and prevent the transmission of infectious bacteria. Nanoparticles induce increased ROS production, facilitating cell wall and membrane disruption. They can potentially ameliorate bacterial toxin secretion as well. Nanotubes combat antibiotic-resistant bacteria via a multifaceted approach, including membrane disruption, ROS generation, metal ion release, DNA damage, and antibiotic synergy. Industries could focus on the optimization of scalable green synthesis methods to uncover future potential and address remaining challenges in the future.

REFERENCES

Abedi, M., Ghasemi, Y., & Nemati, M. M. (2024). Nanotechnology in toothpaste: Fundamentals, trends, and safety. *Heliyon, 10*(3), e24949. DOI: 10.1016/j.heliyon.2024.e24949 PMID: 38317872

Abid, N., Khan, A. M., Shujait, S., Chaudhary, K., Ikram, M., Imran, M., Haider, J., Khan, M., Khan, Q., & Maqbool, M. (2022). Synthesis of nanomaterials using various top-down and bottom-up approaches, influencing factors, advantages, and disadvantages: A review. *Advances in Colloid and Interface Science, 300*, 102597. DOI: 10.1016/j.cis.2021.102597 PMID: 34979471

Acay, H., Güler Güney, İ., Yildirim, A., Derviş, S., & Dereli, E. (2024). Green Synthesis of *Pleurotus Eryngii* -Derived Nanomaterials for Phytopathogen Control. *Chemistry & Biodiversity*, *21*(12), e202401972. DOI: 10.1002/cbdv.202401972 PMID: 39155528

Agreles, M. A. A., Cavalcanti, I. D. L., & Cavalcanti, I. M. F. (2022). Synergism between metallic nanoparticles and antibiotics. *Applied Microbiology and Biotechnology, 106*(11), 3973–3984. DOI: 10.1007/s00253-022-12001-1 PMID: 35670851

Al-Badaii, F.. (2024). Green Synthesis of Zinc Oxide Nanoparticles Using Allium Sativum Extract: Evaluation of Antibacterial Activity Against Nosocomial Bacteria, *Thamar University Journal of Natural &. Applied Sciences (Basel, Switzerland), 9*(1).

Alam, R., Khan, M. A., Khan, R. A., Ghoshal, S., & Mondal, M. I. H. (2008). R., K.M.A., K.R.A., G.S., & M.M.I.H. Alam, Study on the Physico-mechanical Properties of Photo-cured Chitosan Films with Oligomer and Acrylate Monomer. *Journal of Polymers and the Environment, 16*(3), 213–219. DOI: 10.1007/s10924-008-0099-2

Alavi, M., & Rai, M. (2019). Recent advances in antibacterial applications of metal nanoparticles (MNPs) and metal nanocomposites (MNCs) against multidrug-resistant (MDR) bacteria. *Expert Review of Anti-Infective Therapy, 17*(6), 419–428. DOI: 10.1080/14787210.2019.1614914 PMID: 31046483

Ali, S., Chen, X., Ajmal Shah, M., Ali, M., Zareef, M., Arslan, M., Ahmad, S., Jiao, T., Li, H., & Chen, Q. (2021). The avenue of fruit wastes to worth for synthesis of silver and gold nanoparticles and their antimicrobial application against foodborne pathogens: A review. *Food Chemistry, 359*, 129912. DOI: 10.1016/j.foodchem.2021.129912 PMID: 33934027

Alias, R., Mahmoodian, R., Genasan, K., Vellasamy, K. M., Hamdi Abd Shukor, M., & Kamarul, T. (2020). Mechanical, antibacterial, and biocompatibility mechanism of PVD grown silver–tantalum-oxide-based nanostructured thin film on stainless steel 316L for surgical applications. *Materials Science and Engineering C, 107*, 110304. DOI: 10.1016/j.msec.2019.110304 PMID: 31761210

Amal, M. I.. Antibacterial activity of copper oxide nanoparticles prepared by mechanical milling, *IOP Conf Ser Mater Sci Eng* 578 (2019) 012039. DOI: 10.1088/1757-899X/578/1/012039

Andrade, F., Jenipher, C., Gurav, N., Nadaf, S., Khan, M. S., Mahajan, N., Bhagwat, D., Kalaskar, M., Chikhale, R., Bhole, R., Lalsare, S., Baheti, A., Ayyanar, M., & Gurav, S. (2024). Endophytic fungi-assisted biomass synthesis of eco-friendly formulated silver nanoparticles for enhanced antibacterial, antioxidant, and antidiabetic activities. *Journal of Drug Delivery Science and Technology*, *97*, 105749. DOI: 10.1016/j.jddst.2024.105749

Angsantikul, P., Fang, R. H., & Zhang, L. (2018). Toxoid Vaccination against Bacterial Infection Using Cell Membrane-Coated Nanoparticles. *Bioconjugate Chemistry*, *29*(3), 604–612. DOI: 10.1021/acs.bioconjchem.7b00692 PMID: 29241006

Anu Mary Ealia, S., & Saravanakumar, M. P. A review on the classification, characterisation, synthesis of nanoparticles and their application, *IOP Conf Ser Mater Sci Eng* 263 (2017) 032019. DOI: 10.1088/1757-899X/263/3/032019

Araújo, I. M. S., Silva, R. R., Pacheco, G., Lustri, W. R., Tercjak, A., Gutierrez, J., Júnior, J. R. S., Azevedo, F. H. C., Figuêredo, G. S., Vega, M. L., Ribeiro, S. J. L., & Barud, H. S. (2018). Hydrothermal synthesis of bacterial cellulose–copper oxide nanocomposites and evaluation of their antimicrobial activity. *Carbohydrate Polymers*, *179*, 341–349. DOI: 10.1016/j.carbpol.2017.09.081 PMID: 29111060

Asanithi, P., Chaiyakun, S., & Limsuwan, P. (2012). Growth of Silver Nanoparticles by DC Magnetron Sputtering. *Journal of Nanomaterials*, *2012*(1), 963609. DOI: 10.1155/2012/963609

Atabaki, H. (2024). Synthesis of iron oxide magnetic nanoparticles and chitosan biopolymer in aqueous solutions. *Inorganic Chemistry Communications*, *162*, 112161. DOI: 10.1016/j.inoche.2024.112161

Awwad, A. M., & Salem, N. M. (2012). Green Synthesis of Silver Nanoparticles byMulberry LeavesExtract. *Nanoscience and Nanotechnology*, *2*(4), 125–128. DOI: 10.5923/j.nn.20120204.06

Banik, N., & Kaur, P. (2024). *Biopolymeric nanoparticles in controlled release drug delivery*. DOI: 10.1063/5.0193703

Bishoyi, A. K., Sahoo, C. R., & Padhy, R. N. (2023). Recent progression of cyanobacteria and their pharmaceutical utility: An update. *Journal of Biomolecular Structure & Dynamics*, *41*(9), 4219–4252. DOI: 10.1080/07391102.2022.2062051 PMID: 35412441

Bruna, T., Maldonado-Bravo, F., Jara, P., & Caro, N. (2021). Silver Nanoparticles and Their Antibacterial Applications. *International Journal of Molecular Sciences*, *22*(13), 7202. DOI: 10.3390/ijms22137202 PMID: 34281254

Camacho, A. I., Irache, J. M., de Souza, J., Sánchez-Gómez, S., & Gamazo, C. (2013). Nanoparticle-based vaccine for mucosal protection against Shigella flexneri in mice. *Vaccine*, *31*(32), 3288–3294. DOI: 10.1016/j.vaccine.2013.05.020 PMID: 23727423

Chatzikleanthous, D., O'Hagan, D. T., & Adamo, R. (2021). Lipid-Based Nanoparticles for Delivery of Vaccine Adjuvants and Antigens: Toward Multicomponent Vaccines. *Molecular Pharmaceutics*, *18*(8), 2867–2888. DOI: 10.1021/acs.molpharmaceut.1c00447 PMID: 34264684

Chauhan, R. P. Processes for Nanoparticle Synthesis, *in* (2024): pp. 69–100. DOI: 10.4018/979-8-3693-4397-5.ch003

Chen, W., Zhang, Q., Luk, B. T., Fang, R. H., Liu, Y., Gao, W., & Zhang, L. (2016). Coating nanofiber scaffolds with beta cell membrane to promote cell proliferation and function. *Nanoscale*, *8*(19), 10364–10370. DOI: 10.1039/C6NR00535G PMID: 27139582

Chen, Y., Chen, M., Zhang, Y., Lee, J. H., Escajadillo, T., Gong, H., Fang, R. H., Gao, W., Nizet, V., & Zhang, L. (2018). Broad-Spectrum Neutralization of Pore-Forming Toxins with Human Erythrocyte Membrane-Coated Nanosponges. *Advanced Healthcare Materials*, *7*(13), 1701366. DOI: 10.1002/adhm.201701366 PMID: 29436150

Chlumsky, O., Purkrtova, S., Michova, H., Sykorova, H., Slepicka, P., Fajstavr, D., Ulbrich, P., Viktorova, J., & Demnerova, K. (2021). Antimicrobial Properties of Palladium and Platinum Nanoparticles: A New Tool for Combating Food-Borne Pathogens. *International Journal of Molecular Sciences*, *22*(15), 7892. DOI: 10.3390/ijms22157892 PMID: 34360657

Cinteza, L. O., Scomoroscenco, C., Voicu, S. N., Nistor, C. L., Nitu, S. G., Trica, B., Jecu, M.-L., & Petcu, C. (2018). Chitosan-Stabilized Ag Nanoparticles with Superior Biocompatibility and Their Synergistic Antibacterial Effect in Mixtures with Essential Oils. *Nanomaterials (Basel, Switzerland)*, *8*(10), 826. DOI: 10.3390/nano8100826 PMID: 30322127

Crane, J. K. (2020). Metal Nanoparticles in Infection and Immunity. *Immunological Investigations*, *49*(7), 794–807. DOI: 10.1080/08820139.2020.1776724 PMID: 32524902

Darwish, M., Mafla-Gonzalez, C., Kolenovic, B., Deremer, A., Centeno, D., Liu, T., Kim, D.-Y., Cattabiani, T., Drwiega, T. J., Kumar, I., Li, C., & Traba, C. (2022). Rapid synthesis of metal nanoparticles using low-temperature, low-pressure argon plasma chemistry and self-assembly. *Green Chemistry*, *24*(20), 8142–8154. DOI: 10.1039/D2GC02592B PMID: 37153712

Das, V., & Kingsley, D. (2023). In silico and in vitro investigation of the role of Asparagus racemosus lead compound Shatavarin IV and associated silver nanoparticles. *Research Journal of Biotechnology*, *18*(12), 200–217. DOI: 10.25303/1811rjbt0200217

Davies, P., McCarty, S., & Hamberg, K. (2017). Silver-containing foam dressings with Safetac: a review of the scientific and clinical data. Journal of wound care, 26(Sup6a), S1-S32.

Dell'Aglio, M., De Giacomo, A., Manno, D., Mallardi, A., Provenzano, C., Marra, M., Nocito, F., Serra, A., Quarta, G., & Paola Caricato, A. (2024). Boron nanoparticles (BNPs) produced by ns-laser ablation in water: Synthesis and characterization. *Applied Surface Science*, *661*, 160089. DOI: 10.1016/j.apsusc.2024.160089

Deus, D., Kehrenberg, C., Schaudien, D., Klein, G., & Krischek, C. (2017). Effect of a nano-silver coating on the quality of fresh turkey meat during storage after modified atmosphere or vacuum packaging. *Poultry Science*, *96*(2), 449–457. DOI: 10.3382/ps/pew308 PMID: 27647930

Dey, N., Kamatchi, C., Vickram, A. S., Anbarasu, K., Thanigaivel, S., Palanivelu, J., Pugazhendhi, A., & Ponnusamy, V. K. (2022). Role of nanomaterials in deactivating multiple drug resistance efflux pumps – A review. *Environmental Research*, *204*, 111968. DOI: 10.1016/j.envres.2021.111968 PMID: 34453898

Dheyab, M. A., Aziz, A. A., Al-Mafarjy, S. S., Suardi, N., Razak, N. N. A. N. A., Ramizy, A., & Jameel, M. S. (2023). Exploring the anticancer potential of biogenic inorganic gold nanoparticles synthesized via mushroom-assisted green route. *Inorganic Chemistry Communications*, *157*, 111363. DOI: 10.1016/j.inoche.2023.111363 dos Santos, C. A., Ingle, A. P., & Rai, M. (2020). The emerging role of metallic nanoparticles in food. *Applied Microbiology and Biotechnology*, *104*(6), 2373–2383. DOI: 10.1007/s00253-020-10372-x PMID: 31989225

Duncan, B., Le, N. D. B., Alexander, C., Gupta, A., Yesilbag Tonga, G., Yazdani, M., Landis, R. F., Wang, L.-S., Yan, B., Burmaoglu, S., Li, X., & Rotello, V. M. (2017). Sensing by Smell: Nanoparticle–Enzyme Sensors for Rapid and Sensitive Detection of Bacteria with Olfactory Output. *ACS Nano*, *11*(6), 5339–5343. DOI: 10.1021/acsnano.7b00822 PMID: 28423269

El-Sherbiny, I. M., & Sedki, M. Green Synthesis of Chitosan-Silver/Gold Hybrid Nanoparticles for Biomedical Applications, *in* (2019): pp. 79–84.

Fan, X.-Y., & Lowrie, D. B. (2021). Where are the RNA vaccines for TB? *Emerging Microbes & Infections*, *10*(1), 1217–1218. DOI: 10.1080/22221751.2021.1935328 PMID: 34036874

Fernández, J., Piano, S., Bartoletti, M., & Wey, E. Q. (2021). Management of bacterial and fungal infections in cirrhosis: The MDRO challenge. *Journal of Hepatology*, *75*, S101–S117. DOI: 10.1016/j.jhep.2020.11.010 PMID: 34039482

Franck, C. O., Fanslau, L., Bistrovic Popov, A., Tyagi, P., & Fruk, L. (2021). Biopolymer-based Carriers for DNA Vaccine Design. *Angewandte Chemie International Edition*, *60*(24), 13225–13243. DOI: 10.1002/anie.202010282 PMID: 32893932

Fu, C., & Chen, Q. (2025). The future of pharmaceuticals: Artificial intelligence in drug discovery and development. *Journal of Pharmaceutical Analysis*, •••, 101248. DOI: 10.1016/j.jpha.2025.101248

Gao, F., Shao, T., Yu, Y., Xiong, Y., & Yang, L. (2021). Surface-bound reactive oxygen species generating nanozymes for selective antibacterial action. *Nature Communications*, *12*(1), 745. DOI: 10.1038/s41467-021-20965-3 PMID: 33531505

Gao, W., Fang, R. H., Thamphiwatana, S., Luk, B. T., Li, J., Angsantikul, P., Zhang, Q., Hu, C.-M. J., & Zhang, L. (2015). Modulating Antibacterial Immunity via Bacterial Membrane-Coated Nanoparticles. *Nano Letters*, *15*(2), 1403–1409. DOI: 10.1021/nl504798g PMID: 25615236

Ghorbani, H. (2014). A Review of Methods for Synthesis of Al Nanoparticles. *Oriental Journal of Chemistry*, *30*(4), 1941–1949. DOI: 10.13005/ojc/300456

Girija, A. R., Balasubramanian, S., & Cowin, A. J. (2022). Nanomaterials-based Drug Delivery Approaches for Wound Healing. *Current Pharmaceutical Design*, *28*(9), 711–726. DOI: 10.2174/1381612828666220328121211 PMID: 35345993

Görke, M., Okeil, S., Menzel, D., Semenenko, B., & Garnweitner, G. (2024). Tuning the Properties of Iron Oxide Nanoparticles in Thermal Decomposition Synthesis: A Comparative Study of the Influence of Temperature, Ligand Length and Ligand Concentration. *Particle & Particle Systems Characterization*, *41*(10), 2400059. DOI: 10.1002/ppsc.202400059

Gounani, Z., Asadollahi, M. A., Pedersen, J. N., Lyngsø, J., Skov Pedersen, J., Arpanaei, A., & Meyer, R. L. (2019). Mesoporous silica nanoparticles carrying multiple antibiotics provide enhanced synergistic effect and improved biocompatibility. *Colloids and Surfaces. B, Biointerfaces*, *175*, 498–508. DOI: 10.1016/j.colsurfb.2018.12.035 PMID: 30572158

Govindaraju, K., Kiruthiga, V., Kumar, V. G., & Singaravelu, G. (2009). Extracellular Synthesis of Silver Nanoparticles by a Marine Alga, *Sargassum Wightii* Grevilli and Their Antibacterial Effects. *Journal of Nanoscience and Nanotechnology*, *9*(9), 5497–5501. DOI: 10.1166/jnn.2009.1199 PMID: 19928252

Gow, N. A. R., Johnson, C., Berman, J., Coste, A. T., Cuomo, C. A., Perlin, D. S., Bicanic, T., Harrison, T. S., Wiederhold, N., Bromley, M., Chiller, T., & Edgar, K. (2022). The importance of antimicrobial resistance in medical mycology. *Nature Communications*, *13*(1), 5352. DOI: 10.1038/s41467-022-32249-5 PMID: 36097014

Gritsenko, L., Kedruk, Y., Paltusheva, Z., & Syritski, V. (2023). Structural properties of ZnO nanopowders synthesized by thermal decomposition. *Physical Sciences and Technology*, *10*(3-4), 80–86.

Gudikandula, K., & Charya Maringanti, S. (2016). Synthesis of silver nanoparticles by chemical and biological methods and their antimicrobial properties. *Journal of Experimental Nanoscience*, *11*(9), 714–721. DOI: 10.1080/17458080.2016.1139196

Hamilton, S., & Kingston, B. R. (2024). Applying artificial intelligence and computational modeling to nanomedicine. *Current Opinion in Biotechnology*, *85*, 103043. DOI: 10.1016/j.copbio.2023.103043 PMID: 38091874

Hartmann, C. A., Rode, H., & Kramer, B. (2016). Acticoat™ stimulates inflammation, but does not delay healing, in acute full-thickness excisional wounds. *International Wound Journal*, *13*(6), 1344–1348. DOI: 10.1111/iwj.12525 PMID: 26561384

Hatamie, S., Nouri, M., Karandikar, S. K., Kulkarni, A., Dhole, S. D., Phase, D. M., & Kale, S. N. (2012). Complexes of cobalt nanoparticles and polyfunctional curcumin as antimicrobial agents. *Materials Science and Engineering C*, *32*(2), 92–97. DOI: 10.1016/j.msec.2011.10.002

Hazarika, K. P., & Borah, J. P. (2024). Study of biopolymer encapsulated Eu doped Fe3O4 nanoparticles for magnetic hyperthermia application. *Scientific Reports*, *14*(1), 9768. DOI: 10.1038/s41598-024-60040-7 PMID: 38684710

Byon, H. R., Lim, H. S., Song, H. J., & Choi, H. C. (2007). A synthesis of high purity single-walled carbon nanotubes from small diameters of cobalt nanoparticles by using oxygen-assisted chemical vapor deposition process. *Bulletin of the Korean Chemical Society*, *28*(11), 2056–2060.

Hu, C.-M. J., Fang, R. H., Copp, J., Luk, B. T., & Zhang, L. (2013). A biomimetic nanosponge that absorbs pore-forming toxins. *Nature Nanotechnology*, *8*(5), 336–340. DOI: 10.1038/nnano.2013.54 PMID: 23584215

Huang, H., Liu, N., Wang, X., Zhong, M., & Huang, X. (2022). Application of Hydrothermal and Solvothermal Method in Synthesis of MoS2. *Revista de Chimie*, *73*(4), 26–35. DOI: 10.37358/RC.22.4.8544

Huang, L., Wan, J., Wei, X., Liu, Y., Huang, J., Sun, X., Zhang, R., Gurav, D. D., Vedarethinam, V., Li, Y., Chen, R., & Qian, K. (2017). Plasmonic silver nanoshells for drug and metabolite detection. *Nature Communications*, *8*(1), 220. DOI: 10.1038/s41467-017-00220-4 PMID: 28790311

Huang, Y., Guo, X., Wu, Y., Chen, X., Feng, L., Xie, N., & Shen, G. (2024). Nanotechnology's frontier in combatting infectious and inflammatory diseases: Prevention and treatment. *Signal Transduction and Targeted Therapy*, *9*(1), 34. DOI: 10.1038/s41392-024-01745-z PMID: 38378653

Huang, Y., Zou, L., Wang, J., Jin, Q., & Ji, J. (2022). Stimuli-responsive nanoplatforms for antibacterial applications. *Wiley Interdisciplinary Reviews. Nanomedicine and Nanobiotechnology*, *14*(3), e1775. DOI: 10.1002/wnan.1775 PMID: 35142071

Ip, M., Lui, S. L., Poon, V. K. M., Lung, I., & Burd, A. (2006). Antimicrobial activities of silver dressings: An in vitro comparison. *Journal of Medical Microbiology*, *55*(1), 59–63. DOI: 10.1099/jmm.0.46124-0 PMID: 16388031

Iravani, S.. (2014). Synthesis of silver nanoparticles: Chemical, physical and biological methods. *Research in Pharmaceutical Sciences*, *9*(6), 385–406. PMID: 26339255

Jadoun, S., Arif, R., Jangid, N. K., & Meena, R. K. (2021). Green synthesis of nanoparticles using plant extracts: A review. *Environmental Chemistry Letters*, *19*(1), 355–374. DOI: 10.1007/s10311-020-01074-x

Jafarzadeh, S.. (2023). Green synthesis of nanomaterials for smart biopolymer packaging: Challenges and outlooks. *Journal of Nanostructure in Chemistry*.

Jamkhande, P. G., Ghule, N. W., Bamer, A. H., & Kalaskar, M. G. (2019). Metal nanoparticles synthesis: An overview on methods of preparation, advantages and disadvantages, and applications. *Journal of Drug Delivery Science and Technology, 53*, 101174. DOI: 10.1016/j.jddst.2019.101174

Joseph, M. M., Nair, J. B., & Arya, J. S. (2025). Integrated Utilization of Functional Nanomaterials for COVID-19 Monitoring, Prevention, and Diagnostic Strategies. *Research on Biomedical Engineering, 41*(1), 23. DOI: 10.1007/s42600-025-00404-8

Kaabo, H. E.. (2024). Penicillium oxalicum-mediated the green synthesis of silica nanoparticles: Characterization and environmental applications. *Biomass Conversion and Biorefinery.*

Kadam, D., Momin, B., Palamthodi, S., & Lele, S. S. (2019). Physicochemical and functional properties of chitosan-based nano-composite films incorporated with biogenic silver nanoparticles. *Carbohydrate Polymers, 211*, 124–132. DOI: 10.1016/j.carbpol.2019.02.005 PMID: 30824072

Kadam, D., Momin, B., Palamthodi, S., & Lele, S. S. (2019). Physicochemical and functional properties of chitosan-based nano-composite films incorporated with biogenic silver nanoparticles. *Carbohydrate Polymers, 211*, 124–132. DOI: 10.1016/j.carbpol.2019.02.005 PMID: 30824072

Kang, J.. (2017). Orthopedic Applications of Silver and Silver Nanoparticles. In *Orthopedic Biomaterials* (pp. 63–83). Springer International Publishing. DOI: 10.1007/978-3-319-73664-8_3

Karthik, C. S., Chethana, M. H., Manukumar, H. M., Ananda, A. P., Sandeep, S., Nagashree, S., Mallesha, L., Mallu, P., Jayanth, H. S., & Dayananda, B. P. (2021). Synthesis and characterization of chitosan silver nanoparticle decorated with benzodioxane coupled piperazine as an effective anti-biofilm agent against MRSA: A validation of molecular docking and dynamics. *International Journal of Biological Macromolecules, 181*, 540–551. DOI: 10.1016/j.ijbiomac.2021.03.119 PMID: 33766592

Kavitha, T., Haider, S., Kamal, T., & Ul-Islam, M. (2017). Thermal decomposition of metal complex precursor as route to the synthesis of Co3O4 nanoparticles: Antibacterial activity and mechanism. *Journal of Alloys and Compounds, 704*, 296–302. DOI: 10.1016/j.jallcom.2017.01.306

Khare, T., Mahalunkar, S., Shriram, V., Gosavi, S., & Kumar, V. (2021). Embelin-loaded chitosan gold nanoparticles interact synergistically with ciprofloxacin by inhibiting efflux pumps in multidrug-resistant Pseudomonas aeruginosa and Escherichia coli. *Environmental Research*, *199*, 111321. DOI: 10.1016/j.envres.2021.111321 PMID: 33989619

Kim, D., Kwon, S.-J., Wu, X., Sauve, J., Lee, I., Nam, J., Kim, J., & Dordick, J. S. (2018). Selective Killing of Pathogenic Bacteria by Antimicrobial Silver Nanoparticle—Cell Wall Binding Domain Conjugates. *ACS Applied Materials & Interfaces*, *10*(16), 13317–13324. DOI: 10.1021/acsami.8b00181 PMID: 29619821

Koh, S. K., Lee, J. H., Lee, C., & Koh, K. (2016). Nano-Scale Particle Formation by Dynamic Mixing Method in Physical Vapor Deposition. *Key Engineering Materials*, *708*, 14–19. DOI: 10.4028/www.scientific.net/KEM.708.14

Kuo, F.-C., Chen, B., Lee, M. S., Yen, S.-H., & Wang, J.-W. (2017). AQUACEL® Ag Surgical Dressing Reduces Surgical Site Infection and Improves Patient Satisfaction in Minimally Invasive Total Knee Arthroplasty: A Prospective, Randomized, Controlled Study. *BioMed Research International*, *2017*, 1–8. DOI: 10.1155/2017/1262108 PMID: 28831390

Kvítek, O., Hendrych, R., Kolská, Z., & Švorčík, V. (2014). Grafting of Gold Nanoparticles on Glass Using Sputtered Gold Interlayers. *Journal of Chemistry*, *2014*, 1–6. DOI: 10.1155/2014/450413

Labille, J.. (2020). Assessing Sunscreen Lifecycle to Minimize Environmental Risk Posed by Nanoparticulate UV-Filters – A Review for Safer-by-Design Products. *Frontiers in Environmental Science*, •••, 8.

Le, T. C., Yin, H., Chen, R., Chen, Y., Zhao, L., Casey, P. S., Chen, C., & Winkler, D. A. (2016). An Experimental and Computational Approach to the Development of ZnO Nanoparticles that are Safe by Design. *Small*, *12*(26), 3568–3577. DOI: 10.1002/smll.201600597 PMID: 27167706

Lee, J., Arun Kumar, S., Jhan, Y. Y., & Bishop, C. J. (2018). Engineering DNA vaccines against infectious diseases. *Acta Biomaterialia*, *80*, 31–47. DOI: 10.1016/j.actbio.2018.08.033 PMID: 30172933

Lee, J. H., Jeong, D., & Kanmani, P. (2019). Study on physical and mechanical properties of the biopolymer/silver based active nanocomposite films with antimicrobial activity. *Carbohydrate Polymers*, *224*, 115159. DOI: 10.1016/j.carbpol.2019.115159 PMID: 31472865

Li, M., Yu, D.-H., & Cai, H. (2008). The Synthetic Antimicrobial Peptide KLKL $_5$ KLK Enhances the Protection and Efficacy of the Combined DNA Vaccine against *Mycobacterium tuberculosis*. *DNA and Cell Biology*, *27*(8), 405–413. DOI: 10.1089/dna.2007.0693 PMID: 18694298

López-Ruiz, M., Navas, F., Fernández-García, P., Martínez-Erro, S., Fuentes, M. V., Giráldez, I., Ceballos, L., Ferrer-Luque, C. M., Ruiz-Linares, M., Morales, V., Sanz, R., & García-Muñoz, R. A. (2022). L-arginine-containing mesoporous silica nanoparticles embedded in dental adhesive (Arg@MSN@DAdh) for targeting cariogenic bacteria. *Journal of Nanobiotechnology*, *20*(1), 502. DOI: 10.1186/s12951-022-01714-0 PMID: 36457046

Lorenzi, J. C., Trombone, A. P. F., Rocha, C. D., Almeida, L. P., Lousada, R. L., Malardo, T., Fontoura, I. C., Rossetti, R. A. M., Gembre, A. F., Silva, A. M., Silva, C. L., & Coelho-Castelo, A. A. M. (2010). Intranasal vaccination with messenger RNA as a new approach in gene therapy: Use against tuberculosis. *BMC Biotechnology*, *10*(1), 77. DOI: 10.1186/1472-6750-10-77 PMID: 20961459

Luo, L., Huang, W., Zhang, J., Yu, Y., & Sun, T. (2024). Metal-Based Nanoparticles as Antimicrobial Agents: A Review. *ACS Applied Nano Materials*, *7*(3), 2529–2545. DOI: 10.1021/acsanm.3c05615

Mahmoudi, Z., Soleymani, F., Mesgari Abbasi, S., Khalaj, G., & Najafi, A. (2024). Sol-gel synthesis and characterization of mesoporous TiB2 nano powder via Titanium isopropoxide /trimethyl borate precursors. *Ceramics International*, *50*(11), 18081–18089. DOI: 10.1016/j.ceramint.2024.02.304

Majerič, P., Friedrich, B., & Rudolf, R. (2015). Au-nanoparticle synthesis via ultrasonic spray pyrolysis with a separate evaporation zone. *Materiali in Tehnologije*, *49*(5), 791–796. DOI: 10.17222/mit.2014.264

Maruggi, G., Chiarot, E., Giovani, C., Buccato, S., Bonacci, S., Frigimelica, E., Margarit, I., Geall, A., Bensi, G., & Maione, D. (2017). Immunogenicity and protective efficacy induced by self-amplifying mRNA vaccines encoding bacterial antigens. *Vaccine*, *35*(2), 361–368. DOI: 10.1016/j.vaccine.2016.11.040 PMID: 27939014

Mayer, R. L., Verbeke, R., Asselman, C., Aernout, I., Gul, A., Eggermont, D., Boucher, K., Thery, F., Maia, T. M., Demol, H., Gabriels, R., Martens, L., Bécavin, C., De Smedt, S. C., Vandekerckhove, B., Lentacker, I., & Impens, F. (2022). Immunopeptidomics-based design of mRNA vaccine formulations against Listeria monocytogenes. *Nature Communications*, *13*(1), 6075. DOI: 10.1038/s41467-022-33721-y PMID: 36241641

Medarametla, R. T., Kumar, D. J. N. S., Gopaiah, D. K. V., Harshad, S. K., Nannesha, P., Prasad, P. R. D., Mouli, P., & Pravallika, R. L. (2024). Utilization of artificial intelligence and computational modeling in nanomedicine. *International Journal of Pharmacy and Pharmaceutical Sciences*, *6*(2), 106–109. DOI: 10.33545/26647222.2024.v6.i2b.130

Mellbye, B., & Schuster, M. (2011). The Sociomicrobiology of Antivirulence Drug Resistance: A Proof of Concept. *mBio*, *2*(5), e00131-11. DOI: 10.1128/mBio.00131-11 PMID: 21990612

Meza-Segura, M., Birtley, J. R., Maldonado-Contreras, A., Mueller, C., Simin, K. J., Stern, L. J., & McCormick, B. A. (2021). SepA Enhances *Shigella* Invasion of Epithelial Cells by Degrading Alpha-1 Antitrypsin and Producing a Neutrophil Chemoattractant. *mBio*, *12*(6), e02833-21. DOI: 10.1128/mBio.02833-21 PMID: 34724811

Micoli, F., & MacLennan, C. A. (2020). Outer membrane vesicle vaccines. *Seminars in Immunology*, *50*, 101433. DOI: 10.1016/j.smim.2020.101433 PMID: 33309166

Miikkulainen, V., Leskelä, M., Ritala, M., & Puurunen, R. L. (2013). Crystallinity of inorganic films grown by atomic layer deposition: Overview and general trends. *Journal of Applied Physics*, *113*(2), 021301. DOI: 10.1063/1.4757907

Mikušová, V., & Mikuš, P. (2021). Advances in Chitosan-Based Nanoparticles for Drug Delivery. *International Journal of Molecular Sciences*, *22*(17), 9652. DOI: 10.3390/ijms22179652 PMID: 34502560

Mocan, T., Matea, C. T., Pop, T., Mosteanu, O., Buzoianu, A. D., Suciu, S., Puia, C., Zdrehus, C., Iancu, C., & Mocan, L. (2017). Carbon nanotubes as anti-bacterial agents. *Cellular and Molecular Life Sciences : CMLS*, *74*(19), 3467–3479. DOI: 10.1007/s00018-017-2532-y PMID: 28536787

Modabberasl, A., Jaberolansar, E., Kameli, P., & Nikmanesh, H. (2024). Hydrothermal as a synthesis method for characterization of structural, morphological and magnetic properties of Co–Al ferrite nanoparticles. *Materials Chemistry and Physics*, *314*, 128832. DOI: 10.1016/j.matchemphys.2023.128832

Mohammadjani, N., Karimi, S., Moetasam Zorab, M., Ashengroph, M., & Alavi, M. (2023). Comparative molecular docking and toxicity between carbon-capped metal oxide nanoparticles and standard drugs in cancer and bacterial infections. *BioImpacts*, *14*, 27778. DOI: 10.34172/bi.2023.27778 PMID: 38505671

Mohammed, H. A., Sahi, N. M., Ahmed, R. T., & Al-Rubaye, A. (2022). Antimicrobial Activity of Some Nanoparticles Synthesized by Laser Ablation Technique against Some Bacteria Isolated from Oral Cavity. *Medical Journal of Babylon, 19*(4), 601–608. DOI: 10.4103/MJBL.MJBL_147_22

Muhammad, A., Champeimont, J., Mayr, U. B., Lubitz, W., & Kudela, P. (2012). Bacterial ghosts as carriers of protein subunit and DNA-encoded antigens for vaccine applications. *Expert Review of Vaccines, 11*(1), 97–116. DOI: 10.1586/erv.11.149 PMID: 22149712

Mwenze, N. M., Juma, M., Maaza, M., Birech, Z., & Dhlamini, M. S. (2023). Laser liquid ablation for silver nanoparticles synthesis and conjugation with hydroxychloroquine for Covid-19 treatment. *Materials Today: Proceedings*. Advance online publication. DOI: 10.1016/j.matpr.2023.08.195

Nadagouda, M. N., Speth, T. F., & Varma, R. S. (2011). Microwave-Assisted Green Synthesis of Silver Nanostructures. *Accounts of Chemical Research, 44*(7), 469–478. DOI: 10.1021/ar1001457 PMID: 21526846

Nawaz, K., ... Algal-Mediated Biosynthesis of Nanoparticles and Their Potential Therapeutic Applications, *in* (2021): pp. 171–210. DOI: 10.1007/978-3-030-81557-8_8

Nguyen, L., & Pieters, J. (2005). The Trojan horse: Survival tactics of pathogenic mycobacteria in macrophages. *Trends in Cell Biology, 15*(5), 269–276. DOI: 10.1016/j.tcb.2005.03.009 PMID: 15866031

Nguyen, V. N., Nguyen, V. B., Tran, M. D., Doan, M. D., Nguyen, D. S., Nguyen, T. H., Doan, C. T., Tran, T. N., Wang, S. L., & Nguyen, A. D. (2024). Enhancing the antibacterial activity of ampicillin loaded into chitosan/starch nanocomposites against AMR Staphylococcus aureus. *Carbohydrate Research, 545*, 109274. DOI: 10.1016/j.carres.2024.109274 PMID: 39303315

Osman, N., Devnarain, N., Omolo, C. A., Fasiku, V., Jaglal, Y., & Govender, T. (2022). Surface modification of nano-drug delivery systems for enhancing antibiotic delivery and activity. *Wiley Interdisciplinary Reviews. Nanomedicine and Nanobiotechnology, 14*(1), e1758. DOI: 10.1002/wnan.1758 PMID: 34643067

Paredes da Rocha, N.. (2023). Highly water-soluble dapsone nanocrystals: Towards innovative preparations for an undermined drug. *International Journal of Pharmaceutics, 630*, 122428. DOI: 10.1016/j.ijpharm.2022.122428 PMID: 36436741

Pedersen, H., & Elliott, S. D. (2014). Studying chemical vapor deposition processes with theoretical chemistry. *Theoretical Chemistry Accounts*, *133*(5), 1476. DOI: 10.1007/s00214-014-1476-7

Pelgrift, R. Y., & Friedman, A. J. (2013). Nanotechnology as a therapeutic tool to combat microbial resistance. *Advanced Drug Delivery Reviews*, *65*(13–14), 1803–1815. DOI: 10.1016/j.addr.2013.07.011 PMID: 23892192

Perveen, R., Shujaat, S., Qureshi, Z., Nawaz, S., Khan, M. I., & Iqbal, M. (2020). Green versus sol-gel synthesis of ZnO nanoparticles and antimicrobial activity evaluation against panel of pathogens. *Journal of Materials Research and Technology*, *9*(4), 7817–7827. DOI: 10.1016/j.jmrt.2020.05.004

Poater, A., Saliner, A. G., Solà, M., Cavallo, L., & Worth, A. P. (2010). Computational methods to predict the reactivity of nanoparticles through structure–property relationships. *Expert Opinion on Drug Delivery*, *7*(3), 295–305. DOI: 10.1517/17425240903508756 PMID: 20201736

Ponja, S. D., Sehmi, S. K., Allan, E., MacRobert, A. J., Parkin, I. P., & Carmalt, C. J. (2015). Enhanced Bactericidal Activity of Silver Thin Films Deposited via Aerosol-Assisted Chemical Vapor Deposition. *ACS Applied Materials & Interfaces*, *7*(51), 28616–28623. DOI: 10.1021/acsami.5b10171 PMID: 26632854

Prabakaran, S., & Rajan, M. (2021). *Biosynthesis of nanoparticles and their roles in numerous areas*. DOI: 10.1016/bs.coac.2021.02.001

Prasad Yadav, T., Manohar Yadav, R., & Pratap Singh, D. (2012). Mechanical Milling: A Top Down Approach for the Synthesis of Nanomaterials and Nanocomposites. *Nanoscience and Nanotechnology*, *2*(3), 22–48. DOI: 10.5923/j.nn.20120203.01

Raja Rajamanikkam, S. C. R., Anbalagan, G., Subramanian, B., Suresh, V., & Sivaperumal, P. (2024). Green Synthesis of Copper and Copper Oxide Nanoparticles From Brown Algae Turbinaria Species' Aqueous Extract and Its Antibacterial Properties. *Cureus*. Advance online publication. DOI: 10.7759/cureus.57366 PMID: 38694645

Rama, P., Mariselvi, P., Sundaram, R., & Muthu, K. (2023). Eco-friendly green synthesis of silver nanoparticles from Aegle marmelos leaf extract and their antimicrobial, antioxidant, anticancer and photocatalytic degradation activity. *Heliyon*, *9*(6), e16277. DOI: 10.1016/j.heliyon.2023.e16277 PMID: 37255978

Ramesh, S. (2013). Sol-Gel Synthesis and Characterization of Nanoparticles. *Journal of Nanoscience*, *2013*, 1–8. DOI: 10.1155/2013/929321

Rashdan, S.. (2013). Nanoparticles for biomedical applications: current status, trends and future challenges. In *Biomaterials and Medical Tribology* (pp. 1–132). Elsevier. DOI: 10.1533/9780857092205.1

Regiel-Futyra, A., Kus-Liśkiewicz, M., Sebastian, V., Irusta, S., Arruebo, M., Kyzioł, A., & Stochel, G. (2017). Development of noncytotoxic silver–chitosan nanocomposites for efficient control of biofilm forming microbes. *RSC Advances*, *7*(83), 52398–52413. DOI: 10.1039/C7RA08359A PMID: 29308194

Rhim, J. W., Wang, L. F., & Hong, S. I. (2013). Preparation and characterization of agar/silver nanoparticles composite films with antimicrobial activity. *Food Hydrocolloids*, *33*(2), 327–335. DOI: 10.1016/j.foodhyd.2013.04.002

Rincón-Granados, K. L., Vázquez-Olmos, A. R., Rodríguez-Hernández, A.-P., Vega-Jiménez, A., Ruiz, F., Garibay-Febles, V., & Ximénez-Fyvie, L.-A. (2021). Facile solid-state synthesis and study in vitro of the antibacterial activity of NiO and NiFe2O4 nanoparticles. *Materialia*, *15*, 100955. DOI: 10.1016/j.mtla.2020.100955

Román, L. E., Gomez, E. D., Solís, J. L., & Gómez, M. M. (2020). Antibacterial Cotton Fabric Functionalized with Copper Oxide Nanoparticles. *Molecules (Basel, Switzerland)*, *25*(24), 5802. DOI: 10.3390/molecules25245802 PMID: 33316935

Rudra, S. (2024). Harnessing Nature's Power for Eco-Friendly Metal Nanoparticle Synthesis and Applications. *Authorea Preprints*.

Salah, N., Habib, , Khan, , Memic, , Azam, , Al-Hamedi, , Zahed, , & Habib, . (2011). High-energy ball milling technique for ZnO nanoparticles as antibacterial material. *International Journal of Nanomedicine*, •••, 863. DOI: 10.2147/IJN.S18267 PMID: 21720499

Sasaninia, K., Kelley, M., Abnousian, A., Badaoui, A., Alexander, L., Sheren, N., Owens, J., Rajurkar, S., Razo-Botello, B., Chorbajian, A., Yoon, S., Dhama, S., Avitia, E., Ochoa, C., Yutani, R., & Venketaraman, V. (2023). Topical Absorption of Glutathione–Cyclodextrin Nanoparticle Complex in Healthy Human Subjects Improves Immune Response against Mycobacterium avium Infection. *Antioxidants*, *12*(7), 1375. DOI: 10.3390/antiox12071375 PMID: 37507915

Sathiyaseelan, A., Saravanakumar, K., Zhang, X., Naveen, K. V., & Wang, M.-H. (2023). Ampicillin-resistant bacterial pathogens targeted chitosan nano-drug delivery system (CS-AMP-P-ZnO) for combinational antibacterial treatment. *International Journal of Biological Macromolecules*, *237*, 124129. DOI: 10.1016/j.ijbiomac.2023.124129 PMID: 36958450

Schwendener, R. A., ... Liposome-Based Vaccines, *in* (2010): pp. 163–175. DOI: 10.1007/978-1-60327-360-2_11

Serov, N., & Vinogradov, V. (2022). Artificial intelligence to bring nanomedicine to life. *Advanced Drug Delivery Reviews, 184*, 114194. DOI: 10.1016/j.addr.2022.114194 PMID: 35283223

Shah, P., & Gavrin, A. (2006). Synthesis of nanoparticles using high-pressure sputtering for magnetic domain imaging. *Journal of Magnetism and Magnetic Materials, 301*(1), 118–123. DOI: 10.1016/j.jmmm.2005.06.023

Shankar, S., & Rhim, J.-W. (2015). Amino acid mediated synthesis of silver nanoparticles and preparation of antimicrobial agar/silver nanoparticles composite films. *Carbohydrate Polymers, 130*, 353–363. DOI: 10.1016/j.carbpol.2015.05.018 PMID: 26076636

Sharma, B., Purkayastha, D. D., Hazra, S., Thajamanbi, M., Bhattacharjee, C. R., Ghosh, N. N., & Rout, J. (2014). Biosynthesis of fluorescent gold nanoparticles using an edible freshwater red alga, Lemanea fluviatilis (L) CAg and antioxidant activity of biomatrix loaded nanoparticles. *Bioprocess and Biosystems Engineering, 37*(12), 2559–2565. DOI: 10.1007/s00449-014-1233-2 PMID: 24942533

Shende, S., Ingle, A. P., Gade, A., & Rai, M. (2015). Green synthesis of copper nanoparticles by Citrus medica Linn (Idilimbu) juice and its antimicrobial activity. *World Journal of Microbiology & Biotechnology, 31*(6), 865–873. DOI: 10.1007/s11274-015-1840-3 PMID: 25761857

Shojaei, M., Shokuhfar, A., & Zolriasatein, A. (2021). Synthesis and characterization of CuAlS2 nanoparticles by mechanical milling. *Materials Today. Communications, 27*, 102243. DOI: 10.1016/j.mtcomm.2021.102243

Shraouba, A., & Makkia, G. (2022). Impact of Some Essential Oils and Nanoparticles in Chitosan Films to Control Pathogenic Bacteria and Storage Keeping Quality of Meat Products. *Annals of Agricultural Sciences, Moshtohor, 60*(4), 1175–1192. DOI: 10.21608/assjm.2022.284130

Simmons, J. D., Stein, C. M., Seshadri, C., Campo, M., Alter, G., Fortune, S., Schurr, E., Wallis, R. S., Churchyard, G., Mayanja-Kizza, H., Boom, W. H., & Hawn, T. R. (2018). Immunological mechanisms of human resistance to persistent Mycobacterium tuberculosis infection. *Nature Reviews. Immunology, 18*(9), 575–589. DOI: 10.1038/s41577-018-0025-3 PMID: 29895826

Singaravelu, G., Arockiamary, J. S., Kumar, V. G., & Govindaraju, K. (2007). A novel extracellular synthesis of monodisperse gold nanoparticles using marine alga, Sargassum wightii Greville. *Colloids and Surfaces. B, Biointerfaces*, *57*(1), 97–101. DOI: 10.1016/j.colsurfb.2007.01.010 PMID: 17350236

Singh, A. V., Ansari, M. H. D., Rosenkranz, D., Maharjan, R. S., Kriegel, F. L., Gandhi, K., Kanase, A., Singh, R., Laux, P., & Luch, A. (2020). Artificial Intelligence and Machine Learning in Computational Nanotoxicology: Unlocking and Empowering Nanomedicine. *Advanced Healthcare Materials*, *9*(17), 1901862. DOI: 10.1002/adhm.201901862 PMID: 32627972

Singh, P., Kim, Y.-J., Zhang, D., & Yang, D.-C. (2016). Biological Synthesis of Nanoparticles from Plants and Microorganisms. *Trends in Biotechnology*, *34*(7), 588–599. DOI: 10.1016/j.tibtech.2016.02.006 PMID: 26944794

Jalali, T., Ghanavati, F., & Osfouri, S. (2024). Green synthesis of ZnO nanoparticles using marine brown algae (Cystoseira) extract comprising sol–gel, and combustion techniques based on dye-sensitized solar cells application. *International Journal of Modern Physics B*, *38*(14), 2450178.

Tai, C. Y., Tai, C.-T., Chang, M.-H., & Liu, H.-S. (2007). Synthesis of Magnesium Hydroxide and Oxide Nanoparticles Using a Spinning Disk Reactor. *Industrial & Engineering Chemistry Research*, *46*(17), 5536–5541. DOI: 10.1021/ie060869b

Tan, K., Li, R., Huang, X., & Liu, Q. (2018). Outer Membrane Vesicles: Current Status and Future Direction of These Novel Vaccine Adjuvants. *Frontiers in Microbiology*, *9*, 9. DOI: 10.3389/fmicb.2018.00783 PMID: 29755431

Thamphiwatana, S., Angsantikul, P., Escajadillo, T., Zhang, Q., Olson, J., Luk, B. T., Zhang, S., Fang, R. H., Gao, W., Nizet, V., & Zhang, L. (2017). Macrophage-like nanoparticles concurrently absorbing endotoxins and proinflammatory cytokines for sepsis management. *Proceedings of the National Academy of Sciences of the United States of America*, *114*(43), 11488–11493. DOI: 10.1073/pnas.1714267114 PMID: 29073076

Tian, B., Liu, Y., & Chen, D. (2021). Adhesion behavior of silica nanoparticles with bacteria: Spectroscopy measurements based on kinetics, and molecular docking. *Journal of Molecular Liquids*, *343*, 117651. DOI: 10.1016/j.molliq.2021.117651

Tripathi, V. S. Hydrothermal Method for Synthesis of Materials, *in* (2021): pp. 131–152. DOI: 10.1007/978-981-16-1807-9_5

Vardar, Ö., Mehmetoğlu Al, A., & Yıldırım, Y. (2024). Coffee Active Ingredient Loaded Biopolymer Nanoparticles: Synthesis and Characterization, *Celal Bayar Üniversitesi. Fen Bilimleri Dergisi*, *20*(2), 72–81.

Wahab, S., Salman, A., Khan, Z., Khan, S., Krishnaraj, C., & Yun, S.-I. (2023). Metallic Nanoparticles: A Promising Arsenal against Antimicrobial Resistance—Unraveling Mechanisms and Enhancing Medication Efficacy. *International Journal of Molecular Sciences*, *24*(19), 14897. DOI: 10.3390/ijms241914897 PMID: 37834344

Wang, S., & Gao, L. (2019). Laser-driven nanomaterials and laser-enabled nanofabrication for industrial applications. In *Industrial Applications of Nanomaterials* (pp. 181–203). Elsevier. DOI: 10.1016/B978-0-12-815749-7.00007-4

Wang, Y., Zhang, Z., Luo, J., Han, X., Wei, Y., & Wei, X. (2021). mRNA vaccine: A potential therapeutic strategy. *Molecular Cancer*, *20*(1), 33. DOI: 10.1186/s12943-021-01311-z PMID: 33593376

Wang, Z., Zhu, J., Chen, L., Deng, K., & Huang, H. (2023). Multifunctional Gold–Silver–Carbon Quantum Dots Nano-Hybrid Composite: Advancing Antibacterial Wound Healing and Cell Proliferation. *ACS Applied Materials & Interfaces*, *15*(34), 40241–40254. DOI: 10.1021/acsami.3c07625 PMID: 37599603

Webster, T., Wang, Q., & Larese-Casanova, P. (2015). Inhibition of various gram-positive and gram-negative bacteria growth on selenium nanoparticle coated paper towels. *International Journal of Nanomedicine*, •••, 2885. DOI: 10.2147/IJN.S78466 PMID: 25926733

Woźniak-Budych, M. J., Staszak, K., & Staszak, M. (2023). Copper and Copper-Based Nanoparticles in Medicine—Perspectives and Challenges. *Molecules (Basel, Switzerland)*, *28*(18), 6687. DOI: 10.3390/molecules28186687 PMID: 37764463

Wu, Y., Gao, H., Liu, J., & Liang, H. (2023). Chitosan nanoparticles efficiently enhance the dispersibility, stability and selective antibacterial activity of insoluble isoflavonoids. *International Journal of Biological Macromolecules*, *232*, 123420. DOI: 10.1016/j.ijbiomac.2023.123420 PMID: 36708890

Yang, D., Chen, Z., Gao, Z., Tammina, S. K., & Yang, Y. (2020). Nanozymes used for antimicrobials and their applications. *Colloids and Surfaces. B, Biointerfaces*, *195*, 111252. DOI: 10.1016/j.colsurfb.2020.111252 PMID: 32679446

Zhang, M., Huang, Y., Zhuang, Y., Chen, Y., & Zhou, Y. (2023). Antimicrobial copper ion-graphene oxide composite to inhibit *Pseudomonas Aeruginosa* keratitis in rabbits. *MedComm - Biomaterials and Applications*, *2*(3), e56. DOI: 10.1002/mba2.56

Zhang, Q., Yang, Z., Ding, B., Lan, X., & Guo, Y.Q. ZHANG et al. (2010). Preparation of copper nanoparticles by chemical reduction method using potassium borohydride. *Transactions of Nonferrous Metals Society of China*, *20*, s240–s244. DOI: 10.1016/S1003-6326(10)60047-7

Zhang, X., Sun, H., Tan, S., Gao, J., Fu, Y., & Liu, Z. (2019). Hydrothermal synthesis of Ag nanoparticles on the nanocellulose and their antibacterial study. *Inorganic Chemistry Communications*, *100*, 44–50. DOI: 10.1016/j.inoche.2018.12.012

Zhao, Z., Yan, R., Yi, X., Li, J., Rao, J., Guo, Z., Yang, Y., Li, W., Li, Y.-Q., & Chen, C. (2017). Bacteria-Activated Theranostic Nanoprobes against Methicillin-Resistant *Staphylococcus aureus* Infection. *ACS Nano*, *11*(5), 4428–4438. DOI: 10.1021/acsnano.7b00041 PMID: 28350437

Zou, X., Cai, S., Wang, T., Zheng, S., Cui, X., Hao, J., Chen, X., Liu, Y., Zhang, Z., & Li, Y. (2023). Natural antibacterial agent-based nanoparticles for effective treatment of intracellular MRSA infection. *Acta Biomaterialia*, *169*, 410–421. DOI: 10.1016/j.actbio.2023.08.004 PMID: 37557944

Chapter 4 Sustainable and Eco-Friendly Nanomaterials: Innovation for Eco-Friendly Green Healthcare Solutions

Anita Restu Puji Raharjeng
https://orcid.org/0000-0002-8308-4574
Universitas Islam Negeri Raden Fatah Palembang, Palembang, Indonesia

Evika Sandi Savitri
Universitas Islam Negeri Maulana Malik Ibrahim, Malang, Indonesia

Ruqiah Ganda Putri Panjaitan
https://orcid.org/0000-0002-2194-8808
Tanjungpura University, Pontianak, Indonesia

ABSTRACT

This book chapter elucidates key concepts such as the molecular mechanisms of life, biomolecular synthesis, bioenergetics, and chemical interactions within biological systems. This integrated approach is designed to support a science curriculum that meets contemporary needs, emphasizing the exploration of real-world phenomena through laboratory experiments, digital simulations, and cutting-edge technological applications. This book chapter also highlights the importance of global issues such as climate change, waste management, and public health in the context of biology and chemistry. With a research-driven methodology and problem-based learning approaches, it offers practical guidance for educators, students, and researchers to effectively apply molecular science in various academic and industrial contexts. Through educational innovation and cross-disciplinary integration, Molecular Revolution aims to inspire transformation in science teaching and learning, build-

DOI: 10.4018/979-8-3373-1305-4.ch004

ing a strong foundation for future generations to address global challenges with knowledge and empathy.

1. INTRODUCTION

The need for sustainable innovations has gained widespread attention in recent decades due to growing environmental challenges. The healthcare industry, while primarily focused on improving human health and well-being, has a significant environmental footprint that cannot be ignored. Traditional healthcare systems contribute to a range of environmental issues, including the generation of large amounts of hazardous medical waste, high consumption of non-renewable resources, and significant greenhouse gas emissions (Hamad et al., 2014; Stoner, 1986). Hospitals, for instance, are energy-intensive institutions that produce vast quantities of waste, including disposable medical tools, pharmaceutical byproducts, and single-use plastics (McGain, 2015). Furthermore, the carbon footprint associated with the global supply chain of medical devices, pharmaceuticals, and healthcare infrastructure compounds the environmental burden.

These challenges call for a fundamental transformation of how healthcare services are designed and delivered. Sustainability in healthcare requires innovative solutions that minimize environmental impact while maintaining or improving patient outcomes. One of the most promising areas of innovation is the use of sustainable and eco-friendly nanomaterials. Nanotechnology, with its ability to manipulate materials at the atomic and molecular levels, offers revolutionary possibilities for creating solutions that are not only efficient but also environmentally conscious (Malik et al., 2023). Nanomaterials exhibit unique properties, such as high surface area, tunable chemical and physical characteristics, and biocompatibility, making them ideal candidates for addressing a wide range of healthcare needs (Kyriakides et al., 2021).

The application of eco-friendly nanomaterials holds immense potential in redefining healthcare practices (Aithal et al., 2021a). For instance, nanomaterials can enhance the delivery and efficacy of drugs, allowing for targeted therapies that reduce dosage requirements and minimize side effects (A. P. Singh et al., 2019). Biodegradable nanomaterials can replace conventional non-degradable plastics in medical devices, reducing the accumulation of medical waste (Kothawade et al., 2024). Similarly, nanotechnology can be used to develop antimicrobial coatings for surgical instruments and hospital surfaces, minimizing the risk of healthcare-associated infections while reducing the need for chemical disinfectants that can harm the environment (Alhmoud, 2024a).

This chapter aims to explore the pivotal role of sustainable and eco-friendly nanomaterials in transforming healthcare into a greener and more sustainable system. It delves into the environmental challenges posed by traditional healthcare practices and highlights how nanotechnology can address these issues. The chapter will also discuss the synthesis and design of sustainable nanomaterials, their diverse applications in healthcare, and the environmental and ethical considerations associated with their use. By bridging the gap between advanced nanotechnology and environmental sustainability, this chapter seeks to provide valuable insights into how innovative nanomaterials can contribute to a healthier planet and population.

Ultimately, this chapter emphasizes the importance of integrating sustainability into the core of healthcare innovation. As the global demand for healthcare services continues to rise, finding eco-friendly solutions becomes not just an opportunity but an imperative. Sustainable nanomaterials represent a crucial step toward achieving this goal, paving the way for a future where healthcare is both effective and environmentally responsible (Solomon et al., 2024)

2. UNDERSTANDING SUSTAINABLE AND ECO-FRIENDLY NANOMATERIALS

Nanomaterials are materials engineered at the nanoscale, typically ranging from 1 to 100 nanometers, and they possess unique physical, chemical, and biological properties (Findik, 2021). These properties, such as high surface area-to-volume ratio, tunable optical and electronic behavior, and enhanced reactivity, have made nanomaterials a cornerstone of innovation across diverse fields, including healthcare, energy, and environmental science (Liberty et al., 2024). However, the growing production and use of nanomaterials have raised concerns about their environmental impact and long-term sustainability (Kabir et al., 2018). This has led to the emergence of sustainable and eco-friendly nanomaterials, which are designed to minimize harm to the environment and human health while maintaining high performance and functionality.

2.1. Definition of Sustainable and Eco-Friendly Nanomaterials

Sustainable and eco-friendly nanomaterials refer to materials that are developed using processes and resources that adhere to principles of environmental sustainability (Aithal et al., 2021b; Sfameni et al., 2023). These materials prioritize the use of renewable or naturally derived resources, minimize energy-intensive and toxic production methods, and aim to reduce waste and ecological disruption during their life cycle (Ramadan et al., 2024). In healthcare, eco-friendly nanomaterials are particularly valued for their potential to address critical medical challenges while aligning with environmental conservation goals (Pokrajac et al., 2021).

2.2. Criteria for Sustainability in Nanomaterials

2.2.1. Use of Renewable Raw Materials

One of the core principles of sustainability in nanomaterials is the reliance on renewable or naturally abundant resources (Gilbertson et al., 2015). For instance, nanomaterials synthesized from plant extracts, microbial sources, or biodegradable polymers such as cellulose and chitosan exemplify this criterion (Das et al., 2017). By using renewable inputs, the dependency on finite resources like fossil fuels and rare metals is reduced, contributing to resource conservation.

2.2.2. Energy-Efficient and Low-Toxicity Production Processes

Sustainable nanomaterials are produced through energy-efficient methods that minimize carbon emissions and waste generation (Chakrabartty et al., 2022). Green synthesis techniques, which utilize natural reducing agents like plant extracts or enzymes, have gained popularity as an alternative to traditional chemical synthesis methods that often involve hazardous solvents and high energy consumption (Ahmed et al., 2022). These methods not only reduce environmental pollution but also improve the biocompatibility of the resulting nanomaterials, making them safer for medical and environmental applications.

2.2.3. Safety for Humans and the Environment

A key aspect of sustainable nanomaterials is their low toxicity and minimal environmental impact (Saleem et al., 2020). Materials that are biodegradable or that degrade into non-toxic byproducts are preferred, especially in healthcare applications where long-term exposure or accumulation in biological systems can pose risks. For example, nanoparticles made from natural biopolymers or biosynthesized metals are often safer alternatives to conventional synthetic nanomaterials that may persist in the environment or bioaccumulate in living organisms (Saratale et al., 2018).

2.3. Examples of Sustainable and Eco-Friendly Nanomaterials

2.3.1. Carbon-Based Nanomaterials

Carbon-based nanomaterials, such as graphene and carbon nanotubes (CNTs), have shown significant promise in sustainable applications (Nasrollahzadeh et al., 2021). These materials can be derived from renewable biomass sources and exhibit exceptional mechanical strength, electrical conductivity, and chemical stability. For instance, graphene, a two-dimensional material made of carbon atoms, is widely used in medical sensors, drug delivery systems, and tissue engineering (Goenka et al., 2014). Similarly, CNTs offer potential in advanced diagnostics and as carriers for therapeutic agents due to their high surface area and customizable functional groups (Loh et al., 2018).

2.3.2. Green-Synthesized Metallic Nanomaterials

Metallic nanoparticles, such as silver and zinc nanoparticles, have been extensively utilized in healthcare for their antimicrobial, anti-inflammatory, and wound-healing properties (Mendes et al., 2022). However, traditional methods of synthesizing these nanoparticles often involve toxic chemicals and generate hazardous waste (Bystrzejewska-Piotrowska et al., 2009). Green synthesis methods, which use plant extracts, bacteria, or fungi as reducing agents, have emerged as a sustainable alternative. For example, biosynthesized silver nanoparticles (AgNPs) produced using plant-based methods are widely used in antimicrobial coatings for medical devices, offering both efficacy and reduced environmental toxicity (Thomas et al., 2024). Zinc oxide nanoparticles (ZnO NPs), synthesized using similar methods, are biodegradable and exhibit strong UV-blocking and antimicrobial properties, making them ideal for use in cosmetics and wound dressings (Irede et al., 2024).

2.3.3. Biopolymers such as Chitosan and Cellulose

Biopolymers like chitosan and cellulose represent another category of sustainable nanomaterials (Mallakpour et al., 2021). Derived from renewable resources, such as crustacean shells (chitosan) and plant biomass (cellulose), these materials are biodegradable, non-toxic, and biocompatible. Chitosan nanoparticles are extensively used in drug delivery systems due to their ability to encapsulate therapeutic agents and release them in a controlled manner (Nagpal et al., 2010). Similarly, cellulose nanocrystals and nanofibers are employed in wound dressings, tissue scaffolds, and biosensors due to their excellent mechanical properties and versatility (Soroush et al., 2022).

3. GREEN SYNTHESIS OF NANOMATERIALS

The synthesis of nanomaterials is a critical aspect of nanotechnology, determining not only the properties and applications of the materials but also their environmental impact. Traditional methods for producing nanomaterials often involve energy-intensive processes and hazardous chemicals, raising concerns about their sustainability and potential toxicity to humans and ecosystems (Mazari et al., 2021). In response, green synthesis has emerged as a promising alternative, offering eco-friendly approaches that align with the principles of sustainability. This chapter delves into the methods, principles, and examples of green synthesis in nanomaterials, highlighting its significance in reducing environmental footprints while ensuring efficiency and safety.

1.1. Eco-Friendly Approaches to Nanomaterial Synthesis

Green synthesis refers to the production of nanomaterials using methods that minimize environmental harm, reduce chemical waste, and prioritize the use of renewable and non-toxic resources (Soltys et al., 2021). It emphasizes the use of natural agents, low-energy processes, and environmentally benign solvents to achieve high-quality nanomaterials. Two of the most prominent strategies in green synthesis are the use of natural biological agents and the implementation of waste-reducing technologies (El-Sayyad et al., 2024).

1.1.1. Utilizing Natural Agents for Synthesis

One of the key innovations in green synthesis is the use of biological entities such as plant extracts, microorganisms, and enzymes as reducing and stabilizing agents (Bahrulolum et al., 2021). These natural agents not only eliminate the need for hazardous chemicals but also offer a biocompatible approach to nanomaterial production.

1.1.2. Plant Extracts

Plants are rich in bioactive compounds, including polyphenols, alkaloids, terpenoids, and flavonoids, which can act as reducing agents to convert metal salts into nanoparticles (Savitri et al., 2024; Shafey, 2020). For instance, plant extracts derived from leaves, flowers, or roots can effectively reduce silver ions (Ag^{+}) to silver nanoparticles (AgNPs) while stabilizing them to prevent aggregation (Saifuddin et al., 2024). This process is simple, cost-effective, and scalable, making it a popular choice for synthesizing antimicrobial nanoparticles.

1.1.3. Microorganisms

Microbes such as bacteria, fungi, and algae have demonstrated remarkable potential in nanoparticle biosynthesis. These organisms naturally produce enzymes and metabolites that can facilitate the reduction of metal salts into nanoparticles. For example, *Bacillus subtilis* has been used to synthesize gold nanoparticles, while *Fusarium oxysporum* has shown promise in producing silver nanoparticles (Sikkander et al., 2024; Srinath et al., 2018) (Srinath et al., 2018). The microbial route is particularly advantageous due to its ability to operate at ambient temperatures and pressures, reducing energy consumption (Rabaey et al., 2010).

1.1.4. Enzymes

Enzymatic synthesis involves using isolated enzymes to catalyze the formation of nanoparticles. Enzymes such as nitrate reductase and laccase can precisely control the size and shape of nanoparticles, ensuring high reproducibility and efficiency (Elegbede et al., 2021). This method is especially useful for creating biocompatible nanoparticles for medical applications.

1.2. Reducing Chemical Waste Through Green Technology

Green synthesis also incorporates waste-minimizing technologies to make nanoparticle production cleaner and more sustainable (Fatiqin et al., 2021).

3.2.1. Solvent-Free and Aqueous Methods

Many green synthesis protocols avoid organic solvents, relying instead on water as a reaction medium (Cseri et al., 2018). This eliminates the generation of hazardous solvent waste and makes the process safer for both humans and the environment.

3.2.2. Energy-Efficient Processes

Technologies such as microwave-assisted synthesis and sonochemical methods (using ultrasound energy) reduce reaction times and energy inputs compared to traditional heating methods (Adhi et al., 2024). These techniques not only improve the sustainability of nanoparticle production but also enhance the uniformity and quality of the resulting nanomaterials.

1.3. Examples of Green Synthesis Processes

3.3.1 Biosynthesis of Silver Nanoparticles Using Plant Extracts

Silver nanoparticles (AgNPs) are widely recognized for their antimicrobial and catalytic properties, making them valuable in healthcare and environmental applications (Beyene et al., 2017). Green synthesis of AgNPs using plant extracts is a well-documented process. For instance, extracts from *Azadirachta indica* (neem) leaves have been used to synthesize AgNPs by reducing silver nitrate ($AgNO_3$) to metallic silver (Ghazali et al., 2022). The bioactive compounds in the extract serve as both reducing and capping agents, ensuring stable nanoparticle formation (Javed et al., 2020). This method is highly efficient, as it eliminates the need for hazardous chemicals and generates minimal waste.

3.3.2. Enzyme- and Microbe-Based Synthesis

Enzyme-driven nanoparticle synthesis offers a high degree of control over nanoparticle size and morphology. For example, nitrate reductase enzymes from fungi have been utilized to synthesize gold nanoparticles with consistent size distributions (Hamedi et al., 2017). Similarly, microbial synthesis has been applied to produce zinc oxide nanoparticles (ZnO NPs) using *Rhizopus oryzae*. These ZnO NPs exhibit strong antimicrobial properties and are biodegradable, making them ideal for use in biomedicine and food packaging (Chong et al., 2023).

3.3.3. Microwave-Assisted Green Synthesis

Microwave-assisted techniques further enhance green synthesis by accelerating reaction times and improving nanoparticle yield. For example, gold nanoparticles (AuNPs) can be synthesized in minutes using aqueous plant extracts under microwave irradiation (Francis et al., 2018). This approach combines the benefits of green chemistry with advanced energy-efficient technologies, offering rapid and scalable production.

4. APPLICATIONS OF ECO-FRIENDLY NANOMATERIALS IN HEALTHCARE

Nanomaterials have revolutionized modern healthcare with their unique properties, including high surface-to-volume ratio, biocompatibility, and tunable chemical characteristics. Eco-friendly nanomaterials, in particular, are transforming healthcare by offering sustainable solutions that reduce environmental impact while enhancing the quality of medical care (Alhmoud, 2024b). From disease diagnosis and treatment to infection control and tissue regeneration, these materials are addressing critical challenges in healthcare. This section explores the diverse applications of eco-friendly nanomaterials in diagnostics, therapeutics, antimicrobial strategies, and tissue engineering.

4.1. Diagnosis and Treatment

Nanomaterials have significantly improved the precision and efficiency of disease diagnosis and treatment. By leveraging their unique physical and chemical properties, eco-friendly nanomaterials are enabling earlier detection of diseases and more effective therapeutic interventions.

4.1.1. Disease Diagnostics (Biosensors and Imaging)

Eco-friendly nanomaterials are integral to advanced diagnostic tools, such as biosensors and imaging systems. Biosensors utilizing nanomaterials, such as graphene, gold nanoparticles, or quantum dots, offer high sensitivity and specificity for detecting biomarkers associated with diseases like cancer, diabetes, or infectious diseases. For instance:

- Graphene-based biosensors are used to detect glucose levels in diabetic patients with high accuracy and rapid response times (Szunerits et al., 2018).
- Gold nanoparticles enhance the sensitivity of imaging techniques like computed tomography (CT) and magnetic resonance imaging (MRI), improving the detection of tumors at early stages (Luo et al., 2021).

By integrating biodegradable or green-synthesized nanomaterials into diagnostic devices, the environmental impact of healthcare technologies can be significantly reduced without compromising their performance or accuracy. This approach is exemplified in various real-world applications, particularly during critical global health events.

- **Case Study- COVID-19 Nanobiosensors:** During the COVID-19 pandemic, several biotech firms developed nanomaterial-based biosensors for rapid testing. For example, Cardea Bio (USA) developed a graphene-based biosensor capable of detecting viral RNA in real-time with high sensitivity (Ban et al., 2023). These nanobiosensors reduced testing time to under 10 minutes and required minimal sample preparation.

- **Industry Application- Nanoimaging in Oncology:** Bracco Imaging (Italy) uses iron oxide nanoparticles for enhanced MRI contrast agents, helping clinicians visualize tumors more precisely without the toxicity risks of traditional agents (Scarciglia et al, 2025).

4.1.2. Nanomedicine for Targeted Drug Delivery

Nanomedicine leverages nanomaterials to deliver drugs precisely to affected tissues, minimizing side effects and improving therapeutic efficacy. Eco-friendly nanocarriers, such as those made from chitosan or cellulose nanocrystals, are increasingly used for targeted drug delivery. These biodegradable materials ensure that the drug reaches its intended site while reducing residual waste in the body. For example:

- Chitosan nanoparticles have been used to encapsulate anti-cancer drugs, delivering them specifically to tumor cells while sparing healthy tissues (Lunawat et al., 2024).
- Lipid-based nanoparticles, often derived from plant oils, are used to deliver vaccines and therapeutics in a controlled manner, ensuring sustained release and reducing the frequency of doses (Sheoran et al., 2022).

These advancements in eco-friendly drug delivery systems are not just theoretical—they have already been translated into real-world applications that demonstrate both clinical efficacy and sustainability. The following case study and industry application highlight how nanotechnology is being successfully integrated into mainstream healthcare:

- Case Study: *Doxil – Liposomal Doxorubicin*

Doxil, a nanotechnology-based chemotherapy drug by Johnson & Johnson, uses PEGylated liposomes to encapsulate doxorubicin. This reduces side effects and increases delivery specificity to cancer cells (Gabizon et al., 2025). It's FDA-approved and considered a milestone in nanomedicine.

- Industry Application: *Smart Drug Delivery in Diabetes*

MIT researchers and Novo Nordisk collaborated on glucose-responsive nanoparticles for insulin delivery that release insulin only when blood sugar is high, mimicking pancreatic behavior (Volpatti et al., 2019).

5. ANTIMICROBIAL AND STERILIZATION APPLICATIONS

Antimicrobial resistance is a growing concern in healthcare, and eco-friendly nanomaterials offer innovative solutions to combat infections while reducing the use of chemical disinfectants and antibiotics.

5.1. Silver and Gold Nanoparticles as Antimicrobial Agents

Silver nanoparticles (AgNPs) and gold nanoparticles (AuNPs) synthesized through green methods, such as using plant extracts, exhibit potent antimicrobial properties against bacteria, viruses, and fungi.

- AgNPs are widely used in wound dressings, medical device coatings, and disinfectant sprays to prevent infections. Their ability to disrupt microbial membranes and inhibit biofilm formation makes them highly effective (Deshmukh et al., 2019).
- AuNPs, in addition to being biocompatible, are utilized in diagnostics and antimicrobial applications, especially for drug-resistant pathogens (Rabiee et al., 2022).

The practical implementation of green-synthesized silver and gold nanoparticles has extended far beyond laboratory research, offering real-world solutions in both medical and industrial fields. The following examples illustrate how these nanomaterials are being adopted to enhance product performance and public health:

- **Case Study: Nanosilver in Wound Dressings**

Companies like Smith & Nephew have commercialized Acticoat™, a wound dressing infused with nanosilver. It's widely used in burn treatment centers globally due to its sustained antimicrobial action (Fong et al, 2006).

- **Industry Application: Food Packaging**

Tetra Pak has researched using nano-silver coatings to create antimicrobial surfaces inside packaging to increase shelf-life and reduce spoilage in dairy and juice products (Yang et al., 2025).

5.2. Nanotechnology in Medical Coatings

Nanotechnology-based coatings have become essential in ensuring the sterility of medical equipment and surfaces. For instance:

- Eco-friendly nanomaterial coatings, such as zinc oxide nanoparticles or graphene oxide, are applied to surgical instruments, implants, and hospital surfaces to prevent microbial colonization (Mohite et al., 2024).
- These coatings reduce the need for chemical disinfectants, lowering the environmental burden of healthcare-associated waste and protecting patients from healthcare-associated infections (HAIs) (Jose et al., 2023).

6. WOUND HEALING AND TISSUE REGENERATION

Tissue damage and chronic wounds pose significant challenges in healthcare, and eco-friendly nanomaterials have opened new avenues for effective wound management and tissue engineering.

6.1. Hydrogels for Wound Healing

Nanomaterial-based hydrogels are emerging as advanced solutions for wound healing due to their ability to maintain a moist environment, deliver therapeutic agents, and promote tissue repair.

- Hydrogels made from biopolymers such as chitosan and alginate are biodegradable and biocompatible, ensuring minimal environmental impact (Kanmani et al., 2017).
- Silver nanoparticles embedded in hydrogels enhance antimicrobial activity, reducing the risk of wound infections. For instance, chitosan-based hydrogels loaded with growth factors have been successfully used to accelerate the healing of diabetic wounds, where tissue repair is typically impaired (Liu et al., 2018).

6.2. Scaffolds for Tissue Engineering

Nanobiopolymers such as cellulose nanofibers and collagen-based scaffolds are transforming tissue engineering by providing a framework for cell growth and tissue regeneration.

- These scaffolds mimic the extracellular matrix (ECM) in the human body, promoting the adhesion, proliferation, and differentiation of cells.
- For example, cellulose nanofiber scaffolds are used to repair damaged skin or cartilage, while collagen-based scaffolds have been employed for bone regeneration (Mbese et al., 2021).

The biodegradable nature of these materials ensures that they degrade naturally after fulfilling their purpose, leaving no harmful residues in the body or environment.

7. ENVIRONMENTAL IMPACT AND CHALLENGES

While nanomaterials offer transformative solutions across industries, including healthcare, their environmental impact remains a pressing concern. The unique properties that make nanomaterials valuable—such as high reactivity, small size, and persistence—can also pose risks to ecosystems and human health. The environmental challenges associated with nanomaterials stem from their potential toxicity, persistence in the environment, and difficulty in managing their end-of-life stages. This section explores the environmental risks posed by nanomaterials, the challenges in recycling them, and strategies to mitigate their impact.

7.1. Environmental Risks of Nanomaterials

Nanomaterials can unintentionally affect ecosystems due to their small size and high reactivity. These risks include toxicity to organisms, bioaccumulation, and environmental persistence.

7.1.1. Degradation and Toxicity to Ecosystems

7.1.1.1. Persistence and Bioaccumulation

Many nanomaterials, especially those derived from metals (e.g., silver, titanium dioxide), do not readily degrade in the environment (Dahl et al., 2014). When released into soil, water, or air, these particles can accumulate in organisms and ecosystems, disrupting natural processes. For example, silver nanoparticles (AgNPs), widely used for their antimicrobial properties, can persist in aquatic environments, harming beneficial microorganisms and aquatic life.

7.1.1.2. Toxicity to Living Organisms

Nanomaterials can interact with cells and tissues in ways that traditional materials cannot. For instance, some nanoparticles generate reactive oxygen species (ROS), which can damage cells and DNA, leading to oxidative stress in plants, animals, and humans (Horie et al., 2021). Study by Yamini et al (2023) have shown that exposure nanomaterials to carbon nanotubes or zinc oxide nanoparticles can negatively impact aquatic species and soil microorganisms, potentially disrupting food chains.

7.1.2. Challenges in Recycling Nanomaterials

7.1.2.1. Complexity in Recovery

Nanomaterials are often incorporated into composite materials or coatings, making their separation and recovery challenging. For example, nanoparticles embedded in paints, plastics, or textiles are difficult to extract at the end of the product's life cycle (Mitrano et al., 2015).

7.1.2.2. Lack of Recycling Infrastructure

Current waste management systems are not equipped to handle nanomaterials. Many nanomaterials end up in landfills or wastewater, where they may leach into the environment, further complicating waste management (Part et al., 2018). Examples of nanomaterials that contaminate soil and water include the following:

- ✓ Carbon Nanotubes (CNTs), used in electronics, composites, and sensors (Li et al., 2008).
- ✓ Graphene, applied in electronic devices, paints, and superconducting materials (Sattar, 2019).
- ✓ Carbon Black, utilized in printing inks, tires, and dyes (Pfaff, 2022).
- ✓ Silver Nanoparticles (AgNPs), commonly used in antimicrobial products such as clothing, cosmetics, and medical tools (H. Aritonang et al., 2022).
- ✓ Gold Nanoparticles (AuNPs), widely employed in biomedicine, biosensors, and cosmetics (Herlan et al., 2015).
- ✓ Titanium Dioxide (TiO_2), found in sunscreen, paints, and textiles (Sabar, 2013).
- ✓ Zinc Oxide (ZnO), used in sunscreens and cosmetics (Amin et al., 2020).
- ✓ Iron Oxide Nanoparticles, applied in magnetic and medical applications such as MRI .
- ✓ Alumina (Aluminum Oxide), used in coatings, electronics, and catalysts (Tamalia, 2016)
- ✓ Dendrimers, utilized in drug delivery systems (Aristadewi et al., 2021).

- ✓ Nanogels, applied in pharmaceutical and cosmetic products (Ariani, 2020).
- ✓ Silica Nanoparticles (SiO_2), found in paints, coatings, and absorbent materials (Putri, 2016)
- ✓ Quantum Dots, used in display technology, optical devices, and bio-imaging (Fatimah, 2020).
- ✓ Nano-Ceramics, employed in heat-resistant materials, filters, and coatings (N. B. Singh et al., 2022).
- ✓ Nanocellulose, utilized in paper, composites, and biomedical applications (Putri, 2016)
- ✓ Organic-Inorganic Hybrids, commonly used in energy devices such as batteries and solar panels (S. Aritonang et al., 2024).

7.2. Strategies to Mitigate Environmental Impact

Despite these challenges, there are promising strategies to minimize the environmental footprint of nanomaterials and ensure their sustainable use.

7.2.1. Standardizing Green Nanomaterial Production

7.2.1.1. Eco-Friendly Synthesis Methods

The adoption of green synthesis methods, such as using plant extracts or enzymes, can reduce the use of toxic chemicals during production (Bellanthudawa et al., 2023). By focusing on biodegradable and non-toxic raw materials, industries can create nanomaterials that are safer for the environment.

7.2.1.2. Life Cycle Assessment (LCA)

Implementing LCA can help manufacturers evaluate the environmental impact of nanomaterials from production to disposal. This holistic approach ensures that the benefits of nanomaterials outweigh their ecological costs.

7.2.1.3. Developing Biodegradable Nanomaterials

Encouraging the use of biopolymers like chitosan or cellulose to create nanostructures can ensure that nanomaterials break down naturally in the environment without leaving harmful residues.

7.2.2. Monitoring Environmental Impact with Ecotoxicity Testing

7.2.2.1. Comprehensive Ecotoxicity Studies

Testing the effects of nanomaterials on different organisms and ecosystems is crucial. This involves studying their interactions with soil, water, air, and biota under real-world conditions (Bernhardt et al., 2010). By understanding how nanomaterials behave in various environments, researchers can design safer alternatives.

7.2.2.2. Regulatory Frameworks

Governments and international organizations need to establish strict guidelines for nanomaterial use and disposal. These frameworks should include mandatory ecotoxicity testing, environmental monitoring, and transparent reporting by manufacturers.

7.2.2.3. Nanomaterial Risk Assessment Tools

Developing advanced tools and models to predict the long-term behavior of nanomaterials in the environment can help mitigate risks before they occur. For example, simulation models can estimate how nanoparticles disperse in water or soil and their potential for bioaccumulation (Baalousha et al., 2016).

8. THE IMPORTANCE OF SUSTAINABLE NANOMATERIALS FOR GREEN HEALTHCARE SOLUTIONS

Traditional healthcare systems, while advancing human health, often leave a significant ecological footprint. Medical waste, energy-intensive manufacturing processes, and the overuse of chemical agents contribute to environmental degradation (Dharmaraj et al., 2021). Sustainable nanomaterials provide an opportunity to address these issues, offering solutions that align healthcare advancements with environmental preservation.

8.1. Reducing Environmental Impact

Nanomaterials synthesized using eco-friendly methods, such as plant extracts or enzymatic reactions, eliminate the need for toxic reagents and minimize waste production (Seth et al., 2024). This reduces the risk of environmental contamination and promotes a circular economy in healthcare. Materials like biodegradable polymers and naturally derived nanoparticles ensure that residues from medical applications degrade safely, posing no harm to ecosystems (Bellanthudawa et al., 2023).

8.2. Enhancing Healthcare Efficiency

Sustainable nanomaterials also contribute to improving healthcare delivery. For instance, drug delivery systems made from biodegradable nanocarriers ensure precise targeting of affected tissues, minimizing drug wastage and side effects. Similarly, eco-friendly nanomaterials in biosensors and imaging devices enhance the accuracy of disease diagnosis, enabling early intervention and better patient outcomes (Halagali et al., 2025).

8.3. Alignment with Global Sustainability Goals

The integration of sustainable nanomaterials into healthcare aligns with global efforts to achieve sustainability, such as the United Nations' Sustainable Development Goals (SDGs) (Pokrajac et al., 2021). Specifically, these materials support goals related to health (SDG 3), responsible consumption and production (SDG 12), and climate action (SDG 13).

9. THE CALL TO DRIVE ECO-FRIENDLY INNOVATION IN HEALTHCARE

The transition to green healthcare solutions requires a collective effort from researchers, industries, policymakers, and healthcare professionals. Sustainable nanomaterials are a promising foundation, but their widespread adoption hinges on continued innovation, interdisciplinary collaboration, and policy support.

9.1. Encouraging Research and Development

Investments in research and development are critical to unlocking the full potential of sustainable nanomaterials. Scientists must explore new methods for green synthesis, develop multifunctional nanomaterials, and enhance their scalability for industrial applications. Collaborative projects involving materials scientists, biologists, and environmental experts can generate holistic solutions that address both healthcare needs and environmental concerns.

9.2. Integrating Sustainability into Healthcare Policies

Policymakers play a crucial role in fostering the adoption of sustainable nanomaterials. Regulations should incentivize the use of eco-friendly materials in healthcare products and establish guidelines for their safe disposal or recycling. Moreover, international standards for evaluating the environmental impact of nanomaterials can ensure their responsible use across borders.

As reported at https://www.brin.go.id/news/112929/mencari- Solusi-sirklik-Ekonomi-untuk-limbah-medis, the Covid-19 pandemic that has hit the world, including Indonesia, requires people to use protective equipment. personal care (masks) and other health equipment, which gives rise to mask waste, with a very large amount of waste. Research shows that a lot of mask waste ends up in river estuaries, becoming a new environmental problem.

One of the main materials contained in medical masks and other personal protective equipment, including head coverings and hazmat suits, is the plastic material polypropyelene or polypropylene (PP), which can easily be found to contain virgin polymers and virgin polypropyelene by proving it using the recrystallization method.

Research Professor in Chemistry, Agus Haryono, explained that polypropylene is widely used in everyday life. He gave an example, for packaging various food products, drinks and automotive spare parts. Polypropylene is a polymer that has good properties, has a fairly high average molecular weight, is nonpolar, has high frequency insulation, good heat resistance, abrasion resistance and high enough elasticity so that it is comfortable to wear as PPE. Polypropylene is a material that has mechanical strength that does not break down quickly, and is strong against chemicals in general.

It would be very interesting if these materials could be recycled in various ways, such as the recrystallization method or a composite method that mixes them with other biomass, to produce products with economic value, so that there is a circular economy resulting from medical waste that can be utilized.

In the initial stage, sterilization of medical mask waste originating from households and health care facilities is carried out, then continued with recrystallization which produces pure polypropylene, from the resulting polypropylene ore it has the potential to produce, products of economic value, thus forming a circular economic concept from mask waste from various sources. households and health facilities.

9.3. Educating and Engaging Stakeholders

Education and awareness are key to driving change. Healthcare professionals, industry leaders, and the general public must understand the benefits of sustainable nanomaterials and their role in creating a greener healthcare system. Universities and research institutions can offer programs that emphasize sustainability in nanotechnology, equipping the next generation of scientists and engineers to address these challenges.

9.3.1. Raising Awareness Among Health Professionals

Health professionals, including doctors, nurses, and administrators, need to be informed about the environmental impacts of materials used in medical products and devices. Education about the benefits of sustainable nanomaterials—such as lower toxicity, biodegradability, and smaller environmental footprint—can encourage their adoption in clinical practice. Additionally, health professionals should also be trained on how to handle, dispose of, or recycle these materials to minimize potential risks to human health and the environment.

9.3.2. Engage Industry Leaders

Industry leaders, including executives, manufacturers, and policymakers, play a critical role in pushing sustainable nanomaterials in the healthcare sector. These stakeholders must be educated about the long-term economic, environmental, and social benefits of adopting green technologies. Seminars, conferences and collaborative partnerships with research institutions can help bridge knowledge gaps and encourage the integration of sustainability in product design and manufacturing processes.

9.3.3. Public Awareness and Engagement

The general public, both as consumers and supporters of the health system, also needs to be educated about environmentally friendly practices in the health sector. Engaging the public through campaigns highlighting the importance of environmentally friendly ingredients in health products can encourage more conscious choices. This awareness may create demand for greener products and put pressure on healthcare providers to adopt sustainable practices.

9.3.4. The Role of Universities and Research Institutions

Universities and research institutions have an important role to play in shaping the future of sustainable health. These institutions can offer sustainability-focused programs and courses in nanotechnology, training the next generation of scientists and engineers to develop innovative and environmentally friendly solutions. By encouraging research that emphasizes the environmental and health benefits of sustainable nanomaterials, universities can equip students with the knowledge and skills necessary to overcome the challenges of the future.

9.3.5. Collaboration and Knowledge Sharing

To overcome the complex challenges of integrating sustainability in the health sector, collaboration between stakeholders is essential. Academia, industry, government, and the public must work together to share knowledge, resources, and best practices. This collaborative approach can accelerate the development and adoption of sustainable nanomaterials and other green innovations in health.

9.4. Expanding Applications Beyond Healthcare

While healthcare is a major beneficiary of sustainable nanomaterials, their potential extends to other sectors, such as agriculture, energy, and water treatment. By exploring these applications, the impact of green nanotechnology can be amplified, contributing to broader environmental and social benefits.

9.4.1. Agriculture

Sustainable nanomaterials can play an important role in agriculture by increasing the efficiency of use of resources such as water and fertilizer. For example, nanoparticles can be used to deliver nutrients or pesticides more precisely to plants, reducing waste and negative impacts on the environment. Additionally, nanomaterials can be used to develop more sophisticated crop monitoring systems, increasing agricultural yields and reducing the use of harmful chemicals.

9.4.2. Energy

In the energy sector, sustainable nanomaterials have the potential to improve energy efficiency through the development of alternative fuels, energy storage and more efficient solar panels. For example, nanomaterials can be used to improve the conductivity and performance of solar panels, making them more efficient at generating energy from the sun. Nanomaterial-based energy storage technology can also help in overcoming the storage challenges of renewable energy, such as wind and solar power, which require better storage solutions.

9.4.3. Water Treatment

In water treatment, sustainable nanomaterials can be used to filter pollutants and remove harmful substances from water more efficiently. Nanofiltration and nanocatalysis technology can be used to treat water by reducing the use of harmful chemicals, thereby creating a more environmentally friendly process. Nanomaterials can also help in the desalination of seawater, providing a solution to the problem of water shortages in areas that depend on seawater sources.

9.4.4. Wider Environmental and Social Benefits

By expanding the application of sustainable nanomaterials to other sectors, we can magnify their positive impact on the environment. For example, in the agricultural sector, reducing the use of chemicals can protect soil and biodiversity. In the energy sector, improving energy efficiency can reduce carbon emissions and dependence on fossil fuels. In the field of water treatment, nanomaterial technology can increase access to clean water and reduce water pollution.

10. FUTURE CHALLENGES AND CONSIDERATIONS

Addressing the environmental impact of nanomaterials requires coordinated efforts between researchers, industry stakeholders, and policymakers.

10.1. Future Perspectives and Innovations

The future of sustainable nanomaterials lies in continuous innovation and interdisciplinary collaboration. As the demand for greener and more efficient healthcare solutions grows, researchers and industries are focusing on advancing nanotechnology to address global sustainability challenges. By integrating cutting-edge technologies, such as artificial intelligence (AI), with nanotechnology, and fostering collaborations across disciplines, sustainable nanomaterials are poised to revolutionize healthcare systems (Halagali et al., 2025). This section explores the key trends in sustainable nanomaterial research, the role of AI in enhancing their applications, and the importance of interdisciplinary efforts in achieving sustainable healthcare solutions.

10.2. Future Trends in Sustainable Nanomaterials Research

Sustainable nanomaterials are evolving to meet the dual objectives of technological advancement and environmental preservation. Several emerging research trends are shaping the future of this field:

10.2.1. Development of Biodegradable and Renewable Nanomaterials

There is a growing focus on creating nanomaterials from renewable and biodegradable sources to minimize their environmental impact. Study by (Matei et al., 2022) are exploring the use of natural polymers, such as cellulose, chitosan, and lignin, to create nanomaterials that degrade safely in the environment. These materials are particularly promising for applications in drug delivery, wound healing, and tissue engineering.

10.2.2. Multifunctional Nanomaterials

Future nanomaterials are expected to perform multiple functions simultaneously, such as targeted drug delivery combined with real-time monitoring and controlled release. For example, (Bhaskar et al., 2010) are developing nanocarriers that can deliver drugs to specific cells while providing imaging capabilities for tracking the treatment process.

10.2.3. Circular Economy in Nanotechnology

Another significant trend is the adoption of circular economy principles in nanomaterial production and disposal. This involves designing nanomaterials that can be easily recycled or repurposed after their initial use, reducing waste and conserving resources (Abd Elkodous et al., 2022).

10.2.4. Sustainable Production Techniques

Green synthesis methods are being further refined to reduce the use of hazardous chemicals and energy. Innovations such as bioinspired synthesis (Zan et al., 2016a), enzyme-mediated processes (Chen et al., 2017). and low-energy production technologies (Hussein, 2023) are gaining traction. These methods not only improve sustainability but also enhance the biocompatibility of nanomaterials, making them safer for medical applications.

10.3. Integration of AI and Nanotechnology

Artificial intelligence (AI) is playing an increasingly important role in advancing nanotechnology by optimizing design, synthesis, and application processes (Oviedo et al., 2022). The integration of AI with nanotechnology offers several opportunities to create more effective and environmentally friendly healthcare solutions:

10.3.1. AI-Driven Nanomaterial Design

AI can accelerate the discovery and development of sustainable nanomaterials by predicting the properties and behaviors of potential candidates before they are synthesized (Jia et al., 2021). Machine learning algorithms analyze vast datasets to identify optimal compositions, sizes, and structures for specific applications, reducing the need for trial-and-error experiments (Zhou et al., 2019).

10.3.2. Optimizing Green Synthesis

AI algorithms can help optimize green synthesis processes by identifying the most efficient and eco-friendly routes for nanomaterial production (Konstantopoulos et al., 2022). This includes selecting natural reducing agents (Segler et al., 2018), predicting reaction conditions (Venkatasubramanian et al., 2022), and minimizing energy consumption (Putha, 2020).

10.3.3. Enhancing Drug Delivery Systems

AI-powered models can improve the design of nanocarriers for targeted drug delivery by predicting their interactions with biological systems (Kapoor et al., 2024). This ensures that nanocarriers deliver drugs precisely to affected tissues, minimizing side effects and maximizing therapeutic outcomes.

10.3.4. Environmental Monitoring and Risk Assessment

AI can also be used to monitor the environmental impact of nanomaterials (Vasoya, 2023). By analyzing data from ecotoxicity studies and environmental simulations, AI systems can predict the long-term effects of nanomaterials on ecosystems (Zan et al., 2016b) and suggest mitigation strategies (Chirra, 2022).

Figure 1. The interconnections of eco-friendly nanomaterials: Environmental impact, healthcare applications, and future challenges

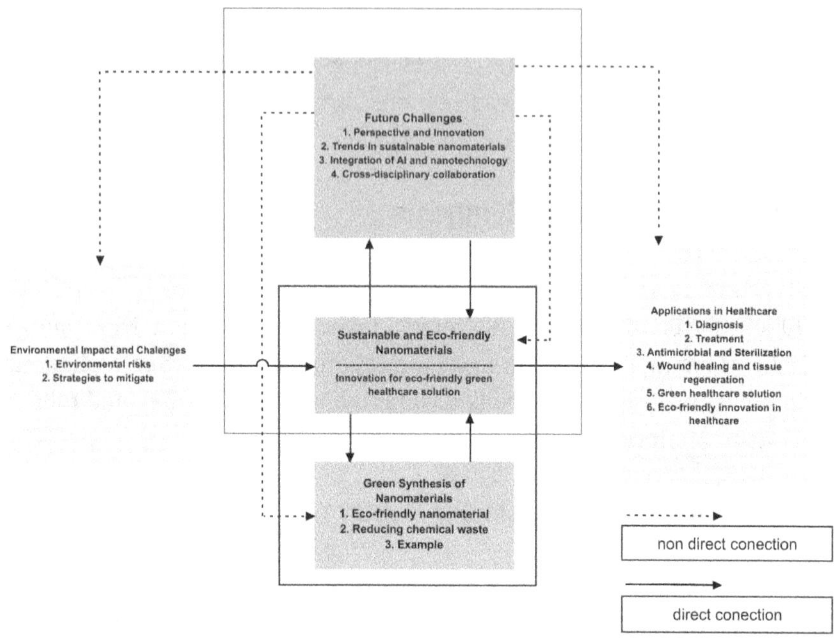

Figure 1 illustrates the interconnections between eco-friendly nanomaterials and various related aspects, including their environmental impact, applications in healthcare, green synthesis methods, and future challenges.

1. Sustainable and Eco-Friendly Nanomaterials lie at the core, serving as a hub for innovation in green healthcare solutions.
2. Environmental Impact and Challenges highlight potential risks associated with nanomaterials and strategies for mitigation, feeding into the need for sustainable approaches.
3. Applications in Healthcare demonstrate the practical use of nanomaterials in diagnosis, treatment, antimicrobial solutions, wound healing, and green healthcare innovations.
4. Green Synthesis of Nanomaterials emphasizes eco-friendly production processes, reducing chemical waste, and specific examples of implementation.
5. Future Challenges explore the perspectives of innovation, trends in sustainable materials, integration of AI, and cross-disciplinary collaboration to advance the field.

The chart uses direct and indirect connections to show how these aspects interact to drive sustainable innovation. All of these aspects are elaborated upon in detail in this book chapter, providing a comprehensive understanding of the role of eco-friendly nanomaterials in addressing environmental and healthcare challenges.

CONCLUSION

As we navigate the complexities of the 21st century, the integration of biology and chemistry offers a transformative lens to address pressing global challenges and revolutionize science education. Through a molecular perspective, we can foster a deeper understanding of natural phenomena, bridge the gap between scientific theory and practical applications, and inspire innovative solutions to societal issues such as climate change, sustainable resource management, and healthcare advancements.

This book has explored how a multidisciplinary approach to molecular science can enrich educational frameworks, empowering students and educators alike to engage in critical thinking, collaborative problem-solving, and sustainable innovation. From molecular mechanisms and biomolecular synthesis to cutting-edge technologies and their applications, the topics presented underscore the need for a holistic approach to science education—one that not only builds scientific knowledge but also nurtures ethical and environmental awareness.

As the molecular revolution unfolds, educators, researchers, policymakers, and industry leaders must collaborate to ensure that science education remains relevant, inclusive, and forward-thinking. By incorporating real-world contexts, digital tools, and hands-on learning into the curriculum, we can cultivate a generation of learners who are scientifically literate and equipped to contribute meaningfully to a sustainable and equitable future.

The journey of integrating biology and chemistry is far from complete. It is a shared responsibility to continue driving innovation, embracing cross-disciplinary approaches, and embedding sustainability at the core of scientific pursuits. As we move forward, let this book serve as both a guide and a call to action—a commitment to transforming science education and harnessing the power of molecular science for the betterment of humanity and the planet.

REFERENCES

Abd Elkodous, M., Hamad, H. A., Abdel Maksoud, M. I., Ali, G. A., El Abboubi, M., Bedir, A. G., Eldeeb, A. A., Ayed, A. A., Gargar, Z., Zaki, F. S., Farage, D. A., Matsuda, A., Abdelnour, M. R., Sabra, B. A., Elsayed, A., Abdelrazek, T. A., Abdelhameed, S. T., Gharieb, M. A., Rabee, M. M., & Kawamura, G. (2022). Cutting-edge development in waste-recycled nanomaterials for energy storage and conversion applications. *Nanotechnology Reviews*, *11*(1), 2215–2294. DOI: 10.1515/ntrev-2022-0129

Adhi, T. P., Aqsha, A., & Indarto, A. (2024). Comparative Studies on Thermal, Microwave-Assisted, and Ultrasound-Promoted Preparations. In *Green Chemical Synthesis with Microwaves and Ultrasound* (pp. 337–380). Wiley., DOI: 10.1002/9783527844494.ch12

Ahmed, S. F., Mofijur, M., Rafa, N., Chowdhury, A. T., Chowdhury, S., Nahrin, M., Islam, A. B. M. S., & Ong, H. C. (2022). Green approaches in synthesising nanomaterials for environmental nanobioremediation: Technological advancements, applications, benefits and challenges. *Environmental Research, 204*, 111967. DOI: 10.1016/j.envres.2021.111967 PMID: 34450159

Aithal, S., & Aithal, P. S. (2021a). Green and Eco-friendly Nanotechnology Concepts and Industrial Prospects. In *Technology, and Social Sciences (IJMTS) A Refereed International Journal of Srinivas University* (Vol. 6, Issue 1). DOI: 10.47992/IJMTS.2581.6012.0127

Aithal, S., & Aithal, P. S. (2021b). Green and Eco-friendly Nanotechnology Concepts and Industrial Prospects. *Technology, and Social Sciences (IJMTS) A Refereed International Journal of Srinivas University, 6*. DOI: 10.5281/zenodo.4496913

Alhmoud, S. H. (2024a). Sustainability of Development and Application of Nanomaterials in Healthcare within Hospital Settings. *SSRG International Journal of Civil Engineering*, *11*(6), 79–97. DOI: 10.14445/23488352/IJCE-V11I6P110

Alhmoud, S. H. (2024b). Sustainability of Development and Application of Nanomaterials in Healthcare within Hospital Settings. *International Journal of Civil Engineering*, *11*(6), 79–97. DOI: 10.14445/23488352/IJCE-V11I6P110

Amin, A., & Ananda, S. R. (2020). Sintesis dan Karakterisasi Nanopartikel Zn Menggunakan Kitosan Sebagai Reduktor. *Fullerene Journal of Chemistry*, *5*(2), 102. DOI: 10.37033/fjc.v5i2.208

Ariani, L. W. (2020). *Formulasi Dan Stabilitas Fisik Sediaan Nanogel Minyak Biji Matahari*. Sekolah Tinggi Ilmu Farmasi Semarang.

Aristadewi, P. A., Gorintha, A. W., & Ivena, A. (2021). Potensi Kombinasi Amido-Bridged Nucleic Acid Modified Antisense Oligonucleotides Dengan Polyamidoamine Dendrimer Generasi 4 Tertarget A-Synuclein Sebagai Terapi Parkinson. *Al-Iqra Medical Journal : Jurnal Berkala Ilmiah Kedokteran*, *4*(1), 10–18. DOI: 10.26618/aimj.v4i1.4985

Aritonang, H., Dewa G., & Widya Astuty Lolo. (2022). *BIOSINTESIS NANOPARTIKEL PERAK (Ag) MENGGUNAKAN EKSTRAK DAUN AFRIKA (VERNONIA AMYGDALINA) DAN POLIETILEN GLIKOL 6000 SERTA APLIKASINYA SEBAGAI DETEKTOR ION LOGAM BERAT* (Issue 18101101045).

Aritonang, S., Al Fajri, Z., Azida, P. W., & Sandri, A. Muhammad, & Dintyra, D. (2024). Teknologi Tenda Militer Portabel Berbasis Tenaga Surya Dalam Mobilisasi Taktis Tempur. *Rekayasa Material, Manufaktur Dan Energi, 7*(1), 73–81. https://creativecommons.org/licenses/by-sa/4.0/

Baalousha, M., Cornelis, G., Kuhlbusch, T. A. J., Lynch, I., Nickel, C., Peijnenburg, W., & van den Brink, N. W. (2016). Modeling nanomaterial fate and uptake in the environment: Current knowledge and future trends. *Environmental Science. Nano*, *3*(2), 323–345. DOI: 10.1039/C5EN00207A

Bahrulolum, H., Nooraei, S., Javanshir, N., Tarrahimofrad, H., Mirbagheri, V. S., Easton, A. J., & Ahmadian, G. (2021). Green synthesis of metal nanoparticles using microorganisms and their application in the agrifood sector. *Journal of Nanobiotechnology*, *19*(1), 1–26. DOI: 10.1186/s12951-021-00834-3 PMID: 33771172

Ban, D. K., Hajian, R., Winton, A. J., Eom, R., Gupta, A., Kane, A. A., Liu, S., Sampath, R., Farrell, M. L., Coppock, M. B., Goldsmith, B., & Aran, K. (2023). A single multiomics transistor for electronic detection of SARS-Cov2 variants antigen and viral RNA without amplification. *Advanced Materials Technologies*, *8*(11), 2201945. DOI: 10.1002/admt.202201945

Bellanthudawa, B. K. A., Nawalage, N. M. S. K., Handapangoda, H. M. A. K., Suvendran, S., Wijayasenarathne, K. A. S. H., Rathnasuriya, M. L. D., Wickramasinghe, P. G. M. U., Aberathna, A. A. A. U., Tennakoon, A., & Perera, I. J. J. U. N. (2023). A perspective on biodegradable and non-biodegradable nanoparticles in industrial sectors: Applications, challenges, and future prospects. *Nanotechnology for Environmental Engineering*, *8*(4), 975–1013. DOI: 10.1007/s41204-023-00344-7

Bernhardt, E. S., Colman, B. P., Hochella, M. F., Cardinale, B. J., Nisbet, R. M., Richardson, C. J., & Yin, L. (2010). An Ecological Perspective on Nanomaterial Impacts in the Environment. *Journal of Environmental Quality*, *39*(6), 1954–1965. DOI: 10.2134/jeq2009.0479 PMID: 21284292

Beyene, H. D., Werkneh, A. A., Bezabh, H. K., & Ambaye, T. G. (2017). Synthesis paradigm and applications of silver nanoparticles (AgNPs), a review. *Sustainable Materials and Technologies*, *13*(January), 18–23. DOI: 10.1016/j.susmat.2017.08.001

Bhaskar, S., Tian, F., Stoeger, T., Kreyling, W., de la Fuente, J. M., Grazú, V., Borm, P., Estrada, G., Ntziachristos, V., & Razansky, D. (2010). Multifunctional Nanocarriers for diagnostics, drug delivery and targeted treatment across blood-brain barrier: Perspectives on tracking and neuroimaging. *Particle and Fibre Toxicology*, *7*(1), 1–25. DOI: 10.1186/1743-8977-7-3 PMID: 20199661

Bystrzejewska-Piotrowska, G., Golimowski, J., & Urban, P. L. (2009). Nanoparticles: Their potential toxicity, waste and environmental management. *Waste Management (New York, N.Y.)*, *29*(9), 2587–2595. DOI: 10.1016/j.wasman.2009.04.001 PMID: 19427190

Chakrabartty, I., Hakeem, K. R., Mohanta, Y. K., & Varma, R. S. (2022). Greener nanomaterials and their diverse applications in the energy sector. *Clean Technologies and Environmental Policy*, *24*(10), 3237–3252. DOI: 10.1007/s10098-022-02368-0

Chen, M., Zeng, G., Xu, P., Lai, C., & Tang, L. (2017). How Do Enzymes 'Meet' Nanoparticles and Nanomaterials? *Trends in Biochemical Sciences*, *42*(11), 914–930. DOI: 10.1016/j.tibs.2017.08.008 PMID: 28917970

Chirra, B. R. (2022). AI-Driven Vulnerability Assessment and Mitigation Strategies for CyberPhysical Systems. *Revista de Inteligencia Artificial En Medicina, 13*(1), 471–493. https://redcrevistas.com/index.php/Revista

Chong, W. J., Shen, S., Li, Y., Trinchi, A., Pejak Simunec, D., Kyratzis, I., Sola, A., & Wen, C. (2022, May). (Louis), Sola, A., & Wen, C. (2023). Biodegradable PLA-ZnO nanocomposite biomaterials with antibacterial properties, tissue engineering viability, and enhanced biocompatibility. *Smart Materials in Manufacturing*, *1*, 100004. DOI: 10.1016/j.smmf.2022.100004

Cseri, L., Razali, M., Pogany, P., & Szekely, G. (2018). Organic Solvents in Sustainable Synthesis and Engineering. In *Green Chemistry* (pp. 513–553). Elsevier., DOI: 10.1016/B978-0-12-809270-5.00020-0

Dahl, M., Liu, Y., & Yin, Y. (2014). Composite titanium dioxide nanomaterials. *Chemical Reviews*, *114*(19), 9853–9889. DOI: 10.1021/cr400634p PMID: 25011918

Das, R. K., Pachapur, V. L., Lonappan, L., Naghdi, M., Pulicharla, R., Maiti, S., Cledon, M., Dalila, L. M. A., Sarma, S. J., & Brar, S. K. (2017). Biological synthesis of metallic nanoparticles: Plants, animals and microbial aspects. *Nanotechnology for Environmental Engineering*, *2*(1), 1–21. DOI: 10.1007/s41204-017-0029-4

Deshmukh, S. P., Patil, S. M., Mullani, S. B., & Delekar, S. D. (2019). Silver nanoparticles as an effective disinfectant: A review. *Materials Science and Engineering C, 97*(July 2018), 954–965. DOI: 10.1016/j.msec.2018.12.102

Dharmaraj, S., Ashokkumar, V., Pandiyan, R., Halimatul Munawaroh, H. S., Chew, K. W., Chen, W. H., & Ngamcharussrivichai, C. (2021). Pyrolysis: An effective technique for degradation of COVID-19 medical wastes. *Chemosphere*, *275*, 130092. DOI: 10.1016/j.chemosphere.2021.130092 PMID: 33984908

El-Sayyad, G. S., Elfadil, D., Mosleh, M. A., Hasanien, Y. A., Mostafa, A., Abdelkader, R. S., Refaey, N., Elkafoury, E. M., Eshaq, G., Abdelrahman, E. A., Malash, M. N., Rizk, S. H., Gobara, M., Nada, H. G., Hashem, A. H., Attia, M. S., Noreddin, A. M., Abdel Maksoud, M. I. A., Ghobashy, M. M., & El-Batal, A. I. (2024). Eco-friendly Strategies for Biological Synthesis of Green Nanoparticles with Promising Applications. *BioNanoScience*, *14*(3), 3617–3659. DOI: 10.1007/s12668-024-01494-x

El Shafey, A. M. (2020). Green synthesis of metal and metal oxide nanoparticles from plant leaf extracts and their applications: A review. *Green Processing and Synthesis*, *9*(1), 304–339. DOI: 10.1515/gps-2020-0031

Elegbede, J. A., & Lateef, A. (2021). *Microbial Enzymes in Nanotechnology and Fabrication of Nanozymes: A Perspective.*, DOI: 10.1007/978-981-33-4777-9_7

Fatimah, S. (2020). Sintesis dan Analisis Fotoluminisens Carbon Dots dari Kandungan Karbohidrat Musa Cavendishii Berbasis Pemanasan Microwave. *Dewantara Journal of Technology*, *1*(1), 8–11.

Fatiqin, A., Amrulloh, H., Simanjuntak, W., Apriani, I., Amelia, R. A. H. T., Syarifah, Sunarti, R. N., & Raharjeng, A. R. P. (2021). *Characteristics of nano-size MgO prepared using aqueous extract of different parts of Moringa oleifera plant as green synthesis agents*. 040001. DOI: 10.1063/5.0041999

Findik, F. (2021). Nanomaterials and their Applications. *Periodicals of Engineering and Natural Sciences*, *9*(3), 62–75. DOI: 10.21533/pen.v9i3.1837

Francis, S., Koshy, E., & Mathew, B. (2018). Microwave aided synthesis of silver and gold nanoparticles and their antioxidant, antimicrobial and catalytic potentials. *Journal of Nanostructures*, *8*(1), 55–66. DOI: 10.22052/JNS.2018.01.007

Gabizon, A. A., Gabizon-Peretz, S., Modaresahmadi, S., & La-Beck, N. M. (2025). Thirty years from FDA approval of pegylated liposomal doxorubicin (Doxil/Caelyx): An updated analysis and future perspective. *BMJ Oncology*, *4*(1), e000573. DOI: 10.1136/bmjonc-2024-000573 PMID: 39885941

Ghazali, S. Z., Mohamed Noor, N. R., & Mustaffa, K. M. F. (2022). Anti-plasmodial activity of aqueous neem leaf extract mediated green synthesis-based silver nitrate nanoparticles. *Preparative Biochemistry & Biotechnology*, *52*(1), 99–107. DOI: 10.1080/10826068.2021.1913602 PMID: 33890844

Gilbertson, L. M., Zimmerman, J. B., Plata, D. L., Hutchison, J. E., & Anastas, P. T. (2015). Designing nanomaterials to maximize performance and minimize undesirable implications guided by the Principles of Green Chemistry. *Chemical Society Reviews*, *44*(16), 5758–5777. DOI: 10.1039/C4CS00445K PMID: 25955514

Goenka, S., Sant, V., & Sant, S. (2014). Graphene-based nanomaterials for drug delivery and tissue engineering. *Journal of Controlled Release*, *173*, 75–88. DOI: 10.1016/j.jconrel.2013.10.017 PMID: 24161530

Halagali, P., Nayak, D., Rathnanand, M., Tippavajhala, V. K., Sharma, H., & Biswas, D. (2025). Synergizing sustainable green nanotechnology and AI/ML for advanced nanocarriers: A paradigm shift in the treatment of neurodegenerative diseases. In *The Neurodegeneration Revolution* (pp. 373–397). Elsevier., DOI: 10.1016/B978-0-443-28822-7.00017-9

Hamad, T. A., Agll, A. A., Hamad, Y. M., & Sheffield, J. W. (2014). Solid waste as renewable source of energy: Current and future possibility in Libya. *Case Studies in Thermal Engineering*, *4*, 144–152. DOI: 10.1016/j.csite.2014.09.004

Hamedi, S., Ghaseminezhad, M., Shokrollahzadeh, S., & Shojaosadati, S. A. (2017). Controlled biosynthesis of silver nanoparticles using nitrate reductase enzyme induction of filamentous fungus and their antibacterial evaluation. *Artificial Cells, Nanomedicine, and Biotechnology*, *45*(8), 1588–1596. DOI: 10.1080/21691401.2016.1267011 PMID: 27966375

Horie, M., & Tabei, Y. (2021). Role of oxidative stress in nanoparticles toxicity. *Free Radical Research*, *55*(4), 331–342. DOI: 10.1080/10715762.2020.1859108 PMID: 33336617

Hussein, H. (2023). The state of the art of nanomaterials and its applications in energy saving. *Bulletin of the National Research Center*, *47*(1), 7. Advance online publication. DOI: 10.1186/s42269-023-00984-4

Irede, E. L., Awoyemi, R. F., Owolabi, B., Aworinde, O. R., Kajola, R. O., Hazeez, A., Raji, A. A., Ganiyu, L. O., Onukwuli, C. O., Onivefu, A. P., & Ifijen, I. H. (2024). Cutting-edge developments in zinc oxide nanoparticles: Synthesis and applications for enhanced antimicrobial and UV protection in healthcare solutions. *RSC Advances*, *14*(29), 20992–21034. DOI: 10.1039/D4RA02452D PMID: 38962092

Javed, R., Zia, M., Naz, S., Aisida, S. O., Ain, N., & Ao, Q. (2020). Role of capping agents in the application of nanoparticles in biomedicine and environmental remediation: Recent trends and future prospects. *Journal of Nanobiotechnology*, *18*(1), 1–15. DOI: 10.1186/s12951-020-00704-4 PMID: 33225973

Jia, Y., Hou, X., Wang, Z., & Hu, X. (2021). Machine Learning Boosts the Design and Discovery of Nanomaterials. *ACS Sustainable Chemistry &amp. ACS Sustainable Chemistry & Engineering*, *9*(18), 6130–6147. DOI: 10.1021/acssuschemeng.1c00483

Jose, A., Gizdavic-Nikolaidis, M., & Swift, S. (2023). Antimicrobial Coatings: Reviewing Options for Healthcare Applications. *Applied Microbiology (Basel, Switzerland)*, *3*(1), 145–174. DOI: 10.3390/applmicrobiol3010012

Kabir, E., Kumar, V., Kim, K.-H., Yip, A. C. K., & Sohn, J. R. (2018). Environmental impacts of nanomaterials. *Journal of Environmental Management*, *225*, 261–271. DOI: 10.1016/j.jenvman.2018.07.087 PMID: 30096714

Kanmani, P., Aravind, J., Kamaraj, M., Sureshbabu, P., & Karthikeyan, S. (2017). Environmental applications of chitosan and cellulosic biopolymers: A comprehensive outlook. *Bioresource Technology*, *242*, 295–303. DOI: 10.1016/j.biortech.2017.03.119 PMID: 28366689

Kapoor, D. U., Sharma, J. B., Gandhi, S. M., Prajapati, B. G., Thanawuth, K., Limmatvapirat, S., & Sriamornsak, P. (2024). AI-driven design and optimization of nanoparticle-based drug delivery systems. *Science. Engineering and Health Studies*, *18*(December), 24010003. Advance online publication. DOI: 10.69598/sehs.18.24010003

Konstantopoulos, G., Koumoulos, E. P., & Charitidis, C. A. (2022). Digital Innovation Enabled Nanomaterial Manufacturing; Machine Learning Strategies and Green Perspectives. *Nanomaterials (Basel, Switzerland)*, *12*(15), 1–57. DOI: 10.3390/nano12152646 PMID: 35957077

Kothawade, S. N., Pande, V. V., Suryawanshi, J., Kumar, A., Kumar, P., & Kumar, A. (2024). Biodegradable and Non-Biodegradable Sustainable Biomaterials. In *Advances in Sustainable Biomaterials* (pp. 92–116). CRC Press. DOI: 10.1201/9781003434313-6

Kyriakides, T. R., Raj, A., Tseng, T. H., Xiao, H., Nguyen, R., Mohammed, F. S., Halder, S., Xu, M., Wu, M. J., Bao, S., & Sheu, W. C. (2021). Biocompatibility of nanomaterials and their immunological properties. *Biomedical Materials (Bristol, England)*, *16*(4), 1–49. DOI: 10.1088/1748-605X/abe5fa PMID: 33578402

Li, C., Thostenson, E. T., & Chou, T.-W. (2008). Sensors and actuators based on carbon nanotubes and their composites: A review. *Composites Science and Technology*, *68*(6), 1227–1249. DOI: 10.1016/j.compscitech.2008.01.006

Liberty, J. T., Anil, A., Ijimdiya, S. J., Kwaji, M. J., & Ijimdiya, R. U. (2024). Harnessing the potential of nanostructured materials for sustainable development. *Nano-Structures & Nano-Objects*, *38*, 101216. DOI: 10.1016/j.nanoso.2024.101216

Liu, H., Wang, C., Li, C., Qin, Y., Wang, Z., Yang, F., Li, Z., & Wang, J. (2018). A functional chitosan-based hydrogel as a wound dressing and drug delivery system in the treatment of wound healing. *RSC Advances*, *8*(14), 7533–7549. DOI: 10.1039/C7RA13510F PMID: 35539132

Loh, K. P., Ho, D., Chiu, G. N. C., Leong, D. T., Pastorin, G., & Chow, E. K. (2018). Clinical Applications of Carbon Nanomaterials in Diagnostics and Therapy. *Advanced Materials*, *30*(47), 1802368. Advance online publication. DOI: 10.1002/adma.201802368 PMID: 30133035

Lunawat, A. K., Thakur, S., Das Kurmi, B., Das Gupta, G., Patel, P., & Raikwar, S. (2024). Revolutionizing cancer treatment: The role of chitosan nanoparticles in therapeutic advancements. *Journal of Drug Delivery Science and Technology*, *96*, 105661. DOI: 10.1016/j.jddst.2024.105661

Luo, D., Wang, X., Burda, C., & Basilion, J. P. (2021). Recent development of gold nanoparticles as contrast agents for cancer diagnosis. *Cancers (Basel)*, *13*(8), 1825. Advance online publication. DOI: 10.3390/cancers13081825 PMID: 33920453

Malik, S., Muhammad, K., & Waheed, Y. (2023). Nanotechnology: A Revolution in Modern Industry. *Molecules (Basel, Switzerland)*, *28*(2), 661. Advance online publication. DOI: 10.3390/molecules28020661 PMID: 36677717

Mallakpour, S., Sirous, F., & Hussain, C. M. (2021). A journey to the world of fascinating ZnO nanocomposites made of chitosan, starch, cellulose, and other biopolymers: Progress in recent achievements in eco-friendly food packaging, biomedical, and water remediation technologies. *International Journal of Biological Macromolecules*, *170*, 701–716. DOI: 10.1016/j.ijbiomac.2020.12.163 PMID: 33388319

Matei, E., Predescu, A. M., Râpă, M., urcanu, A. A., Mate , I., Constantin, N., & Predescu, C. (2022). Natural Polymers and Their Nanocomposites Used for Environmental Applications. *Nanomaterials (Basel, Switzerland)*, *12*(10), 1707. Advance online publication. DOI: 10.3390/nano12101707 PMID: 35630932

Mazari, S. A., Ali, E., Abro, R., Khan, F. S. A., Ahmed, I., Ahmed, M., Nizamuddin, S., Siddiqui, T. H., Hossain, N., Mubarak, N. M., & Shah, A. (2021). Nanomaterials: Applications, waste-handling, environmental toxicities, and future challenges – A review. *Journal of Environmental Chemical Engineering*, *9*(2), 105028. DOI: 10.1016/j.jece.2021.105028

Mbese, Z., Alven, S., & Aderibigbe, B. (2021). Collagen-Based Nanofibers for Skin Regeneration and Wound. *Polymers*, *13*(24), 4368. DOI: 10.3390/polym13244368 PMID: 34960918

McGain, F. (2015). *Environmental Sustainability in Hospitals: An Exploration Within Anaesthetic and Intensive Care Settings*.

Mendes, C., Thirupathi, A., Corrêa, M. E. A. B., Gu, Y., & Silveira, P. C. L. (2022). The Use of Metallic Nanoparticles in Wound Healing: New Perspectives. *International Journal of Molecular Sciences*, *23*(23), 15376. Advance online publication. DOI: 10.3390/ijms232315376 PMID: 36499707

Mitrano, D. M., Motellier, S., Clavaguera, S., & Nowack, B. (2015). Review of nanomaterial aging and transformations through the life cycle of nano-enhanced products. *Environment International*, *77*, 132–147. DOI: 10.1016/j.envint.2015.01.013 PMID: 25705000

Mohite, P., Munde, S., & Uddin, Md. J., Pawar, A., & Singh, S. (2024). Biocompatible Coating of Medical Devices for Protection Against Biofilms. In *Medical Applications for Biocompatible Surfaces and Coatings* (pp. 336–363). Royal Society of Chemistry. DOI: 10.1039/9781837675555-00336

Nagpal, K., Shailendra, K, S., & Dina, N. (2010). *Chitosan Nanoparticles: A Promising System in Novel Drug Delivery. 58*(November).

Nasrollahzadeh, M., Sajjadi, M., Iravani, S., & Varma, R. S. (2021). Carbon-based sustainable nanomaterials for water treatment: State-of-art and future perspectives. *Chemosphere*, *263*, 128005. DOI: 10.1016/j.chemosphere.2020.128005 PMID: 33297038

Oviedo, L. R., Oviedo, V. R., Martins, M. O., Fagan, S. B., & da Silva, W. L. (2022). Nanoarchitectonics: The role of artificial intelligence in the design and application of nanoarchitectures. *Journal of Nanoparticle Research*, *24*(8), 157. DOI: 10.1007/s11051-022-05535-y

Part, F., Berge, N., Baran, P., Stringfellow, A., Sun, W., Bartelt-Hunt, S., Mitrano, D., Li, L., Hennebert, P., Quicker, P., Bolyard, S. C., & Huber-Humer, M. (2018). A review of the fate of engineered nanomaterials in municipal solid waste streams. *Waste Management (New York, N.Y.)*, *75*, 427–449. DOI: 10.1016/j.wasman.2018.02.012 PMID: 29477652

Pfaff, G. (2022). Carbon black pigments. *Physical Sciences Reviews*, *7*(2), 109–125. DOI: 10.1515/psr-2020-0152

Pokrajac, L., Abbas, A., Chrzanowski, W., Dias, G. M., Eggleton, B. J., Maguire, S., Maine, E., Malloy, T., Nathwani, J., Nazar, L., Sips, A., Sone, J., Van Den Berg, A., Weiss, P. S., & Mitra, S. (2021). Nanotechnology for a Sustainable Future: Addressing Global Challenges with the International Network4Sustainable Nanotechnology. *ACS Nano*, *15*(12), 18608–18623. DOI: 10.1021/acsnano.1c10919 PMID: 34910476

Putha, S. (2020). AI-Driven Energy Management in Manufacturing: Optimizing Energy Consumption and Reducing Operational Costs. *Distributed Learning and Broad Applications in Scientific Research, 6*, 313–353. https://dlabi.org/index.php/journal/article/view/107

Putri, A. L. (2016). *Identifikasi Produk Korosi Baja SS304 Coating PANi / SiO 2 Pada Larutan Salinitas Tinggi NaCl 3, 5 M.*

Rabaey, K., & Rozendal, R. A. (2010). Microbial electrosynthesis — Revisiting the electrical route for microbial production. *Nature Reviews. Microbiology*, *8*(10), 706–716. DOI: 10.1038/nrmicro2422 PMID: 20844557

Rabiee, N., Ahmadi, S., Akhavan, O., & Luque, R. (2022). Silver and Gold Nanoparticles for Antimicrobial Purposes against Multi-Drug Resistance Bacteria. *Materials (Basel)*, *15*(5), 1–25. DOI: 10.3390/ma15051799 PMID: 35269031

Ramadan, B. S., Wibowo, Y. G., Anwar, D., & Maryani, A. T. (2024). *A Review of Life Cycle Assessment of Nanomaterials-Based Adsorbent for Environmental Remediation.* https://doi.org/DOI: 10.30955/gnj.006216

Sabar, S. (2013). *Immobilized TiO2/chitosan Layered System Incorporating Reactive Red 4 Dye for the Photocatalytic Degradation of Phenol.* Universiti Sains Malaysia.

Saifuddin, N. N., Matussin, S. N., Fariduddin, Q., & Khan, M. M. (2024). Potentials of roots, stems, leaves, flowers, fruits, and seeds extract for the synthesis of silver nanoparticles. *Bioprocess and Biosystems Engineering*, *47*(8), 1119–1137. DOI: 10.1007/s00449-024-03044-x PMID: 38904717

Saleem, H., & Zaidi, S. (2020). Sustainable Use of Nanomaterials in Textiles and Their Environmental Impact. *Materials (Basel)*, *13*(22), 5134. DOI: 10.3390/ma13225134 PMID: 33203051

Saratale, R. G., Saratale, G. D., Shin, H. S., Jacob, J. M., Pugazhendhi, A., Bhaisare, M., & Kumar, G. (2018). New insights on the green synthesis of metallic nanoparticles using plant and waste biomaterials: Current knowledge, their agricultural and environmental applications. *Environmental Science and Pollution Research International*, *25*(11), 10164–10183. DOI: 10.1007/s11356-017-9912-6 PMID: 28815433

Savitri, E. S., Rahmawaty, A. E., & Minarno, E. B. (2024). Antioxidant, anti-collagenase, and antibacterial activities of Fucus vesiculosus silver nanoparticles. *Narra J*, *4*(3), e882. DOI: 10.52225/narra.v4i3.882 PMID: 39816101

Scarciglia, A., Papi, C., Romiti, C., Leone, A., Di Gregorio, E., & Ferrauto, G. (2025). *Gadolinium-Based Contrast Agents (GBCAs) for MRI: A Benefit–Risk Balance Analysis from a Chemical, Biomedical, and Environmental Point of View*. Global Challenges., DOI: 10.1002/gch2.202400269

Segler, M. H. S., Preuss, M., & Waller, M. P. (2018). Planning chemical syntheses with deep neural networks and symbolic AI. *Nature*, *555*(7698), 604–610. DOI: 10.1038/nature25978 PMID: 29595767

Seth, R., & Meena, A. (2024). Enzymes-based nanomaterial synthesis: An eco-friendly and green synthesis approach. *Clean Technologies and Environmental Policy*. Advance online publication. DOI: 10.1007/s10098-024-02854-7

Sfameni, S., Rando, G., & Plutino, M. R. (2023). Sustainable Secondary-Raw Materials, Natural Substances and Eco-Friendly Nanomaterial-Based Approaches for Improved Surface Performances: An Overview of What They Are and How They Work. *International Journal of Molecular Sciences*, *24*(6), 5472. DOI: 10.3390/ijms24065472 PMID: 36982545

Sheoran, S., Arora, S., Samsonraj, R., Govindaiah, P., & vuree, S. (2022). Lipid-based nanoparticles for treatment of cancer. *Heliyon*, *8*(5), e09403. DOI: 10.1016/j.heliyon.2022.e09403 PMID: 35663739

Sikkander, A. M., Yasmeen, K., & Haseeb, M. (2024). *The biological synthesis, characterization, and therapeutic utility of Fusarium oxysporum silver nanoparticles*. DOI: 10.21203/rs.3.rs-4649729/v1

Singh, A. P., Biswas, A., Shukla, A., & Maiti, P. (2019). Targeted therapy in chronic diseases using nanomaterial-based drug delivery vehicles. *Signal Transduction and Targeted Therapy*, *4*(1), 33. DOI: 10.1038/s41392-019-0068-3 PMID: 31637012

Singh, N. B., Guin, M., & Tomar, R. (2022). Nanostructured ceramics. In *Ceramic Science and Engineering* (pp. 545–573). Elsevier., DOI: 10.1016/B978-0-323-89956-7.00013-9

Solomon, P. S., Adenekan, O. A., & Obasi, S. C. (2024). Sustainable nanomaterials' role in green supply chains and environmental sustainability. *Engineering Science & Technology Journal*, *5*(5), 1678–1694. DOI: 10.51594/estj.v5i5.1136

Soltys, L., Olkhovyy, O., Tatarchuk, T., & Naushad, M. (2021). Green Synthesis of Metal and Metal Oxide Nanoparticles: Principles of Green Chemistry and Raw Materials. *Magnetochemistry (Basel, Switzerland)*, *7*(11), 145. DOI: 10.3390/magnetochemistry7110145

Soroush, E., Mohammadpour, Z., Kharaziha, M., Bakhsheshi-Rad, H. R., & Berto, F. (2022). Polysaccharides-based nanofibrils: From tissue engineering to biosensor applications. *Carbohydrate Polymers*, *291*, 119670. DOI: 10.1016/j.carbpol.2022.119670 PMID: 35698424

Srinath, B. S., Namratha, K., & Byrappa, K. (2018). Eco-Friendly Synthesis of Gold Nanoparticles by *Bacillus subtilis* and Their Environmental Applications. *Advanced Science Letters*, *24*(8), 5942–5946. DOI: 10.1166/asl.2018.12224

Stoner, B. P. (1986). UNDERSTANDING MEDICAL SYSTEMS: TRADITIONAL, MODERN, AND SYNCRETIC HEALTH CARE ALTERNATIVES IN MEDICALLY PLURALISTIC SOCIETIES. *Medical Anthropology Quarterly*, *17*(2), 44–48. DOI: 10.1111/j.1937-6219.1986.tb01021.x

Szunerits, S., & Boukherroub, R. (2018). *Graphene-based biosensors.*

Tamalia, N. (2016). *Pengaruh Penambahan Alumina (0, 10 Dan 15 Wt%) Terhadap Karakteristik Termal (Dta-Tga) Dan Konduktivitas Termal Bahan Keramik Cordierite Berbasis Silika Sekam Padi*. Unila.

Tang, F., Li, L., & Chen, D. (2012). Mesoporous Silica Nanoparticles: Synthesis, Biocompatibility and Drug Delivery. *Advanced Materials*, *24*(12), 1504–1534. DOI: 10.1002/adma.201104763 PMID: 22378538

Thomas, S., Gonsalves, R. A., Jose, J., Zyoud, S. H., Prasad, A. R., & Garvasis, J. (2024). Plant-based synthesis, characterization approaches, applications and toxicity of silver nanoparticles: A comprehensive review. *Journal of Biotechnology*, *394*, 135–149. DOI: 10.1016/j.jbiotec.2024.08.009 PMID: 39159752

Venkatasubramanian, V., & Mann, V. (2022). Artificial intelligence in reaction prediction and chemical synthesis. *Current Opinion in Chemical Engineering*, *36*, 100749. DOI: 10.1016/j.coche.2021.100749

Volpatti, L. R., Matranga, M. A., Cortinas, A. B., Delcassian, D., Daniel, K. B., Langer, R., & Anderson, D. G. (2019). Glucose-responsive nanoparticles for rapid and extended self-regulated insulin delivery. *ACS Nano*, *14*(1), 488–497. DOI: 10.1021/acsnano.9b06395 PMID: 31765558

Yang, T., & Skirtach, A. G. (2025). Nanoarchitectonics of Sustainable Food Packaging: Materials, Methods, and Environmental Factors. *Materials (Basel)*, *18*(5), 1167. DOI: 10.3390/ma18051167 PMID: 40077396

Zan, G., & Wu, Q. (2016a). Biomimetic and Bioinspired Synthesis of Nanomaterials/Nanostructures. *Advanced Materials*, *28*(11), 2099–2147. DOI: 10.1002/adma.201503215 PMID: 26729639

Zan, G., & Wu, Q. (2016b). Biomimetic and Bioinspired Synthesis of Nanomaterials/Nanostructures. *Advanced Materials*, *28*(11), 2099–2147. DOI: 10.1002/adma.201503215 PMID: 26729639

Zhou, T., Song, Z., & Sundmacher, K. (2019). Big Data Creates New Opportunities for Materials Research: A Review on Methods and Applications of Machine Learning for Materials Design. *Engineering (Beijing)*, *5*(6), 1017–1026. DOI: 10.1016/j.eng.2019.02.011

Chapter 5
Biodegradable Materials and Pioneering Sustainable Solutions in Dental Care and Engineering

Jenny Jacob
https://orcid.org/0000-0001-8336-0500
Mar Athanasios College for Advanced Studies, Thiruvalla, India

M. Unnimaya
https://orcid.org/0009-0009-0136-5371
MES M K Mackar Pillai College For Advanced Studies, Edathala, India

Beegam L. Ramlath
St. Berchmans College, Changanassery, India

Treesa Varghese
https://orcid.org/0009-0005-4579-3889
Mar Athanasios College for Advanced Studies, Tiruvalla, India

ABSTRACT

Biomaterials have been developed in the medical field as an innovation evolved for sustainable therapeutic and surgical approaches. These materials comprise natural and synthetic polymers which degrades naturally to nontoxic by-products within biological systems. They can offer temporary structural support and encourage tissue regeneration, which makes them useful in regenerative medicine, drug deliv-

DOI: 10.4018/979-8-3373-1305-4.ch005

ery systems, and temporary medical implants. This chapter includes biodegradable engineering and dental care materials, representing new and sustainable options for temporary and permanent implants. Nanocomposites doped with nanoparticles such as hydroxyapatite and bioactive glasses can improve mechanical strength, biocompatibility, and bioactivity, proving more prominent in dental implants, as integration with the tissue is crucial here. Continued study is positioning such materials to dramatically change how sustainable and effective dental care is achieved, marrying the clinician's needs with the demands of environmental stewardship.

1. INTRODUCTION

Biomaterials are those materials that can be used for interaction in biological systems, while biodegradable materials are considered simply non-toxic. The non-toxic nature of biomaterials includes its biodegradable process which happens naturally without intervention (Lakshmi Reddy et al., 2024). Biodegradable biomaterials provide a safer, sustainable solution to biomedical devices, medical implants, prosthetics, and tissue-engineered devices (Jagur-Grodzinski, 2006; Teo et al., 2016). Biomaterials can also be categorized as bio-inert or biodegradable based on their interaction within the biological system (Godavitarne et al., 2017). Bio-inert materials like stainless steel, cobalt-chromium alloys, and titanium do not provoke a response from the host when introduced into biological tissue and are frequently utilized in contemporary orthopedic surgery. While the primary benefit lies in mechanical strength, there are several notable drawbacks, such as the impact of stress shielding, potential failure of metal components necessitating further surgical intervention, the release of metal ions into adjacent tissues, and the distortion of imaging techniques (Hosseini et al., 2021). The identified limitations have prompted the creation of safer biodegradable alternatives that can break down and be replaced by the body naturally (Shu, 2025).

Biodegradable materials are eco-friendly and can advance sustainability in health care. Medical procedures have drastically changed with the use of biodegradable sutures, which degrade naturally, reducing discomfort in patient care. Reducing medical waste can lower the impact on the environment and positively enhance patient outcomes. The use of bone grafts with resorbability can help in tissue regeneration, eliminating the requirements for additional procedures and reducing long-term pollution (Zafar et al., 2020). Additional surgery would not be necessary to remove these biodegradable implants, which ultimately reduces environmental consequences (Hosseini et al., 2021). Extensive studies have been conducted on the use of polylactic-co-glycolic acid (PLGA) implants successfully in tissue engineering and drug delivery (Kerimoglu and Alarçin, 2012; Makadia and Siegel, 2011). PLA and polycaprolactone (PCL) were studied as small carriers with minimal toxicity for delivering drugs, and they were found to release the drugs in a controlled manner while working very well in the body. Biocomposites have been used as biodegradable materials for tissue repair and regeneration, particularly biomedical scaffolds fabricated with electrospinning, which are injectable and minimally invasive (Liao et al., 2024; Cheng et al., 2025; Vahidi et al., 2024)

Dentistry is progressively adopting biodegradable materials owing to their various benefits, such as diminished environmental effects, superior biocompatibility, increased patient comfort, fewer follow-up operations, and a reduced necessity for subsequent surgeries (Chen et al., 2021). Maxillofacial surgery and dental surgery are increasingly using biodegradable polymers for bone regeneration, particularly in periodontal cases. These polymers can reduce the facial and dental distortions that are inevitable with the non-degradable traditional dental materials (Conte et al., 2018). In the proper context of wound healing in dental surgery, these biopolymers can also act as a scaffold, providing regenerative tissue, while in the context of drug delivery, they allow medicines to be released under a controlled and targeted regime (Powell & Pring, 2024). In tissue engineering and regenerative medicine, the material allows cell growth and nutrient synthesis and ultimately helps heal the skin, bone, and cartilage (Dong et al., 2019).

Figure 1. Applications of biomaterials

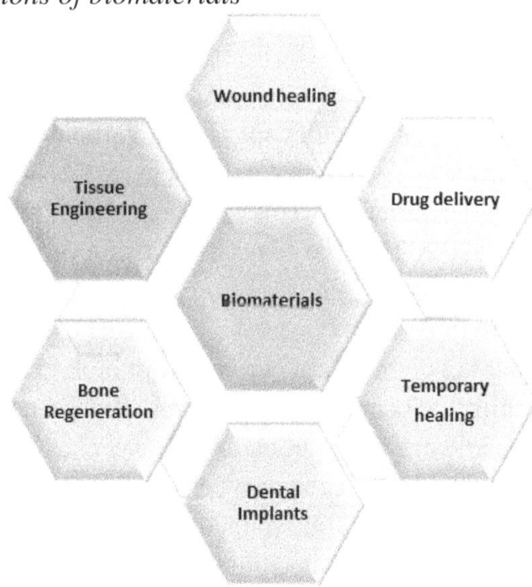

2. PROPERTIES AND TYPES OF BIODEGRADABLE MATERIALS

Diverse categories of biodegradable biomaterials extend across a diverse number of medical applications, be it for use as a scaffold or even for medical packaging. They include both natural and synthetic materials like collagen, chitosan, and polylactic acid, along with more advanced materials made from small particles like silicon and magnesium mixed with hydroxyapatites (Vladescu et al., 2018). Composites and bioceramics, such as calcium phosphate and bioactive glasses, are essential for helping bones heal and for tissue engineering. This structured categorization indicates their adaptability across all medical applications, including regenerative medicine to temporary and permanent implants (Veis & Goldberg, 2014).

2.1 Classification of Biodegradable Materials Based on Composition

Biodegradable materials can be categorized based upon their chemical composition as biodegradable polymers, composite materials, bioceramics, and glasses. Each possesses specific physiochemical and biological properties for biomedical and dental applications.

2.1.1 Biodegradable Polymers

Biodegradable polymers are materials broken down by living entities, mostly microorganisms, into simpler molecules like water, carbon dioxide, biomass, and inorganic chemicals. Microbial enzymes help these organisms in the process of breaking down the polymer structures (Hosseini et al., 2021; Mohammadi & Dummer, 2011; Modrak et al., 2023). The benefits of using biodegradable polymers are substantial in medicine, especially for sutures, drug delivery, bone grafts, and tissue scaffolding.

Natural biodegradable polymers are derived from biological sources and offer excellent biocompatibility, bioactivity, and controlled degradation, making them ideal for various dental and medical applications (Liu et al., 2019). These polymers act like the natural framework that cells grow on, which is important for repairing tissues, delivering medicine, and healing wounds (Dilshad et al., 2021). Among these, collagen, taken from animal tissues, is commonly used in membranes for guided tissue regeneration (GTR), bone grafts, and as a support for cell growth because it helps with bone formation and healing wounds. Cellulose, the most important structural element of plant cell walls, has applications in dental materials such as fillers, adhesives, and impression materials, mainly because of its mechanical strength and biocompatibility (Doppalapudi et al., 2014).

Chitosan, which comes from the shells of crustaceans, is mainly used in wound dressings, gum disease treatment, and delivering drugs because it can fight bacteria, help stop bleeding, and is safe for the body (Vroman & Tighzert, 2009). As denatured collagen gelatin is utilized frequently in the drug delivery system for tissue engineering scaffolds as well as for wound dressings, there is provision of support to cellular attachment as well as its further proliferation (Brunski et al., 1998). Alginate, obtained from brown seaweed, is used in impression materials, wound dressings, and as a tissue engineering scaffold because of its gelling property and biocompatibility (Vroman & Tighzert, 2009). Lastly, hyaluronic acid is a natural part of the connective tissues that help in gum treatment and tissue repair, and it is found in mouthwashes and gels because it helps reduce inflammation, keeps things moist, and aids in healing wounds (Dilshad et al., 2021). These natural materials break down easily and provide safe, eco-friendly options instead of synthetic ones, playing an important role in improving dental care, healing wounds, and the study of biomaterials (Doppalapudi et al., 2014).

Synthetic biopolymers are currently preferred due to the ease of synthesis and applicability. PLA and polyglycolic acids (PGA) are biocompatible and can degrade under controlled conditions (Rocha et al., 2016). PLA sourced from corn starch and sugarcane is biodegradable to lactic acid, making it suitable for guided tissue regeneration (GTR) membranes, resorbable sutures, and bone screws. PGA from sugarcane and sugar beet degrades through hydrolysis to glycolic acid, a key material for resorbable sutures, tissue scaffolds, and composite materials (Liu et al., 2019).

Table 1. Classification of synthetic biodegradable polymers

Name of Polymer	Degradation products	Uses
Polydioxanone (PDO)	P-dioxanone	Sutures
Polycaprolactone (PCL)	Hydroxycaproic acid	Long-term drug delivery systems and tissue engineering scaffolds
Polyhydroxyalkanoates (PHA)	Water and carbon dioxide	Bone grafts and as scaffolds for tissue
Polylactic acid (PLA)	Lactic acid	GTR membranes Resorbable sutures Bone screws
Polyglycolic acid (PGA)	Glycolic acid	Resorbable sutures Tissue scaffolds Composite materials
Polylactic-co-Glycolic Acid (PLGA)	Lactic acid and glycolic acid	Drug delivery systems and resorbable sutures

2.1.2 Bioceramics

Bioceramics are specialty ceramic materials in dentistry that are biocompatible and designed for tissue regeneration. These materials have targeted mechanical strength, bioactivity, and customizability, which qualifies them for several uses in orthopedics, tissue engineering, and drug delivery apart from dentistry. Common bioceramic materials are hydroxyapatite, tricalcium phosphate cement, bioactive glass, and calcium silicate cement, like mineral trioxide aggregate (MTA) (Mohammadi and Dummer, 2011). These materials are greatly used in dental implants to increase the chances of osseointegration, increase fixation, and reduce rejection (Raghavendra et al., 2017) in periodontics and endodontics. Hydroxyapatite and bioactive glass are also used for osseous regeneration and tissue engineering in bone grafting procedures. Bioceramics are also used in dental restoratives such as crowns, bridges, and dentures because of their high strength, resistance against wear, and natural aesthetics (Dong et al., 2023). Their role in tissue engineering is of great significance, as it promotes the formation of new tissues, aids regenerative processes, and makes them applicable to both soft and hard tissues (Jitaru et al., 2016).

Table 2. List of applications of bioceramic material

Area of interest	Bioceramics role
Dental implants	Enhance osteointegration and reduce the risk of rejection
Bone grafting	Bone regeneration and tissue engineering
Dental restoratives	Crowns, bridges, and dentures
Tissue engineering	Support the growth of new tissue and promote regeneration
Orthodontic brackets	Aesthetic and biocompatible alternative to traditional metal brackets
Dental cements	Luting and restorative procedures
Tooth whitening	Whitening toothpaste and mouthwashes
Dental membranes	Guided tissue regeneration
Maxillofacial reconstruction	Reconstruction Reconstruct facial defects and trauma
Periodontal treatment	Periodontal regeneration and tissue repair

2.1.3 Biodegradable Composites

Biodegradable composites are materials consisting of a polymer-based matrix reinforced with natural fibers (Tomer et al., 2020). For tissue engineering applications, composites have already been made from various biodegradable polymeric materials (Abraham et al., 2023). Based on where they come from, these materials can be divided into two main categories: natural polymers and synthetic polymers. Natural biodegradable polymers include proteins like silk and polysaccharides like alginate, chitosan, and derivatives of hyaluronic acid. Synthetic polymers encompass PLA, PGA, poly(-caprolactone) (PCL), and poly(3-hydroxybutyrate) (PHB) (Kadambi et al., 2021). The majority of natural polymers are water soluble in nature; resorbability enables them to form gels with excellent physical and mechanical properties to support dental applications. In addition, they also have excellent biocompatibility and biodegradability, along with outstanding structural strength, which induces cell proliferation and differentiation.

Synthetic biodegradable polymers are hydrophobic in nature with poor water absorption capacity. Even so, the strong structure of synthetic polymers and their ability to create pores can be adjusted for useful uses in dentistry, especially for things like filling root canals, engineering tissues, and guiding tissue growth. The absence of cell recognition sequences in synthetic polymers offers special benefits for dental materials, such as less bacteria sticking to them, controlled breakdown, and increased strength.

In living systems, the breakdown of polymeric biomaterials usually happens when weak connections in the polymer structure are broken down, either by water (for synthetic polymers) or by enzymes (for natural polymers). The speed at which synthetic polymers break down can be affected by things like their chemical makeup, structure, size, variety of sizes, how solid they are, their shape (like how porous they are and their surface area), how the chains are arranged, and how much they attract water, making these factors some of the more predictable traits of synthetic polymers (Tomer et al., 2020).

PLA composite materials have important advantages in biomedical applications because they can be molded into any shape, which is a beneficial feature for 3D printing applications, such as resorbable sutures, bone screws, and GTR membranes. Nanocomposites, like hydroxyapatite-based dental implants and bioactive glass coatings, are safe for the body, do not harm living cells, and can fight off germs while also providing physical protection, which makes them very useful in medicine. Starch-based composites are renewable, biodegradable, cheap, and plentiful, making them a sustainable choice for medical applications, such as tissue scaffolds and drug delivery carriers (Karacan et al., 2017). Another key biodegradable material is polyglycolide (PGA), which can break down completely in the human body without needing special enzymes and is beneficial for different medical uses, like stitches that dissolve and materials for bone grafts.

Using biodegradable bionanocomposites in dentistry shows outstanding potential because they have special features like breaking down at a controlled rate, being more compatible with the body, and having better strength. They are composed of natural or synthetic biodegradable polymers integrated with nanoscale materials

(1 to 100 nm in size). These eco-friendly materials offer excellent biodegradability and biocompatibility, making them ideal for biomimetic applications. Unlike regular composites, nanocomposites have better strength because they have a lot of surface area compared to their size, which helps them get into bacterial cells and break down the outer layer of sugars that bacteria produce. Adding these tiny materials to the tooth helps rebuild its structure and slows down bacterial growth, which lowers the chances of getting new cavities.

Extracellular matrix (ECM) is a tissue-specific, highly complex three-dimensional network composed of several macromolecules and plays a vital role in cell differentiation and tissue homeostasis mechanisms. The addition of ECM significantly enhances their biocompatibility and enhances cell interaction (Gothard et al., 2015; Harvestine et al., 2016). These materials are commonly utilized for tissue engineering and regenerative medicine. Nano-fiber scaffolds based on ECM for articular cartilage regeneration are one of the promising applications of this material (Goldberg and Smith 2004).

2.2 Properties of Biodegradable Materials

Mechanical, chemical, physical, and degradation-related characteristics primarily govern the selection and utilization of biodegradable materials in the engineering and dental fields (Ramezani & Ripin, 2023).

2.2.1 Mechanical Properties

Mechanical properties dictate the performance of biodegradable materials and are of particular relevance for load-bearing applications, such as dental implants, bone scaffolds, and orthopedic fixations (Hynes & Naba, 2011). Mechanical strength of these biomaterials are important for handling pulling and pushing forces. Materials that have both of these strengths and are lighter than plastics, making them good choices for dental screws and temporary support devices. To lessen stress shielding, a bioactive material should be as flexible as the surrounding tissue. Fracture toughness and fatigue resistance are also important, especially for devices that experience repeated stress, like those used for chewing in the mouth. Flexibility and the ability to change shape are more important in soft tissue uses because the materials need to fit and move with changing tissue surfaces, like collagen or electrospun polymer membranes (Engler et al., 2006). Another good way to improve how biodegradable materials work is by changing the polymer chemistry, such as using different kinds of poly(lactic-co-glycolic acid)s (PLGA), where you can modify the mix of polylactide and polyglycolic acid, or by adding composite systems with bioceramic particles or nanofillers to strengthen them (Paduano et al., 2016).

2.2.2 Physical Properties

Physical properties play an important role in the processing of biodegradable materials during fabrication and in their performance in a physiological environment. Density and porosity are key factors in tissue engineering because porosity helps cells move and allows nutrients and fluids to flow, as well as supports the growth of blood vessels. If the porosity is too high, it can weaken the material. Surface roughness and the shape of a material affect how cells behave when in contact, like cell growth and development. These attributes remain important for the integration of dental and orthopedic implants (Dong et al., 2019). Natural polymers (e.g., collagen and chitosan) are often hydrophilic and conducive to favorable biological interfaces, while synthetic polymers are usually hydrophobic and need surface modification to assist with wettability. Thermal properties like melting temperature and glass transition temperature (Tg) are important during processing methods and dictate the material's structural integrity and formability (Sudhakar et al., 2024). Together, these physical properties also promote the material's degradation profile, swelling, or biointeractions when in hydrated or body-like conditions.

2.2.3 Chemical Properties

The chemical attributes of biodegradable substances are essential to their degradation methods, biological environment reactions, and potential commercial adaptations. The chemical bond arrangements decide how the material breaks down—like hydrolysis for aliphatic polyesters such as PLA and PLGA, enzymes for natural polymers like collagen or chitosan. In synthetic polymers, the hydrolysis of ester bonds yields biocompatible by-products such as lactic and glycolic acid. Some parts of the materials, like carboxyl, amine, and hydroxyl groups, make it easier for them to react and connect with bioactive molecules, drug molecules, or crosslinking agents, which can alter how the scaffold functions in medical applications. Biodegradable materials respond differently to changes in pH; materials like calcium phosphates and extracellular matrix-based (ECM) scaffolds break down at different speeds depending on the pH, which is particularly important in inflamed or infected tissues where the pH can vary. Some biodegradable materials also release ions; for instance, bioactive glasses and magnesium-based alloys will let go of ions like calcium (Ca^{2+}), magnesium (Mg^{2+}), and silicon (Si^{4+}), which can help with tissue healing and have properties that fight infections and adjust the immune response.

2.3 Regulatory Considerations and Standards for Biodegradable Dental Materials

The safety and effectiveness of biodegradable materials for dental applications depend on adherence to rigorous regulatory systems (Modrák et al., 2023). National and international regulatory bodies closely monitor these materials as they are intended for use in or on the human body, particularly in the sensitive oral environment. This process ensures verification of biocompatibility and functional performance as well as safe and gradual material degradation (Vasquez & Forest, 2014).

Dental biomaterials in the United States are regulated by the Food and Drug Administration (FDA) through its Center for Devices and Radiological Health (CDRH). Usually, depending on their use and degree of risk, these materials are categorized as Class II or III medical devices (Schmalz & Reichl, 2021). New or high-risk devices need stricter Premarket Approval (PMA), but materials that are similar to existing ones might be able to use the easier 510(k) premarket notification process by showing they are very similar. If one is to be compliant, the Medical Device Regulation (MDR 2017/745) has to be followed in the EU (Svempe, 2024). The technical papers, risk assessments, and clinical evaluation reports are examined by a notified body before granting CE certification (Schröttner & Baumgartner, 2023).

A crucial step in the process of regulatory approval is biocompatibility testing, which ensures the material will not react harmfully or toxically when it comes into contact with human tissue. Manufacturers must adhere to the ISO 10993 series' standardized testing criteria (Al-Zyoud et al., 2023). Usually beginning with cytotoxicity tests, especially vital or dental materials due to their prolonged mouth exposure (Shahi et al., 2019), genotoxicity tests using Ames test or micronucleus test (Landsiedel et al., 2022) and in vivo biocompatibility studies help assess the material's interactions with living tissues. These studies provide knowledge of how the material breaks down, whether any byproducts of the materials are harmful,, and whether the host tissue properly incorporates it (Veronesi et al., 2020).

A biodegradable dental material has to meet particular mechanical criteria to function well under oral stress conditions. Standards including ISO 14801 and ISO 10477 direct these assessments for dental implants and prostheses. Techniques like contact angle measurements, atomic force microscopy (AFM), and scanning electron microscopy (SEM) help researchers examine surface properties, including porosity, surface roughness, and how well surfaces attract water, all of which influence how well cells stick and integrate with the material (Hanna et al., 2024). Using the ISO and ASTM (American Society for Testing and Materials) criteria, developers can better fit their material testing to globally recognized standards. For example, ISO 7405 governs the evaluation of preclinical dental materials; ISO 10993 governs the evaluation of biological materials. ASTM also provides methods for assessing the physical and degradation characteristics of biodegradable polymers. Following these guidelines helps to get regulatory approval and increases the credibility of the material in the clinical and commercial sectors (Halamoda-Kenzaoui et al., 2019).

3. ROLE OF BIODEGRADABLE MATERIALS IN DENTAL CARE

3.1 Bioresorbable Fixation and Support Devices

Bioresorbable fixation and support devices offer a new way to help with dental and facial surgeries by giving temporary support that breaks down as the soft tissue heals. These support devices include mini-implants, miniplates and biomembranes.

3.1.1 Bioresorbable Mini-Implant

Non-degradable materials used as permanent implants can cause serious problems, such as infections, when they stay in the body for a long time (Ahmed et al., 2024). This concern has led to an emphasis on the use of bioresorbable biomaterials for medical surgery, reducing the physical pain of the patient as well as the recovery of the implant device (Morsada et al., 2021). These techniques can utilize both passive and wearable and implantable devices. Recent studies on resorbable implants indicate that they are often surrounded by bony tissue, sometimes accompanied by a thin fibrous layer. Mg-Ca alloys exhibit degradation within a three-month period post-bone formation (Chang et al., 2017; Kartik et al., 2021). Applying protective coatings, including calcium phosphate, fluorinated materials, or polymers, is an effective strategy to mitigate the degradation of magnesium alloys. PLA and PGA implants have been extensively used for soft tissue implants in sports injuries and have been found to be self-reinforcing (Maitra et al., 1998). The time required for the implant degradation remains the most important characteristic to be studied. Changing the PLA/PGA ratio can effectively change how quickly the implants break down, how they are removed from the body, and their strength and flexibility (Kartik et al., 2021). Dentistry uses orthodontic wires and brackets, which require long-term usage and can cause angular friction. Nickel/titanium wires can exhibit heat activation, causing permanent deformation, while in contrast, the addition of copper can resist any such deformations (Prakasham et al., 2017; Pietrzak et al., 1996). This technology can be further extended to stents with magnesium, zinc, iron, and cobalt-chromium for treating coronary artery diseases (Gasik et al., 2021).

3.1.2 Bioresorbable Miniplates and Metal Biomembranes

Rigid plates and screws are typically used for complicated face fractures. These metal implants, however, may cause corrosion, electrolysis, hypersensitivity, and possible carcinogenic concerns in addition to interfering with imaging methods like CT and MRI scans. The development of bioresorbable osteo-fixation materials is becoming more and more popular as a solution to these problems (Dutta et al., 2020). Most bioresorbable plates today are mainly made from synthetic semi-crystalline poly-4 (alpha hydroxy acid) and its copolymers. Alpha-hydroxy acid, or poly-4, has special qualities that make it ideal for biodegradation in contrast to titanium. Because they break down naturally, have beneficial mechanical properties, can help create bone, are compatible with the body, and fight bacteria, biodegradable metals are being closely examined for use in tissue regeneration (Zheng et al., 2014). Magnesium-based biomembranes can combine the safe features and gradual breakdown of natural tissues with the strength of metal alloys (Chen et al., 2021).

Figure 2. Applications of magnesium in biomembrane

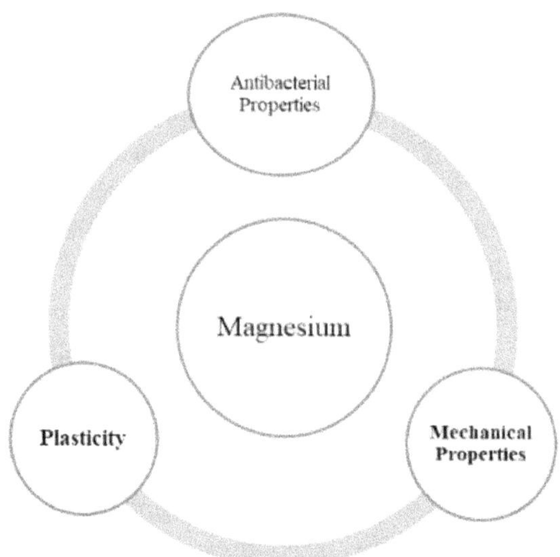

3.2 Orthodontic and Prosthodontic Applications

3.2.1 Biodegradable Aligners

Aligners are used in orthodontics to align and straighten teeth so that they can gradually clear out after long-time use. People consider it an aesthetic alternative to the traditional use of metal wires and braces. Clear aligner therapy (CAT) is now a suitable option for fixing crooked teeth, crowded teeth, and problems that come back after braces (Bichu et al., 2023; Macrì et al., 2024). Innovative compostable and completely biodegradable alternatives, like GT FLEX, are becoming available in addition to traditional BPA-free and recyclable aligner materials. Compared to conventional commercial aligners, these materials are designed to provide more strength and flexibility (Mallakpour et al., 2021).

3.2.2 Biodegradable Denture Base Material

PMMA has traditionally been the primary material used for tooth and denture bases. However, research on substitute materials has been spurred by their drawbacks, which include staining susceptibility, noise during mastication, poor impact strength, short shelf life, and variable performance (Dutta et al., 2020; Mallakpour et al., 2021). Denture bases that are more resilient and patient-friendly by the integration of these materials into the PMMA matrix can increase tensile strength, impact strength, compressive strength, and microhardness.

3.3 Biodegradable Surgical and Periodontal Materials

Giving sustainable alternatives to traditional, non-resorbable materials, biodegradable materials are a revolutionary development in engineering and dental treatment. Ongoing studies and cross-disciplinary cooperation nevertheless propel development despite manufacturing, scalability, and regulatory acceptability hurdles.

3.3.1 Biodegradable Sutures

Suture anchor designs and materials have advanced significantly during the last few decades (Dennis et al., 2016). Originally made of non-biodegradable metals and polymers, they have seen a significant shift recently toward biodegradable polymers (Faris et al., 2022). Benefits of the biodegradable polymer anchors include enhanced postsurgical imaging, less migration risk, less complicated revision surgery, no removal procedure, and gradual breakdown over time (Nouri et al., 2023). These anchors, however, are less fixable than metal anchors and are prone to rapid disintegration, inflammatory reactions, and unfavorable local tissue reactions (Khiste et al., 2013). Future researchers can make the biodegradable suture anchors thinner and smaller due to their high strength and bone-like flexibility. When used to close wounds, biodegradable sutures can break down at a pace that corresponds with the tissue's natural healing process (Randhawa et al., 2024). They aid in wound care, medication delivery, and healing (Chen et al., 2021).

3.3.2 Biodegradable Membranes for Guided Tissue Regeneration

Guided Tissue Regeneration (GTR) is a common dental procedure that uses special membranes that break down over time to help new cells grow and repair soft and bone tissue. Biodegradable membranes help bone and periodontal ligament cells grow back slowly, but they also make it take longer for skin cells to move into the damaged area. These biodegradable membranes provide structure during essential wound healing and resorb without harm. Some biodegradable membranes contain bioactive compounds, nanoparticles, or antibacterial agents to increase healing, infection risk, and efficacy.

3.4 Endodontic Applications

Endodontics is increasingly utilizing biodegradable materials for the creation of an apical barrier, root canal filling, and pulp regeneration. Natural and manmade polymers such as collagen, chitosan, and PLGA promote stem cell activity and eventually degrade after the assistance of tissue repair. These materials also function as carriers for bioactive materials or antimicrobials, thus enhancing healing and eliminating the need for surgical removal.

3.4.1 Biodegradable Filler for Roots

Nanofillers are novel materials that help other materials enhance their mechanical properties. By being added to other materials, these nanofillers help nanocomposite materials keep their best density while also strengthening them, improving them at handling heat, resistant to fire, and able to absorb water (Jagadeesh et al., 2021; Ilalova et al., 2023). Resilon is a root canal filling material made of radiopaque fillers, bioactive glass, and a methacrylate resin base that was first presented in 2004 as an alternative to guttapercha. The purpose of this thermoplastic polymer is to create a monolithic seal inside the canal by bonding with the root dentin (Modrák et al., 2023). Both biotic and abiotic degradation of Resilon have been the subject of research. Assessing Resilon's biodegradability by microbes is crucial because it is a polymer blend that contains bioactive glass and mineral fillers. Microorganisms in dental sludge can break down the polycaprolactone part of Resilon, which easily reacts with alkaline substances and enzymes.

3.4.2 Biodegradable Intracanal Medication

Because of its antibacterial qualities, calcium hydroxide ($Ca(OH)_2$) has been utilized as an intracanal drug in endodontics for many years. Over time, many attempts have been made to overcome its drawbacks, including the decreased antibacterial efficacy brought on by dentine buffering, which lowers the drug's alkalinity (Tomer et al., 2020). Traditional intracanal medications are unable to reach every location due to the anatomical complexity of root canal networks (Zafar et al., 2020). Nanotechnology-based improvements in drug delivery systems have been suggested as a solution (Modrák et al., 2023). After being improved and tested, $Ca(OH)_2$-loaded PLGA nanoparticles (NPs) showed a strong negative charge, were smaller than 200 nm on average, had a low level of size variation, and were excellent at holding onto the drug. These nanoparticles showed improved penetration into dentinal tubules and sustained drug release, which makes them a viable substitute for intracanal antibacterial therapy (Chang et al., 2017; Dong et al., 2019). Ester hydrolysis is the mechanism by which PLGA biodegrades (Chang et al., 2017). Lactide-rich PLGA copolymers degrade more slowly, absorb less water, and have reduced hydrophilicity (Kartik et al., 2021).

4. EMERGING TECHNOLOGIES: NANOCOMPOSITES IN DENTAL IMPLANTS

Traditional ways of making and combining biodegradable nanocomposites usually have problems like weak strength, uneven breakdown rates, limited ability to fight bacteria, and poor attachment to dental tissues, which limits how well they work in dental implants (Zhang et al., 2021). To address the challenges of conventional approaches, a number of advanced fabrication techniques, such as electrospinning, 3D bioprinting, and nanostructuring, may be adopted. Additionally, advanced fabrication techniques create small structures of biodegradable nanocomposites that are stronger, work better with the body, release drugs steadily, and fight bacteria, making them a better choice for dental implants (Velu et al., 2020). Methods to modify the surface, such as applying a hydroxyapatite coating, using bioactive glass, or incorporating silver or zinc oxide nanoparticles, enhance the material's performance and its effectiveness against germs. These nanocomposites can blend with dental tissues by copying the extracellular matrix and helping them grow back slowly as the material breaks down (Kang et al., 2021). Optimized fabrication and integration strategies ensure a temporary structural support while being perfectly replaced by a natural one, hence making them a very effective and sustainable solution in modern dental care (Ramezani & Ripin, 2023).

4.1 Types of Nanocomposites and their Fabrication Methods

Nanocomposites in dental implants are categorized into polymer-based, ceramic-based, and metallic-based systems, each offering distinct advantages and limitations. Polymer-based nanocomposites are appreciated for their flexibility and aesthetic appeal but often lack the mechanical strength when compared with metal- and ceramic-based composites (Carrouel et al., 2020). Ceramic-based nanocomposites provide excellent biocompatibility and wear resistance, though their brittleness can limit use in high-stress applications. These types of nanocomposites, including hydroxyapatite and zirconia, provide high bioactivity and excellent osteointegration (Ramezani & Ripin, 2023). Metallic-based nanocomposites offer superior strength and corrosion resistance, making them suitable for load-bearing applications, but may pose risks of toxicity due to metal ion release. Metallic nanocomposites incorporate silver and titanium dioxide, which are antibacterial agents to prevent the infection while improving the mechanical properties. This material combination allows for the creation of highly advanced, biofunctional dental implants that have a better healing outcome and long-term performance (Armentano et al., 2010). A novel biodegradable composite consisting of polycaprolactone and magnesium allows for the adjustment of the compressive moduli of the composites to align with the spectrum of human cancellous bone due to the incorporation of magnesium micro-particles. The silane-coated Mg/PCL composites exhibit superior cytocompatibility and promote osteoblastic development (Tomer et al., 2020). Biomaterials will assume a more proactive function post-implantation, rather than merely serving as a tissue engineering scaffold.

4.1.1 Electrospun Method

Electrospinning is a highly versatile, efficient technique for producing porous nanofibers with high surface area and tunable properties widely used in biomedical applications, due to its ability to create fibers with nanoscale diameters and controlled porosity (Velu et al., 2020). Electrospun materials provides adequate support with satisfactory rigidity, making them excellent for biomedical and tissue engineering application (Kang et al., 2021). Studies have shown that cells seeded on electrospun meshes with high porosity tend to proliferate and differentiate more rapidly than those on scaffolds with lower porosity (Lowery et al., 2010). A range of polymer and composite materials have been electrospun to create scaffolds aimed at regenerating dental tissues, including oral mucosa, periodontium, dentin, and skeletal tissues (Zafar et al., 2016).

4.1.2 Solvent Casting Method

Solvent casting is one of the most widely used and simple fabrication techniques for biodegradable nanocomposites in dental implants. This method involves the dissolution of polymers and nanoparticles in a suitable solvent to form a homogeneous solution, which is then poured into molds or onto a substrate. As the solvent gradually evaporates, it leaves behind a solidified composite material (Souza et al., 2015). This technique allows for uniform nanoparticle dispersion within the polymer matrix, improving mechanical strength, bioactivity, and controlled degradation (Yoshinari et al., 2001). Solvent casting is particularly useful for creating thin films, membranes, and porous scaffolds that support cell attachment, bone regeneration, and drug delivery in dental applications (LaBagnara, 1995).

4.1.3 Sol-Gel Technologies

As the most predominant method for nanocomposites, Sol-Gel technique involves the transformation of a precursor solution (sol) containing monomers into a solid form through subsequent gelification (gel) (Sudhakar et al., 2024). This method facilitates the uniform dispersion of nanoparticles within the polymer, either through colloidal suspension prior to gelification or by in situ particle formation during the gelation phase by incorporating appropriate precursors for filler nucleation. The polymerization process driven by solvent evaporation enables the molding of the final composite into thin films (Suárez et al., 2021).

4.1.4 Thermally Induced Phase Separation Method

Thermally Induced Phase Separation (TIPS) or Freeze-drying method is another most versatile and an easy-to-tune fabrication process capable of producing porous polymeric scaffold and it has been largely used for its capability to produce highly porous and interconnected scaffolds (Velu et al., 2020) . TIPS technique relies on temperature changes to trigger the phase separation of a polymer solution, resulting in a multi-phase system. Incorporation of suitable inorganic fillers into the solution can improve both bioactivity and mechanical properties of the scaffold. Polini et al., (2013) demonstrated the protocol for gelatin and bioactive glass (BG)-based nanocomposites using TIPS method. These scaffolds exhibit tunable silica content and demonstrate good biological properties, including biodegradation stability and biocompatibility. TIPS technique has also been adopted to develop hybrid nanocomposite materials using gelatin and tunable silica shows good biocompatibility, biodegradation stability and apatite-forming ability. Use of the TIPS method aided formation nanocomposites using amorphous calcium phosphate (ACP) and PLA enhance osteoblastic adhesion and differentiation, making them suitable for bone tissue engineering (Bienek and Skrtic, 2017). Additionally, polyurethane and carbon nanotube composite - based scaffolds also fabricated using TIPS, offers enhanced mechanical properties and are suitable for various biomedical applications (Jell et al., 2007).

4.1.5 3D-Bioprinting

3D bioprinting is an advanced fabrication method that provides detailed control over the design of the implant, so that it may be designed for tailored porosity, mechanical strength, and bioactivity (Mohammadi & Dummer, 2011). The method is characterized by layer-by-layer deposition of biodegradable materials such as PLA, PGA, and bioactive nanocomposites, thus ensuring high structural accuracy and patient-specific customization. Implants may be designed to have optimal degradation rates, enhanced osseointegration, and improved load-bearing capacity by adjusting printing parameters. Additionally, 3D printing facilitates the incorporation of bioactive nanoparticles, such as hydroxyapatite and silver, which improve bone regeneration and antibacterial properties, making it a promising approach for next-generation dental implants (Powell and Pring, 2024).

4.1.6 In-Situ Polymerization

In-situ polymerization is a fabrication technique where nanoparticles are uniformly dispersed within a polymer matrix, leading to enhanced mechanical stability and controlled degradation. This process involves polymerizing monomers around pre-dispersed nanoparticles, ensuring strong interfacial bonding and homogeneity within the composite structure (Dutta et al., 2020). The method allows for fine-tuned nanoparticle loading, enabling implants to exhibit improved strength, flexibility, and bioactivity. In dentistry, in situ polymerization is very useful in scaffold and coating applications for implants that require biodegradability, osteoconductivity, and antibacterial resistance for long-term success (Souza et al., 2015).

4.2 Integration of Nanocomposites with Dental Tissues

The main role of surface modification techniques for biodegradable dental implants is to enhance biocompatibility, osseointegration, and antibacterial properties (Ramezani and Ripin, 2023). Hydroxyapatite coating enhances the bonding of implants to bone tissue; thus, there is faster healing and regeneration. Plasma treatments involve modification of the surface chemistry with increased cell adhesion and absorption of proteins in order to get better tissue interaction (Armentano et al., 2010). Functionalization of the antibacterial nanoparticle also avoids infections by using silver (Ag) and zinc oxide (ZnO), thus reducing the chance of implant failure. Surface treatments are also crucial to ascertain long-term stability, improvement in healing, and enhanced functionality of biodegradable dental implants (Chang et al., 2017).

Figure 3. Manufacturing methods of nanocomposite for dental implants

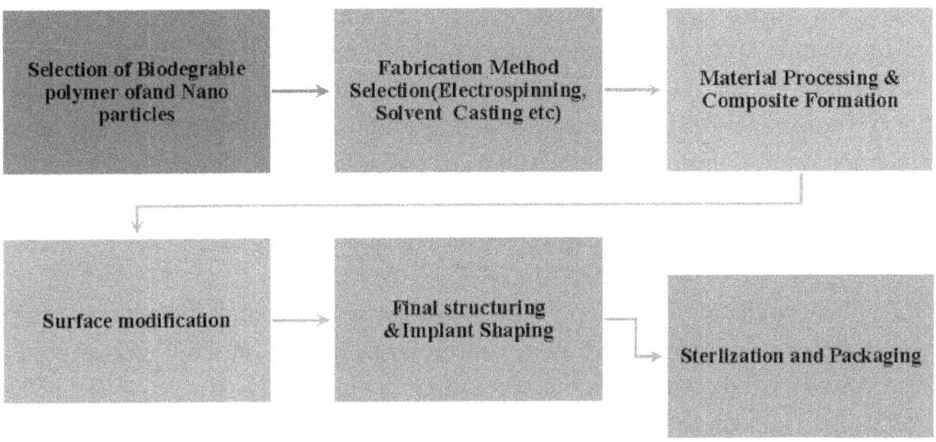

4.2.1 Surface Modification to Improve Osseointegration

Surface modification enhances the osseointegration of biodegradable nanocomposite dental implants (Zheng et al., 2014). The techniques involved in surface modification methods are plasma treatment, hydroxyapatite coating, and bioactive glass deposition that can improve the interface between the implant and osseous tissue. The plasma treatment increases the surface energy of the implant material and hence increases the adhesion of osteocytes and proteins. It increases the surface roughness to allow better integration with the surrounding tissues (Chen et al., 2021). Hydroxyapatite (HA) coatings closely resemble the mineral composition of natural bone significantly enhancing the bonding between the implant and bone tissue, leading to osteointegration and enhancing the life of the implant. The bioactive glass deposition method releases ions such as calcium, phosphate, and silicon, which advance osteogenesis and enhance the integration of the implant with nearby bone (Zafar et al., 2020).

4.2.2 Functionalization with Growth Factors and Proteins

Functionalization with growth factors and proteins modifies nanocomposite surfaces with bioactive molecules to directly promote tissue regeneration and to assist the osseointegration process (Modrák et al., 2023). Inevitably, collagen or BMPs (Bone Morphogenetic Proteins) coated on nanocomposite implants work towards the regeneration of bone through the stimulation of osteoblast differentiation and the acceleration of bone healing processes (Kunduru et al., 2016). BMPs, specifically, are a series of growth factors responsible for some key activities in new bone formation at the implantation site. Chitosan and gelatin are natural polymers recognized for their suitability and enhancing the integration of soft tissues (Shu, 2025). These materials help form a fibrous capsule around the implant, aiding tissue repair and limiting inflammation (Kunduru et al., 2016; Shu, 2025).

4.2.3 Nanoparticle Layering for Antibacterial Effects

Applying antibacterial nanoparticles to the surface of dental implants may help reduce the risks of infection, a common problem in implantology (Aktas et al., 2024). Silver is revered for its intense antimicrobial effects. Silver nanoparticles inhibit bacterial settlement and biofilm formation, which would have led to infections around the implant site (Lakshmi Reddy et al., 2024). The antimicrobial properties of these nanoparticles ZnO (antibacterial) and TiO_2 (providing a self-cleaning effect by photocatalytic activity) would also prevent infections and improve the lifespan of the implant.

4.2.4 Controlled Degradation for Gradual Tissue Replacement

Biocompatibility coupled with slow degradation is the hallmark of biodegradable nanocomposite materials for dental implants. Controlled degradation means the natural bone replaces the implant slowly and gradually, reducing the chances of implant rejection or failure. Nanocomposites like PLGA are controlled for the degradation rate to allow time for the bone to replace the implant. While degrading, the ions or molecules released by the implant material may enhance further growth of bone or healing (Chen et al., 2021; Zheng et al., 2014).

Figure 4. Healing process of nanocomposite dental implants

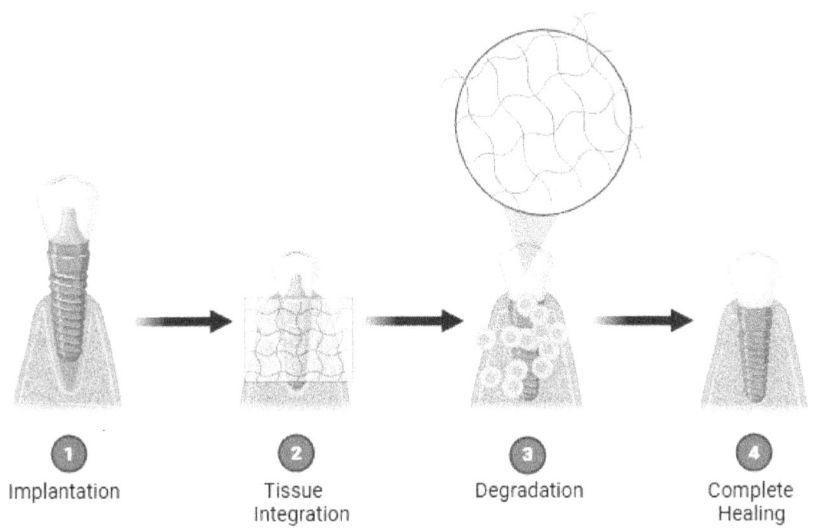

4.3 Properties of Nanocomposites

Nanocomposites, which consist of a polymer matrix integrated with nanoscale fillers such as hydroxyapatite (HA), bioactive glass, graphene oxide, carbon nanotubes, and metallic nanoparticles, show superior and tunable properties when compared to their base materials. One of the most valuable benefits is the improvement in mechanical properties, such as tensile strength, modulus, and fracture toughness, which are important for dental applications that bear load, such as bone grafts or implant coatings. The introduction of nanofillers increases the surface area-to-volume ratio of the entire composite, allowing improved whether cell adhesion, proliferation, or differentiation, resulting in improved biocompatibility, bioactivity, and osteoconductivity. Nanocomposites allow for modified degradation rates as nanoparticles slow or accelerate matrix degradation depending on their composition and dispersion. Additionally, many nanofillers, including silver, zinc oxide, and chitosan-based nanostructures, can impart antibacterial activity, which is important for preventing infection in dental implants or wound healing membranes. Increased thermal and electrical conductivity and barrier properties can also be attained, making nanocomposite fit for sensors and drug delivery platforms. Overall, nanocomposites show a multifunctional platform with a synergistic balance of biological and physicochemical property balances that are also easily adjustable for advanced dental and biomedical applications. Table 3 includes clinical trials conducted in dental care research that are relevant to the work.

Table 3. Clinical trials conducted in dental care research

Sl No	Reference	Description
1.	Elabd et al., 2024	A randomized controlled trial looked at adding 1% titanium dioxide nanoparticles to the acrylic baseplates of twin block orthodontic functional appliances. The study aimed to enhance the antimicrobial properties of the appliances without compromising their mechanical performance or clinical effectiveness.
2.	Demirci et al., 2018	In restorative dentistry, nanofilled resin composites like Filtek Supreme XT and nanohybrid composites such as Ceram X Duo are widely used due to their improved mechanical properties, esthetics, and wear resistance. These materials offer enhanced polishability and longevity, making them suitable for both anterior and posterior restorations.
3.	Burke et al., 2017	In restorative dentistry, Filtek Supreme XTE™ incorporates nanofillers to enhance its mechanical strength, polish retention, and esthetic qualities, making it a highly durable and visually appealing material for both anterior and posterior restorations.
4.	Bechara et al., 2017	Calcium is important for dental implants because it helps the bone attach and grow around the implant, making it more stable and successful over time.
5.	Danelon et al., 2019	Enamel remineralization using HMPnano (nano-hydroxyapatite and polyphosphate-based agents) serves as an effective preventive measure by restoring mineral content, enhancing enamel strength, and reducing the risk of caries through biomimetic repair of early demineralized lesions.
6.	Mangano et al., 2017	Calcium phosphate-coated dental implants with nanostructured surfaces, such as NCI implants, demonstrated significantly higher bone-implant contact (BIC) compared to other implants, indicating enhanced early bone healing and successful osseointegration under immediate loading conditions.

5. FAILURE MECHANISMS OF BIODEGRADABLE DENTAL MATERIALS

In dentistry, although environmentally advantageous, biodegradable materials have obstacles, including insufficient durability for prolonged use, which may lead to restoration failures (LaBagnara, 1995). Their erratic deterioration can jeopardize the integrity of dental procedures, and the amalgamation of elevated expenses and specialist management further complicates their application. Dental implants are supplementing dentures as the preferred treatment for tooth loss (Vasconcelos et al., 2016; Vishwakarma et al., 2016). Dental implants, known as "artificial tooth roots," are metallic posts surgically embedded in the upper or lower jaw beneath the gingiva to hold artificial crowns as replacements for absent teeth (Ding et al., 2018).

The osseointegration healing period for dental implants situated in the alveolar bone spans three to six months. Successful osseointegration post-implantation is crucial for the effective functioning of the dental implant (Lotz et al., 2020). Inadequate implant-bone contact contributes to the gradual loss of marginal bone during osseointegration under compromised local or systemic settings (Gulati et al., 2023). A deterioration in systemic health, history of periodontitis, bacterial buildup, or trauma may lead to implant failure (both early and late), ultimately requiring implant removal (Zhang et al., 2021). Early failure pertains to the inability of dental implants to attain osseointegration, while late failure denotes the loss of either the established osseointegration or the functionality of dental implants (Verron et al., 2010). Surgical stress, insufficient primary stability, and perioperative contamination are the key causes leading to early implant failure. Conversely, peri-implantitis and overloading are the primary factors associated with late implant failure (Diz et al., 2013). Furthermore, a transmucosal segment that infiltrates the soft tissue between the bone and the prosthesis is a defining feature of dental implants. Consequently, robust and continuous soft-tissue integration (STI) is essential for the long-term functionality of dental implants, alongside adequate osseointegration (Diz et al., 2013).

Mechanical debridement techniques and laser treatments are the predominant non-surgical approaches for managing peri-implantitis (Mehdikhani-Nahrkhalaji et al., 2012). Surgical approaches encompass reconstruction surgery alongside debridement (Kang et al., 2021). Initial clinical indicators of infection, discomfort or tenderness, a non-dull sound following percussion, radiographic evidence, implant mobility, and hemorrhage upon probing are essential for diagnosing implant failure (Liu et al., 2021). The pursuit of improved bone regeneration under challenging conditions has driven the advancement of modern dental implants from the perspective of implant manufacturing (Das et al., 2019).

Local or systemic disorders and other contributing factors can affect the long-term efficacy of implant therapy (Nasar, 2019). Consequently, numerous characteristics can be recognized as contraindications for implant implantation (Ramezani and Ripin, 2023). Bone abnormalities, such as osteogenesis imperfecta and osteoporosis, may impede the regeneration of alveolar bone. Additional risk factors that affect the success of implant surgery encompass uncontrolled diabetes, smoking, human immunodeficiency virus (HIV), chronic renal diseases, inadequate dental hygiene, and a history of periodontal disease (Hakim et al., 2024).

6. CHALLENGES IN BIODEGRADABLE BIOMATERIALS

The predominant challenges arise from the design of most standard tests, which are intended for permanent implant materials, biodegradable polymers, or ceramics. A prevalent prerequisite for standardization, by International Organization for Standardization (ISO) or American Society for Testing and Materials (ASTM) regulations are the provision of experimental methodologies that exhibit high reproducibility across various laboratories and organizations (Hosseini et al., 2021). Table 4 describes the major challenges of biodegradable materials in detail.

6.1 Economic and Environmental impact

While biodegradable materials have transformative capabilities in a clinical and engineering context, their uptake has been constrained due to various technical, economic, environmental, and social obstacles. Overcoming these barriers is important for successful translation from research to regular clinical and industrial practice.

Table 4. Major challenges of biodegradable materials

Sl No	Major Challenges of Biodegradable Materials	Description
1	High production cost	Expensive synthesis and processing steps
2	Scaling up difficulties	Hard to maintain quality in large-scale production
3	Limited raw material availability	Dependence scarce of natural sources
4	Waste and energy during processing	Energy-intensive and solvent-heavy process
5	Lifecycle uncertainty	Unclear degradation pathway and byproducts
6	Recycling and disposal challenge	Inefficient breakdown in some disposal conditions

6.2 Patient Perspectives

Biodegradable biomaterials in dental and medical applications depend on patient acceptability. Patients value the properties of non-invasiveness and biological resorption that biodegradable implants offer, most importantly if a second surgical removal procedure is completely avoided. The novelty of a newly developed biomaterial may create uncertainty in long-term safety, possibility of local inflammatory response, or potential for incomplete degradation. In the dental care the use of biodegradable materials may be perceived as experimental due to the lack of effective patient education, and, evidence-based patient outcomes.

6.3 Market Analysis

Barriers to commercialization of biodegradable materials pose unique challenges, including high innovation costs, a slow rate of clinical acceptance, and a heavily regulated approval component. There is low market penetration in lower- and middle-income regions due to costs and technical infrastructure. There is reluctance to accept biomaterials when they are competing against permanent materials like titanium that have an attractive price. Additionally, widespread adoption by clinicians will depend on clear clinical applicability standards and accessible long-term outcome data.

7. FUTURE STUDIES IN BIODEGRADABLE BIOMATERIALS

Future research and development in biomaterials may focus on "multifunctional capabilities," such as offering temporary implant materials that combine the structural properties of classic metallic biomaterials with innovative biological functions characteristic of advanced metallic biomaterials. Furthermore, the amalgamation of different biomaterials, particularly biodegradable ceramics and polymers, utilizing sophisticated production techniques, will represent a viable avenue for the future advancement of biomaterials.

In addition to offering mechanical support during the early degradation phase, the ongoing chemical synthesis of diverse biodegradation products will elicit a response from the host and, more significantly, facilitate the body's self-healing processes (Dong et al., 2019). The mechanical, chemical, and biological interactions converge and evolve over time and space, culminating in the complete repair and regeneration of tissues. Biodegradable metals are undoubtedly emerging as the next generation of metallic biomaterials (Suárez et al., 2021). Numerous uncertainties persist with BM, and extensive research and development efforts are required to commercialize BM medical devices. By teaming up material scientists and medical professionals, new biomaterial options with unexpected qualities will be created, which could help improve both basic research and real-world uses.

8. CONCLUSION

Biodegradable materials represent an exceptional advancement in engineering and dentistry, providing eco-friendly alternatives to conventional non-resorbable materials. Their innate biocompatibility, adaptable degradation rates, and ability to stimulate tissue regeneration make them suitable for numerous structural and biological applications. Better strength, biological activity, and resistance to bacteria from new developments in polymers, bioceramics, composites, and nanocomposites show promise for creating useful biomaterials that support healing. Despite challenges associated with manufacturing, scalability, and regulatory acceptance, continued research and interdisciplinary collaboration foster progress. Biodegradable materials have the potential to revolutionize sector-specific, sustainable solutions in health care and beyond as technologies advance.

REFERENCES

Abraham, A. M., & Venkatesan, S. (2023). A review on application of biomaterials for medical and dental implants. Proceedings of the Institution of Mechanical Engineers, *Part L: Journal of Materials: Design and Applications, 237*(2), 249-273. DOI: 10.1177/14644207221121981

Aghion, E. (2018). Biodegradable metals. *Metals*, *8*(10), 804. DOI: 10.3390/met8100804

Ahmed, Y., Ankah, N. K., Ogunlakin, N., Toor, I. U., & Farooq, W. (2024). Exploring the future of metallic implants: A review of biodegradable and non-biodegradable solutions. *Corrosion Reviews*. Advance online publication. DOI: 10.1515/corrrev-2024-0125

Aktas, O. C., Puchert, K., Vurucu, E. E., Ersöz, B., Veziroglu, S., & Sen, S. (2024). A review on nanocomposite coatings in dentistry. *Journal of Materials Science*, *59*(38), 17991–18008. DOI: 10.1007/s10853-024-09915-8

Al-Zyoud, W., Haddadin, D., Hasan, S. A., Jaradat, H., & Kanoun, O. (2023). Biocompatibility testing for implants: A novel tool for selection and characterization. *Materials (Basel)*, *16*(21), 6881. DOI: 10.3390/ma16216881 PMID: 37959478

Armentano, I., Dottori, M., Fortunati, E., Mattioli, S., & Kenny, J. M. (2010). Biodegradable polymer matrix nanocomposites for tissue engineering: A review. *Polymer Degradation & Stability*, *95*(11), 2126–2146. DOI: 10.1016/j.polymdegradstab.2010.06.007

Bechara, S., Lukosiunas, A., Dolcini, G. A., & Kubilius, R. (2017). A short-term clinical study on fixed full arches supported by tapered implants that have a knife-edge thread design and a surface with nanostructures and calcium. *BioMed Research International*, *2017*(1), 4170537. PMID: 28246595

Bichu, Y. M., Alwafi, A., Liu, X., Andrews, J., Ludwig, B., Bichu, A. Y., & Zou, B. (2023). Advances in orthodontic clear aligner materials. *Bioactive Materials*, *22*, 384–403. DOI: 10.1016/j.bioactmat.2022.10.006 PMID: 36311049

Bienek, D. R., & Skrtic, D. (2017). Utility of amorphous calcium phosphate-based scaffolds in dental/biomedical applications. *Biointerface Research in Applied Chemistry*, *7*(1), 1989. PMID: 29225960

Burke, F. J. T., Crisp, R. J., Palin, W. M., Sands, P., Thompson, O., Jones, J., James, A., & Osborne-Smith, K. (2017). A randomised controlled trial of a nanofilled composite at three years: Did selective enamel etching have an effect? *The European Journal of Prosthodontics and Restorative Dentistry*, *25*(1), 35–41. PMID: 28569449

Carrouel, F., Viennot, S., Ottolenghi, L., Gaillard, C., & Bourgeois, D. (2020). Nanoparticles as anti-microbial, anti-inflammatory, and remineralizing agents in oral care cosmetics: A review of the current situation. *Nanomaterials (Basel, Switzerland)*, *10*(1), 140. DOI: 10.3390/nano10010140 PMID: 31941021

Chang, B., Ahuja, N., Ma, C., & Liu, X. (2017). Injectable scaffolds: Preparation and application in dental and craniofacial regeneration. *Materials Science and Engineering R Reports*, *111*, 1–26. DOI: 10.1016/j.mser.2016.11.001 PMID: 28649171

Chen, I. H., Lee, T. M., & Huang, C. L. (2021). Biopolymers hybrid particles used in dentistry. *Gels (Basel, Switzerland)*, *7*(1), 31. DOI: 10.3390/gels7010031 PMID: 33809903

Cheng, F., Song, D., Li, H., Ravi, S. K., & Tan, S. C. (2025). Recent progress in biomedical scaffold fabricated via electrospinning: Design, fabrication and tissue engineering application. *Advanced Functional Materials*, *35*(1), 2406950. DOI: 10.1002/adfm.202406950

Conte, R., Di Salle, A., Riccitiello, F., Petillo, O., Peluso, G., & Calarco, A. (2018). Biodegradable polymers in dental tissue engineering and regeneration. *AIMS Materials Science*, *5*(6), 1073–1101. DOI: 10.3934/matersci.2018.6.1073

Danelon, M., Garcia, L. G., Pessan, J. P., Passarinho, A., Camargo, E. R., & Delbem, A. C. (2019). Effect of fluoride toothpaste containing nano-sized sodium hexametaphosphate on enamel remineralization: An in situ study. *Caries Research*, *53*(3), 260–267. DOI: 10.1159/000491555 PMID: 30278457

Das, R., & Bhattacharjee, C. (2019). Titanium-based nanocomposite materials for dental implant systems. In *Applications of Nanocomposite Materials in Dentistry* (pp. 271–284). Woodhead Publishing. DOI: 10.1016/B978-0-12-813742-0.00016-X

Demirci, M., Tuncer, S., Sancakli, H. S., Tekçe, N., & Baydemir, C. (2018). Five-year clinical evaluation of a nanofilled and a nanohybrid composite in class IV cavities. *Operative Dentistry*, *43*(3), 261–271. DOI: 10.2341/16-358-C PMID: 29533716

Dilshad, E., Waheed, H., Ali, U., Amin, A., & Ahmed, I. (2021). General structure and classification of bioplastics and biodegradable plastics. *Bioplastics for Sustainable Development*, 61-82.

Ding, X., Zhang, Y., Ling, J., & Lin, C. (2018). Rapid mussel-inspired synthesis of PDA-Zn-Ag nanofilms on TiO2 nanotubes for optimizing the antibacterial activity and biocompatibility by doping polydopamine with zinc at a higher temperature. *Colloids and Surfaces. B, Biointerfaces*, *171*, 101–109. DOI: 10.1016/j.colsurfb.2018.07.014 PMID: 30015139

Diz, P., Scully, C., & Sanz, M. (2013). Dental implants in the medically compromised patient. *Journal of Dentistry*, *41*(3), 195–206. DOI: 10.1016/j.jdent.2012.12.008 PMID: 23313715

Dong, L., Tong, X., Li, X., Zhou, J., Wang, S., & Liu, B. (2019). Some developments and new insights of environmental problems and deep mining strategy for cleaner production in mines. *Journal of Cleaner Production*, *210*, 1562–1578. DOI: 10.1016/j.jclepro.2018.10.291

Dong, Q., Lele, A. D., Zhao, X., Li, S., Cheng, S., Wang, Y., Cui, M., Guo, M., Brozena, A. H., Lin, Y., Li, T., Xu, L., Qi, A., Kevrekidis, I. G., Mei, J., Pan, X., Liu, D., Ju, Y., & Hu, L. (2023). Depolymerization of plastics by means of electrified spatiotemporal heating. *Nature*, *616*(7957), 488–494. DOI: 10.1038/s41586-023-05845-8 PMID: 37076729

Doppalapudi, S., Jain, A., Khan, W., & Domb, A. J. (2014). Biodegradable polymers—An overview. *Polymers for Advanced Technologies*, *25*(5), 427–435. DOI: 10.1002/pat.3305

Dutta, P., Giri, S., & Giri, T. K. (2020). Xyloglucan as green renewable biopolymer used in drug delivery and tissue engineering. *International Journal of Biological Macromolecules*, *160*, 55–68. DOI: 10.1016/j.ijbiomac.2020.05.148 PMID: 32450326

Elabd, G. M., Eldars, W., Shamaa, M. S., & Tawfik, M. A. (2024). Evaluation of the antibacterial effect of titanium dioxide nanoparticles combined with acrylic laminates for functional orthodontic appliances: A randomized controlled clinical trial. *BMC Oral Health*, *24*(1), 20. DOI: 10.1186/s12903-023-03805-2 PMID: 38178135

Engler, A. J., Sen, S., Sweeney, H. L., & Discher, D. E. (2006). Matrix elasticity directs stem cell lineage specification. *Cell*, *126*(4), 677–689. DOI: 10.1016/j.cell.2006.06.044 PMID: 16923388

Faris, A., Khalid, L., Hashim, M., Yaghi, S., Magde, T., Bouresly, W., Hamdoon, Z., Uthman, A. T., Marei, H., & Al-Rawi, N. (2022). Characteristics of suture materials used in Oral Surgery: Systematic review. *International Dental Journal*, *72*(3), 278–287. DOI: 10.1016/j.identj.2022.02.005 PMID: 35305815

Gasik, M., Lambert, F., & Bacevic, M. (2021). Biomechanical properties of bone and mucosa for design and application of dental implants. *Materials (Basel), 14*(11), 2845. DOI: 10.3390/ma14112845 PMID: 34073388

Godavitarne, C., Robertson, A., Peters, J., & Rogers, B. (2017). Biodegradable materials. *Orthopaedics and Trauma, 31*(5), 316–320. DOI: 10.1016/j.mporth.2017.07.011

Goldberg, M., & Smith, A. J. (2004). Cells and extracellular matrices of dentin and pulp: A biological basis for repair and tissue engineering. *Critical Reviews in Oral Biology and Medicine, 15*(1), 13–27. DOI: 10.1177/154411130401500103 PMID: 14761897

Gothard, D., Smith, E. L., Kanczler, J. M., Black, C. R., Wells, J. A., Roberts, C. A., White, L. J., Qutachi, O., Peto, H., Rashidi, H., Rojo, L., Stevens, M. M., El Haj, A. J., Felicity, R. A., Rose, J., Shakesheff, K. M., & Oreffo, R. O. (2015). In vivo assessment of bone regeneration in alginate/bone ECM hydrogels with incorporated skeletal stem cells and single growth factors. *PLoS One, 10*(12), e0145080. DOI: 10.1371/journal.pone.0145080 PMID: 26675008

Gulati, K., Chopra, D., Kocak-Oztug, N. A., & Verron, E. (2023). Fit and forget: The future of dental implant therapy via nanotechnology. *Advanced Drug Delivery Reviews, 199*, 114900. DOI: 10.1016/j.addr.2023.114900 PMID: 37263543

Hakim, L. K., Yari, A., Nikparto, N., Mehraban, S. H., Cheperli, S., Asadi, A., Darehdor, A. A., Nezaminia, S., Dortaj, D., Nazari, Y., Dehghan, M., Hojjat, P., Mohajeri, M., & Jebelli, M. S. H. (2024). The current applications of nano and biomaterials in drug delivery of dental implant. *BMC Oral Health, 24*(1), 126. DOI: 10.1186/s12903-024-03911-9 PMID: 38267933

Halamoda-Kenzaoui, B., Holzwarth, U., Roebben, G., Bogni, A., & Bremer-Hoffmann, S. (2019). Mapping of the available standards against the regulatory needs for nanomedicines. *Wiley Interdisciplinary Reviews. Nanomedicine and Nanobiotechnology, 11*(1), e1531. DOI: 10.1002/wnan.1531 PMID: 29923692

Hanna, E. G., Amine, S., Prasad, B., & Younes, K. (2024). Exploring polyetheretherketone in dental implants and abutments: A focus on biomechanics and finite element methods. *Reviews on Advanced Materials Science, 63*(1), 20240031. DOI: 10.1515/rams-2024-0031

Harvestine, J. N., Vollmer, N. L., Ho, S. S., Zikry, C. A., Lee, M. A., & Leach, J. K. (2016). Extracellular Matrix-Coated Composite Scaffolds Promote Mesenchymal Stem Cell Persistence and Osteogenesis. *Biomacromolecules, 17*(11), 3524–3531. DOI: 10.1021/acs.biomac.6b01005 PMID: 27744699

Hosseini, E. S., Dervin, S., Ganguly, P., & Dahiya, R. (2021). Biodegradable Materials for Sustainable Health Monitoring Devices. *ACS Applied Bio Materials*, *4*(1), 163–194. DOI: 10.1021/acsabm.0c01139 PMID: 33842859

Hynes, R. O., & Naba, A. (2011). Overview of the Matrisome—An inventory of extracellular matrix constituents and functions. *Cold Spring Harbor Perspectives in Biology*, *4*(1), a004903. PMID: 21937732

Jagadeesh, P., Puttegowda, M., Mavinkere Rangappa, S., & Siengchin, S. (2021). A review on extraction, chemical treatment, characterization of natural fibers and its composites for potential applications. *Polymer Composites*, *42*(12), 6239–6264. DOI: 10.1002/pc.26312

Jitaru, S., Hodisan, I., Timis, L., Lucian, A., & Bud, M. (2016). The use of bioceramics in endodontics-literature review. *Clujul Medical*, *89*(4), 470. PMID: 27857514

Kadambi, P., Luniya, P., & Dhatrak, P. (2021). Current advancements in polymer/polymer matrix composites for dental implants: A systematic review. *Materials Today: Proceedings*, *46*, 740–745. DOI: 10.1016/j.matpr.2020.12.396

Kang, M. S., Lee, J. H., Hong, S. W., Lee, J. H., & Han, D. W. (2021). Nanocomposites for enhanced osseointegration of dental and orthopedic implants revisited: Surface functionalization by carbon nanomaterial coatings. *Journal of Composites Science*, *5*(1), 23. DOI: 10.3390/jcs5010023

Karacan, I., Macha, I. J., Choi, G., Cazalbou, S., & Ben-Nissan, B. (2017). Antibiotic containing poly lactic acid/hydroxyapatite biocomposite coatings for dental implant applications. *Key Engineering Materials*, *758*, 120–125. DOI: 10.4028/www.scientific.net/KEM.758.120

Kartik, A., Akhil, D., Lakshmi, D., Panchamoorthy Gopinath, K., Arun, J., Sivaramakrishnan, R., & Pugazhendhi, A. (2021). A critical review on production of biopolymers from algae biomass and their applications. *Bioresource Technology*, *329*, 124868. DOI: 10.1016/j.biortech.2021.124868 PMID: 33707076

Kerimoglu, O., & Alarçin, E. (2012). Poly (lactic-co-glycolic acid) based drug delivery devices for tissue engineering and regenerative medicine. *ANKEM Dergisi*, *26*(2), 86–98. DOI: 10.5222/ankem.2012.086

Khiste, S. V., Ranganath, V., & Nichani, A. S. (2013). Evaluation of tensile strength of surgical synthetic absorbable suture materials: An in vitro study. *Journal of Periodontal & Implant Science*, *43*(3), 130–135. DOI: 10.5051/jpis.2013.43.3.130 PMID: 23837127

LaBagnara, J.Jr. (1995). A review of absorbable suture materials in head & neck surgery and introduction of monocryl: A new absorbable suture. *Ear, Nose, and Throat Journal*, *74*(6), 409–415. DOI: 10.1177/014556139507400609 PMID: 7628331

Lakshmi Reddy, K. M., Reddy, D. S., Pradeep, K., & Marna, A. K. (2024). Biodegradable materials in dentistry: A comprehensive review of current trends. *International Journal of Dental Materials*, *06*(03), 70–76. DOI: 10.37983/IJDM.2024.6304

Landsiedel, R., Honarvar, N., Seiffert, S. B., Oesch, B., & Oesch, F. (2022). Genotoxicity testing of nanomaterials. *Wiley Interdisciplinary Reviews. Nanomedicine and Nanobiotechnology*, *14*(6), e1833. DOI: 10.1002/wnan.1833 PMID: 36416021

Liao, J., Timoshenko, A. B., Cordova, D. J., Astudillo Potes, M. D., Gaihre, B., Liu, X., Elder, B. D., Lu, L., & Tilton, M. (2024). Propelling Minimally Invasive Tissue Regeneration With Next-Era Injectable Pre-Formed Scaffolds. *Advanced Materials*, *36*(33), 2400700. DOI: 10.1002/adma.202400700 PMID: 38842622

Liu, L. X., Chen, W., Zhang, H. B., Wang, Q. W., Guan, F., & Yu, Z. Z. (2019). Flexible and multifunctional silk textiles with biomimetic leaf-like MXene/silver nanowire nanostructures for electromagnetic interference shielding, humidity monitoring, and self-derived hydrophobicity. *Advanced Functional Materials*, *29*(44), 1905197. DOI: 10.1002/adfm.201905197

Liu, Z., Liu, X., & Ramakrishna, S. (2021). Surface engineering of biomaterials in orthopedic and dental implants: Strategies to improve osteointegration, bacteriostatic and bactericidal activities. *Biotechnology Journal*, *16*(7), 2000116. DOI: 10.1002/biot.202000116 PMID: 33813785

Lotz, E. M., Cohen, D. J., Schwartz, Z., & Boyan, B. D. (2020). Titanium implant surface properties enhance osseointegration in ovariectomy induced osteoporotic rats without pharmacologic intervention. *Clinical Oral Implants Research*, *31*(4), 374–387. DOI: 10.1111/clr.13575 PMID: 31953969

Lowery, J. L., Datta, N., & Rutledge, G. C. (2010). Effect of fiber diameter, pore size and seeding method on growth of human dermal fibroblasts in electrospun poly (ε-caprolactone) fibrous mats. *Biomaterials*, *31*(3), 491–504. DOI: 10.1016/j.biomaterials.2009.09.072 PMID: 19822363

Macrì, M., D'Albis, V., Marciani, R., Nardella, M., & Festa, F. (2024). Towards Sustainable Orthodontics: Environmental Implications and Strategies for Clear Aligner Therapy. *Materials (Basel)*, *17*(17), 4171. DOI: 10.3390/ma17174171 PMID: 39274561

Maitra, R. S., Brand, J. C.Jr, & Caborn, D. N. (1998). Biodegradable implants. *Sports Medicine and Arthroscopy Review*, *6*(2), 103–111. DOI: 10.1097/00132585-199804000-00006

Makadia, H. K., & Siegel, S. J. (2011). Poly lactic-co-glycolic acid (PLGA) as biodegradable controlled drug delivery carrier. *Polymers*, *3*(3), 1377–1397. DOI: 10.3390/polym3031377 PMID: 22577513

Mallakpour, S., Sirous, F., & Hussain, C. M. (2021). A journey to the world of fascinating ZnO nanocomposites made of chitosan, starch, cellulose, and other biopolymers: Progress in recent achievements in eco-friendly food packaging, biomedical, and water remediation technologies. *International Journal of Biological Macromolecules*, *170*, 701–716. DOI: 10.1016/j.ijbiomac.2020.12.163 PMID: 33388319

Mangano, F. G., Iezzi, G., Shibli, J. A., Pires, J. T., Luongo, G., Piattelli, A., & Mangano, C. (2017). Early bone formation around immediately loaded implants with nanostructured calcium-incorporated and machined surface: A randomized, controlled histologic and histomorphometric study in the human posterior maxilla. *Clinical Oral Investigations*, *21*(8), 2603–2611. DOI: 10.1007/s00784-017-2061-y PMID: 28154996

Mehdikhani-Nahrkhalaji, M., Fathi, M. H., Mortazavi, V., Mousavi, S. B., Hashemi-Beni, B., & Razavi, S. M. (2012). Novel nanocomposite coating for dental implant applications in vitro and in vivo evaluation. *Journal of Materials Science. Materials in Medicine*, *23*(2), 485–495. DOI: 10.1007/s10856-011-4507-0 PMID: 22127403

Modrák, M., Trebuňová, M., Balogová, A. F., Hudák, R., & Živčák, J. (2023). Biodegradable Materials for Tissue Engineering: Development, Classification and Current Applications. *Journal of Functional Biomaterials*, *14*(3), 159. DOI: 10.3390/jfb14030159 PMID: 36976083

Mohammadi, Z., & Dummer, P. M. H. (2011). Properties and applications of calcium hydroxide in endodontics and dental traumatology. *International Endodontic Journal*, *44*(8), 697–730. DOI: 10.1111/j.1365-2591.2011.01886.x PMID: 21535021

Morsada, Z., Hossain, M. M., Islam, M. T., Mobin, M. A., & Saha, S. (2021). Recent progress in biodegradable and bioresorbable materials: From passive implants to active electronics. *Applied Materials Today*, *25*, 101257. DOI: 10.1016/j.apmt.2021.101257

Nasar, A. (2019). Hydroxyapatite and its coatings in dental implants. In *Applications of Nanocomposite Materials in Dentistry* (pp. 145–160). Woodhead Publishing. DOI: 10.1016/B978-0-12-813742-0.00008-0

Nouri, A., Shirvan, A. R., Li, Y., & Wen, C. (2023). Biodegradable metallic suture anchors: A review. *Smart Materials in Manufacturing*, *1*, 100005. DOI: 10.1016/j.smmf.2022.100005

Paduano, F., Marrelli, M., White, L. J., Shakesheff, K. M., & Tatullo, M. (2016). Odontogenic Differentiation of Human Dental Pulp Stem Cells on Hydrogel Scaffolds Derived from Decellularized Bone Extracellular Matrix and Collagen Type I. *PLoS One*, *11*(2), e0148225. DOI: 10.1371/journal.pone.0148225 PMID: 26882351

Pietrzak, W. S., Sarver, D., & Verstynen, M. (1996). Bioresorbable implants—Practical considerations. *Bone*, *19*(1), S109–S119. DOI: 10.1016/S8756-3282(96)00139-1 PMID: 8831002

69. Powell, J., & Pring, T. (2024). The impact of social media influencers on health outcomes: Systematic review. *Social Science & Medicine*, *340*, 340. DOI: 10.1016/j.socscimed.2023.116472 PMID: 38070305

Raghavendra, S. S., Jadhav, G. R., Gathani, K. M., & Kotadia, P. (2017). Bioceramics in endodontics–a review. *Journal of Istanbul University Faculty of Dentistry*, *51*(3, Suppl 1), 128–137. PMID: 29354316

Ramezani, M., & Ripin, Z. M. (2023). An Overview of Enhancing the Performance of Medical Implants with Nanocomposites. *Journal of Composites Science*, *7*(5), 199. DOI: 10.3390/jcs7050199

Randhawa, R. K., Dubey, T., Pansuriya, I., Mishra, T., Tanwar, M., Kumar, A., & Singh, R. (2024). Assessment of the Mechanical Properties of Different Suture Materials for Oral Surgery: An In Vitro Tensile Strength Study. *Cureus*, *16*(8), e65952. DOI: 10.7759/cureus.65952 PMID: 39221394

Rocha, W. F., & Sheen, D. A. (2016). Classification of biodegradable materials using QSAR modelling with uncertainty estimation. *SAR and QSAR in Environmental Research*, *27*(10), 799–811. DOI: 10.1080/1062936X.2016.1238010 PMID: 27710037

Schmalz, G., & Reichl, F. X. (2021). Regulation of Dental Materials. In *Regulatory Toxicology* (pp. 1153–1183). Springer International Publishing. DOI: 10.1007/978-3-030-57499-4_126

Schröttner, J., & Baumgartner, C. (2023). The notified body: the conformity assessment body for medical devices in Europe. In *Medical Devices and In Vitro Diagnostics: Requirements in Europe* (pp. 39–61). Springer International Publishing. DOI: 10.1007/978-3-031-22091-3_1

Shahi, S., Özcan, M., Maleki Dizaj, S., Sharifi, S., Al-Haj Husain, N., Eftekhari, A., & Ahmadian, E. (2019). A review on potential toxicity of dental material and screening their biocompatibility. *Toxicology Mechanisms and Methods*, *29*(5), 368–377. DOI: 10.1080/15376516.2019.1566424 PMID: 30642212

Shu, R., Guan, Y., & Liu, B. (2025). Preparation of nitrogen-doped reduced graphene oxide/zinc ferrite@ nitrogen-doped carbon composite for broadband and highly efficient electromagnetic wave absorption. *Journal of Materials Science and Technology*, *214*, 16–26. DOI: 10.1016/j.jmst.2024.07.006

Souza, J. C. M., Barbosa, S. L., Ariza, E. A., Henriques, M., Teughels, W., Ponthiaux, P., Celis, J. P., & Rocha, L. A. (2015). How do titanium and Ti6Al4V corrode in fluoridated medium as found in the oral cavity? An in vitro study. *Materials Science and Engineering C*, *47*, 384–393. DOI: 10.1016/j.msec.2014.11.055 PMID: 25492211

Suárez, L., Castellano, J., Díaz, S., Tcharkhtchi, A., & Ortega, Z. (2021). Article are natural-based composites sustainable? *Polymers*, *13*(14), 2326. DOI: 10.3390/polym13142326 PMID: 34301085

Sudhakar, M. P., Nallasamy, V. D., Dharani, G., & Buschmann, A. H. (2024). Applications of seaweed biopolymers and its composites in dental applications. *Journal of Applied Biology and Biotechnology*, *12*(1), 62–68.

Svempe, L. (2024). Exploring impediments imposed by the Medical Device Regulation EU 2017/745 on software as a medical device. *JMIR Medical Informatics*, *12*(1), e58080. DOI: 10.2196/58080 PMID: 39235850

Teo, A. J., Mishra, A., Park, I., Kim, Y. J., Park, W. T., & Yoon, Y. J. (2016). Polymeric biomaterials for medical implants and devices. *ACS Biomaterials Science & Engineering*, *2*(4), 454–472. DOI: 10.1021/acsbiomaterials.5b00429 PMID: 33465850

Tomer, D., Kumari, D. S., Rastogi, D. D., Cecilia, D. L. L., Singh, D. S., & Tyagi, D. A. (2020). Bioceramics in Endodontics - A Review. *International Journal of Applied Dental Sciences*, *6*(3), 588–594. DOI: 10.22271/oral.2020.v6.i3i.1012

Vahidi, M., Rizkalla, A. S., & Mequanint, K. (2024). Extracellular Matrix-Surrogate Advanced Functional Composite Biomaterials for Tissue Repair and Regeneration. *Advanced Healthcare Materials*, *13*(27), 2401218. DOI: 10.1002/adhm.202401218 PMID: 39036851

Vasconcelos, D. M., Santos, S. G., Lamghari, M., & Barbosa, M. A. (2016). The two faces of metal ions: From implants rejection to tissue repair/regeneration. []. Elsevier Ltd.]. *Biomaterials*, *84*, 262–275. DOI: 10.1016/j.biomaterials.2016.01.046 PMID: 26851391

Vasquez, P. A., & Forest, M. G. (2014). *Complex Fluids and Soft Structures in the Human Body*. Springer.

Veis, A., & Goldberg, M. (2014). Pulp extracellular matrix. In Goldberg, M. (Ed.), *The Dental Pulp: Biology, Pathology, and Regenerative Therapies* (pp. 35–46). Springer. DOI: 10.1007/978-3-642-55160-4_3

Velu, R., Calais, T., Jayakumar, A., & Raspall, F. (2020). A comprehensive review on bio-nanomaterials for medical implants and feasibility studies on fabrication of such implants by additive manufacturing technique. *Materials (Basel)*, *13*(1), 92. DOI: 10.3390/ma13010092 PMID: 31878040

Veronesi, F., Maglio, M., Brogini, S., & Fini, M. (2020). In vivo studies on osteoinduction: A systematic review on animal models, implant site, and type and postimplantation investigation. *Journal of Biomedical Materials Research. Part A*, *108*(9), 1834–1866. DOI: 10.1002/jbm.a.36949 PMID: 32297695

Verron, E., Masson, M., Khoshniat, S., Duplomb, L., Wittrant, Y., Baud'Huin, M., Badran, Z., Bujoli, B., Janvier, P., Scimeca, J. C., Bouler, J. M., & Guicheux, J. (2010). Gallium modulates osteoclastic bone resorption in vitro without affecting osteoblasts. *British Journal of Pharmacology*, *159*(8), 1681–1692. DOI: 10.1111/j.1476-5381.2010.00665.x PMID: 20397300

Vishwakarma, A., Bhise, N. S., Evangelista, M. B., Rouwkema, J., Dokmeci, M. R., Ghaemmaghami, A. M., Vrana, N. E., & Khademhosseini, A. (2016). Engineering Immunomodulatory Biomaterials To Tune the Inflammatory Response. *Trends in Biotechnology*, *34*(6), 470–482. DOI: 10.1016/j.tibtech.2016.03.009 PMID: 27138899

Vladescu, A., Cotrut, C. M., Azem, F. A., Bramowicz, M., Pana, I., Braic, V., Birlik, I., Kiss, A., Braic, M., Abdulgader, R., Booysen, R., Kulesza, S., & Monsees, T. K. (2018). Sputtered Si and Mg doped hydroxyapatite for biomedical applications. *Biomedical Materials (Bristol, England)*, *13*(2), 025011. DOI: 10.1088/1748-605X/aa9718 PMID: 29381477

Vroman, I., & Tighzert, L. (2009). Biodegradable polymers. *Materials (Basel)*, *2*(2), 307–344. DOI: 10.3390/ma2020307

Yoshinari, M., Oda, Y., Kato, T., & Okuda, K. (2001). Influence of surface modifications to titanium on antibacterial activity in vitro. *Biomaterials*, *22*(14), 2043–2048. DOI: 10.1016/S0142-9612(00)00392-6 PMID: 11426884

Zafar, M., Najeeb, S., Khurshid, Z., Vazirzadeh, M., Zohaib, S., Najeeb, B., & Sefat, F. (2016). Potential of electrospun nanofibers for biomedical and dental applications. *Materials (Basel)*, *9*(2), 73. DOI: 10.3390/ma9020073 PMID: 28787871

Zafar, M. S., Amin, F., Fareed, M. A., Ghabbani, H., Riaz, S., Khurshid, Z., & Kumar, N. (2020). Biomimetic aspects of restorative dentistry biomaterials. *Biomimetics*, *5*(3), 34. DOI: 10.3390/biomimetics5030034 PMID: 32679703

Zhang, Y., Gulati, K., Li, Z., Di, P., & Liu, Y. (2021). Dental implant nano-engineering: Advances, limitations and future directions. *Nanomaterials (Basel, Switzerland)*, *11*(10), 2489. DOI: 10.3390/nano11102489 PMID: 34684930

Zheng, Y. F., Gu, X. N., & Witte, F. (2014). Biodegradable metals. *Materials Science and Engineering R Reports*, *77*, 1–34. DOI: 10.1016/j.mser.2014.01.001

Chapter 6
Harnessing Biomaterials to Overcome Challenges in Cancer Immunotherapy

Vivek Pazhamalai
https://orcid.org/0000-0003-2088-7545
Vels Institute of Science, Technology and Advanced Studies, Chennai, India

Meenupriya Venkatesan
Vels Institute of Science, Technology and Advanced Studies, Chennai, India

Jayasri Rajkumar
Vels Institute of Science, Technology and Advanced Studies, Chennai, India

S. S. Meenambiga
https://orcid.org/0000-0002-5445-525X
Vels Institute of Science, Technology and Advanced Studies, Chennai, India

S. Ivo Romauld
https://orcid.org/0000-0003-0610-0646
Vels Institute of Science, Technology and Advanced Studies, Chennai, India

K. Rajakumari
https://orcid.org/0000-0002-8102-9512
Vels Institute of Science, Technology and Advanced Studies, Chennai, India

V. Gowthami
Vels Institute of Science, Technology and Advanced Studies, Chennai, India

ABSTRACT

The intrinsic immune system activity awakens and trains the patient's immune system to destroy tumor cells. Immunotherapy has become a standard method for treating cancer since it is a more potent and secure option than conventional therapies like surgery, radiotherapy, and chemotherapy. Chimeric antigen receptor-modified T cells, immune checkpoint blockades, and cancer vaccines are the three primary forms of cancer immunotherapy that have been developed recently. Chemotherapy, radiation therapy, and surgery continue to be the mainstays of cancer treatment de-

DOI: 10.4018/979-8-3373-1305-4.ch006

spite decades of advancements. Lung cancer, melanoma, advanced bladder, kidney, and other advanced tumors have all been successfully treated with immunotherapy. Immunotherapy is used to cure illnesses by regulating an overactive or underactive immune system. Biomaterials efficiency will be increased with the help of immune system engineering and targeted drug delivery. Chapter highlights the recent advancement in tailored biomaterials for cancer immunotherapy.

1. INTRODUCTION

Globally, cancer is one of the leading causes of death. Every year, there are over 10 million new cases, and over 6 million people will pass away from the illness. There are numerous reasons for the recent rise in cancer cases. Another important factor is changing one's lifestyle, particularly with relation to diet, alcohol consumption, and tobacco use, (Yoo & Shin, 2003). Cancer is a disorder when body tissue is destroyed by uncontrollably dividing aberrant cells which spreads to other parts of the body. It is a major global health challenge as it affects millions of people each year. The most prevalent cancers in men are bladder, colon and rectum, lung and bronchus, and prostate, in that order. The breast, lung and bronchus, colon and rectum, uterine corpus, and thyroid are the areas in women where cancer is most common. This demonstrates that breast cancer in women and prostate cancer in males make up a sizable percentage of all cancer cases, (Siegel, Miller, & Jemal, 2019). An abnormal mass of tissue called a neoplasm, neo means new and plasia means tissue or cells. neoplasm, which in Greek literally translates to "new tissue." This suggests that tumors are essentially newly formed cell growths, develops when cells divide and expand more than they should or do not die when they should. There are two types of neoplasms known as malignant (cancerous) and benign (non- cancerous), (Sirica, 1989).

In order to stop cancer and tumor growth, the immune system is crucial. Immunotherapy has showed considerable promise in treating a variety of cancer types, with many cases showing promise for a cure. The body's immune system is used in this method to identify and combat cancer cells, (Zhang & Zhang, 2020). Immunotherapy has become a viable substitute for conventional cancer therapies such as radiation and chemotherapy because of a number of important benefits such as Focused strategy More accurately than with conventional treatments, immunotherapy enables physicians to target cancer cells. These treatments can kill cancer cells only while leaving healthy tissue intact by boosting the immune system, (Tan, Li, & Zhu, 2020). In order to treat illnesses, immunotherapy is utilized to regulate an overactive or underactive immune system. Biomaterials can help with immune system engineering and targeted medicine delivery, which can increase its effectiveness. However, we also need to take into account how these substances impact the immune system, (Dai, Fan, & Wang, 2022).

Biomaterials are substances created with the intention of interacting with biological systems. These substances are bioactive and readily assimilated into human tissue. The extent of their biodegradability can be considered quite significant and effective. They are frequently employed in the production of human body parts, tissue engineering, medications, and other manufacturing processes. Biomaterials and sustainability work together to assist the creation of new sustainable materials through the use of cutting-edge technical methods. Biomaterials are environmentally friendly and it is produced from various biological resources, (Biswal, BadJena, & Pradhan, 2020).

Since ancient Egypt, anecdotal evidence of spontaneous tumor regressions following infections has supported the idea that the immune system can be used to combat cancer. William Coley created one of the earliest immune-based cancer treatments in the late 1800s by injecting bacterial toxins to trigger the body's defenses against malignancies, (Dobosz & Dzieciatkowski, 2019). Significant advancements were made in the 1990s and 2000s with the identification of immunological checkpoints and the creation of checkpoint inhibitors. Another effective immunotherapy strategy that surfaced in the 2010s was CAR T-cell treatment, (Decker et al., 2017). Interest in employing biomaterials to improve immunotherapy has grown in recent years. The use of biomaterials such as hydrogels, micelles, and nanoparticles to more efficiently administer immunotherapeutic is being investigated. Utilizing biomaterials customized for each patient's biopsies, individualized immunotherapy techniques may be possible. The best biomaterial systems for various tumor types are still difficult to build, (Yang et al., 2020).

Different immunotherapy techniques have different mechanisms of action and aim to improve the recipient's immune function. Based on their capacity to induce memory immunological responses, immunotherapies are sometimes divided into two categories: passive (adoptive) and active immunotheapies, (Dahri et al., 2023). Active immunotherapy produces immunological memory and a long-lasting response by actively stimulating an immune response. The reactions might be specific, which refers to generating immune responses against particular antigens, or non-specific, which is referred to as a general immune system response via cell signalling molecules, (Beheshtizadeh et al., 2021). Direct antibody delivery is known as passive immunotherapy since it does not stimulate the immune system and instead promotes the development of immunological memory, (Tostanoski, Gosselin, & Jewell, 2016).

2. BIOMATERIALS IN CANCER IMMUNOTHERAPY

The term "cancer immunotherapy" refers to methods of treating cancer that alter the host immune system or use immune system components. Regulatory agencies have approved 17 immunologic products due to their anticancer properties. These consist of the cytokines, interleukin-2 and interferon-α, the nonspecific immune stimulants levamisole and BCG, monoclonal antibodies, radiolabeled antibodies, immunotoxins, nonmyeloablative allogeneic transplants with donor lymphocyte infusions, and the anti-prostate cancer cell-based treatment sipuleucel-T, (Dillman, 2011).

In terms of survival and quality of life, cancer immunotherapy has significantly improved patient outcomes when compared to earlier standards of care such as chemotherapy, radiation, and surgery. With many cancer types, immunotherapy has now solidly established itself as a novel pillar of cancer care, from the metastatic stage to the adjuvant and neoadjuvant settings, (Esfahani et al., 2020). The goal of cancer immunotherapy is to reorient the target from the tumor cells to the patient's immune system in order to facilitate its mobilization and improve the antitumor immune response's activation. This aids the immune system in identifying, attacking, and ultimately getting rid of the tumor cells, (Miller & Sadelain, 2015). Melanoma, lung cancer, kidney cancer, bladder cancer, head and neck cancer, liver cancer, Hodgkin lymphoma, and Merkel cell carcinoma are among the types of cancer for which immune checkpoint inhibitors have been authorized for use in treating select patients. The development of genetically modified immune cells, the identification of various cancer immune checkpoints, the growing knowledge of the function of cytokines in triggering the antitumor response, and advancements in genetic engineering technology have all altered the field of cancer treatment and brought the possibility of a definitive cure closer than ever, (Kciuk & Yahya, 2023). In order to be eligible for immunotherapy therapies, patients usually need to fulfill certain requirements. Surgery, chemotherapy, radiation, and hormone therapy are examples of conventional therapies that are either unavailable or extremely harmful to patients, (Padmanabhan, Meskin, & Al Moustagfa, 2021). The list of tumors that immunotherapy can treat is always changing as more treatments are assessed in clinical trials. Frequently, immunotherapy is used in conjunction with targeted medicines or chemotherapy, (Cook et al., 2016). The use of immunotherapy in cancer in its early stages, either before to or following surgery, is growing. In certain instances, immunotherapy is currently being utilized to treat brain metastases, (Sampson et al., 2020).

The complex ecology that surrounds a tumor and is made up of different cells and non-cellular elements is known as the tumor microenvironment. These cells are essential for tumor development, invasion, and treatment response, (Arneth, 2019). The efficacy of traditional treatments like surgery, radiation, and chemotherapy may be surpassed by cancer immunotherapy, which has been referred to as the fourth pillar of tumor therapy, (Shi et al., 2018). There are five main types of cancer immunotherapies such as the regulation of immune checkpoints, oncolytic virus therapies, cancer vaccines, cytokine therapies, and adoptive cell transfer.

2.1 Immune Checkpoints Inhibitors

In the field of cancer immunotherapy, the identification of immune checkpoint proteins like PD-1/PDL-1 and CTLA-4 marks a major advancement. Humanized monoclonal antibodies that target these immune checkpoint proteins have therefore been used with efficacy in treating patients with non-small lung cancer, head and neck malignancies, renal cell carcinoma, and metastatic melanoma, (Shiravand et al., 2022). ICIs are cancer immunotherapies that work by focusing on immunologic receptors on the surface of T-lymphocytes to increase anti-cancer immune responses. Therefore, in 2011, when ipilimumab was approved, ICIs were seen as a revolutionary treatment option that revolutionized the treatment of cancer, (Robert, 2020) (Ledford, 2011). ICIs function differently from conventional therapeutic approaches by boosting the host immune system's ability to combat tumor cells, (Cai et al., 2021). These immunological checkpoints are a collection of pathways that affect immune cell activity, both stimulatory and inhibitory, (Pardoll, 2012). The most popular immunotherapeutic medicines in the past ten years have been antibodies that target immunological inhibitory receptors, including CTLA-4, PD-1, and PD-L. There are a number of antibodies and small molecules in clinical development that target different immune checkpoint proteins, such as CD39, CD73, B7H3, the adenosine A2A receptor, and CD47, (Chrétien et al., 2019).

2.2 Oncolytic Virus Therapies

Interest in oncolytic virus immunotherapy is growing quickly in the field of cancer immunotherapy. Therapy with oncolytic viruses (OVs) is an intriguing treatment option because of the low toxicity at the end of treatment and the simultaneous action of direct oncolysis and immune activation. Several OVs have undergone clinical trials to evaluate their safety and effectiveness, yet the FDA has only approved one OV to date, (De Graaf et al., 2020). Using genetically modified viruses, viro immunotherapy is also referred to as oncolytic virotherapy is a type of cancer immunotherapy that targets and kills cancer cells while triggering the immune system to target tumor cells, (Volovat et al., 2024) (Zeng et al., 2021). The examples of oncolytic viruses used in viro immunotherapy include vaccine virus (VV) is a naturally occurring member of the Poxviridae family that targets cancer. It has been designed to take many different forms, such as: (JX-594) Pexa-Vec: In phase I and

II clinical trials, an oncolytic VV equipped with GM-CSF and TK gene disruption is being studied for the treatment of soft-tissue sarcoma, advanced breast cancer, and renal cell carcinoma. Another oncolytic viruses is the herpes simplex virus (HSV). Newcastle disease virus (NDV) is an oncolytic virus that is a paramyxovirus. Reovirus is a double-stranded RNA virus that takes advantage of cancer cells' weakened antiviral defenses to multiply in those cells. Seneca Valley virus (SVV) is an Oncolytic virotherapy employs this picornavirus. The measles virus (MV) is a paramyxovirus that has been modified to act as an oncolytic. Poliovirus is another example of Oncolytic virotherapy employs this picornavirus. An encapsulated RNA virus that functions as an oncolytic platform is the Vesicular Stomatitis Virus (VSV), (Jafari et al., 2022). Adenoviruses, especially serotype 5 (group C) adenovirus, are the most often utilized backbone for oncolytic viral creation. Some examples are as follows such as in clinical trials, Ad5:0, an attenuated adenovirus with neither E1 or E4 genes, has demonstrated encouraging outcomes. A modified adenovirus called Delta24-RGD replicates specifically in glioma cells because E1A no longer binds to the Rb protein. Adenoviruses: Widely used in oncolytic virotherapy because of their capacity to infect cells regardless of the state of cell division, (Hemminki, Dos Santos, & Hemminki, 2020). These viruses, which can be naturally occurring or manufactured, proliferate only in cancer cells while avoiding normal tissues. Directly destroying cancer cells and triggering anti-tumor immune responses are two of the ways they function. Numerous of these viruses are being studied in clinical trials for different kinds of cancer.

2.3 Cancer Vaccine

The goal of cancer vaccines is to stimulate the immune system to identify and fight cancer cells. Preventing tumor growth, recurrence, or metastasis while improving the immune system's ability to recognize and eradicate cancer cells are their main goals. In order to target particular tumor-associated antigens (TAAs), cancer vaccines trigger an immune response. Cancer cells are destroyed as a result of this immunological response, which includes the activation of T cells, B cells, and other immune cells, (Kaczmarek et al., 2023). Traditionally, vaccinations based on cells are made from isolated tumor antigens or complete, dead cancer cells. Microbial vector vaccines are the vaccinations that deliver tumor antigens using bacteria or viruses as vectors. Peptide vaccines: Made up of brief tumor antigen sequences. Genes that encode tumor antigens are the basis for genetic vaccinations, (Verma et al., 2023).

2.4 Cytokine Therapies

Cytokines are molecular messengers that facilitate communication between immune system cells, resulting in a coordinated, strong, yet self-limited response to a target antigen. Over the past 20 years, there has been an increase in efforts to describe cytokines and take advantage of their extensive signaling networks in order to develop cancer treatments, in tandem with the growing interest in using the immune system to destroy cancer, (Lee & Margolin, 2011). Cytokines are polypeptides or glycoproteins that have a molecular weight of less than 30 kDa and give various cell types signals for growth, differentiation, and inflammation or anti-inflammation, (Berraondo et al., 2019). Interferon-α is family of cytokines has been utilized to treat solid tumors and a number of hematological malignancies at high dosages to take advantage of their direct pro-apoptotic/anti-proliferative action on tumor cells since IFN-α was originally approved in 1986 for the treatment of hairy cell leukemia. These elevated levels of IFN-α also have anti-tumor effects because they have a strong antiangiogenic effect on the tumor vasculature, (Spaapen et al., 2014). Additionally approved for use as an adjuvant therapy for melanoma was PEGylated IFN-α, (Herndon et al., 2012). Current clinical trials are investigating a number of cytokines, such as GM-CSF IFN gamma (IFNγ), IL-7, IL-12, IL-15, and IL-21.Recently, IL-15 finished its first clinical trials as a single drug.The difficulties associated with cytokine monotherapy are being addressed by ongoing trials that examine cytokines in conjunction with other biological agents, (Conlon, Miljkovic, & Waldmann, 2019). Targeting cytokine pathways has recently demonstrated encouraging therapeutic potential, providing novel approaches to immune system modulation, tumor development inhibition, and treatment resistance. Our knowledge and use of cytokine- and chemokine-targeted treatments for cancer patients are greatly enhanced by ongoing clinical trials, (Yi et al., 2024).

2.5 Adoptive Cell Transfer

The treatment known as adoptive cell therapy (ACT) uses the anti-tumor-active T cells that cancer patients have naturally, which are then grown in vitro and reinfused into the patient. It entails finding ex vivo autologous or allogeneic lymphocytes that exhibit anticancer activity and administering them to cancer patients.Just a handful of anti-tumor cells with suitable characteristics need to be found and grown. Tests conducted in vitro can pinpoint the precise populations and effector roles needed for cancer regression. In the lab, cells can be stimulated without the presence of endogenous inhibitory molecules. Before cell transfer, the host environment can be changed to create the best possible conditions, (Rosenberg et al., 2008). Recently, ACT has been linked to a steady rate of long-lasting regressions in patients with renal cell carcinoma and melanoma. It also has significant potential in a number of other oncological contexts, (Galluzzi et al., 2012).

Since biomaterials allow for the local delivery of immunomodulatory drugs, they are becoming more and more significant in the advancement of cancer immunotherapy. Novel delivery methods for cancer immunotherapies are being developed using engineered biomaterials, such as implantable, injectable, and transdermal materials, (Cai et al., 2020). For the delivery of localized immunotherapy, a variety of tailored biomaterials are being investigated. Materials like as PLG, alginate, and hyaluronic acid are used to create implantable scaffolds. Systems of injectable hydrogels Transdermal arrays of microneedles These can be engineered to recruit immune cells, regulate release kinetics, and establish advantageous tumor microenvironments, (Chao, Chen, & Liu, 2020). Instances of biomaterial-based strategies examples are Dendritic cells are recruited using PLG scaffolds loaded with GM-CSF. Anti-PD-L1 and chemotherapeutics in hydrogel systems Microneedle patches that administer tumor lysate and checkpoint inhibitors. In preclinical models, these methods have demonstrated potential by improving local immune responses in contrast to conventional systemic injections. In conclusion, biomaterials are making it possible for immunotherapies to be delivered more precisely and efficiently, resolving major issues in the treatment of cancer by enhancing localization and lowering systemic adverse effects. In order to fully grasp the potential of biomaterials in immunotherapy, ongoing research endeavors to enhance their characteristics and delivery methods, (Cunningham, Lapointe, & Lerouge, 2022) (Zhang, Billingsley, & Mitchell, 2018).

2.6 Benefits

It aims in Targeted delivery that Biomaterials can enhance targeting by conjugating ligands or antibodies to receptors expressed on target tissues or cells, (Leach, Young, & Hartgerink, 2019). Biomaterials can improve pharmacokinetics and reduce toxicity through controlled release profiles. Biologic cargo can be protected by biomaterials from enzymatic degradation and extreme pH levels, (Chen, Chen, & Liu, 2019). Better tumor targeting, The EPR effect allows materials to collect at tumors preferentially. The medicine can be released gradually over time or when it reaches target tissues, including tumors, to reduce systemic toxicity. Combination therapy is the use of biomaterials to produce multiple therapeutic molecules. It helps in Reprogramming immune cells as some biomaterials are naturally immunogenic, they may be exploited to polarize immunity. Many immunological signals can be constructed via self-assembly techniques, which eliminate the requirement for artificial carriers, (Gammon, Dold, & Jewell, 2016).

2.7 Innovations and Ongoing Clinical Trials

There are several cancer vaccines based on biomaterials undergoing clinical testing. For instance, the FDA authorized sipuleucel-T (Provenge), an autologous dendritic cell vaccine that encapsulates GM-CSF linked to prostate cancer antigen PAP, in 2010. CTLA-4 inhibition is currently being investigated in conjunction with this vaccine in phase II trials, (Pardoll, 2012) (Sharma & Allison, 2015). A phase II clinical trial is under underway to examine GVAX, a whole cell pancreatic cancer vaccine that uses tumor cells that express GM-CSF, in conjunction with nivolumab, a PD-1 checkpoint inhibitor, (Wrzeskinski, Wan, & Flavell, 2007).

DNA vaccines are now undergoing phase I and II clinical studies for a number of malignancies, including cervical, prostate, lymphoma, and melanoma. Although several have so far demonstrated very modest effectiveness, advancements in delivery techniques such as electroporation and gene gunning are being investigated further, (Tiptiri-Kourpeti et al., 2016). Additionally, clinical trials for mRNA-based cancer vaccines are beginning. In order to increase the effectiveness of DNA vaccines, attempts are being made to optimize their delivery through the use of biomaterial-based vehicles, (Pardi et al., 2018). Research on advanced biomaterials to enhance cancer modeling is being funded by the NIH/NCI through SBIR grants. This implies that new biomaterials are still being developed for use in cancer applications. Although numerous preclinical trials of early-stage biomaterial-based immunotherapy techniques have demonstrated promise, it is still difficult to translate these into clinical success. Which biomaterial-based strategies provide patients with long-term advantages will be determined in part by ongoing research. The sector is still developing quickly, with new materials and delivery systems being created to solve lingering issues, (Peer et al., 2020) (Avula & Grodzinski, 2024).

3. DRUG DELIVERY SYSTEMS (DDS)

3.1 Implantable Biomaterials

Implantable biomaterial scaffolds that are preloaded with cells, bioactive substances, or immunological agents can be placed subcutaneously or into resected tissue space by a minor surgical operation. It is possible to recruit immune cells into scaffolds and activate them for additional biological programming by releasing immunoregulatory agents gradually, (Li et al., 2020)

Some of the examples of engineered polymeric biomaterials which is used as scaffolds in implantable delivery systems include poly(lactide-co glycolide) (PLG), alginate (ALG), polyglyconate and porcine gelatin, collagen, and hyaluronic acid (HA), (Cai et al., 2020).

3.2 Injectable Biomaterials

Transformable gel-like biomaterials known as injectable biomaterial scaffolds can be injected into the site of a tumor or resection to generate a potent local or systemic immune response against the tumor, (Villard et al., 2019). The degradable hydrogel which is injectable and forms in-situ (via a Michael-type addition reaction) was created that may simultaneously deliver microparticles co-loaded with DNA and siRNA and DC-attracting chemokines. At the injection location, such as muscle, the released chemokines draw in naïve immature DCs, which phagocytose the DNA/siRNA-loaded microparticles extracted from the disintegrating gel and become activated, (Singh et al., 2011).

3.3 Transdermal Delivery System

The physicochemical characteristics of medicinal substances plays a crucial role for transdermal immunotherapy, because the way that medicinal drugs are administered has a significant impact on their bioavailability. One accessible, painless, and non-invasive method of administering medications is transdermal administration. Because it avoids the gastrointestinal tract and shields medications from first-pass metabolism, it is an effective method for systemic delivery, (Dahri et al., 2023) Additionally, this removes the need for intrusive, uncomfortable needles that produce medical waste, increase the risk of infection, and require medically trained personnel to administer, (Bird & Ravindra, 2020).

4. TYPES OF BIOMATERIALS IN IMMUNOTHERAPY

Architecture, aerodynamics, mechanical engineering, materials science, and other technical fields are constantly inspired by biological structures to solve their problems. The comparatively small number of basic elements found in natural materials are utilized to create a wide range of minerals and polymers, (Fratzl, 2007). Classification of biomaterial is illustrated in table 1. The four main classification of materials that comprise biomaterials are metals, polymers, ceramics (including carbons, glass-ceramics, and glasses), and natural materials (including those derived from plants and animals), (Ige, Umoru, & Aribo, 2012) The biomedical industry makes extensive use of polymeric materials. Natural polymers are also necessary because of their biocompatibility and biodegradability, even though synthetic polymers are far simpler to employ in the biomedical area. Blending synthetic and natural polymers is another way to generate polymeric materials for biomedical uses. In comparison to a number of naturally occurring polymers, synthetic polymers exhibit superior mechanical and thermal stability. The primary biopolymers utilized in the production of materials for biomedical purposes are elastin, collagen, chitin, chitosan, keratin and silk —all naturally occurring polymers obtained from animal tissues. Additionally, there is a class of natural polymers that come from plants, including pectinc, cellulose, and starch, (Bhatia & Bhatia, 2016).

Table 1. Classification of biomaterials

Types of polymers	Examples
Natural polymers	Collagen, chitin
Synthetic polymers	Plga, carbon quantum dots

4.1 Collagen

Collagen is a natural protein present in the skin, connective tissues, and bone. It is widely utilized as a cosmetic ingredient. collagen-based biomaterials is considered to be both adaptable and compatible with human tissues have attracted a lot of attention for the replacement and repair of bodily tissues such bones, tendons, skin, vascular grafts, heart valves, and teeth, (Sionkowska, 2011). Recent research has demonstrated that collagen can influence the activity and phenotype of many types of tumor infiltrating immune cells, including tumor-associated macrophages (TAMs) and T cells, (Radhakrishnan et al., 2020). Collagen is an intriguing biomaterial due to its many general characteristics, including its low antigenicity, strong mechanical strength of the fibers, suitability as a cell growth substrate, and adjustable stability through chemical or physical cross-linking, (Goh & Holmes, 2017).

4.2 Chitin

Found in the walls of fungi and the shells of crustaceans, chitosan is a partially deacetylated derivative of chitin, one of the most prevalent polymers in nature. It is made up of widely dispersed β-(1-4)-linked D-glucosamine (glucosamine) and N-acetyl-d-glucosamine (N-acetylglucosamine) structural units that resemble glycosaminoglycan, a crucial component of the cell surface and bone matrix, (Liang et al., 2022). Chitosan has been employed as an immunotherapeutic agent carrier to increase antitumor response, control the immune system, and improve bioavailability. Because of its readily adaptable structure, chitosan can be used to create a wide variety of delivery vectors for improved immunotherapy, (Cao & Wang, 2009). Biomaterials are also biologically derived materials employed for their structural rather than biological qualities. The food sector also uses biotechnologically modified carbohydrates as bulking agents and as lubricants for biomedical applications. Biomaterials generated from natural sources have only recently been investigated as potential promoters and facilitators of healing and regeneration. Everything from tendon and ligament restoration to wound dressings is being done now with biomaterials of all kinds, (Huang & Zeng, 2020).The materials that have been utilized for artificial antigen presenting cells (aAPCs) include biological or biomimetic materials like cell membranes or liposomes, inorganic materials like carbon nanotubes or iron oxide, and polymeric materials like polystyrene or poly(lactic-co-glycolic acid) (PLGA). Material choice plays a crucial role in determining the function of artificial antigen presenting cells(aAPC) because material choice creates significant impact on properties of the particle such as membrane fluidity, nanoscale organization of ligands, stability, stiffness, degradability, surface area, ease of encapsulation of soluble factors and response to magnetic field. dendritic cells which is also known as the most potent professional APCs (Antigen presenting cells) are capable of combining both adaptive and innate immunity. Antigen Presenting Cells in particular dendritic cells must seize the antigens inorder to induce the cytotoxic CD8+T – cells (CTC) immune response which is directed against cancerous cells.

4.3 Lipid Based Materials

Lipid- based nanomaterials like liposomes have been discovered to distribute antigens and adjuvants directly to dendritic cells in vivo, (Karanth & Murthy, 2007). Liposomes, which are commonly known as lipid-based vesicles, are seen as one of the most adaptable and flexible drug delivery vehicles, (De Leo et al., 2021). A phospholipid bilayer forms the nanosized bubbles known as liposomes, which is also known as the primary lipid- based nanobiomaterials. The surface of liposomes was altered to include extremely pH-sensitive polymers, which increased the tumor's therapeutic effects and encouraged the release of Th1 cytokines from dendritic cells, (Chelu & Musuc, 2023) (Makadia & Siegel, 2011). These pH-sensitive liposomes is used to double-stimulate Dendritic Cells and enhance antitumor immunity when combined with adjuvants that target Dendritic Cells, (Xiong et al., 2021).They have proven to be more effective than synthetic polymers due to their high biocompatibility, ready biodegradability, excellent drug loading capacity and rapid absorption which helps them in site specific drug targeting and delivery, (Ginjupalli et al., 2017).

4.4 Polymer Based Biomaterials

The most widely used multifunctional materials in biomedicine are polymers. Using micellar structures or polymer-drug conjugates, they have been utilized to provide a range of treatments. Some polymers have special photochemical characteristics that make them useful for cancer treatment. To improve antitumor immunity, several polymer-based substances have been employed as adjuvants or neoantigen carriers, such as poly(lactic-co-glycolic) acid (PLGA), and polyethyleneimine, (Patil et al., 2024).

4.5 PLGA Poly(Lactic-Co-Glycolic)

Saturated aliphatic polyesters, such as poly(glycolic acid) (PGA), polylactic acid (PLA), and the copolymer poly(lactic-co - glycolic acid) (PLGA), are widely employed to create 3D scaffolds used in tissue engineering because of their biocompatibility and biodegradability, (Brugnera et al., 2022). As a highly crystalline, hydrophilic polymer that degrades relatively quickly in aqueous solutions or in vivo, PGA is widely used in injectable microspheres, biological adhesives and glues, oral surgery, and medication delivery, (Davis et al., 2022). Using polymer-based materials, medicines with different hydrophilic and hydrophobic qualities can be delivered simultaneously to enhance conventional treatments like gene editing, photodynamic therapy (PDT), chemotherapy, and radiotherapy. This shows how the substances have the ability to produce antitumor immunity and immunogenic cell death, (Yuan et al., 2024).

4.6 Synthetic Biomaterials

One interesting method for locally delivering immunotherapeutic drugs is the use of synthetic scaffolds. Scaffolds, when positioned strategically throughout the body, can increase the concentration of the substance at the place of interest while decreasing adverse effects, (Cai, Zhu, & Qi, 2020). Synthetic biomaterials are biomaterials which is created in labs which offer more durability and strength than natural biomaterials, (Li et al., 2024).

4.7 Metals

The main purpose of metallic biomaterials is to replace damaged hard tissues. Numerous biomedical applications use different kinds of high-strength alloys that contain harmless components. The remarkable shape of memory and super elastic capabilities of NiTi (Nitinol) alloys have led to the development of functional devices based on these materials. In addition to super elastic bone staples for orthopaedics and super elastic orthodontic wires for dentistry, the alloy is utilized in the production of self-expandable stents for cardiovascular surgery, (Jana & Dev, 2022). The required biocompatibility, bioactivity, surface integrity, and wear resistance are made into patient-specific medical implants, such as bone plates, screws, cranial, or dental devices, (Escriche-Navarro *et al.*, 2022). Among metal-based materials utilized in immunotherapy, the most commonly adopted strategy involves delivery of immunomodulators, including adjuvants, cytokines, neoantigens, and checkpoint inhibitors, (Yan et al., 2020). According to recent research, the main obstacles to immunotherapy include the tumor immunosuppressive microenvironment, poor response rates to current therapies, and severe side effects. Through Tumor Microenvironment reversal, immune adjuvant activity, and the induction of novel models of programmed cell death, metal-based biomaterials can improve the effectiveness of immunotherapy, (Pei, Lei, & Cheng, 2023).

4.8 Inorganic Biomaterials

The efficient delivery of drugs with improved bioavailability and fewer side effects is being studied extensively using biodegradable inorganic drug nanocarriers. High biosafety for in vivo applications requires a drug nanocarrier with both high biocompatibility and good biodegradability. Examples of several inorganic drug carriers include silica, metal oxides, and carbon-based compounds, (Hess, Medintz, & Jewell, 2019).

4.9 Carbon Quantum Dots

Typically spherical in shape and less than 10 nm in size, carbon quantum dots (CQDs) are carbon-based nanoparticles that exhibit photoluminescence. Distinct physicochemical characteristics, remarkable biocompatibility, environmental friendliness, and simplicity of surface functionalization are all displayed by these nanoparticles. Due to their small size, CQDs can approximate the glomerular filtration barrier, which makes them appropriate as mediators of reactive oxygen species (ROS) production and carriers for the transport of drugs, (Mowery & Chen, 2024). Hence researchers have been using Carbon Quantum Dots extensively in cancer cell imaging, cancer targeted drug delivery and in immunotherapies in recent years, (Pérez-Herrero et al., 2024).

4.10 Mesoporous Silica-Based Materials

It has been reported in recent years that mesoporous silica-based nanomaterials can function as adjuvants, an immunological substance that can activate APC and trigger an immune response. These nanoparticles can trigger both tumoral and cell-mediated immune responses, which sets them apart from conventional adjuvants. They can also be used as nanocarriers to deliver antigens in cancer vaccines, (Uhrich et al., 1999).

5. APPLICATIONS OF BIOMATERIALS IN CANCER IMMUNOTHERAPY

5.1 Drug Delivery Systems

The FDA has approved many immunotherapy-based medications to treat primary and metastatic tumors, however due to primary and acquired resistances, only a tiny percentage of the population can benefit from these medications. Additionally, the short half-lives of the molecules involved, the challenges of delivering them to the target sites, and some serious side effects linked to these approaches make it difficult to translate immunotherapy from the bench to clinical practice, (Ribas & Wolchok, 2018). Drug delivery methods may be able to directly target cancer cells, which would lessen acquired resistance and off-target side effects. Additionally, they lower the necessary dosage, which lowers toxicity, and they can increase effectiveness and enable immune response tunability. Drug delivery systems can extend the shelf life of pharmaceuticals, resulting in scalable products, and, if required, can protect the therapy from immune system identification or degradation. Additionally, they have the ability to modify drug release rates, which can benefit patients in a variety of ways, (Choi et al., 2024).

5.2 Immune Checkpoint Blockade Therapy

Long-lasting tumor responses in cancer patients have been caused by immune checkpoints, which restrict antitumor responses. By inhibiting the PD-1 or CTLA-4 pathway, this is accomplished. Even when the condition is under control, one-third of individuals experience relapses. Although the mechanisms of acquired resistance are not well understood, they may be addressed by changes in interferon-γ signaling pathways and antigen presentation, (Yu et al., 2024). The development of immune checkpoint blockade (ICB) treatments has accelerated the expansion of cancer immunotherapy, especially after cytotoxic T-lymphocyte-associated protein 4 (CTLA-4) inhibitors such as ipilimumab were initially approved. The therapy options for a variety of cancers have expanded as a result of the thorough investigations into numerous immune checkpoint antibodies. With fewer than 15% responsiveness and significant side effects in certain individuals, the clinical response to these antibody-based ICB treatments is still quite small, (Lin et al., 2024).

5.3 CAR-T Cell Therapy

The process of CAR-T treatment involves altering the patient's own T cells to express particular receptors that can identify and eliminate cancerous tumor cells, (De Graaf et al., 2020). Recent years have seen a tremendous advancement in the study of using biomaterials to improve the effectiveness of cell immunotherapy, (Chao & Liu, 2023). In order to address abnormal vascular distribution, hypoxia, acidity, and heterogeneity, biomaterial-based delivery systems have been created to alter and enhance TME (Tumor Microenvironment). Additionally, they encourage the infiltration of different immune cells and boost the activity of immune cells that fight tumors, which improves the effectiveness of immunotherapies, (Roma-Rodrigues et al., 2019). CAR-T cells bind to several types of biomaterials loaded with various functional biomolecules to enhance synergistic immunotherapy in solid tumors, (Lai et al., 2021).

5.4 Modulating Tumor Microenvironment

Immunotherapy response is significantly influenced by the immunosuppressive tumor microenvironment (TME). The tumor microenvironment (TME) of solid tumors can inhibit immune cell function and stop infiltration. Through the use of biomaterials-based techniques that target, react to, and modify the TME's physico-chemical characteristics—such as hypoxia, acidity, elevated reactive oxygen species, a dense extracellular matrix, and aberrant vasculature—the immunosuppressive aspects of the TME can be altered, (Emens et al., 2024). Biomaterials are essential for improving cancer treatment by focusing on the TME. Mesoporous silica NPs and metal oxide NPs are examples of inorganic NPs that allow for precise drug administration and immunomodulation in the TME. Natural and manufactured biopolymers are examples of organic biomaterials that provide flexible platforms for immune cell targeting. These techniques consist of Treg cell modulation, Tumor Associated Macrophages (TAM), DC, and NK, (Chu et al., 2024).

6. CHALLENGES AND OPPORTUNITIES

6.1 Challenges

Methods of antitumor action are the processes driving the toxicity and effectiveness of anticancer drugs in human versus animal models are not well understood. Better biomarkers are needed to predict toxicity and response. Resistance to therapy Tumors that are resistant to treatment acquire immune system escape mechanisms. Understanding the mechanisms of resistance is still challenging. Targeting and delivering are the challenges of efficiently transporting pharmaceuticals to their designated places. Single-target techniques are not very effective or specific. The toxicity Serious adverse events (irAEs) connected to the immune system could occur. Reducing toxicity is necessary to optimize anticancer efficacy. Modeling before clinical use of Current animal models only partially mirror human immune systems and malignancies. We need more pre-clinical models that are therapeutically useful. Standards and data exchange of the sector's progress is hampered by a lack of data exchange. We need standard concepts and frameworks to study ir-toxicity, (Whiteside et al., 2016) (Peterson, Denlinger, & Yang, 2022).

6.2 Opportunities

Synergistic effects when combining several immunotherapy treatments are the possibility of increased efficacy through logical combinations. Personalized immunotherapy based on individual profile is possible with the discovery of new immunologic biomarkers for response monitoring. Discovery of tumor antigens that is the Recognition of neoantigens from cancer mutations where the better creation of vaccines based on antigens specific to tumors. Advances in cellular therapy are the ability to produce, transport, and distribute therapeutic cells more efficiently. The possibility of cellular medicines becoming more widely available. In addition to other therapies, Synergy between immunotherapy and traditional treatments, such as radiation Potentiation of immunotherapy may have abscopal consequences. Focusing on immune-suppressive processes leads to the discovery of new checkpoints and inhibitory pathways are found, and inhibitors that target these pathways are developed, (Remesh, 2012) (Uranga, Nurgali, & Abalo, 2023).

6.3 Safety and Long-Term Effects

Most pharmacological anticancer drugs affect the cell growth process. The rapid proliferation of certain normal cells, including bone marrow cells, oral mucosal cells, and hair follicles, must be mentioned in addition to cancer cells, (Trill, 2013). This explains the serious adverse effects of cancer chemotherapy, (Berger et al., 2010) (Lewandowska et al., 2020). Anticancer medications harm the epithelium protecting the gastrointestinal system, resulting in the most frequent adverse effects, nausea and vomiting, (Chen, Yu, & Yang, 2008). As a result of intestinal epithelium damage, diarrhea is another common adverse effect, (Gammon, Dold, & Jewell, 2016). Alopecia and hair loss are common side effects of chemotherapy, but thankfully, they are treatable, (Aguado et al., 2018). Cancer chemotherapy also frequently causes anxiety, sleep issues, sexual dysfunction, and exhaustion, (Maciejko, Smalley, & Goldman, 2017). These problems can be solved by using biomaterials for cancer immunotherapy.

6.4 Advances in Personalized Medicines

As the need for precision medicine grows, the "one-size-fits-all" method of creating medical treatments and equipment is becoming less and less effective. Although biomaterials offer a lot of potential to revolutionize precision medicine, the intricacy of each patient frequently means that combining several uses into one device is necessary to effectively customize individualized treatments, (Song, Musetti, & Huang, 2017). The field of personalized medicine has changed to adapt to the new cancer immunotherapy to overcome the constraints of individualized cancer treatment, new platform technologies have been developed by reprogramming patient-autologous T-cells, novel approaches are being employed to customize immunotherapy. Immunotherapeutics are being delivered locally via engineered biomaterials such as transdermal, injectable, and implantable. The goal of these biomaterial-based strategies is to increase safety and effectiveness by triggering anticancer immunity only when necessary. Biomaterials enable spatially regulated release of immunomodulators and enhanced drug accumulation at target sites, (Goldberg, 2019).

7. EMERGING TRENDS IN NANOTECHNOLOGY AND BIOMATERIALS IN CANCER IMMUNOTHERAPY

Materials that have at least one dimension between 1 and 1000 nm are called nanomaterials, while in practice they could be anywhere between 1 and 200 nm. Over the last three decades, there has been significant progress in the use of different nanomaterials for cancer treatment and diagnosis, (Chen et al., 2020). Pioneers in the field of cancer immunotherapy were granted the 2018 Nobel Prize in Physiology or Medicine because it has been clinically proven that using a patient's coordinated and adaptive immune system to combat their particular tumor is effective. Because tumors can evade the immune system in a number of ways, the percentage of patients who react to immunotherapy is still limited around 15% objective response rate across indications, (Dong et al., 2020).

Administration systems based on nanoparticles that is Nanoparticles are being investigated extensively for the regulated and targeted administration of immunotherapeutic drugs straight to malignancies. Researchers are taking advantage of the capacity to alter the surface of nanoparticles in order to enhance their targeting and interaction with molecular and cellular targets. Self-assembled nanostructures are Novel strategies which are being investigated for photodynamic therapy, such as the self-assembly of pyro pheophorbide derivatives, (Kandasamy, Karuppasamy, & Krishnan, 2023). Optogenetic approaches like light-sensitive immunomodulator-loaded hydrogel implants are being studied for perioperative immunotherapy. In DNA nanocarriers, Research is being conducted on loading exosomes with therapeutic agents and altering their surfaces for improved targeting. The development of novel DNA-based carriers that co-encapsulates many treatments (such as doxorubicin and CpG) for chemoimmunotherapy is underway, (Xiao et al., 2023). Targeting the tumor microenvironment that is Targeting primary and metastatic cancers by taking advantage of physical characteristics like stiffness is becoming more and more popular. Optogenetic up conversion systems are being investigated for the regulated release of cells with immunomodulatory engineering. In Phage-based vaccination platforms, new vaccine strategies are being developed using M13 bacteriophage-based systems, (Yan et al., 2019).

Combination therapies are equipped by Many as people are interested in using nanocarriers to combine immunotherapy with other treatments like radiation therapy, photothermal therapy (PTT), and chemotherapy. Before clinical translation, there is an increasing need to evaluate these biomaterial-based techniques' safety and effectiveness in more detail. The continuous attempts to overcome obstacles in cancer immunotherapy by using novel biomaterials and nanotechnology techniques are reflected in these trends. Discipline is still developing quickly as scientists look at novel substances, ways to distribute them, and ways to combine them to enhance therapy results, (Shams et al., 2022).

7.1 Nanomaterials for Antigen Delivery

Antigen-presenting cells such as dendritic cells are receiving tumor antigens via nanoparticles (NPs) such as polymeric NPs, liposomes, exosomes, metal NPs, mesoporous silica NPs, carbon nanotubes, and virus-like particles. Targeting DCs in lymph nodes, NPs can alter the tumor microenvironment and trigger downstream effector T cells. Various NP types have special qualities that make them ideal for delivering antigens, including vast surface areas, controlled release, and targeting abilities, (Fan et al., 2018).

7.2 Nanomaterials for Vaccine Carriers

As vaccine carriers, PLGA NPs, dendrimers, micelles, liposomes, exosomes, metal NPs, MSNs, CNTs, and VLPs are being investigated to improve immunogenicity. Nano vaccines offer prolonged antigen release and are more efficient than standard vaccines at targeting immune cells. Numerous Nano vaccines have demonstrated potential treating a range of cancer types in preclinical investigations, (Kaur et al., 2024).

7.3 Nanomaterials for Checkpoint Inhibitors

To increase efficacy while lowering toxicity, checkpoint inhibitors like anti-CTLA-4 and anti-PD-1 antibodies are being coupled with nanoparticles. NPs coupled with anti-CTLA-4 and anti-PD-1/PD-L1 antibodies are two examples. Compared to free antibodies, certain nano combinations exhibit better tumor targeting and immune activation, (Parhi, Mohanty, & Sahoo, 2012).

7.4 Targeting Immune Cells

Targeting different immune cells, such as dendritic cells, T cells, regulatory T cells, and myeloid-derived suppressor cells, is done with nanoparticles in cancer immunotherapy. For instance, macrophages linked to ovarian tumors have been targeted by large anionic liposomes. Immuno-checkpoint blockade in conjunction with hybrid nanoparticles has demonstrated potential in regulating T cells.

7.5 Combination Therapies

Combining several therapeutic modalities, including immunotherapy, photodynamic therapy, and chemotherapy, is being investigated in nanoparticle-based combination therapies. To treat ovarian cancer, for example, biodegradable photo responsive nanoparticles have been developed for photothermal, photodynamic, and chemotherapy treatments.

8. CONCLUSION

It is true that biomaterial-based immunotherapeutic approaches have demonstrated significant promise in cancer immunotherapy treatments, further research is required to improve the biomaterials design in order to provide more individualized treatment plans for cancer patients with distinct characteristics. In this chapter various immunotherapy approaches and its cutting-edge biomaterials that could be used to increase therapeutic efficacy and lessen side effects. Despite the rapid advancements in cancer immunotherapy, the use of biomaterials to create the best systems for different tumor types is still in its infancy. Biomaterials are hoped to be more broadly and creatively developed for cancer immunotherapy, increasing its effectiveness and lowering immune-related side effects. Biomaterials are essential in CAR T-cell treatment, cancer immunotherapy, vaccines, and tumor regulation associated with checkpoint blockade. A wide variety of biomaterials, including macroscale particles, viruses, bacteria, tiny chemicals, and nanosized organic and inorganic particles, have been developed to improve antitumor immune responses. Utilizing these formulations enhances treatment efficacy of tumor and offers many benefits and functions to increase antitumor immunity. Biomaterials adaptability in creating individualized therapies has enormous potential for more focused and efficient cancer treatments.

REFERENCES

Aguado, B. A., Grim, J. C., Rosales, A. M., Watson-Capps, J. J., & Anseth, K. S. (2018). Engineering precision biomaterials for personalized medicine. *Science Translational Medicine*, *10*(424), eaam8645. DOI: 10.1126/scitranslmed.aam8645 PMID: 29343626

Arneth, B. (2019). Tumor microenvironment. *Medicina*, *56*(1), 15. DOI: 10.3390/medicina56010015 PMID: 31906017

Avula, L. R., & Grodzinski, P. (2024). How organ-on-a-chip is advancing cancer research and oncology-a cancer hallmarks' perspective. *Frontiers in Lab on a Chip Technologies*, *3*, 1487377. DOI: 10.3389/frlct.2024.1487377

Beheshtizadeh, N., Asgari, Y., Nasiri, N., Farzin, A., Ghorbani, M., Lotfibakhshaiesh, N., & Azami, M. (2021). A network analysis of angiogenesis/osteogenesis-related growth factors in bone tissue engineering based on in-vitro and in-vivo data: A systems biology approach. *Tissue & Cell*, *72*, 101553. DOI: 10.1016/j.tice.2021.101553 PMID: 33975231

Berger, A. M., Abernethy, A. P., Atkinson, A., Barsevick, A. M., Breitbart, W. S., Cella, D., Cimprich, B., Cleeland, C., Eisenberger, M. A., Escalante, C. P., Jacobsen, P. B., Kaldor, P., Ligibel, J. A., Murphy, B. A., O'Connor, T., Pirl, W. F., Rodler, E., Rugo, H. S., Thomas, J., & Wagner, L. I. (2010). Cancer-related fatigue. *Journal of the National Comprehensive Cancer Network : JNCCN*, *8*(8), 904–931. DOI: 10.6004/jnccn.2010.0067 PMID: 20870636

Berraondo, P., Sanmamed, M. F., Ochoa, M. C., Etxeberria, I., Aznar, M. A., Pérez-Gracia, J. L., Rodríguez-Ruiz, M. E., Ponz-Sarvise, M., Castañón, E., & Melero, I. (2019). Cytokines in clinical cancer immunotherapy. *British Journal of Cancer*, *120*(1), 6–15. DOI: 10.1038/s41416-018-0328-y PMID: 30413827

Bhatia, S., & Bhatia, S. (2016). Natural polymers vs synthetic polymer. *Natural polymer drug delivery systems: nanoparticles, plants, and algae*, 95-118

Bird, D., & Ravindra, N. M. (2020). Transdermal drug delivery and patches—An overview. *Medical Devices & Sensors*, *3*(6), e10069. DOI: 10.1002/mds3.10069

Biswal, T., BadJena, S. K., & Pradhan, D. (2020). Sustainable biomaterials and their applications: A short review. *Materials Today: Proceedings*, *30*, 274–282. DOI: 10.1016/j.matpr.2020.01.437

Brugnera, M., Vicario-de-la-Torre, M., Andrés-Guerrero, V., Bravo-Osuna, I., Molina-Martínez, I. T., & Herrero-Vanrell, R. (2022). Validation of a rapid and easy-to-apply method to simultaneously quantify co-loaded dexamethasone and melatonin PLGA microspheres by HPLC-UV: Encapsulation efficiency and in vitro release. *Pharmaceutics*, *14*(2), 288. DOI: 10.3390/pharmaceutics14020288 PMID: 35214021

Cai, A. Y., Zhu, Y. J., & Qi, C. (2020). Biodegradable inorganic nanostructured biomaterials for drug delivery. *Advanced Materials Interfaces*, *7*(20), 2000819. DOI: 10.1002/admi.202000819

Cai, L., Xu, J., Yang, Z., Tong, R., Dong, Z., Wang, C., & Leong, K. W. (2020). Engineered biomaterials for cancer immunotherapy. *MedComm*, *1*(1), 35–46. DOI: 10.1002/mco2.8 PMID: 34766108

Cai, L., Xu, J., Yang, Z., Tong, R., Dong, Z., Wang, C., & Leong, K. W. (2020). Engineered biomaterials for cancer immunotherapy. *MedComm*, *1*(1), 35–46. DOI: 10.1002/mco2.8 PMID: 34766108

Cai, X., Zhan, H., Ye, Y., Yang, J., Zhang, M., Li, J., & Zhuang, Y. (2021). Current progress and future perspectives of immune checkpoint in cancer and infectious diseases. *Frontiers in Genetics*, *12*, 785153. DOI: 10.3389/fgene.2021.785153 PMID: 34917131

Cao, Y., & Wang, B. (2009). Biodegradation of silk biomaterials. *International Journal of Molecular Sciences*, *10*(4), 1514–1524. DOI: 10.3390/ijms10041514 PMID: 19468322

Chao, Y., Chen, Q., & Liu, Z. (2020). Smart injectable hydrogels for cancer immunotherapy. *Advanced Functional Materials*, *30*(2), 1902785. DOI: 10.1002/adfm.201902785

Chao, Y., & Liu, Z. (2023). Biomaterials tools to modulate the tumour microenvironment in immunotherapy. *Nature Reviews Bioengineering*, *1*(2), 125–138. DOI: 10.1038/s44222-022-00004-6

Chelu, M., & Musuc, A. M. (2023). Advanced biomedical applications of multifunctional natural and synthetic biomaterials. *Processes (Basel, Switzerland)*, *11*(9), 2696. DOI: 10.3390/pr11092696

Chen, J., Fan, T., Xie, Z., Zeng, Q., Xue, P., Zheng, T., Chen, Y., Luo, X., & Zhang, H. (2020). Advances in nanomaterials for photodynamic therapy applications: Status and challenges. *Biomaterials*, *237*, 119827. DOI: 10.1016/j.biomaterials.2020.119827 PMID: 32036302

Chen, M. L., Yu, C. T., & Yang, C. H. (2008). Sleep disturbances and quality of life in lung cancer patients undergoing chemotherapy. *Lung Cancer (Amsterdam, Netherlands)*, *62*(3), 391–400. DOI: 10.1016/j.lungcan.2008.03.016 PMID: 18468718

Chen, Q., Chen, M., & Liu, Z. (2019). Local biomaterials-assisted cancer immunotherapy to trigger systemic antitumor responses. *Chemical Society Reviews*, *48*(22), 5506–5526. DOI: 10.1039/C9CS00271E PMID: 31589233

Choi, Y., Seok, S. H., Yoon, H. Y., Ryu, J. H., & Kwon, I. C. (2024). Advancing cancer immunotherapy through siRNA-based gene silencing for immune checkpoint blockade. *Advanced Drug Delivery Reviews*, *209*, 115306. DOI: 10.1016/j.addr.2024.115306 PMID: 38626859

Chrétien, S., Zerdes, I., Bergh, J., Matikas, A., & Foukakis, T. (2019). Beyond PD-1/PD-L1 inhibition: What the future holds for breast cancer immunotherapy. *Cancers (Basel)*, *11*(5), 628. DOI: 10.3390/cancers11050628 PMID: 31060337

Chu, Z., Wang, W., Zheng, W., Fu, W., Wang, Y., Wang, H., & Qian, H. (2024). Biomaterials with cancer cell-specific cytotoxicity: Challenges and perspectives. *Chemical Society Reviews*, *53*(17), 8847–8877. DOI: 10.1039/D4CS00636D PMID: 39092634

Conlon, K. C., Miljkovic, M. D., & Waldmann, T. A. (2019). Cytokines in the treatment of cancer. *Journal of Interferon & Cytokine Research*, *39*(1), 6–21. DOI: 10.1089/jir.2018.0019 PMID: 29889594

Cook, A. M., Lesterhuis, W. J., Nowak, A. K., & Lake, R. A. (2016). Chemotherapy and immunotherapy: Mapping the road ahead. *Current Opinion in Immunology*, *39*, 23–29. DOI: 10.1016/j.coi.2015.12.003 PMID: 26724433

Cunningham, N., Lapointe, R., & Lerouge, S. (2022). Biomaterials for enhanced immunotherapy. *APL Bioengineering*, *6*(4), 041502. DOI: 10.1063/5.0125692 PMID: 36561511

Dahri, M., Beheshtizadeh, N., Seyedpour, N., Nakhostin-Ansari, A., Aghajani, F., Seyedpour, S., Masjedi, M., Farjadian, F., Maleki, R., & Adibkia, K. (2023). Biomaterial-based delivery platforms for transdermal immunotherapy. *Biomedicine and Pharmacotherapy*, *165*, 115048. DOI: 10.1016/j.biopha.2023.115048 PMID: 37385212

Dahri, M., Beheshtizadeh, N., Seyedpour, N., Nakhostin-Ansari, A., Aghajani, F., Seyedpour, S., Masjedi, M., Farjadian, F., Maleki, R., & Adibkia, K. (2023). Biomaterial-based delivery platforms for transdermal immunotherapy. *Biomedicine and Pharmacotherapy*, *165*, 115048. DOI: 10.1016/j.biopha.2023.115048 PMID: 37385212

Dai, H., Fan, Q., & Wang, C. (2022, December). Recent applications of immunomodulatory biomaterials for disease immunotherapy. In Exploration (Vol. 2, No. 6, p. 20210157). DOI: 10.1002/EXP.20210157

Davis, R., Singh, A., Jackson, M. J., Coelho, R. T., Prakash, D., Charalambous, C. P., Ahmed, W., da Silva, L. R. R., & Lawrence, A. A. (2022). A comprehensive review on metallic implant biomaterials and their subtractive manufacturing. *International Journal of Advanced Manufacturing Technology*, *120*(3), 1473–1530. DOI: 10.1007/s00170-022-08770-8 PMID: 35228769

De Graaf, J. F., Huberts, M., Fouchier, R. A. M., & van den Hoogen, B. G. (2020). Determinants of the efficacy of viro-immunotherapy: A review. *Cytokine & Growth Factor Reviews*, *56*, 124–132. DOI: 10.1016/j.cytogfr.2020.07.001 PMID: 32919831

De Leo, V., Milano, F., Agostiano, A., & Catucci, L. (2021). Recent advancements in polymer/liposome assembly for drug delivery: From surface modifications to hybrid vesicles. *Polymers*, *13*(7), 1027. DOI: 10.3390/polym13071027 PMID: 33810273

Decker, W. K., da Silva, R. F., Sanabria, M. H., Angelo, L. S., Guimarães, F., Burt, B. M., Kheradmand, F., & Paust, S. (2017). Cancer immunotherapy: Historical perspective of a clinical revolution and emerging preclinical animal models. *Frontiers in Immunology*, *8*, 829. DOI: 10.3389/fimmu.2017.00829 PMID: 28824608

Dillman, R. O. (2011). Cancer immunotherapy. *Cancer Biotherapy & Radiopharmaceuticals*, *26*(1), 1–64. DOI: 10.1089/cbr.2010.0902 PMID: 21355777

Dobosz, P., & Dzieciątkowski, T. (2019). The intriguing history of cancer immunotherapy. *Frontiers in Immunology*, *10*, 2965. DOI: 10.3389/fimmu.2019.02965 PMID: 31921205

Dong, X., Yang, A., Bai, Y., Kong, D., & Lv, F. (2020). Dual fluorescence imaging-guided programmed delivery of doxorubicin and CpG nanoparticles to modulate tumor microenvironment for effective chemo-immunotherapy. *Biomaterials*, *230*, 119659. DOI: 10.1016/j.biomaterials.2019.119659 PMID: 31831223

Emens, L. A., Romero, P. J., Anderson, A. C., Bruno, T. C., Capitini, C. M., Collyar, D., Gulley, J. L., Hwu, P., Posey, A. D.Jr, Silk, A. W., & Wargo, J. A. (2024). Challenges and opportunities in cancer immunotherapy: A Society for Immunotherapy of Cancer (SITC) strategic vision. *Journal for Immunotherapy of Cancer*, *12*(6), e009063. DOI: 10.1136/jitc-2024-009063 PMID: 38901879

Escriche-Navarro, B., Escudero, A., Lucena-Sánchez, E., Sancenón, F., García-Fernández, A., & Martínez-Máñez, R. (2022). Mesoporous silica materials as an emerging tool for cancer immunotherapy. *Advancement of Science*, *9*(26), 2200756. DOI: 10.1002/advs.202200756 PMID: 35866466

Esfahani, K., Roudaia, L., Buhlaiga, N. A., Del Rincon, S. V., Papneja, N., & Miller, W. H. (2020). A review of cancer immunotherapy: From the past, to the present, to the future. *Current Oncology (Toronto, Ont.)*, *27*(12, s2), 87–97. DOI: 10.3747/co.27.5223 PMID: 32368178

Fan, Q., Chen, Z., Wang, C., & Liu, Z. (2018). Toward biomaterials for enhancing immune checkpoint blockade therapy. *Advanced Functional Materials*, *28*(37), 1802540. DOI: 10.1002/adfm.201802540

Fratzl, P. (2007). Biomimetic materials research: What can we really learn from nature's structural materials? *Journal of the Royal Society, Interface*, *4*(15), 637–642. DOI: 10.1098/rsif.2007.0218 PMID: 17341452

Galluzzi, L., Vacchelli, E., Eggermont, A., Fridman, W. H., Galon, J., Sautès-Fridman, C., Tartour, E., Zitvogel, L., & Kroemer, G. (2012). Trial Watch: Adoptive cell transfer immunotherapy. *OncoImmunology*, *1*(3), 306–315. DOI: 10.4161/onci.19549 PMID: 22737606

Gammon, J. M., Dold, N. M., & Jewell, C. M. (2016). Improving the clinical impact of biomaterials in cancer immunotherapy. *Oncotarget*, *7*(13), 15421–15443. DOI: 10.18632/oncotarget.7304 PMID: 26871948

Gammon, J. M., Dold, N. M., & Jewell, C. M. (2016). Improving the clinical impact of biomaterials in cancer immunotherapy. *Oncotarget*, *7*(13), 15421–15443. DOI: 10.18632/oncotarget.7304 PMID: 26871948

Ginjupalli, K., Shavi, G. V., Averineni, R. K., Bhat, M., Udupa, N., & Upadhya, P. N. (2017). Poly (α-hydroxy acid) based polymers: A review on material and degradation aspects. *Polymer Degradation & Stability*, *144*, 520–535. DOI: 10.1016/j.polymdegradstab.2017.08.024

Goh, K. L., & Holmes, D. F. (2017). Collagenous extracellular matrix biomaterials for tissue engineering: Lessons from the common sea urchin tissue. *International Journal of Molecular Sciences*, *18*(5), 901.

Ressler, A. (2022). Chitosan-based biomaterials for bone tissue engineering applications: a short review

Goldberg, M. S. (2019). Improving cancer immunotherapy through nanotechnology. *Nature Reviews. Cancer*, *19*(10), 587–602. DOI: 10.1038/s41568-019-0186-9 PMID: 31492927

Hemminki, O., Dos Santos, J. M., & Hemminki, A. (2020). Oncolytic viruses for cancer immunotherapy. *Journal of Hematology & Oncology*, *13*(1), 1–15. DOI: 10.1186/s13045-020-00922-1 PMID: 32600470

Herndon, T. M., Demko, S. G., Jiang, X., He, K., Gootenberg, J. E., Cohen, M. H., Keegan, P., & Pazdur, R. (2012). US Food and Drug Administration Approval: Peginterferon-alfa-2b for the adjuvant treatment of patients with melanoma. *The Oncologist*, *17*(10), 1323–1328. DOI: 10.1634/theoncologist.2012-0123 PMID: 23002124

Hess, K. L., Medintz, I. L., & Jewell, C. M. (2019). Designing inorganic nanomaterials for vaccines and immunotherapies. *Nano Today*, *27*, 73–98. DOI: 10.1016/j.nantod.2019.04.005 PMID: 32292488

Huang, Y., & Zeng, J. (2020). Recent development and applications of nanomaterials for cancer immunotherapy. *Nanotechnology Reviews*, *9*(1), 367–384. DOI: 10.1515/ntrev-2020-0027

Ige, O. O., Umoru, L. E., & Aribo, S. (2012). Natural products: A minefield of biomaterials. *International Scholarly Research Notices*, *2012*(1), 983062.

Jafari, M., Kadkhodazadeh, M., Shapourabadi, M. B., Goradel, N. H., Shokrgozar, M. A., Arashkia, A., Abdoli, S., & Sharifzadeh, Z. (2022). Immunovirotherapy: The role of antibody based therapeutics combination with oncolytic viruses. *Frontiers in Immunology*, *13*, 1012806. DOI: 10.3389/fimmu.2022.1012806 PMID: 36311790

Jana, P., & Dev, A. (2022). Carbon quantum dots: A promising nanocarrier for bioimaging and drug delivery in cancer. *Materials Today. Communications*, *32*, 104068. DOI: 10.1016/j.mtcomm.2022.104068

Kaczmarek, M., Poznańska, J., Fechner, F., Michalska, N., Paszkowska, S., Napierała, A., & Mackiewicz, A. (2023). Cancer vaccine therapeutics: Limitations and effectiveness—A literature review. *Cells*, *12*(17), 2159. DOI: 10.3390/cells12172159 PMID: 37681891

Kandasamy, G., Karuppasamy, Y., & Krishnan, U. M. (2023). Emerging trends in nano-driven immunotherapy for treatment of cancer. *Vaccines, 11*(2), 458. DOI: 10.3390/vaccines11020458 PMID: 36851335

Karanth, H., & Murthy, R. S. R. (2007). pH-Sensitive liposomes-principle and application in cancer therapy. *The Journal of Pharmacy and Pharmacology, 59*(4), 469–483. DOI: 10.1211/jpp.59.4.0001 PMID: 17430630

Kaur, P., Singh, S. K., Mishra, M. K., Singh, S., & Singh, R. (2024). Nanotechnology for boosting ovarian cancer immunotherapy. *Journal of Ovarian Research, 17*(1), 202. DOI: 10.1186/s13048-024-01507-z PMID: 39402681

Kciuk, M., Yahya, E. B., Mohamed Ibrahim Mohamed, M., Rashid, S., Iqbal, M. O., Kontek, R., Abdulsamad, M. A., & Allaq, A. A. (2023). Recent advances in molecular mechanisms of cancer immunotherapy. *Cancers (Basel), 15*(10), 2721. DOI: 10.3390/cancers15102721 PMID: 37345057

Lai, C., Lin, S., Huang, X., & Jin, Y. (2021). Synthesis and properties of carbon quantum dots and their research progress in cancer treatment. *Dyes and Pigments, 196*, 109766. DOI: 10.1016/j.dyepig.2021.109766

Leach, D. G., Young, S., & Hartgerink, J. D. (2019). Advances in immunotherapy delivery from implantable and injectable biomaterials. *Acta Biomaterialia, 88*, 15–31. DOI: 10.1016/j.actbio.2019.02.016 PMID: 30771535

Ledford, H. (2011). Melanoma drug wins US approval. *Nature, 471*(7340), 561. DOI: 10.1038/471561a PMID: 21455150

Lee, S., & Margolin, K. (2011). Cytokines in cancer immunotherapy. *Cancers (Basel), 3*(4), 3856–3893. DOI: 10.3390/cancers3043856 PMID: 24213115

Lewandowska, A., Rudzki, G., Lewandowski, T., Próchnicki, M., Rudzki, S., Laskowska, B., & Brudniak, J. (2020). Quality of life of cancer patients treated with chemotherapy. *International Journal of Environmental Research and Public Health, 17*(19), 6938. DOI: 10.3390/ijerph17196938 PMID: 32977386

Li, J., Luo, Y., Li, B., Xia, Y., Wang, H., & Fu, C. (2020). Implantable and injectable biomaterial scaffolds for cancer immunotherapy. *Frontiers in Bioengineering and Biotechnology, 8*, 612950. DOI: 10.3389/fbioe.2020.612950 PMID: 33330440

Li, Y., Xu, Z., Qi, Z., Huang, X., Li, M., Liu, S., Yan, Y., & Gao, M. (2024). Application of carbon nanomaterials to enhancing tumor immunotherapy: Current advances and prospects. *International Journal of Nanomedicine, 19*, 10899–10915. DOI: 10.2147/IJN.S480799 PMID: 39479174

Liang, X., Mu, M., Fan, R., Zou, B., & Guo, G. (2022). Functionalized chitosan as a promising platform for cancer immunotherapy: A review. *Carbohydrate Polymers*, *290*, 119452. DOI: 10.1016/j.carbpol.2022.119452 PMID: 35550761

Lin, Y., Chen, Y., Luo, Z., & Wu, Y. L. (2024). Recent advances on biomaterial designs in assisting CAR-T cell therapy towards potential solid tumor treatment. *Nanoscale*, *16*(7), 3226–3242. DOI: 10.1039/D3NR05768B PMID: 38284230

Maciejko, L., Smalley, M., & Goldman, A. (2017). Cancer immunotherapy and personalized medicine: Emerging technologies and biomarker-based approaches. *Journal of Molecular Biomarkers & Diagnosis*, *8*(5). Advance online publication. DOI: 10.4172/2155-9929.1000350 PMID: 29285416

Makadia, H. K., & Siegel, S. J. (2011). Poly lactic-co-glycolic acid (PLGA) as biodegradable controlled drug delivery carrier. *Polymers*, *3*(3), 1377–1397. DOI: 10.3390/polym3031377 PMID: 22577513

Miller, J. F., & Sadelain, M. (2015). The journey from discoveries in fundamental immunology to cancer immunotherapy. *Cancer Cell*, *27*(4), 439–449. DOI: 10.1016/j.ccell.2015.03.007 PMID: 25858803

Mowery, J. L., & Chen, J. (2024). Recent Biomedical Applications of Carbon Quantum Dots in Cancer Treatment. *The Journal of Physical Chemistry. C, Nanomaterials and Interfaces*, *128*(39), 16291–16301. DOI: 10.1021/acs.jpcc.4c04847

Padmanabhan, R., Meskin, N., & Al Moustafa, A. E. (2021). *Mathematical models of cancer and different therapies*. Springer. DOI: 10.1007/978-981-15-8640-8

Pardi, N., Hogan, M. J., Porter, F. W., & Weissman, D. (2018). mRNA vaccines—A new era in vaccinology. *Nature Reviews. Drug Discovery*, *17*(4), 261–279. DOI: 10.1038/nrd.2017.243 PMID: 29326426

Pardoll, D. M. (2012). The blockade of immune checkpoints in cancer immunotherapy. *Nature Reviews. Cancer*, *12*(4), 252–264. DOI: 10.1038/nrc3239 PMID: 22437870

Parhi, P., Mohanty, C., & Sahoo, S. K. (2012). Nanotechnology-based combinational drug delivery: An emerging approach for cancer therapy. *Drug Discovery Today*, *17*(17-18), 1044–1052. DOI: 10.1016/j.drudis.2012.05.010 PMID: 22652342

Patil, S. J., Thorat, V. M., Koparde, A. A., Bhosale, R. R., Bhinge, S. D., Chavan, D. D., & Tiwari, D. D. (2024). Theranostic applications of scaffolds in current biomedical research. *Cureus*, *16*(10), e71694. DOI: 10.7759/cureus.71694 PMID: 39559663

Peer, D., Karp, J. M., Hong, S., Farokhzad, O. C., Margalit, R., & Langer, R. (2020). Nanocarriers as an emerging platform for cancer therapy. Nano-enabled medical applications, 61-91.

Pei, Z., Lei, H., & Cheng, L. (2023). Bioactive inorganic nanomaterials for cancer theranostics. *Chemical Society Reviews*, *52*(6), 2031–2081. DOI: 10.1039/D2CS00352J PMID: 36633202

Pérez-Herrero, E., Lanier, O. L., Krishnan, N., D'Andrea, A., & Peppas, N. A. (2024). Drug delivery methods for cancer immunotherapy. *Drug Delivery and Translational Research*, *14*(1), 30–61. DOI: 10.1007/s13346-023-01405-9 PMID: 37587290

Peterson, C., Denlinger, N., & Yang, Y. (2022). Recent advances and challenges in cancer immunotherapy. *Cancers (Basel)*, *14*(16), 3972. DOI: 10.3390/cancers14163972 PMID: 36010965

Radhakrishnan, S., Nagarajan, S., Bechelany, M., & Kalkura, S. N. (2020). Collagen based biomaterials for tissue engineering applications: A review. *Processes and phenomena on the boundary between biogenic and Abiogenic nature*, 3-22

Remesh, A. (2012). Toxicities of anticancer drugs and its management. *International Journal of Basic and Clinical Pharmacology*, *1*(2), 2319–2003. DOI: 10.5455/2319-2003.ijbcp000812

Ribas, A., & Wolchok, J. D. (2018). Cancer immunotherapy using checkpoint blockade. *Science*, *359*(6382), 1350–1355. DOI: 10.1126/science.aar4060 PMID: 29567705

Robert, C. (2020). A decade of immune-checkpoint inhibitors in cancer therapy. *Nature Communications*, *11*(1), 3801. DOI: 10.1038/s41467-020-17670-y PMID: 32732879

Roma-Rodrigues, C., Mendes, R., Baptista, P. V., & Fernandes, A. R. (2019). Targeting tumor microenvironment for cancer therapy. *International Journal of Molecular Sciences*, *20*(4), 840. DOI: 10.3390/ijms20040840 PMID: 30781344

Rosenberg, S. A., Restifo, N. P., Yang, J. C., Morgan, R. A., & Dudley, M. E. (2008). Adoptive cell transfer: A clinical path to effective cancer immunotherapy. *Nature Reviews. Cancer*, *8*(4), 299–308. DOI: 10.1038/nrc2355 PMID: 18354418

Sampson, J. H., Gunn, M. D., Fecci, P. E., & Ashley, D. M. (2020). Brain immunology and immunotherapy in brain tumours. *Nature Reviews. Cancer*, *20*(1), 12–25. DOI: 10.1038/s41568-019-0224-7 PMID: 31806885

Shams, F., Golchin, A., Azari, A., Mohammadi Amirabad, L., Zarein, F., Khosravi, A., & Ardeshirylajimi, A. (2022). Nanotechnology-based products for cancer immunotherapy. *Molecular Biology Reports*, •••, 1–24. PMID: 34716502

Sharma, P., & Allison, J. P. (2015). Immune checkpoint targeting in cancer therapy: Toward combination strategies with curative potential. *Cell*, *161*(2), 205–214. DOI: 10.1016/j.cell.2015.03.030 PMID: 25860605

Shi, T., Ma, Y., Yu, L., Jiang, J., Shen, S., Hou, Y., & Wang, T. (2018). Cancer immunotherapy: A focus on the regulation of immune checkpoints. *International Journal of Molecular Sciences*, *19*(5), 1389. DOI: 10.3390/ijms19051389 PMID: 29735917

Shiravand, Y., Khodadadi, F., Kashani, S. M. A., Hosseini-Fard, S. R., Hosseini, S., Sadeghirad, H., Ladwa, R., O'Byrne, K., & Kulasinghe, A. (2022). Immune checkpoint inhibitors in cancer therapy. *Current Oncology (Toronto, Ont.)*, *29*(5), 3044–3060. DOI: 10.3390/curroncol29050247 PMID: 35621637

Siegel, R. L., Miller, K. D., & Jemal, A. (2019). Cancer statistics, 2019. *CA: a Cancer Journal for Clinicians*, *69*(1), 7–34. DOI: 10.3322/caac.21551 PMID: 30620402

Singh, A., Qin, H., Fernandez, I., Wei, J., Lin, J., Kwak, L. W., & Roy, K. (2011). An injectable synthetic immune-priming center mediates efficient T-cell class switching and T-helper 1 response against B cell lymphoma. *Journal of Controlled Release*, *155*(2), 184–192. DOI: 10.1016/j.jconrel.2011.06.008 PMID: 21708196

Sionkowska, A. (2011). Current research on the blends of natural and synthetic polymers as new biomaterials. *Progress in Polymer Science*, *36*(9), 1254–1276. DOI: 10.1016/j.progpolymsci.2011.05.003

Sirica, A. E. (1989). Classification of neoplasms. In *The pathobiology of neoplasia* (pp. 25–38). Springer US. DOI: 10.1007/978-1-4684-5523-6_2

Song, W., Musetti, S. N., & Huang, L. (2017). Nanomaterials for cancer immunotherapy. *Biomaterials*, *148*, 16–30. DOI: 10.1016/j.biomaterials.2017.09.017 PMID: 28961532

Spaapen, R. M., Leung, M. Y., Fuertes, M. B., Kline, J. P., Zhang, L., Zheng, Y., Fu, Y.-X., Luo, X., Cohen, K. S., & Gajewski, T. F. (2014). Therapeutic activity of high-dose intratumoral IFN-β requires direct effect on the tumor vasculature. *The Journal of Immunology : Official Journal of the American Association of Immunologists*, *193*(8), 4254–4260. DOI: 10.4049/jimmunol.1401109 PMID: 25217157

Tan, S., Li, D., & Zhu, X. (2020). Cancer immunotherapy: Pros, cons and beyond. *Biomedicine and Pharmacotherapy*, *124*, 109821. DOI: 10.1016/j.biopha.2020.109821 PMID: 31962285

Tiptiri-Kourpeti, A., Spyridopoulou, K., Pappa, A., & Chlichlia, K. (2016). DNA vaccines to attack cancer: Strategies for improving immunogenicity and efficacy. *Pharmacology & Therapeutics*, *165*, 32–49. DOI: 10.1016/j.pharmthera.2016.05.004 PMID: 27235391

Tostanoski, L. H., Gosselin, E. A., & Jewell, C. M. (2016). Engineering tolerance using biomaterials to target and control antigen presenting cells. *Discovery Medicine*, *21*(117), 403–410. PMID: 27355336

Trill, M. D. (2013). Anxiety and sleep disorders in cancer patients. *EJC Supplements : EJC : Official Journal of EORTC, European Organization for Research and Treatment of Cancer*, *11*(2), 216–224. DOI: 10.1016/j.ejcsup.2013.07.009 PMID: 26217130

Uhrich, K. E., Cannizzaro, S. M., Langer, R. S., & Shakesheff, K. M. (1999). Polymeric systems for controlled drug release. *Chemical Reviews*, *99*(11), 3181–3198. DOI: 10.1021/cr940351u PMID: 11749514

Uranga, J. A., Nurgali, K., & Abalo, R. (2023). Gastrointestinal Side Effects of Anticancer Therapy. In *Handbook of Cancer and Immunology* (pp. 1–36). Springer International Publishing. DOI: 10.1007/978-3-030-80962-1_343-1

Verma, C., Pawar, V. A., Srivastava, S., Tyagi, A., Kaushik, G., Shukla, S. K., & Kumar, V. (2023). Cancer Vaccines in the Immunotherapy Era: Promise and Potential. *Vaccines*, *11*(12), 1783. DOI: 10.3390/vaccines11121783 PMID: 38140187

Villard, P., Rezaeeyazdi, M., Colombani, T., Joshi-Navare, K., Rana, D., Memic, A., & Bencherif, S. A. (2019). Autoclavable and injectable cryogels for biomedical applications. *Advanced Healthcare Materials*, *8*(17), 1900679. DOI: 10.1002/adhm.201900679 PMID: 31348620

Volovat, S. R., Scripcariu, D. V., Vasilache, I. A., Stolniceanu, C. R., Volovat, C., Augustin, I. G., Volovat, C. C., Ostafe, M.-R., Andreea-Voichi a, S.-G., Bejusca-Vieriu, T., Lungulescu, C. V., Sur, D., & Boboc, D. (2024). Oncolytic virotherapy: A new paradigm in cancer immunotherapy. *International Journal of Molecular Sciences*, *25*(2), 1180. DOI: 10.3390/ijms25021180 PMID: 38256250

Whiteside, T. L., Demaria, S., Rodriguez-Ruiz, M. E., Zarour, H. M., & Melero, I. (2016). Emerging opportunities and challenges in cancer immunotherapy. *Clinical Cancer Research*, *22*(8), 1845–1855. DOI: 10.1158/1078-0432.CCR-16-0049 PMID: 27084738

Wrzesinski, S. H., Wan, Y. Y., & Flavell, R. A. (2007). Transforming growth factor-β and the immune response: Implications for anticancer therapy. *Clinical Cancer Research, 13*(18), 5262–5270. DOI: 10.1158/1078-0432.CCR-07-1157 PMID: 17875754

Xiao, M., Tang, Q., Zeng, S., Yang, Q., Yang, X., Tong, X., Zhu, G., Lei, L., & Li, S. (2023). Emerging biomaterials for tumor immunotherapy. *Biomaterials Research, 27*(1), 47. DOI: 10.1186/s40824-023-00369-8 PMID: 37194085

Xiong, X., Zhao, J., Su, R., Liu, C., Guo, X., & Zhou, S. (2021). Double enhancement of immunogenic cell death and antigen presentation for cancer immunotherapy. *Nano Today, 39*, 101225. DOI: 10.1016/j.nantod.2021.101225

Yan, S., Luo, Z., Li, Z., Wang, Y., Tao, J., Gong, C., & Liu, X. (2020). Improving cancer immunotherapy outcomes using biomaterials. *Angewandte Chemie, 132*(40), 17484–17495. DOI: 10.1002/ange.202002780 PMID: 32297434

Yan, S., Zhao, P., Yu, T., & Gu, N. (2019). Current applications and future prospects of nanotechnology in cancer immunotherapy. *Cancer Biology & Medicine, 16*(3), 486. DOI: 10.20892/j.issn.2095-3941.2018.0493 PMID: 31565479

Yang, F., Shi, K., Jia, Y. P., Hao, Y., Peng, J. R., & Qian, Z. Y. (2020). Advanced biomaterials for cancer immunotherapy. *Acta Pharmacologica Sinica, 41*(7), 911–927. DOI: 10.1038/s41401-020-0372-z PMID: 32123302

Yi, M., Li, T., Niu, M., Zhang, H., Wu, Y., Wu, K., & Dai, Z. (2024). Targeting cytokine and chemokine signaling pathways for cancer therapy. *Signal Transduction and Targeted Therapy, 9*(1), 176. DOI: 10.1038/s41392-024-01868-3 PMID: 39034318

Yoo, K. Y., & Shin, H. R. (2003). Cancer epidemiology and prevention. *Epidemiology and Health, 25*(1), 1–15. PMID: 11850580

Yu, G., Ye, Z., Yuan, Y., Wang, X., Li, T., Wang, Y., ... & Yan, J. (2024). Recent Advancements in Biomaterials for Chimeric Antigen Receptor T Cell Immunotherapy. *Biomaterials Research, 28*, 0045

Yuan, K., Zhang, C., Pan, X., Hu, B., Zhang, J., & Yang, G. (2024). Immunomodulatory metal-based biomaterials for cancer immunotherapy. *Journal of Controlled Release, 375*, 249–268. DOI: 10.1016/j.jconrel.2024.09.008 PMID: 39260573

Zeng, J., Li, X., Sander, M., Zhang, H., Yan, G., & Lin, Y. (2021). Oncolytic viro-immunotherapy: An emerging option in the treatment of gliomas. *Frontiers in Immunology, 12*, 721830. DOI: 10.3389/fimmu.2021.721830 PMID: 34675919

Zhang, R., Billingsley, M. M., & Mitchell, M. J. (2018). Biomaterials for vaccine-based cancer immunotherapy. *Journal of Controlled Release*, *292*, 256–276. DOI: 10.1016/j.jconrel.2018.10.008 PMID: 30312721

Zhang, Y., & Zhang, Z. (2020). The history and advances in cancer immunotherapy: Understanding the characteristics of tumor-infiltrating immune cells and their therapeutic implications. *Cellular & Molecular Immunology*, *17*(8), 807–821. DOI: 10.1038/s41423-020-0488-6 PMID: 32612154

Chapter 7
Metallic 3D-Printed Scaffolds with Functional Coatings:
Advancing Tissue Regeneration through Bioactive and Antibacterial Surfaces

Jagadeesh Baskaran
https://orcid.org/0000-0003-3081-7030
PSG Institute of Technology and Applied Research, Thanjavur, India

ABSTRACT

The convergence of metal 3D printing and advanced surface engineering offers a transformative approach to tissue engineering, particularly in orthopedic and dental applications. This chapter explores the development of metallic 3D-printed scaffolds enhanced with functional coatings to address biocompatibility, antibacterial resistance, and mechanical robustness. We discuss state-of-the-art techniques in additive manufacturing, surface functionalization strategies, and their synergistic role in promoting tissue regeneration. By integrating bioactive and antibacterial features, these scaffolds provide a sustainable solution for complex tissue engineering challenges, paving the way for next-generation regenerative medicine.

DOI: 10.4018/979-8-3373-1305-4.ch007

INTRODUCTION

Scaffolds are indispensable in tissue engineering as they serve as the foundation for tissue formation and regeneration (Yoo, 2011; Zhang, Fang, Xing, Liu, & Zhou, 2018). Scaffolds provide a three-dimensional (3D) framework that maintains the mechanical integrity of the defect site. This is particularly critical in load-bearing applications such as bone regeneration, where the scaffold must support external forces while the tissue is repaired (Rho, Kuhn-Spearing, & Zioupos, 1998). Key design parameters include porosity, pore size, and interconnectivity, which must balance mechanical strength and space for tissue ingrowth. For instance, scaffolds with porosities ranging from 50% to 90% have been shown to offer sufficient mechanical strength while allowing cell proliferation (Choy, Sun, Leong, & Wei, 2017). Computational modeling and finite element analysis are often employed to optimize scaffold designs, ensuring that the mechanical properties mimic those of the target tissue, such as cortical or trabecular bone (Cheah, Azman, & Bajuri, 2022). Scaffolds act as a substrate for cellular adhesion, which is the initial step in tissue formation. This function is mediated by surface properties such as roughness, wettability, and the presence of bioactive molecules. Surface roughness enhances cell attachment by providing physical anchoring sites, while hydrophilic surfaces improve cell spreading and proliferation.

Functionalization techniques, such as coating scaffolds with extracellular matrix (ECM) proteins like collagen or fibronectin, further enhance cellular adhesion. These proteins mimic the natural cellular environment and facilitate integrin-mediated binding. Scaffolds serve as templates that guide cell migration, differentiation, and organization into functional tissues. This is achieved through their architecture, which influences cellular behavior via mechanotransduction pathways. Gradients in scaffold properties, such as stiffness or bioactive factor concentration, can direct stem cell differentiation into specific lineages (Jagadeesh & Duraiselvam, 2023; Niknam & Akbarzadeh, 2020). For example, stiffer regions of a scaffold may promote osteogenesis, while softer areas support chondrogenesis. Advanced designs incorporate micro- and nanoscale features to mimic the hierarchical structure of native tissues. These features enhance cell-scaffold interactions and promote the deposition of ECM, accelerating tissue regeneration. Emerging technologies include the development of dynamic scaffolds that respond to environmental stimuli. These scaffolds can release growth factors, adjust their mechanical properties, or degrade in a controlled manner to match the pace of tissue formation.

1.1 The Emergence of Metallic 3D Printing in Tissue Engineering

To discuss the use of metallic 3D printing in Tissue Engineering, it is essential to know the historical developments and evolution of additive manufacturing technologies. The origins of additive manufacturing can be traced back to the 1980s. While the concept of automated manufacturing was not new, the notion of "building" objects layer by layer rather than cutting or subtracting from a solid block was groundbreaking.

The first true additive manufacturing process was developed by Dr. Charles Hull in 1983, when he invented Stereolithography (SLA). Hull, a visionary in rapid prototyping, created a method of using ultraviolet (UV) light to cure layers of liquid photopolymer resin into solid objects. This innovation marked the birth of 3D printing as we know it. He patented the technology and founded 3D Systems, one of the first companies dedicated to commercializing SLA technology. Hull's method enabled rapid prototyping, allowing designers to create physical models directly from digital files, dramatically reducing the time and cost of creating prototypes.

Around the same time, Selective Laser Sintering (SLS) was developed by Dr. Carl Deckard at the University of Texas in 1984. This method uses a laser to fuse small particles of powder (typically plastic, metal, or ceramic), which could be used to build more complex, durable prototypes and parts than what was possible with SLA. SLS was a significant milestone, as it allowed for the production of functional parts, not just prototypes.

By the 1990s, the potential of additive manufacturing had caught the attention of industries beyond just prototyping. The technology was evolving to create parts for more demanding applications, such as aerospace, automotive, and medical fields. A range of new AM processes started to emerge during this period. In 1992, Fused Deposition Modeling (FDM) was patented by Scott Crump, who later founded Stratasys, a leading 3D printing company. FDM works by extruding molten thermoplastic material through a heated nozzle, which then solidifies layer by layer. This method was more accessible and cost-effective compared to other processes, making it widely adopted in industrial, educational, and even consumer markets. FDM became one of the most widely used AM techniques, especially with the advent of consumer-grade 3D printers in the 2000s. Also, in the 1990s, Laminated Object Manufacturing (LOM) and Electron Beam Melting (EBM) were developed. LOM uses thin layers of material that are bonded together using heat and pressure, while EBM utilizes an electron beam to melt and fuse metal powder. These techniques allowed for the creation of larger parts and components and helped broaden the range of materials that could be used in AM.

The 2000s saw the proliferation of 3D printing technologies. One of the most significant milestones was the release of the first low-cost, desktop 3D printers, which allowed individuals and small businesses to access the power of AM. The most notable of these was the RepRap project, started by Dr. Adrian Bowyer in 2005. The RepRap project aimed to create a self-replicating 3D printer capable of printing most of its own parts, which would dramatically lower the cost of entry into 3D printing for hobbyists and makers. Meanwhile, major companies like Stratasys and 3D Systems continued to advance the industrial application of AM. Industries such as aerospace, automotive, and medical devices began to recognize the potential of AM for creating lightweight, custom parts that would be difficult or impossible to manufacture using traditional methods. For example, aerospace companies started using 3D printing to produce complex jet engine parts that were both lighter and stronger than conventional counterparts.

The 2010s marked the true maturation of additive manufacturing as it became integrated into full-scale manufacturing processes. Key advancements during this period include:

Metal Additive Manufacturing: While metal 3D printing had been around in the form of technologies like SLS and EBM, it was in the 2010s that metal AM truly took off. Direct Metal Laser Sintering (DMLS) and Selective Laser Melting (SLM) became popular techniques in industries that required high-performance materials. These processes allowed for the creation of fully functional metal parts, which revolutionized sectors like aerospace and healthcare.

Bioprinting: In healthcare, 3D printing made substantial strides in producing prosthetics, implants, and even bioprinted tissue. Technologies like bioinks allowed for the printing of organic materials, leading to developments in creating tissues and organs that could one day be used for transplants.

Advancements in Materials: During this decade, there was an explosion of new materials for 3D printing. In addition to traditional plastics, the range of materials now included metals, ceramics, composites, and even food-grade materials. This expanded the range of possible applications for AM, including in areas like fashion, food production, and consumer goods.

Speed and Precision: Companies focused on increasing the speed and precision of additive manufacturing processes. New developments in Continuous Liquid Interface Production (CLIP), for example, revolutionized SLA by using a continuous flow of liquid resin, resulting in faster print speeds and smoother finishes.

The current decade represents a period of rapid growth and refinement for additive manufacturing. The focus is now on achieving large-scale production while maintaining the benefits of customization and flexibility that AM provides. Here are some key trends shaping the future of AM:

Mass Customization: With advancements in artificial intelligence and machine learning, companies are increasingly able to offer personalized products at scale. For example, dental implants, custom prosthetics, and tailored fashion products are becoming more accessible thanks to AM technologies.
Sustainability: Additive manufacturing holds significant potential in creating more sustainable manufacturing practices. By reducing waste and enabling localized production, AM helps to reduce the carbon footprint associated with traditional manufacturing and global supply chains. Recycling materials and using biodegradable materials is also becoming a significant part of the AM industry. Integration with Industry 4.0: The integration of additive manufacturing with other advanced technologies like the Internet of Things (IoT), robotics, and artificial intelligence (AI) is pushing the boundaries of what AM can do. Figure 1 shows the steps required from obtaining patient data regarding the bone morphology to realizing the implant through metal 3D printing. Metallic 3D printing has revolutionized the field of tissue engineering, offering unprecedented control over the design and fabrication of scaffolds for regenerative medicine. Traditional scaffold manufacturing techniques, such as solvent casting and particulate leaching, lacked the precision and repeatability required to meet the complex demands of tissue engineering applications.

Figure 1. Digital process chain of the metal 3D printing of a medical implant (Reproduced from Edelmann, A., Dubis, M., & Hellmann, R., 2020).

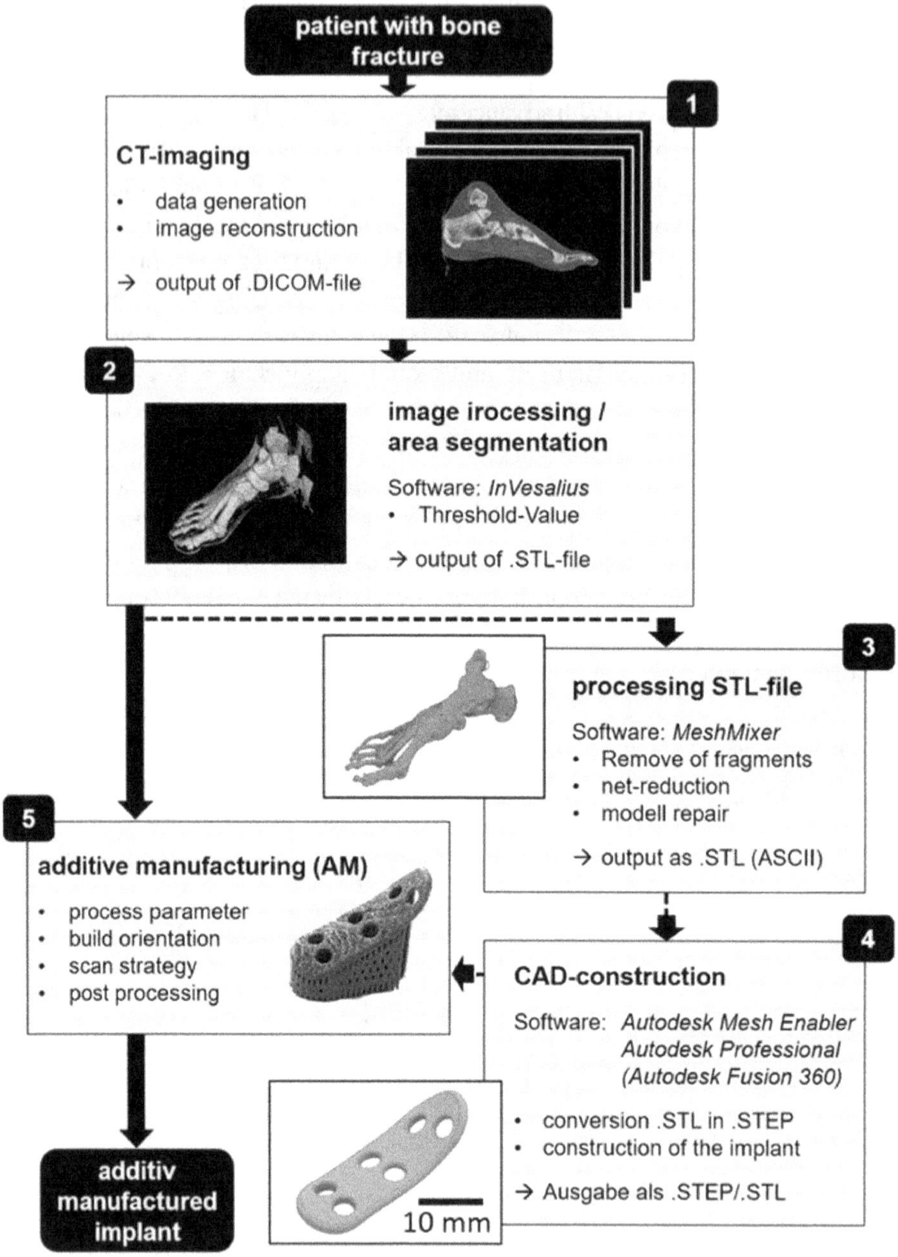

Selective laser melting of patient individualized osteosynthesis plates—digital to physical process chain. Materials, 13(24), 5786.

Metallic 3D printing, particularly powder bed fusion technologies like Selective Laser Melting (SLM) and Electron Beam Melting (EBM), has addressed these limitations(Gibson, Rosen, & Stucker, 2015; Jagadeesh, Duraiselvam, & Prashanth, 2023; Mahamood, Akinlabi, Mahamood, & Akinlabi, 2017). The emergence of metallic 3D printing is characterized by its ability to fabricate highly complex, patient-specific scaffolds(Baskaran, 2024a; Baskaran, Muthukannan, Shukla, & Gokuldoss, 2024; Kannan, Sivakumar, Jagadeesh, & Balaji, 2024). This capability is critical for developing implants that mimic the mechanical properties and porosity of native tissues. Metallic 3D printing is particularly beneficial for load-bearing applications, where the interplay between mechanical strength and biological compatibility is paramount. Advances in computer-aided design (CAD) and finite element modeling (FEM) have further enhanced the potential of metallic 3D printing, enabling the optimization of scaffold geometries to achieve desired biological and mechanical outcomes.

Recent breakthroughs in process optimization, including the fine-tuning of laser or electron beam parameters and post-processing techniques, have significantly improved the quality and performance of metallic scaffolds. These advancements have expanded the scope of applications, from bone regeneration to dental implants and spinal fusion devices. Metallic 3D printing thus represents a transformative technology in tissue engineering, bridging the gap between engineered scaffolds and clinical applications.

1.2 Advantages of Titanium Alloys, Cobalt-Chromium, and Stainless Steel for Load-Bearing Applications

1. Titanium Alloys (e.g., Ti-6Al-4V):

Biocompatibility: Titanium alloys exhibit excellent biocompatibility, making them ideal for integration with biological tissues. They are inert and resist corrosion in physiological environments.

High Strength-to-Weight Ratio: Titanium alloys combine high mechanical strength with low density, reducing the overall weight of implants.

Osteoconductivity: Titanium can support bone ingrowth when coupled with surface modifications, such as hydroxyapatite coatings or surface texturing.

Fatigue Resistance: These alloys withstand cyclic loading, making them suitable for dynamic environments such as joints and spine implants.

2. Cobalt-Chromium Alloys:

Wear Resistance: These alloys exhibit superior wear resistance, a crucial property for applications like hip and knee replacements.

High Modulus: Cobalt-chromium alloys provide excellent mechanical stability, particularly in load-bearing areas.

Corrosion Resistance: Their inherent corrosion resistance enhances longevity and reduces the risk of material degradation in the body.

Machinability and Polishing: These materials can achieve smooth surfaces, which are critical for articulating components in joint replacements.

3. Stainless Steel (e.g., 316L):

Cost-Effectiveness: Stainless steel is more affordable compared to titanium and cobalt-chromium alloys.

Mechanical Strength: It provides sufficient mechanical strength for short-term load-bearing applications, such as temporary fixation devices(Bakhtiarian, Omidvar, Mashhuriazar, Sajuri, & Gur, 2024).

Ease of Fabrication: Stainless steel is easier to process, weld, and shape, making it suitable for a wide range of implant geometries.

Corrosion Resistance: While slightly inferior to titanium and cobalt-chromium, stainless steel still offers acceptable corrosion resistance when passivated.

1.3 Opportunities Presented by Additive Manufacturing in Creating Patient-Specific, Highly Porous Structures with Tunable Mechanical Properties

Additive manufacturing (AM) enables the creation of implants tailored to a patient's anatomy. Utilizing imaging techniques such as CT or MRI, AM can produce scaffolds that precisely match the defect site, improving implant integration and reducing recovery times (Baskaran, 2024a; Baskaran et al., 2024; Hernández-Nava et al., 2017). AM technologies like SLM and EBM allow for the precise control of pore size, shape, and distribution. Porous structures mimic the extracellular matrix, facilitating cell adhesion, proliferation, and vascularization. Interconnected pores ensure efficient nutrient and oxygen diffusion, critical for tissue regeneration. The ability to modulate scaffold porosity and material density enables the customization of mechanical properties (Alaña, Cutolo, Ruiz de Galarreta, & Van Hooreweder, 2021). This is particularly important for load-bearing applications, where the implant must balance structural integrity with stress shielding to promote bone remodeling. Emerging AM technologies are exploring the fabrication of multi-material scaffolds that combine metals with ceramics or polymers (Friel & Harris, 2013; Wu, Song, Di, Niu, & Ma, 2022). This hybrid approach can enhance mechanical performance while introducing bioactive features, such as growth factor delivery. AM minimizes material waste by building scaffolds layer by layer, unlike traditional subtractive manufacturing methods (Baskaran, 2024b). This efficiency reduces costs and accelerates production timelines, especially for patient-specific implants. AM can produce scaffolds with graded properties, transitioning from dense, mechanically robust regions to porous, biologically active zones. This mimics the hierarchical structure of natural tissues like bone. Post-processing techniques such as surface roughening, bioactive coatings, or laser texturing can be seamlessly integrated into AM workflows. These enhancements improve cell adhesion, osteointegration, and overall scaffold performance.

1.4 Motivation for Functional Coatings

Functional coatings have emerged as a versatile and promising strategy to enhance the bioactivity, promote osteointegration, and impart antibacterial properties to medical scaffolds. Bioactivity refers to a material's ability to interact with biological systems, facilitating cellular adhesion, proliferation, and differentiation. Functional coatings can significantly improve the bioactivity of scaffolds by incorporating bioactive molecules, minerals, or polymers. Hydroxyapatite (HA), a naturally occurring mineral found in bone, is widely used as a coating material due to its excellent biocompatibility and similarity to bone mineral. HA coatings enhance osteoblast adhesion and proliferation, creating an environment conducive to new bone formation. Incorporating growth factors such as bone morphogenetic proteins (BMPs) or vascular endothelial growth factors (VEGFs) into scaffold coatings can accelerate tissue regeneration. These coatings release bioactive molecules in a controlled manner, stimulating cell recruitment and differentiation at the defect site. Inspired by mussel adhesive proteins, polydopamine (PDA) coatings facilitate the immobilization of bioactive molecules and nanoparticles on scaffold surfaces. PDA's unique chemistry enhances scaffold interaction with cells and proteins, improving overall bioactivity. Osteointegration, the direct structural and functional connection between living bone and the surface of a load-bearing implant, is critical for the long-term success of bone scaffolds. Functional coatings can enhance osteointegration through:

Mineralization Coatings: Calcium phosphate and bioactive glass coatings promote the deposition of bone-like apatite, forming a strong bond with native bone tissue.

Surface Topography Modulation: Functional coatings can introduce nanoscale or microscale surface features that mimic the extracellular matrix, enhancing osteoblast adhesion and differentiation.

Electroactive Coatings: Conductive polymers such as polypyrrole or polyaniline can be used to create electroactive coatings. These coatings stimulate osteogenic differentiation by providing electrical cues that mimic the natural bioelectric environment of bone.

Infections pose a significant risk to the success of medical scaffolds, often leading to implant failure. Functional coatings can mitigate this risk by imparting antibacterial properties through:

Silver Nanoparticles: Silver nanoparticles (AgNPs) are widely recognized for their broad-spectrum antimicrobial activity. Coating scaffolds with AgNPs provides a sustained release of silver ions, inhibiting bacterial growth while minimizing cytotoxicity.
Antimicrobial Peptide Coatings: Antimicrobial peptides (AMPs) offer a biocompatible alternative to traditional antibiotics. Coating scaffolds with AMPs can effectively target and eliminate bacteria without promoting antibiotic resistance.
Photothermal and Photodynamic Coatings: Functional coatings incorporating photothermal agents (e.g., gold nanoparticles) or photosensitizers (e.g., porphyrins) enable the use of light-based therapies to eradicate bacteria. These coatings are particularly useful in combating biofilm-associated infections.

1.4.1 Multifunctional Coatings

The ultimate goal in scaffold design is to create multifunctional coatings that simultaneously enhance bioactivity, promote osteointegration, and provide antibacterial protection. Advances in nanotechnology, biomaterials science, and surface engineering have enabled the development of such coatings. For example:

Layer-by-Layer (LbL) Assembly: This technique allows the sequential deposition of thin layers of biomaterials, enabling precise control over coating composition and functionality.
Hybrid Coatings: Combining organic and inorganic components, hybrid coatings leverage the strengths of both materials to achieve superior performance.
Stimuli-Responsive Coatings: Coatings that respond to environmental stimuli (e.g., pH, temperature, or mechanical stress) can dynamically regulate the release of bioactive molecules or antimicrobial agents, adapting to the healing process.

2 METAL 3D PRINTING FOR SCAFFOLDS IN TISSUE ENGINEERING

Scaffold production in tissue engineering is a critical process aimed at creating structures that mimic the extracellular matrix, promoting cell attachment, proliferation, and differentiation. Among the advanced AM techniques, SLM and Electron Beam Melting (EBM) have gained prominence due to their ability to fabricate highly intricate, patient-specific scaffolds with controlled porosity and mechanical properties.

2.1 Selective Laser Melting (SLM)

SLM is a laser-based powder bed fusion process that uses a high-energy laser to selectively melt and fuse metallic powders layer by layer. It is particularly suited for producing scaffolds with intricate geometries and fine resolution. High Resolution and Precision: SLM can achieve fine details, enabling the fabrication of scaffolds with complex pore structures (Xiong et al., 2021), which are essential for mimicking the natural extracellular matrix. It works with biocompatible materials such as titanium alloys (e.g., Ti-6Al-4V) and cobalt-chromium alloys, which are widely used in orthopedic and dental applications. The process allows precise control over the pore size, shape, and interconnectivity, which are crucial for nutrient transport, waste removal, and cell migration. Scaffolds produced via SLM exhibit superior mechanical properties, making them suitable for load-bearing applications such as bone regeneration. A schematic of SLM and EBM processes is provided in Figure 2.

Figure 2. Schematic of the SLM and EBM processes

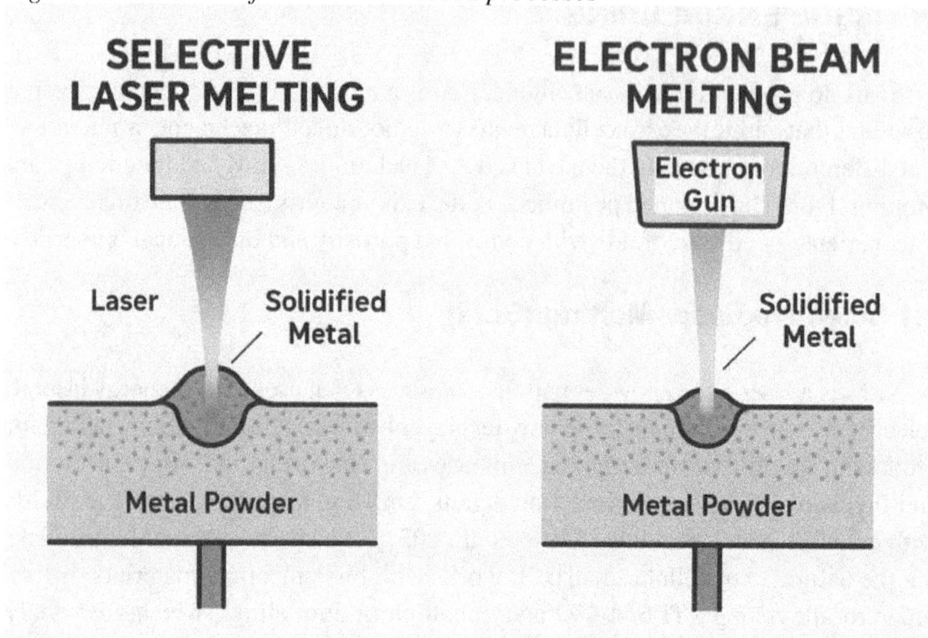

2.1.1 Applications

- Bone Tissue Engineering: SLM is frequently used to fabricate titanium scaffolds for bone defect repair. These scaffolds can be coated with bioactive materials, such as hydroxyapatite, to enhance osteoconductivity.
- Dental Implants: Customized dental scaffolds with microarchitectures designed to integrate seamlessly with jawbone tissue are produced using SLM.

Despite its advantages, SLM has limitations, including high energy consumption and the need for post-processing to remove residual stresses and enhance surface properties for cell adhesion.

2.2 Electron Beam Melting (EBM)

EBM is another powder bed fusion technique, which uses a high-energy electron beam to melt metallic powders layer by layer under a vacuum (Epasto et al., 2019; Gibson et al., 2015; Technologies & Terminology, 2012). The vacuum environment minimizes contamination, making EBM particularly appealing for medical applications. The absence of oxygen in the vacuum environment prevents oxidation of metallic powders, ensuring high-purity scaffolds. The electron beam pre-heats the entire powder bed, reducing residual stresses and warping in the final scaffold. EBM allows for the tuning of scaffold mechanical properties by adjusting process parameters such as beam power and scanning speed. EBM is ideal for processing reactive metals like titanium and its alloys, which are commonly used for their excellent biocompatibility and mechanical properties.

2.2.1 Applications

- Orthopedic Implants: EBM is widely employed to produce porous titanium scaffolds for joint replacement and spinal fusion devices. The interconnected pore structure facilitates osseointegration and vascularization (Hernández-Nava et al., 2017).
- Craniofacial Reconstruction: The technique has been utilized for fabricating patient-specific scaffolds for cranial and facial bone reconstruction, where precise anatomical replication is essential.

Table 1 presents the aspects with which SLM and EBM differ significantly in scaffold production. Minimal residual stresses and very good surface finish make EBM, an attractive technology.

Table 1. Comparison between SLM and EBM in scaffold production

Aspect	SLM	EBM
Energy Source	Laser	Electron Beam
Environment	Inert gas (e.g., argon)	Vacuum
Resolution	Higher resolution for fine details	Slightly lower resolution
Residual Stresses	Higher, requiring post-processing	Lower due to pre-heating
Surface Finish	Rougher, often requiring polishing	Smoother due to pre-heating

3 COMPUTATIONAL MODELLING FOR DESIGN OPTIMIZATION OF SCAFFOLDS

To optimize scaffold performance, computational modeling plays a crucial role, offering insights into how structural design affects mechanical robustness and porosity. The scaffolds must balance mechanical strength and porosity to ensure biocompatibility, nutrient transport, and structural stability. Computational modeling facilitates this balance by enabling the precise design and evaluation of scaffold geometries before fabrication.

3.1 Importance of Mechanical Robustness and Porosity

Mechanical robustness ensures that scaffolds maintain their structural integrity under physiological loads. Porosity, on the other hand, is critical for nutrient diffusion, waste removal, and vascularization. Achieving the right trade-off between these properties is challenging, as increasing porosity often compromises mechanical strength. Computational tools provide a framework to optimize this trade-off systematically. Finite Element Analysis (FEA) is a widely used method for assessing the mechanical performance of scaffolds (Cheah et al., 2022). By dividing the scaffold geometry into finite elements, FEA predicts stress, strain, and deformation under various loading conditions. This helps identify weak points and optimize structural design to improve mechanical robustness. Computational Fluid Dynamics (CFD) models simulate fluid flow through scaffold pores, evaluating parameters like shear stress and nutrient transport. These simulations help optimize pore size and interconnectivity, ensuring adequate diffusion while maintaining structural stability.

Topology optimization algorithms iteratively adjust scaffold designs to achieve desired mechanical and porosity characteristics. These methods often employ objective functions that minimize material usage while maintaining mechanical strength and permeability. Multiscale models integrate microscale features, such as pore architecture, with macroscale mechanical behavior. This approach provides a comprehensive understanding of how local design choices impact overall scaffold performance.

3.2 Strategies to Achieve Graded Porosity for Mimicking Natural Bone

A critical design consideration is achieving graded porosity, which enhances mechanical properties, promotes cell proliferation, and supports vascularization. Natural bone features a gradient in porosity, transitioning from dense cortical bone to highly porous cancellous bone. Mimicking this structure requires advanced strategies to design and fabricate scaffolds with precise porosity gradients. Below, we outline key approaches to achieving graded porosity in metallic scaffolds. Advanced CAD software enables the creation of 3D models with tailored porosity gradients. These tools allow for:

Variable Lattice Structures: Designs incorporating lattice geometries (e.g., gyroids, diamond, and hexagonal structures) with adjustable strut thickness and pore sizes.

Spatial Control: Gradual transitions in porosity can be achieved by interpolating between dense and porous regions.

Topology optimization algorithms distribute material based on mechanical constraints (Rankouhi et al., 2020; Xiao et al., 2021; Xu et al., 2019). This method ensures that:

Load-bearing regions are denser, while non-load-bearing areas feature higher porosity.

Optimal mechanical performance and reduced stress shielding are achieved.

Functionally Graded Materials (FGM) involve compositional or structural variation to create a gradient in properties.

3.3 Biomimetic Approaches

Designing porosity gradients inspired by natural bone structures can ensure functional integration. Techniques include:

Mimicking trabecular patterns for cancellous regions.

Incorporating hierarchical designs for multi-scale porosity.

4 X-RAY MICRO COMPUTED TOMOGRAPHY

Figure 3. Process schematic of X-ray μCT

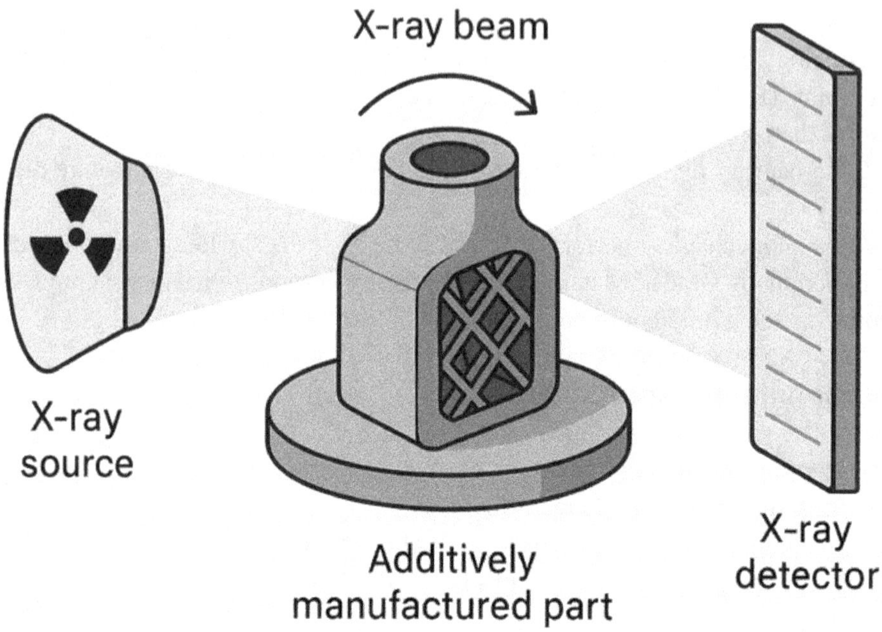

X-ray micro-computed tomography is an advanced imaging technique that enables high-resolution, non-destructive 3D imaging of internal structures of materials. μCT works by passing X-rays through the object from multiple angles, capturing the attenuation of X-rays as they pass through different densities of material. Using sophisticated algorithms, these projections are reconstructed into a 3D model that provides detailed information about the internal microstructure of the sample. The process schematic and reconstruction are provided in figures 3 and 4 respectively.

Figure 4. Reconstruction procedure followed during μCT

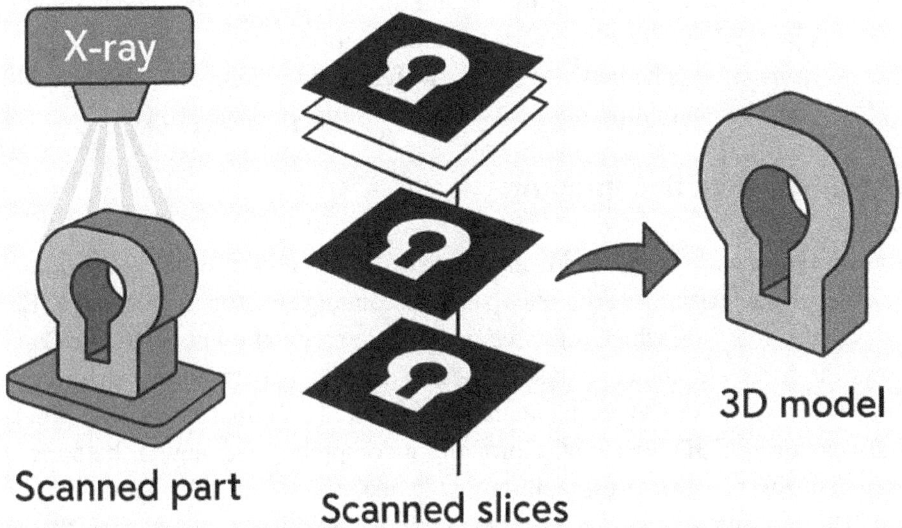

In the context of additive manufacturing, μCT offers a remarkable advantage: it allows for the analysis of complex structures, including internal voids, porosity, and layer-by-layer deposition patterns, without the need to physically section or alter the object. This capability makes μCT particularly valuable for characterizing the intricate geometries of biomedical scaffolds produced by AM technologies. (Abdullah, Abdullah, & Ramlee, 2023; Peto, Ramírez-Cedillo, Hernández, & Siller, 2019)

4.1 Criticality of X-ray μCT in Characterizing Additively Manufactured Scaffolds

4.1.1. *Resolution and Accuracy:* X-ray μCT provides very high spatial resolution, typically in the range of micrometers (1 μm), which is ideal for imaging the fine details of additively manufactured biomedical scaffolds. This resolution allows for a detailed assessment of the scaffold's internal structure, such as:

4.1.2 Porosity: The distribution and size of pores within the scaffold are vital for cell migration and nutrient exchange. μCT can identify both open and closed pores and quantify their sizes and distributions, ensuring that the scaffold meets the required porosity specifications.

4.1.3 Pore Interconnectivity: Scaffolds designed for tissue engineering often require interconnected pores to facilitate cell movement and tissue integration. μCT can visualize and quantify the degree of pore interconnectivity, which is critical for successful tissue ingrowth and vascularization.

4.1.4 Layer-to-Layer Accuracy: In AM processes, the layer-by-layer deposition can sometimes result in irregularities or inconsistencies. μCT allows for the detection of potential flaws such as cracks, voids, or misalignments between layers, which could compromise the scaffold's mechanical properties or its ability to support tissue growth.

4.2 Non-Destructive Imaging

One of the most significant advantages of μCT is its non-destructive nature. Unlike other characterization techniques, such as scanning electron microscopy (SEM) or mechanical testing, which often require sample preparation or destruction, μCT allows the complete, intact analysis of scaffolds. This is particularly important in biomedical applications where maintaining the scaffold's original properties is crucial.

By capturing a 3D image, μCT provides a comprehensive view of both the internal and external structures, facilitating the analysis of the entire scaffold in one scan. This non-invasive analysis is essential when working with materials that are sensitive or where preserving the sample for future testing is required.

4.3 Quantifying Mechanical Properties

While μCT does not directly measure the mechanical properties of scaffolds, it provides critical information for assessing these properties indirectly. The microstructural features observed through μCT, such as porosity, pore size, and geometry, significantly influence the mechanical behavior of the scaffold, including its stiffness, strength, and load-bearing capacity. By combining μCT data with mechanical simulations or testing, researchers can predict how a scaffold will behave under different loading conditions, which is vital for ensuring that the scaffold can support tissue growth and function.

4.4 Comparing Different Materials and Manufacturing Techniques

Additive manufacturing allows for the use of a wide variety of materials in scaffold fabrication, including biodegradable polymers, ceramics, and composite materials. Different AM techniques can lead to variations in the final product's microstructure. μCT can be used to compare and contrast scaffolds made from different materials or using different AM methods. This helps researchers optimize material selection and manufacturing processes to achieve the desired balance of properties such as porosity, mechanical strength, and degradation rate.

4.5 Applications of X-ray μCT in Biomedical Scaffold Characterization

Optimizing Scaffold Design: By providing detailed information on the scaffold's internal and external features, μCT helps researchers refine scaffold designs. For instance, adjusting the scaffold's porosity or pore connectivity based on μCT analysis can lead to improved cell infiltration, tissue growth, and vascularization.

Quality Control and Process Monitoring: During the additive manufacturing process, defects such as incomplete bonding between layers, inconsistent porosity, or material inhomogeneities can occur. μCT serves as a powerful tool for monitoring the quality of scaffolds during and after production. This ensures that scaffolds meet the required standards for biomedical applications.

Post-Manufacturing Evaluation: After a scaffold has been implanted in a biological environment, μCT can be used to assess its degradation over time. As scaffolds break down and are replaced by natural tissue, μCT allows for continuous, non-invasive monitoring of the scaffold's structural integrity and degradation process, ensuring that the degradation rate aligns with the tissue regeneration rate.

Personalized Medicine: In the future, μCT could play a key role in the development of patient-specific scaffolds. By scanning a patient's anatomy, a scaffold can be designed and printed to match the exact shape and structure of the defect or tissue loss. μCT can be used to verify that the scaffold fits the patient's anatomy precisely before implantation.

4.6 Challenges

While X-ray μCT is a powerful tool, it is not without limitations. The resolution of μCT, although high, is still limited compared to techniques like electron microscopy, which can achieve nanoscale resolution. Additionally, imaging large scaffolds with μCT can be time-consuming and computationally demanding. Advances in μCT technology, such as the development of higher-resolution detectors and faster scanning techniques, will likely address these limitations in the future.

The integration of μCT with other techniques, such as micro-mechanical testing or finite element analysis (FEA), will further enhance its ability to predict the behavior of scaffolds in biological environments. Moreover, as 3D printing technologies continue to evolve, μCT will play a central role in ensuring the production of scaffolds that are not only structurally sound but also tailored for specific biomedical applications.

5 FUNCTIONAL COATINGS FOR METALLIC SCAFFOLDS

Processing Techniques for Functional Coatings

The choice of coating technique significantly influences the properties and performance of functional coatings. Common processing methods include:

- Physical Vapor Deposition (PVD): PVD techniques, such as sputtering and evaporation, deposit thin films of biocompatible materials like titanium and hydroxyapatite. These coatings provide excellent adhesion and uniformity.
- Chemical Vapor Deposition (CVD): CVD processes are employed to create coatings with high chemical stability, such as silicon-based or diamond-like carbon coatings, which improve the mechanical properties of scaffolds.
- Electrospinning: This method produces nanofiber coatings that mimic the extracellular matrix. Functional additives, such as growth factors or antimicrobial agents, can be incorporated into the electrospun fibers for enhanced functionality.
- Layer-by-Layer (LbL) Assembly: LbL techniques allow for precise control over coating thickness and composition by alternating the deposition of oppositely charged layers of polymers, nanoparticles, or proteins.
- Spray Coating and Dip Coating: These simple and scalable techniques enable the deposition of functional layers by spraying or immersing scaffolds in a coating solution.

REFERENCES

Abdullah, N. N. A. A., Abdullah, A. H., & Ramlee, M. H. (2023). Current trend of lattice structures designed and analysis for porous hip implants: A short review. *Materials Today: Proceedings*.

Alaña, M., Cutolo, A., Ruiz de Galarreta, S., & Van Hooreweder, B. (2021). Influence of relative density on quasi-static and fatigue failure of lattice structures in Ti6Al4V produced by laser powder bed fusion. *Scientific Reports*, *11*(1), 1–15. DOI: 10.1038/s41598-021-98631-3 PMID: 34588524

Bakhtiarian, M., Omidvar, H., Mashhuriazar, A., Sajuri, Z., & Gur, C. H. (2024). The effects of SLM process parameters on the relative density and hardness of austenitic stainless steel 316L. *Journal of Materials Research and Technology*, *29*, 1616–1629. DOI: 10.1016/j.jmrt.2024.01.237

Baskaran, J. (2024a). Advancements in Metal Additive Manufacturing Technology for Biomedical Applications. In *Trends and Applications in Mechanical Engineering, Composite Materials and Smart Manufacturing* (pp. 1-34): IGI Global. DOI: 10.4018/979-8-3693-1966-6.ch001

Baskaran, J. (2024b). Roadmap to Achieve Sustainable and Eco-Friendly Metal Additive Manufacturing Processes. In *Futuristic Technology for Sustainable Manufacturing* (pp. 185–215). IGI Global. DOI: 10.4018/979-8-3693-1862-1.ch011

Baskaran, J., Muthukannan, D., Shukla, R., & Gokuldoss, P. K. (2024). Manufacturability and deformation studies on a novel metallic lattice structure fabricated by Selective Laser Melting. *Vacuum*, *222*, 113065. DOI: 10.1016/j.vacuum.2024.113065

Cheah, Y. K., Azman, A. H., & Bajuri, M. Y. (2022). Finite-element analysis of load-bearing hip implant design for additive manufacturing. *Journal of Failure Analysis and Prevention*, *22*(1), 1–12. DOI: 10.1007/s11668-021-01304-6

Choy, S. Y., Sun, C.-N., Leong, K. F., & Wei, J. (2017). Compressive properties of Ti-6Al-4V lattice structures fabricated by selective laser melting: Design, orientation and density. *Additive Manufacturing*, *16*, 213–224. DOI: 10.1016/j.addma.2017.06.012

Epasto, G., Palomba, G., D'Andrea, D., Guglielmino, E., Di Bella, S., & Traina, F. (2019). Ti-6Al-4V ELI microlattice structures manufactured by electron beam melting: Effect of unit cell dimensions and morphology on mechanical behaviour. *Materials Science and Engineering A*, *753*, 31–41. DOI: 10.1016/j.msea.2019.03.014

Friel, R. J., & Harris, R. A. (2013). Ultrasonic additive manufacturing–a hybrid production process for novel functional products. *Procedia CIRP*, *6*, 35–40. DOI: 10.1016/j.procir.2013.03.004

Gibson, I., Rosen, D. W., & Stucker, B. (2015). *Additive manufacturing technologies* (2nd ed.). Springer. DOI: 10.1007/978-1-4939-2113-3

Hernández-Nava, E., Tammas-Williams, S., Smith, C., Leonard, F., Withers, P. J., Todd, I., & Goodall, R. (2017). X-ray tomography characterisation of lattice structures processed by selective electron beam melting. *Metals*, *7*(8), 300. DOI: 10.3390/met7080300

Jagadeesh, B., & Duraiselvam, M. (2023). Investigations on the compressive behaviour of novel cell size graded primitive lattice structure produced by Metal Additive Manufacturing. *Materials Letters*, *333*, 133643. DOI: 10.1016/j.matlet.2022.133643

Jagadeesh, B., Duraiselvam, M., & Prashanth, K. (2023). Deformation behavior of metallic lattice structures with symmetrical gradients of porosity manufactured by metal additive manufacturing. *Vacuum*, *211*, 111955. DOI: 10.1016/j.vacuum.2023.111955

Kannan, G. R., Sivakumar, M., Jagadeesh, B., & Balaji, N. (2024). Powder Bed Fusion Process–State of Art. In *Advances in Additive Manufacturing* (pp. 89-107). DOI: 10.1002/9781394238316.ch5

Mahamood, R. M., Akinlabi, E. T., Mahamood, R. M., & Akinlabi, E. T. (2017). Additive manufacturing of funtionally graded materials. *Functionally graded materials*, 47-68.

Niknam, H., & Akbarzadeh, A. (2020). Graded lattice structures: Simultaneous enhancement in stiffness and energy absorption. *Materials & Design*, *196*, 109129. DOI: 10.1016/j.matdes.2020.109129

Peto, M., Ramírez-Cedillo, E., Hernández, A., & Siller, H. R. (2019). Structural design optimization of knee replacement implants for additive manufacturing. *Procedia Manufacturing*, *34*, 574–583. DOI: 10.1016/j.promfg.2019.06.222

Rankouhi, B., Bertsch, K., de Bellefon, G. M., Thevamaran, M., Thoma, D., & Suresh, K. (2020). Experimental validation and microstructure characterization of topology optimized, additively manufactured SS316L components. *Materials Science and Engineering A*, *776*, 139050. DOI: 10.1016/j.msea.2020.139050

Rho, J.-Y., Kuhn-Spearing, L., & Zioupos, P. (1998). Mechanical properties and the hierarchical structure of bone. *Medical Engineering & Physics*, *20*(2), 92–102. DOI: 10.1016/S1350-4533(98)00007-1 PMID: 9679227

Technologies, A. C. F. A. M., & Terminology, A. C. F. A. M. T. S. F. o. (2012). *Standard terminology for additive manufacturing technologies*. Astm International.

Wu, D., Song, C., Di, T., Niu, F., & Ma, G. (2022). Intermetallic regulation mechanism of inconel 718/Ti6Al4V composite by novel follow-up ultrasonic assisted laser additive manufacturing. *Composites. Part B, Engineering*, *235*, 109736. DOI: 10.1016/j.compositesb.2022.109736

Xiao, M., Liu, X., Zhang, Y., Gao, L., Gao, J., & Chu, S. (2021). Design of graded lattice sandwich structures by multiscale topology optimization. *Computer Methods in Applied Mechanics and Engineering*, *384*, 113949. DOI: 10.1016/j.cma.2021.113949

Xiong, Y., Han, Z., Qin, J., Dong, L., Zhang, H., Wang, Y., Chen, H., & Li, X. (2021). Effects of porosity gradient pattern on mechanical performance of additive manufactured Ti-6Al-4V functionally graded porous structure. *Materials & Design*, *208*, 109911. DOI: 10.1016/j.matdes.2021.109911

Xu, Y., Zhang, D., Hu, S., Chen, R., Gu, Y., Kong, X., Tao, J., & Jiang, Y. (2019). Mechanical properties tailoring of topology optimized and selective laser melting fabricated Ti6Al4V lattice structure. *Journal of the Mechanical Behavior of Biomedical Materials*, *99*, 225–239. DOI: 10.1016/j.jmbbm.2019.06.021 PMID: 31400657

Yoo, D. J. (2011). Porous scaffold design using the distance field and triply periodic minimal surface models. *Biomaterials*, *32*(31), 7741–7754. DOI: 10.1016/j.biomaterials.2011.07.019 PMID: 21798592

Zhang, X.-Y., Fang, G., Xing, L.-L., Liu, W., & Zhou, J. (2018). Effect of porosity variation strategy on the performance of functionally graded Ti-6Al-4V scaffolds for bone tissue engineering. *Materials & Design*, *157*, 523–538. DOI: 10.1016/j.matdes.2018.07.064

Chapter 8
Recent Advances in Biomaterials and Device Technologies for Chronic Wound Healing and Tissue Repair

Treesa Varghese
https://orcid.org/0009-0005-4579-3889
Mar Athanasios College for Advanced Studies, Tiruvalla, India

Beegam L. Ramlath
https://orcid.org/0009-0009-1535-8770
St.Berchmans College (Autonomous), Changanassery, India

M. Unnimaya
https://orcid.org/0009-0009-0136-5371
MES M K Mackar Pillay College for Advanced Studies, Edathala, India

Jenny Jacob
https://orcid.org/0000-0001-8336-0500
Mar Athanasios College for Advanced Studies, Tiruvalla, India

ABSTRACT

Wound healing is a highly complicated event, involving re-vascularization, and re-epithelialization, followed by cellular proliferation, and tissue remodeling. Recent technological interventions have great potential in managing a healthy wound environment, thus reducing inflammation and healing time while promoting tissue repair. In addition, these inventions enhance the biocompatibility of wounds and

DOI: 10.4018/979-8-3373-1305-4.ch008

improve the patient's quality of life. Major technological breakthroughs include self-healing hydrogels, hydrocolloids, hydro-fibers, surgical sutures, wearable wound monitoring systems, environment-responsive dressings, negative pressure wound therapy devices, growth-factor-based therapy, gene therapy, stem-cell therapy, and bioengineered skin substitutes. This chapter discusses the recent advancements in wound care technologies, focussing on biomaterials, biomaterial devices, and their applications.

1. INTRODUCTION

Wound management remains one of the most difficult processes as mismanagement can lead to severe complications. Typical complications of wound healing involve the growth of resistant and pathogenic organisms and the formation of abnormal tissues or scar tissues. The process of wound healing is a multilayered procedure ranging from hemostasis to collagen remodeling which are distinct but overlapping phases (Figure 1).

Figure 1. Wound healing stages

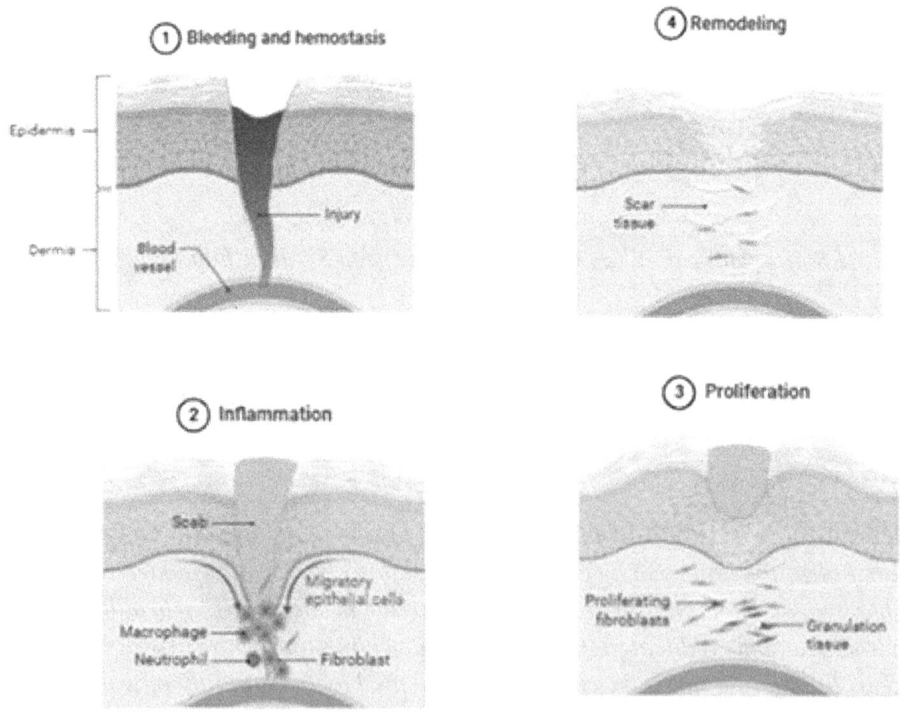

The phases can change based on the etiology and time of healing of the wounds. In general, wounds can be grouped as acute or chronic. Tissue restoration in chronic wounds is complicated and disordered compared to the systematic stages of acute wound healing. In other terms, acute wound healing involves hemostasis, inflammation, proliferation typically followed by tissue remodeling which may finally lead to scar tissue formation without capillaries. Comparatively chronic wounds demonstrate interrupted healing due to the lack of blood flow, continuous microbial growth, infection, cellular abnormality, and the imbalanced release of cytokines and growth factors (Enoch, & Leaper, 2008). The development of wound-healing materials or other assistive technologies that can focus on the healing process has an important role in this segment. These developments allow adaptation to a good cellular environment, prevent microbial growth and thus manage proper wound healing (Hossain et al., 2017).

Along with the modulatory effect of physiological responses on wound recovery, the behavioral pattern of an individual could indirectly influence wound repair. Individuals with greater levels of mental stress are prone to use tobacco or alcohol in heavy doses may experience the minimum of their physical activity and sleeplessness. Additionally, elderly and financially backward patients with chronic wounds face various difficulties when going to medical treatment for wound care. The potential difficulties are related to transportation, physical limitations, and emotional and psychological support (Jain et al., 2025). Hence translational work should be necessary to identify key factors determining most effective and developing new treatment strategies for better wound care management. This chapter points to the recent advances in biomaterials, devices and assistive technologies for chronic wound healing and tissue repair.

2. CHRONIC WOUNDS: PATHOPHYSIOLOGY AND CLINICAL CHALLENGES

Chronic wounds are characterized by a disruption in the normal healing process, where the wound stalls in its recovery, frequently becoming stuck in a prolonged inflammatory state. This midstage delay is commonly linked with many factors including prolonged or persistent infection. These wounds are expressed with higher levels of proinflammatory cytokines, proteolytic enzymes, reactive oxygen species (ROS), and senescent cells. Together, these factors create a hostile environment that disrupts the healing process and makes recovery more challenging (Frykberg & Banks, 2015).

Managing chronic wounds requires a structured approach that starts with thorough assessments of both the patient and the wound. These evaluations help identify underlying issues, like vascular problems or infections, that can hinder progress. Effective treatment for chronic wounds often involves a multidisciplinary strategy including addressing any coexisting medical conditions and together with specialized wound treatment to support the best possible healing outcomes.

3. BIOMATERIALS IN WOUND HEALING

Biomaterials are vital in treating chronic wounds by supporting the healing process through diverse mechanisms. These substances are usually custom designed to interact with biological systems, fostering tissue repair and regeneration. With the rising occurrence of chronic wounds, often linked to conditions such as diabetes and other infections, there is an increasing focus on developing advanced biomaterials that overcome the challenges posed by traditional wound care approaches (Zhang et al., 2020). Different types of biomaterials are available for wound healing and are classified as natural and synthetic biomaterials (Figure 2).

Figure 2. Types of biomaterials

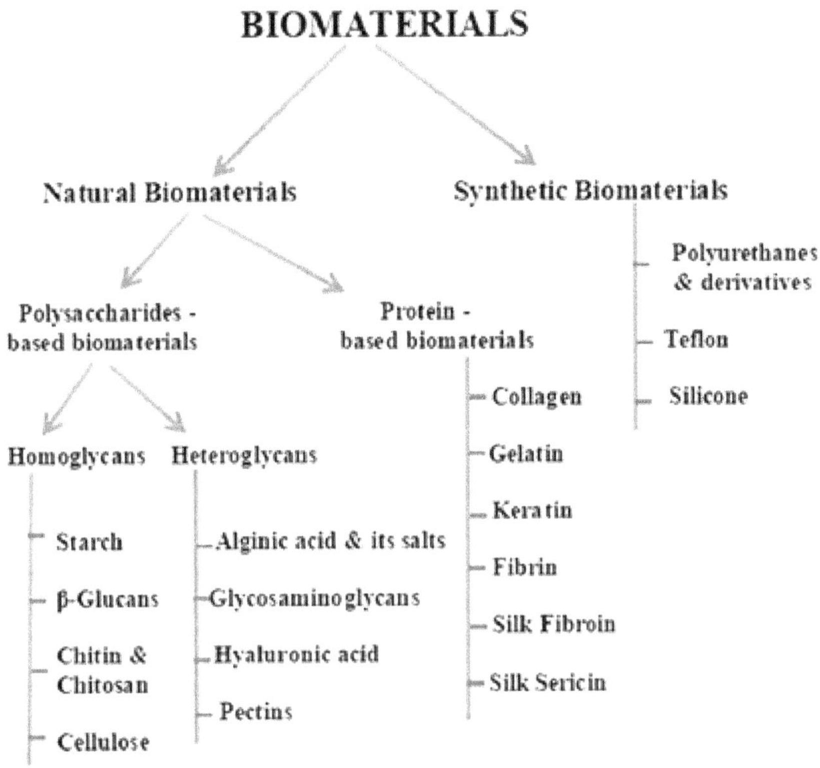

3.1. Natural Biomaterials

Natural biomaterials are materials sourced from nature, including plants and animals, and are extensively used in medical settings to repair, enhance, or replace tissues and organs in the human body. Their increasing usage can be attributed to their remarkable biocompatibility and ability to integrate naturally with biological systems, making them highly suitable for various medical purposes. A significant advantage of these biomaterials is their structural and functional similarity to the extracellular matrix (ECM) found in the human body (Mayet et al., 2014). The calming, defending, and curing abilities of natural substances — comprising their potential to act as anti-inflammatory, anti-microbial, tissue-strengthening, and antioxidative — may help in the wound healing process (Ige et.al., 2012; Mogosanu et al., 2012).

Natural polymers like chitosan, collagen, elastin, and fibrinogen are non-toxic materials that mimic the macromolecules naturally seen in the human body (Mogosanu & Grumezescu, 2014). They are also applied in regenerative medicine for proliferating human epithelial stem cells or generating cultured epithelial tissue substitutes (Guerra et al., 2009). Major types of natural biomaterials are polysaccharide-based biomaterials and protein-based biomaterials.

3.1.1. Natural Polysaccharides for Wound Repair

Polysaccharides offer a promising solution for wound healing due to their natural origin, affordability, and biodegradability. These biomaterials can be grouped into various categories for wound care applications. Basically, they are Homoglycans (starch, β-glycans, cellulose, chitin and chitosan) and Heteroglycans (alginic acid and its salts, glycosaminoglycans, hyaluronic acid and pectins) (Kennedy et al., 2011).

Homoglycans composed of a single type of monosaccharide units are called homoglycans. These bio-based non-toxic materials are used to regulate cellular activities (Jabeen et al., 2024). Starch, a widely available and affordable polysaccharide, occurs naturally in granular form. Comprising amylose and amylopectin, its composition varies by source, impacting its behavior and properties. Insoluble in cold water, starch absorbs moisture reversibly. Renewability, biodegradability, and versatility of starch molecules make it suitable for biomedical applications, including bone substitutes, drug delivery systems, and tissue engineering scaffolds (Sivamaruthi et al., 2022). Researchers examined various β-glucans from yeast, fungi, and grains for their immune-boosting and medicinal properties (Hameed et al., 2024). A highly purified yeast-derived β-glucan demonstrated remarkable benefits, including suppressing fat cell formation, enhancing wound recovery, and reducing skin irritation more effectively than traditional cotton gauze (Majtan & Jesenak, 2018).

Chitin and its derivative chitosan, are amino polysaccharide found in crustacean shells and fungal cell walls. Similar to cellulose, chitin has strong hydrogen bonds, but its insolubility in common solvents makes processing challenging. Chitin has several benefits, including promoting wound healing, enhancing immunity, and demonstrating hemostatic properties (Islam et al., 2017; Singh et al., 2017). As a biocompatible, biodegradable, and non-toxic biomaterial, chitin is well-tolerated by the body, making it a valuable resource for various applications (Islam et al., 2017). Chitosan, derived from chitin, is a linear polysaccharide composed of glucosamine and N-acetylglucosamine units. Its biocompatibility, minimal toxicity, and low risk of blood clotting make it a popular choice in biomedical applications, despite its tendency to cause red blood cell clumping (Jayakumar et.al., 2011).

Cellulose and their chemically modified derivatives offer a promising natural biomaterial for wound care. Its biocompatibility, biodegradability, and antimicrobial properties make it an innovative and safe choice for wound dressing applications (Sulaeva et al., 2015). Bacterial cellulose, with its unique nanoscale structure, exceptional strength, and swelling capabilities, offers a promising natural biomaterial for wound care. Its biocompatibility, biodegradability, and antimicrobial properties make it an innovative and safe choice for wound dressing applications (Czaja et al., 2007).

Heteroglycans are polysaccharides with different kinds of monomer units, showing unique properties of heteroglycans make them valuable in biomedical applications, Heteroglycans offer some benefits like biocompatibility, biodegradability, and specialized physical and chemical characteristics (Rimondo et al., 2019).

Glycosaminoglycans (GAGs) play a vital role in skin and bone regeneration as key components of the extracellular matrix (ECM). Their structure and properties influence the recruitment of precursor cells. Modified nanofibers and engineered polymers mimicking GAGs have been shown to promote tissue repair, reduce inflammation, and enhance wound healing by stimulating blood vessel growth and collagen formation (Melrose et al., 2016).

Hyaluronic acid (HA) is a naturally occurring, highly hydrophilic biomaterial found in connective tissues, skin, cartilage, and other bodily fluids. Its unique structure, composed of glucose and gluconic acid residues, enables it to retain water, provide lubrication, and influence various cellular functions. HA interacts with proteins, growth factors, and tissue components, making it essential for wound healing (Neuman et al., 2015). Its antibacterial properties, biodegradability, and non-toxicity have led to its widespread use in medical and bioengineering applications, including wound care, tissue engineering, ophthalmic surgery, and joint lubrication (Sala et al., 2022).

Pectins, a type of hydrocolloid, are used in wound dressings to promote healing. As a biocompatible and biodegradable natural polymer, pectin has various applications beyond food, including targeted drug delivery, wound care, and tissue engineering (Koshy & Sangeetha, 2024).

3.1.2. Protein-Based Biomaterial

Proteins, also known as polypeptides, are made up of various combinations of 20 amino acids. What sets protein biomaterials apart is that the specific sequence of these amino acids is predetermined during the formation process, giving them unique properties.

Collagen, a fibrous protein plays a vital role in the structure of skin and connective tissue. Its distinctive triple-helix arrangement gives unusual strength and stability to stress. Biomedical applications of collagen are diverse, including sutures, wound dressings, and tissue reconstruction (Mathew-Steiner et al., 2021) Collagen-based dressings offer practical advantages, but their effectiveness depends on processing and stabilization techniques to prevent shrinkage and maintain scaffold structure (Chattopadhyay & Raines, 2014). Gelatin, derived from denatured collagen, is a biocompatible, biodegradable, and non-immunogenic material. Gelatin is widely used in tissue engineering, medicine, and surgery as a scaffold, hemostatic sponge, wound dressing, and adhesive pad due to its unique properties (Naomi et al., 2021).

Keratin, a protein found in vertebrate epithelia, offers unique properties making it an ideal biomaterial. Its biocompatibility, controlled biodegradability, and bioactivity enable various biomedical applications (Ige et al., 2012). Keratin extracted from hair and wool can be used to create biomaterials for wound healing, nerve regeneration, and tissue engineering. Additionally, keratin-based dressings can provide controlled release of antibiotics and growth factors, promoting healing and tissue repair (Vasconcelos & Cavaco-Paulo, 2011; Sierpinski et al., 2007).

Fibrin, a protein formed from fibrinogen, serves as a natural scaffold for wound healing and cell transplantation. Its applications include cartilage repair, cardiac tissue engineering, and hemostatic dressings (Ye et al., 2011). Research has shown promising results using fibrin-based dressings, derived from sources like salmon, to promote smooth tissue healing and minimize immune responses in animal models (Laidmae et al., 2018).

Silk, a natural protein fiber produced by silkworms and spiders, has exceptional mechanical strength and elasticity, making them suitable for biomedical applications. Its structure, composed of repeating amino acid sequences, provides exceptional mechanical strength and elasticity. Silk fibroin, derived from silk fibers, supports cell growth and adhesion, has low thrombogenicity, and elicits minimal inflammation. Its versatility allows it to be prepared in various forms, including gels, films, and scaffolds, for wound healing, skin regeneration, and tissue repair (Lehmann et al., 2022). Coating or blending silk fibroin with other materials can enhance its properties, promoting improved wound care and tissue engineering outcomes (Pollini et al., 2020).

3.2. Synthetic Biomaterials

Synthetic biomaterials have distinct advantages over natural ones, as they can be engineered with precise control to produce consistent and uniform physical, chemical, and stability properties tailored to specific needs (Zhong et al., 2010). These materials, often made from polymers, metals, or ceramics, are designed to replicate the characteristics of natural tissues. A major benefit of synthetic biomaterials is their ability to be tailored, allowing researchers to modify features such as mechanical strength, degradation speed, and compatibility with the body to suit specific medical needs. This adaptability is critical in complex procedures like islet transplantation, where combining synthetic and natural biomaterials can greatly improve the performance of implantable devices (Deng et al., 2022). Nevertheless, there are challenges like controlling immune reactions and ensuring that the materials remain stable in the body over time. To overcome these obstacles, current research is focused on creating composite biomaterials that combine the advantages of synthetic and natural materials (Farasati et al., 2025).

Polyurethanes, formed by combining diol and diisocyanate groups, are versatile synthetic biomaterials known for their biocompatibility, strength, and flexibility (Pivec et al., 2017). They are commonly used in medical devices like catheters and gastric balloons (Davis et al., 2008). Although they can degrade in acidic environments, certain polyurethanes, like Pellethane, are non-toxic and have been used to treat burns and wounds, promoting faster healing (Miri et al., 2023).

Teflon, another synthetic polymer made from tetrafluoroethylene, is a non-toxic and versatile material. They are insoluble in various solvents, easy to sterilize, and can be molded to fit comfortably over injured areas with minimal pressure, making it a suitable choice for medical applications (Shenoy et al., 2024). Silicone is a highly biocompatible material that is non-toxic and hypoallergenic. Its resistance to degradation makes it suitable for use in implantable devices, soft tissue repair, and medical equipment like needles and syringes (Gao et al., 2021).

4. ADVANCED DEVICE TECHNOLOGIES

Modern medical devices are critical in addressing the complex challenges of chronic wound care, supporting recovery, and enhancing patient quality of life. Breakthroughs like bioengineered skin and tissue substitutes mimic the properties of natural skin, providing a framework that promotes cellular growth and tissue repair. Negative-pressure wound therapy (NPWT) applies a vacuum to the wound site, improving circulation and reducing swelling, which speeds up the healing process. Similarly, hyperbaric oxygen therapy (HBO) increases the oxygen supply to damaged tissues, aiding infection control and promoting recovery in stubborn wounds. Studies reveal that advanced treatments, such as allogeneic bilayered cultured skin constructs, significantly outperform traditional methods, leading to faster healing and wound closure for chronic diabetic foot ulcers (Dean et al., 2025). Furthermore, these innovative approaches may offer long-term economic advantages by extending ulcer-free periods and reducing the risk of amputation (Wu, 2010) (Figure 3).

Figure 3. Recent advancements in wound healing

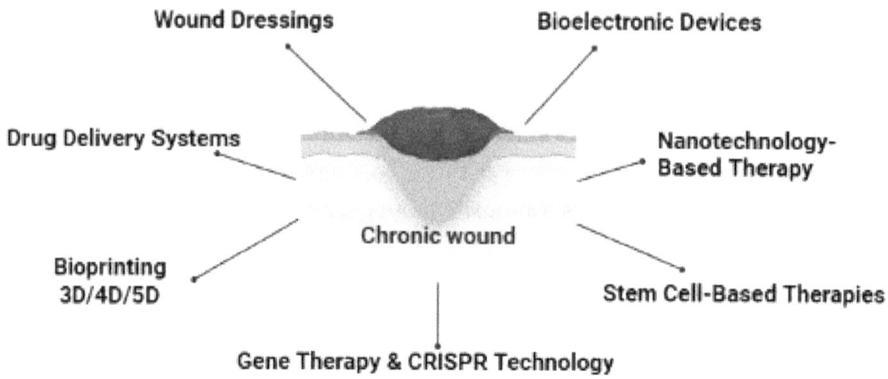

4.1. Wound Dressings

Wound dressings are specifically designed to support tissue repair at the wound site, control and prevent infections, and restore the skin's natural functions (Dong & Guo, 2021). The conventional method for treating chronic wounds involves wound dressings, which need to be regularly changed and carefully monitored by medical professionals. A significant advancement in modern wound dressings is their capability to sustain a moist environment. Dressings that regulate moisture have been proven to accelerate tissue repair, alleviate pain, reduce the risk of infection, and enhance the overall appearance of wounds (Fonder et al., 2008).

Modern wound care is centered around moist wound healing, with innovative dressings such as hydrogels and alginates that are developed to preserve optimal moisture levels crucial for effective recovery. In addition, the incorporation of active ingredients in these dressings raises regulatory challenges, especially in determining their classification as either medical devices or pharmaceutical products based on their primary mechanism of action (Ovington,2007). Furthermore, antimicrobial dressings, which release substances like iodine, have shown considerable success in reducing bacterial loads and facilitating the healing of chronic wounds (Sarheed et.al., 2016). Exogenous collagen is used as a biomaterial and mimics the body's natural tissue, and is effective in encouraging cell recruitment and supporting the repair process (Chattopadhyay & Raines, 2014). Moreover, innovative wound dressing strategies are being developed to target increased protease levels, a condition that can obstruct the healing of chronic wounds. Looking to the future, advancements in wound dressings aim to create products that actively promote recovery by addressing challenges like infections and chemical imbalances that impede the healing process (Ovington, 2007). These advancements in wound dressings, reflect the increasing sophistication in wound care, emphasizing the importance of multifunctional dressings in achieving better healing outcomes.

4.2. Drug Delivery Systems

Another emerging field in wound healing is the drug delivery systems, one of the major challenges faced by the system is the non-functional vasculature in the wound bed, which may interfere with the efficient delivery of medications when given through systemic administration (Saghazadeh et.al., 2018; Johnson, & Wang, 2015). Successful drug delivery to the infected diabetic wounds includes neutralization of reactive free radicals, suppression of infectious bacterial growth, reduction of inflammatory responses, and induction of vascularization and angiogenesis. Furthermore, tissue specific application of drugs to the affected area may reduce the toxic off-target effects along with the enhanced drug efficacy.

There are two types of drug delivery systems – Active Drug Delivery Systems (ADDS) and Passive Drug Delivery Systems (PDDS) (Johnson & Wang, 2015). In ADDS drug release happens in a controlled manner, ensuring a consistent and gradual release over time. This approach is more effective than conventional methods such as hypodermic injections, which may result in high plasma concentrations beyond the therapeutic range, potentially leading to side effects. ADDS also allows for more efficient local treatment by releasing drugs in a controlled, directed manner, overcoming some of the disadvantages of classic treatment methods, but where issues of biocompatibility, scaling up, and regulatory compliance are major issues from a clinical point of view (Lopez-Vidal et al., 2025). Passive drug delivery systems are designed to provide localized and controlled release, ensuring precise spatiotemporal regulation of drug dosage at the wound site. These systems safeguard drugs from metabolic breakdown and help sustain their concentration over prolonged durations (Boateng et. al., 2008). Comparing ADDS and PDDS based on their mechanism of action – delivery of drugs on demand based on reaction to physiological changes like pH or temperature shifts. This capability is especially beneficial for managing infections in chronic wounds. In PDDS – enabling the sequential and targeted release of therapeutic agents, including antibacterial compounds and growth factors is crucial for the efficient healing of chronic wounds (Brown et al., 2006). Polymers are particularly preferred in this stimulus generative system because of their flexible properties that allow the regulation of drug release while reducing the risk of side effects (Srivastava et al., 2015). Application of polymeric biomaterials could offer a sustained- targeted delivery of angiogenic factors into the precise site-specific locations, thus overcoming the huddles due to neuropathy, hyperglycemia, neuropathy. Emerging trends in pharmaceutical science and nanotechnology have a great role in the development of drug delivery systems that can optimize drug release control to the wound areas, improving the healing process.

Use of lipid-based drug delivery systems (liposomes) could encapsulate the targeted drugs and can readily deliver the drug more effectively through subcutaneous injections directly or topically to the wound. They exhibit a diverse membrane lamellarity properties along with their wide range of size (20-1000 nm), thus giving an added advantage to lodge and permit sustained release of specific drugs in the localized areas. Targeted drugs can also be designed to be encapsulated by nanoparticles for the effective tissue-specific drug delivery for acute or chronic wound healing. A wide range of metal, polymer, or lipid-based Nanoparticles (NPs) have been effectively used as targeted drug therapy (Aljmal et al., 2024). Application of surface functionalization and bioactive coatings may offer a new approach to the hallmark challenges associated with the diabetic wounds.

4.3. Bioelectronic Devices

Biomedical devices are vital in improving chronic wound care by supporting continuous assessment and promoting the healing process. These devices are fabricated to analyze the major physiological factors essential to wound recovery, such as temperature, oxygen levels, and pH balance. By infusing bioelectronic technology into wound dressings, real-time information can be acquired, yielding improved healthcare outcomes. This action allows for proper care and reduces the need for frequent hospital visits. The effectiveness and efficiency of bioelectronic devices are mainly due to the choice of materials like paper, polydimethylsiloxane (PDMS), and various other polymers. They are frequently chosen because of their lightweight nature and ability to stretch. Paper substrates are an economical option and provide distinct benefits such as breathability and disposability, making them ideal for single-use applications like wound care (Baniya et al., 2024). In contrast, PDMS offers superior stretchability and closely mimics the mechanical characteristics of human skin, improving patient comfort. Advanced microfabrication techniques are mainly involved in the fabrication of biomaterials due to their flexible and stretchable character (Betancourt & Brannon-Peppas, 2006). These findings facilitate the development of complex designs capable of adapting to the body's dynamic movements, especially in regions with frequent motion. Combining rigid components with flexible connections provides durability without compromising functionality.

5. EMERGING THERAPIES AND INNOVATIONS

The cellular and molecular basis for the rehabilitation mechanism may vary in different types of wounds, hence a singular treatment approach is insufficient for the complete and successful wound healing process. The recent advances and innovations in biomedical technologies have greatly enhanced the current understanding regarding medical evaluation followed by the treatment strategies in the field of wound healing research. Some of the revolutionized developments in this field include the use of bioengineered substitutes for human skin, growth factor(s)-based therapies, stimuli-responsive wound dressings strategies, stem cell therapy, gene therapy, moist wound dressings instead of dry dressings, and nanotherapeutics. Additionally, the fabrication of personalized medicine has been achieved through the development of ECM-based treatment approaches (Hosty et al., 2024), platelet-rich plasma (PRP) therapy (Lacci, & Dardik, 2010), and 3D bioprinting technologies (Cubo-Mateo, & Gelinsky, 2021). However, the evaluation and management of chronic wounds remain a significant challenge. Therefore, wound healing needs new and better solutions that prioritize effectiveness, risk-benefit balance, and cost efficiency. This section will outline and examine some of the emerging and novel treatment methods currently being utilized and investigated for wound healing, highlighting their benefits and challenges.

5.1. Stem Cell-Based Therapies

In the current scenario, recent developments in regenerative medicine have become a cutting-edge field, offering alternative therapeutic approaches to enhance wound healing and restore normal skin structure (Dickinson et al., 2016). Stem cell-based therapy has attracted significant attention for wound healing and skin regeneration due to its unique features, including long-term self-renewal properties and the ability to differentiate into pluripotent cells (Chen et al., 2009). Currently, stem cell therapy and progenitor cell therapy have been getting much more attention, the stem cells located near the wound site contribute to healing due to their plasticity and regenerative capabilities. Additionally, this technology offers significant potential for treating chronic wounds that are unresponsive to conventional methods by leveraging processes such as growth factor interactions, modulation of inflammation, and stimulation of immune responses to promote vascularization and re-epithelialization (Kolle et al., 2013). The autologous stem cells, with their exceptional differentiation potential, ability to support angiogenesis, minimal adverse effects, and capacity to transform into various cell types, make them ideal for enhancing natural healing, promoting cell proliferation, and accelerating wound closure.

The primary sources of stem cells used for wound healing and skin regeneration include adult mesenchymal stem cells (MSCs), embryonic stem cells (ESCs), and induced pluripotent stem cells (iPSCs) (Dash et al., 2018). MSCs are the most promising source, offering benefits such as inflammation modulation, enhanced angiogenesis, granulation tissue formation, antimicrobial effects, scar reduction, and fibroblast promotion, while due to ethical concerns, ESCs are rarely used for wound healing (Mazini et al., 2020).

Scaffold-based strategies, involving the transplantation of stem cells seeded on a three-dimensional scaffold matrix, may greatly enhance the stem cell survival rate and facilitate normal cellular functions (Hamdan et al., 2017). Integration of growth factors within the scaffolds may improve vascularization and wound repair (Goodarzi et al., 2018). Furthermore, adipose tissue-derivedMSCs can be utilized in wound healing therapies because of their minimal invasiveness, high accessibility, and lack of ethical concerns (Heo et al., 2021; Weiliang et al., 2021). Treatment using umbilical cord blood stem cells (UCBSC) has shown excellent therapeutic indexing in diabetic wound healing with greater collagen deposition and hence cellular proliferation potential (Jung et al., 2018).

5.2. Extracellular Matrix (ECM)-Based Therapies

The extracellular matrix (ECM) is a complex three-dimensional network of fibrous proteins like collagen, elastin, laminin, fibronectin, and vitronectin, as well as proteoglycans and glycosaminoglycans, providing structural integrity and mechanical support to tissues (Kusindarta et al., 2018). It also coordinates cellular activities in damaged skin to support tissue repair and regeneration by delivering a variety of cytokines and growth factors (Rasouli et al., 2021; Turner, 2021).

The extracellular matrix has a vital impact on various stages of the wound healing process. Alternatively, together with fibrin, fibronectin forms a provisional extracellular matrix that is developed during the hemostasis phase to facilitate cell adhesion and cellular migration process. During the inflammation phase, the extracellular matrix provides a three-dimensional structural framework that prevents the entry of pathogenic microorganisms. Eventually, during the homeostasis phase, the provisional extracellular matrix disintegrates and is replaced by granulation tissue containing fibronectin to support collagen-1 deposition. As a final event, during the remodeling phase, collagen I is replaced by collagen III to enhance mechanical support. During the repair process, the presence of integrin and non-integrin facilitates proper communication between the components of the extracellular matrix with stem cells and other precursor cells (Rasouli et al., 2021).

Chronic wounds exhibit poor healing due to ECM degradation caused by a prolonged inflammatory phase, the presence of highly activated matrix metalloproteinases, and an abundance of senescent fibroblasts (Sutcliffe et al., 2017). To restore the normal functionality of the chronic wound, several membranous extracellular matrix (ECM)--based scaffolds represent a highly promising biomaterial for skin wound healing therapies. Different types of ECM-based scaffolds include cellular-derived ECM (Assunção et al., 2020), and decellularized ECM (dECM) (Cramer et al., 2020; Jiang et al., 2021). Among them, dECM-based therapeutic strategy is the most powerful approach to overcome the hurdles associated with tissue or organ transplantation. Because the dECM can serve as a reservoir for site-specific bioactive components and improve the cell-matrix interactions, it provides an added advantage for tissue regeneration without inducing any illness due to their toxic effects (Zhang et al., 2011). Furthermore, releasing of fibroblast growth factors from dECM inhibits the degree of contraction and reduces scar formation in tissue wounds(Choi et al., 2013). dECM scaffolds create a biomimetic microenvironment that enhances cell adhesion, proliferation, and differentiation, thereby accelerating wound closure and tissue regeneration with minimal scar formation. Additionally, their immunomodulatory properties help to mitigate excessive inflammation, a key challenge in diabetic wound healing (Milan, et al.2016; Hoganson et al., 2010).

In recent years, fully functional acellular dermal matrices (ADMs) have been commercialized from a variety of sources, including bovine (BADM), porcine (PADM), and human (HADM), (Petrie et al., 2022). The implantation of decellularized human placenta-derived ECM scaffolds has been reported to successfully promote healing in full-thickness wounds while also supporting hair follicle formation while supporting hair follicle sweat gland formation is crucial for active skin regeneration that was absent in earlier clinical products (Su et al., 2019, Choi et al., 2013).

5.3. Platelet-Rich Plasma Based Therapies

Platelet-rich plasma (PRP) is a blood plasma component with platelet concentrations higher than normal levels. These properties make PRP essential for promoting tissue repair and regeneration (Helmy et al., 2021, Qu W et al., 2021). Therapeutic strategy using Platelet-rich plasma is attributed to the fact that the Platelet growth factors (PGFs) play a crucial role in inflammatory, proliferation, and tissue remodeling phases of wound repair and healing mechanisms (Everts et al., 2020).

Application of PRP-based technology for effective wound healing is steadily increasing day by day (Suthar et al., 2017; Jee et al., 2016). PRP-based therapy has been investigated in many human and animal trial models for different types of wounds, including acute cutaneous wounds, burns, chronic skin ulcers, and procedures in cosmetic and plastic surgery using different types of PRP formulations such as solution, gel, or injection (Pallua et al., 2020; Suthar et al., 2017).

5.4 Gene Therapy and CRISPR Technology

Gene therapy is an innovative and promising therapeutic approach, able to provide more precise and personalized treatment possibilities for a wide range of life-threatening diseases. Gene therapy can be used for inactivation of a gene (gene silencing), addition of a gene to a cell (gene augmentation), and modification of existing genetic code (genome editing). The most commonly investigated therapeutic molecules for gene expression modulation include messenger RNA (mRNA) and plasmid DNA (pDNA)for gene overexpression, as well as microRNA (miRNA), small interfering RNA (siRNA), aptamer, and oligonucleotides for post-transcriptional gene silencing (Elnaz Shaabani et al., 2020).

In wound healing, gene therapy enhances wound closure induces many biochemical pathways and by promoting cellular functions. This effective method operates by changing the wound's microenvironment, influencing its natural processes through a mix of biochemical and physical changes (Pang et al., 2021). There must be a carrier system to deliver nucleic acids and other gene products into the targeted intracellular region, whereas their topical application to cutaneous wounds is easy to perform (Desmet et al., 2018).

CRISPR Technology is a modernized gene therapy and genetic research that promotes totally reliable gene editing to enhance the efficacy of cell-based therapies (Henn et al., 2024). Efficient delivery of CRISPR components depends on the various vectors and delivery methods. An alternative approach involves delivering the Cas9 protein and guide RNA as ribonucleoprotein (RNP) complexes, which are transient in nature. This method can reduce off-target effects while maintaining high editing accuracy (Uddin et al., 2020). This is achieved through the CRISPR/Cas9 system, which uses a guide RNA to direct the Cas9 protein to specific DNA sequences, creating double-strand breaks for precise genetic modifications (Cong & Zhang, 2015). Studies by Henn et al. (2024) state that the highest number of differentially expressed genes was found in wound fibroblast cells. Important differentially expressed wound healing-related genes in fibroblasts. Edited dendritic cells had the strongest impact on fibroblast gene expression within the wound bed and showed a stronger signaling activity within their wound environment.

5.5. Bioprinting in Tissue Repair

At present, various therapeutic approaches have been widely used for managing both acute and chronic wounds. Nevertheless, many of these treatments rely on manual techniques, and their success was limited by the extended time required to cure the wounds. To overcome this hurdle, three-dimensional bioprinting (3-D Printing) has evolved in recent years as a prominent solution as an advanced, high-throughput automation technology to resolve the various challenges in tissue regenerative medicine. 3D bioprinting is an automated technology, able to provide effective fabrication strategies for biocompatible artificial skins and closely mimic the native tissue architecture. In 3-D bioprinting, an effective bioprinted skin graft should be able to transport wound exudates and nutritional factors, and must be ready to accommodate various skin cell types, including fibroblasts, keratinocytes, and others, which are organized in specific layers and locations. The biocompatibility, degradability, permeability, and material strength should exactly duplicate the original skin structure, and should be able to withstand the external pressure and forces that are present in in vivo conditions. Furthermore, there should be a synergy between structure and morphology, mechanical behavior, biochemical behavior and biodegradability of scaffolds to regulate cellular behavior and control cell fate (Robin et al., 2017; Murphy & Atala, 2014).

Bioprinting technologies can be categorized into four main groups: laser-based, extrusion-based, inkjet-based, and stereolithography-based. Among these, extrusion-based bioprinting stands out as the most popular method for printing skin, thanks to its unique advantages, including ease of use, affordability, rapid printing speeds, versatility with various biomaterials, and ability to recreate intricate tissue architectures (Matai et al., 2020). Recently, the development of a new and improved hybrid type of next generation bioprinting systems are being explored as promising solutions for Skin Bioprinting, Continuous Liquid Interface Production (CLIP) (Tumbleston et al., 2015), Multi-material Multi-nozzle 3D printing (MM3D) (Skylar-Scott et al., 2019), and Computed Axial Lithography (CAL) (Kelly et al., 2019) are some examples for next-generation bioprinting technologies, in which integrate two or more existing bioprinting techniques integrated into fully functional one.

CLIP-based bioprinting offers significant advantages over conventional UV/laser -based stereolithography (SLA) printing with 100 times faster bioprinting ability. CLIP bioprinters can also be adapted for large-scale multi-layer skin printing using various biocompatible photopolymers, visible light techniques and photo-initiators (Jeong et al., 2024). MM3D bioprinting uses a unique, voxel-based method, replacing traditional layer-based printing. This technique employs a specialized printhead that rapidly switches between multiple materials (Skylar-Scott et al., 2019). This approach benefits skin tissue engineering by maintaining stiffness differences within a single layer and between different layers of skin.

Another crucial factor for successful wound healing and skin tissue engineering in 3D bioprinting is the selection of an appropriate biomaterial ink or bio-ink (Groll et al., 2019; Hospodiuk et al., 2017). Bio-inks are a mix of biomaterials, cells, and nutrients that support growth. In contrast, biomaterial inks have similar components, but without the living cells. A diverse range of biomaterial hydrogels, such as collagen, gelatin, hyaluronic acid, chitosan, cellulose, silk fibroin and alginate have commonly used in skin bioprinting, often in combination with synthetic biopolymers to enhance the mechanical properties of printed constructs (Masri et al., 2021; Donderwinkel, et al., 2017).

Hallmarks in the selection of bio-inks in 3d bioprinting includes, they should exhibit excellent biocompatibility, biodegradability, greater mechanical stability, high availability, good printability along high shape fidelity after bioprinting. The viscoelastic properties of the bio- ink may have a great impact on their extracellular matrix (ECM) remodeling capacity, skin bio-printability, cellular migration, proliferation abilities (Hazur et al., 2021). Furthermore, since bio-inks contain living cells, consideration for the selection of cells may also be crucial since the living cells can influence major immunological responses after implantation. For creating skin tissue, it's best to use either primary skin cells like fibroblasts, keratinocytes, and melanocytes, or stem cells. This helps ensure that the bioprinted skin functions normally, just like natural skin (Masri et al, 2022).

Bioprinting has been applied to heal chronic and persistent wounds that don't respond to traditional treatments, including diabetic foot ulcers, venous ulcers, burn injuries and pressure ulcers (Liu et al., 2020; Admane et al., 2019; Derr et al., 2019). Also, this method serves as an alternative strategy to the conventional one and helps to overcome the issues related with immunological responses during transplantation reaction and surgery complications (Admane et al., 2019).

Two major approaches adapted in Skin 3-D bioprinting for a wound healing procedure are "ex vivo bioprinting" and "in situ bioprinting" (Wallace et al., 2023). An extrusion-, inkjet-, or laser-based bioprinting followed by implantation into the wound area is adapted in vivo bioprinting to construct dermal and epidermal skin layers. Whereas in situ bioprinting is achieved through the imprinting of bio-inks (skin cells entrapped in a biomaterial hydrogel) directly onto the wound site, through in-situ approach using a handheld extrusion bioprinter in order to reconstructs the skin structure directly on the wound (Velasco et al., 2018).

In a novel approach to skin bioprinting, pro-angiogenic peptides were integrated into hydrogel patches to develop 3D-bioprinted skin constructs. The activated bio-inks so developed exhibited excellent printability and vascularization abilities and hence play a significant role in skin regeneration (Jang et al., 2021). Researchers have created a 3D-printed peptide patch that promotes blood vessel growth, aiming to enhance its effectiveness in treating skin wounds. To create a bioprintable material, researchers chemically bonded GelMA (gelatin methacryloyl) and HAMA (hyaluronic acid methacryloyl) to a specific peptide sequence, QHREDGS. The bioprinted patch showed outstanding compatibility with the body and promoted wound healing and blood vessel growth (Guan et al., 2021). Also, a bioprinted tissue co-culture platform "FPM "bio-ink" was developed by Jara et al. (2020) using a mixture of macrophages, plasma-derived fibrinogen, fibronectin, thrombin, and factor XIII. Unlike 3D printing, where structures are printed in fixed form with a combination of materials, 4D printing involves the consideration of time as a variable, so materials are designed to react and change with external stimuli, rendering it suited to applications like self-healing tissue and adaptable prosthetics with changing requirements. The innovative application of 4D printing with portable bioprinters to directly deposit biological macromolecules over wounds allows in situ healing of wounds by using biocompatible materials that can change based on external stimuli, promoting tissue regeneration and enhancing treatment of various wounds (Li et al., 2024). 5D printing goes beyond 3D and 4D printing by not only enabling materials to modify their form based on stimuli but also having embedded information to facilitate intelligent interaction with the environment, rendering it extremely useful for applications such as intelligent biomedical implants and dynamic manufacturing (Lai, J., & Wang, M. 2023).

5.6. Nanotechnology- Based Therapy

Nanotechnology is transforming regenerative medicine with advanced solutions. It utilizes tiny, biocompatible materials for diagnosis, treatment, and delivery. By developing nanoparticles, researchers can create targeted treatments with minimal side effects (Kubinova & Sykova, 2010). The integration of nanotechnology and biomedicine has led to revolutions in biomaterials, biosensors, and therapies. This integration of fields holds great promise for advancing wound care, real-time monitoring, and tissue repair. Initially, nanobiotechnology focused on developing scaffolds for wound treatment (Nosrati et al., 2021), but recent advancements have led to the development of sophisticated systems for gene and drug delivery (Pang et al., 2021), antimicrobial and anti-inflammatory treatments (Sharda et al., 2024), and tissue regeneration (Blanco-Fernandez et al., 2021; Tocco et al., 2012). Nanoparticles enhance wound healing by delivering medications directly to the wound site, reducing side effects. Tiny carriers like liposomes and polymeric nanoparticles release growth factors, antibiotics, and anti-inflammatory agents in a controlled manner, promoting efficient healing (Shi et al., 2024; Suri et al., 2007). In addition, Silver gold, and zinc oxide nanoparticles exhibit potent antimicrobial effects, fighting bacterial infections that often plague chronic wounds. These nanomaterials also help regulate inflammation, preventing excessive swelling that can slow down the healing process (Nor-Azlan, et al., 2020). Certain nanomaterials, such as graphene-based compounds and peptide-coated nanoparticles, promote the growth of new blood vessels, ensuring wounds receive adequate oxygen and nutrients. Additionally, nanofibers and hydrogels that mimic the body's natural tissue structure support cell growth, multiplication, and tissue repair, fostering a conducive environment for healing (Blanco-Fernandez et al., 2021; Tocco et al., 2012).

6. CONCLUSION AND FUTURE PERSPECTIVES

Recent advancements in tissue engineering and regenerative medicine have significantly impacted wound healing, particularly for chronic wounds. Advances in biology and pharmaceutical sciences have led to the creation of new active compounds that enhance tissue regeneration and help restore disrupted physiological functions. To maximize the effectiveness of these treatments, improved drug delivery systems need to be developed and tested to ensure better absorption at the injury site. A major challenge in this field is designing drug carriers that address the complex causes of chronic wounds while supporting the natural healing process.

This article highlights past achievements and exciting new developments in biologics, cell-based therapies, and 3D biomaterials platforms. Stem cell therapies show promise, but cell availability remains a challenge. Combining biologics and cell-based approaches with traditional tissue engineering strategies may enhance wound healing. Emerging technologies like 3D bioprinting, enabled by additive manufacturing, are revolutionizing the field, enabling the creation of complex, realistic products and scalable fabrication processes. However, accessing advanced treatment facilities for patients is a challenging factor, especially for the elderly and financially backward groups.

REFERENCES

Admane, P., Gupta, A. C., Jois, P., Roy, S., Lakshmanan, C. C., Kalsi, G., & Ghosh, S. (2019). Direct 3D bioprinted full-thickness skin constructs recapitulate regulatory signaling pathways and physiology of human skin. *Bioprinting (Amsterdam, Netherlands), 15*, e00051. DOI: 10.1016/j.bprint.2019.e00051

Aljamal, D., Iyengar, P. S., & Nguyen, T. T. (2024). Translational challenges in drug therapy and delivery systems for treating chronic lower extremity wounds. *Pharmaceutics*, *16*(6), 750. DOI: 10.3390/pharmaceutics16060750 PMID: 38931872

Assunção, M., Dehghan-Baniani, D., Yiu, C. H. K., Später, T., Beyer, S., & Blocki, A. (2020). Cell-derived extracellular matrix for tissue engineering and regenerative medicine. *Frontiers in Bioengineering and Biotechnology*, *8*, 602009. DOI: 10.3389/fbioe.2020.602009 PMID: 33344434

Baniya, P., Tebyani, M., Hee, W. S., Li, H., Asefifeyzabadi, N., Yang, H., Zhu, K., Keller, G., Franco, C., Schorger, K., Devarajan, K., Barbee, A., Hernandez, C., Nguyen, T., Lu, F., Gallegos, A., Recendez, C., Isseroff, R. R., Zhao, M., & Teodorescu, M. (2024). Wireless bioelectronic device for wound healing. *bioRxiv*, 12, 629068. DOI: 10.1101/2024.12.18.629068

Betancourt, T., & Brannon-Peppas, L. (2006). Micro-and nanofabrication methods in nanotechnological medical and pharmaceutical devices. *International Journal of Nanomedicine*, *1*(4), 483–495. DOI: 10.2147/nano.2006.1.4.483 PMID: 17722281

Blanco-Fernandez, B., Castano, O., Mateos-Timoneda, M. Á., Engel, E., & Pérez-Amodio, S. (2021). Nanotechnology approaches in chronic wound healing. *Advances in Wound Care*, *10*(5), 234–256. DOI: 10.1089/wound.2019.1094 PMID: 32320364

Boateng, J. S., Matthews, K. H., Stevens, H. N., & Eccleston, G. M. (2008). Wound healing dressings and drug delivery systems: A review. *Journal of Pharmaceutical Sciences*, *97*(8), 2892–2923. DOI: 10.1002/jps.21210 PMID: 17963217

Brown, M. B., Martin, G. P., Jones, S. A., & Akomeah, F. K. (2006). Dermal and transdermal drug delivery systems: Current and future prospects. *Drug Delivery*, *13*(3), 175–187. DOI: 10.1080/10717540500455975 PMID: 16556569

Chattopadhyay, S., & Raines, R. T. (2014). Collagen-based biomaterials for wound healing. *Biopolymers*, *101*(8), 821–833. DOI: 10.1002/bip.22486 PMID: 24633807

Chen, M., Przyborowski, M., & Berthiaume, F. (2009). Stem cells for skin tissue engineering and wound healing. *Critical Reviews in Biomedical Engineering*, *37*(4-5), 399–421. DOI: 10.1615/CritRevBiomedEng.v37.i4-5.50 PMID: 20528733

Choi, J. S., Kim, J. D., Yoon, H. S., & Cho, Y. W. (2013). Full-thickness skin wound healing using human placenta-derived extracellular matrix containing bioactive molecules. *Tissue Engineering. Part A*, *19*(3-4), 329–339. DOI: 10.1089/ten.tea.2011.0738 PMID: 22891853

Cong, L., & Zhang, F. (2015). Genome engineering using CRISPR-Cas9 system. *Methods in Molecular Biology (Clifton, N.J.)*, *1239*, 197–217. DOI: 10.1007/978-1-4939-1862-1_10 PMID: 25408407

Cramer, M. C., & Badylak, S. F. (2020). Extracellular matrix-based biomaterials and their influence upon cell behavior. *Annals of Biomedical Engineering*, *48*(7), 2132–2153. DOI: 10.1007/s10439-019-02408-9 PMID: 31741227

Cubo-Mateo, N., & Gelinsky, M. (2021). Wound and skin healing in space: The 3D bioprinting perspective. *Frontiers in Bioengineering and Biotechnology*, *9*, 720217. DOI: 10.3389/fbioe.2021.720217 PMID: 34760878

Czaja, W. K., Young, D. J., Kawecki, M., & Brown, R. M. (2007). The future prospects of microbial cellulose in biomedical applications. *Biomacromolecules*, *8*(1), 1–12. DOI: 10.1021/bm060620d PMID: 17206781

Dash, B., Xu, Z., Lin, L., Koo, A., Ndon, S., Berthiaume, F., Dardik, A., & Hsia, H. (2018). Stem cells and engineered scaffolds for regenerative wound healing. *Bioengineering (Basel, Switzerland)*, *5*(1), 23. DOI: 10.3390/bioengineering5010023 PMID: 29522497

Davis, F. J., & Mitchell, G. R. (2008). Polyurethane based materials with applications in medical devices. In *Bio-materials and prototyping applications in medicine* (pp. 27–48). Springer US., DOI: 10.1007/978-0-387-47683-4_3

Dean, J., Hoch, C., Wollenberg, B., Navidzadeh, J., Maheta, B., Mandava, A., Knoedler, S., Sherwani, K., Baecher, H., Schmitz, A., Alfertshofer, M., Heiland, M., Kreutzer, K., Koerdt, S., & Knoedler, L. (2025). Advancements in bioengineered and autologous skin grafting techniques for skin reconstruction: A comprehensive review. *Frontiers in Bioengineering and Biotechnology*, *12*, 1461328. DOI: 10.3389/fbioe.2024.1461328 PMID: 39840132

Deng, X., Gould, M., & Ali, M. A. (2022). A review of current advancements for wound healing: Biomaterial applications and medical devices. *Journal of Biomedical Materials Research. Part B, Applied Biomaterials*, *110*(11), 2542–2573. DOI: 10.1002/jbm.b.35086 PMID: 35579269

Derr, K., Zou, J., Luo, K., Song, M. J., Sittampalam, G. S., Zhou, C., Michael, S., Ferrer, M., & Derr, P. (2019). Fully three-dimensional bioprinted skin equivalent constructs with validated morphology and barrier Function. *Tissue Engineering. Part C, Methods*, *25*(6), 334–343. DOI: 10.1089/ten.tec.2018.0318 PMID: 31007132

Desmet, C. M., Préat, V., & Gallez, B. (2018). Nanomedicines and gene therapy for the delivery of growth factors to improve perfusion and oxygenation in wound healing. *Advanced Drug Delivery Reviews*, *129*, 262–284. DOI: 10.1016/j.addr.2018.02.001 PMID: 29448035

Dickinson, L. E., & Gerecht, S. (2016). Engineered biopolymeric scaffolds for chronic wound healing. *Frontiers in Physiology*, *7*, 341. DOI: 10.3389/fphys.2016.00341 PMID: 27547189

Donderwinkel, I., Van Hest, J. C., & Cameron, N. R. (2017). Bio-inks for 3D bioprinting: Recent advances and future prospects. *Polymer Chemistry*, *8*(31), 4451–4471. DOI: 10.1039/C7PY00826K

Dong, R., & Guo, B. (2021). Smart wound dressings for wound healing. *Nano Today*, *41*, 101290. DOI: 10.1016/j.nantod.2021.101290

Enoch, S., & Leaper, D. J. (2008). Basic science of wound healing. [Oxford]. *Surgery (Oxford)*, *26*(2), 31–37. DOI: 10.1016/j.mpsur.2007.11.005

Everts, P., Onishi, K., Jayaram, P., Lana, J. F., & Mautner, K. (2020). Platelet-rich plasma: New performance understandings and therapeutic considerations in 2020. *International Journal of Molecular Sciences*, *21*(20), 7794. DOI: 10.3390/ijms21207794 PMID: 33096812

Farasati Far, B., Jameie, L., Taromi, P., Nahavndi, R., & Jamshidi, E. (2025). Dermal and Oral Wound Healing. In *Green Biomaterials in Tissue Engineering* (pp. 297–329). American Chemical Society., DOI: 10.1021/bk-2025-1497.ch009

Fonder, M. A., Lazarus, G. S., Cowan, D. A., Aronson-Cook, B., Kohli, A. R., & Mamelak, A. J. (2008). Treating the chronic wound: A practical approach to the care of nonhealing wounds and wound care dressings. *Journal of the American Academy of Dermatology*, *58*(2), 185–206. DOI: 10.1016/j.jaad.2007.08.048 PMID: 18222318

Frykberg, R. G., & Banks, J. (2015). Challenges in the treatment of chronic wounds. *Advances in Wound Care*, *4*(9), 560–582. DOI: 10.1089/wound.2015.0635 PMID: 26339534

Gao, Z., Su, C., Wang, C., Zhang, Y., Wang, C., Yan, H., & Hou, G. (2021). Antibacterial and hemostatic bilayered electrospun nanofibrous wound dressings based on quaternized silicone and quaternized chitosan for wound healing. *European Polymer Journal, 159*, 110733. DOI: 10.1016/j.eurpolymj.2021.110733

Goodarzi, P., Larijani, B., Alavi-Moghadam, S., Tayanloo-Beik, A., Mohamadi-Jahani, F., Ranjbaran, N., & Arjmand, B. (2018). Mesenchymal stem cells-derived exosomes for wound regeneration. In B. Arjmand (Ed.), *Cell biology and translational medicine, volume 4: Stem cells and cell based strategies in regeneration* (pp. 119–131). Springer. DOI: 10.1007/5584_2018_251

Groll, J., Burdick, J. A., Cho, D.-W., Derby, B., Gelinsky, M., Heilshorn, S. C., Jüngst, T., Malda, J., Mironov, V. A., Nakayama, K., Ovsianikov, A., Sun, W., Takeuchi, S., Yoo, J. J., & Woodfield, T. B. F. (2019). A definition of bioinks and their distinction from biomaterial inks. *Biofabrication, 11*(1), 013001. DOI: 10.1088/1758-5090/aaec52 PMID: 30468151

Guan, G., Lv, Q., Liu, S., Jiang, Z., Zhou, C., & Liao, W. (2022). 3D-bioprinted peptide coupling patches for wound healing. *Materials Today. Bio*, *13*, 100188. DOI: 10.1016/j.mtbio.2021.100188 PMID: 34977527

Guerra, L., Dellambra, E., Panacchia, L., & Paionni, E. (2009). Tissue engineering for damaged surface and lining epithelia: Stem cells, current clinical applications, and available engineered tissues. *Tissue Engineering. Part B, Reviews, 15*(2), 91–112. DOI: 10.1089/ten.teb.2008.0418 PMID: 19196154

Hamdan, S., Pastar, I., Drakulich, S., Dikici, E., Tomic-Canic, M., Deo, S., & Daunert, S. (2017). Nanotechnology-driven therapeutic interventions in wound healing: Potential uses and applications. *ACS Central Science*, *3*(3), 163–175. DOI: 10.1021/acscentsci.6b00371 PMID: 28386594

Hameed, M. A. K., Alsafah, A. H., & Mahdi, H. T. (2024). Beta-Glucan: An Overview of its Properties, sources, Health Benefits, immunity and Extraction methods. *Journal of Kerbala University*, *21*(2).

Hazur, J., Endrizzi, N., Schubert, D. W., Boccaccini, A. R., & Fabry, B. (2021). Stress relaxation amplitude of hydrogels determines migration, proliferation, and morphology of cells in 3D culture. *Biomaterials Science*, *10*(1), 270–280. DOI: 10.1039/D1BM01089A PMID: 34850787

Helmy, Y., Farouk, N., Dahy, A. A., Abu-Elsoud, A., Khattab, R. F., Mohammed, S. E., Gad, L. A., Altramsy, A., Hussein, E., & Farahat, A. (2021). Objective assessment of Platelet-Rich Plasma (PRP) potentiality in the treatment of Chronic leg Ulcer: RCT on 80 patients with Venous ulcer. *Journal of Cosmetic Dermatology*, *20*(10), 3257–3263. DOI: 10.1111/jocd.14138 PMID: 33880860

Henn, D., Zhao, D., Sivaraj, D., Trotsyuk, A., Fischer, K., Fehlmann, T., Levi, B., Keller, A., Chen, K., Qi, L. S., & Gurtner, G. C. (2024). 14. CRISPR/CAS9 edited dendritic cells accelerate wound healing by targeting wound fibroblasts via growth factor signaling. *Plastic and Reconstructive Surgery. Global Open*, *12*(S4), 10. DOI: 10.1097/01.GOX.0001015148.77646.c2

Heo, J. S., Kim, S., Yang, C. E., Choi, Y., Song, S. Y., & Kim, H. O. (2021). Human adipose mesenchymal stem cell-derived exosomes: A key player in wound healing. *Tissue Engineering and Regenerative Medicine*, *18*(4), 537–548. DOI: 10.1007/s13770-020-00316-x PMID: 33547566

Hoganson, D., O'Doherty, E. M., Owens, G. E., Harilal, D. O., Goldman, S. M., Bowley, C. M., Neville, C. M., Kronengold, R. T., & Vacanti, J. P. (2010). The retention of extracellular matrix proteins and angiogenic and mitogenic cytokines in a decellularized porcine dermis. *Biomaterials*, *31*(26), 6730–6737. DOI: 10.1016/j.biomaterials.2010.05.019 PMID: 20576289

Hospodiuk, M., Dey, M., Sosnoski, D., & Ozbolat, I. T. (2017). The bioink: A comprehensive review on bioprintable materials. *Biotechnology Advances*, *35*(2), 217–239. DOI: 10.1016/j.biotechadv.2016.12.006 PMID: 28057483

Hossain, A., Roy, S., & Guin, P. S. (2017). The importance of advanced biomaterials in modern technology: A review. *Asian Journal of Research in Chemistry*, *10*(4), 441–453. DOI: 10.5958/0974-4150.2017.00073.6

Hosty, L., Heatherington, T., Quondamatteo, F., & Browne, S. (2024). Extracellular matrix-inspired biomaterials for wound healing. *Molecular Biology Reports*, *51*(1), 830. DOI: 10.1007/s11033-024-09750-9 PMID: 39037470

Ige, O. O., Umoru, L. E., & Aribo, S. (2012). Natural products: A minefield of biomaterials. *International Scholarly Research Notices*, *1*, 983062. DOI: 10.5402/2012/983062

Islam, S., Bhuiyan, M. R., & Islam, M. N. (2017). Chitin and chitosan: Structure, properties and applications in biomedical engineering. *Journal of Polymers and the Environment*, *25*(3), 854–866. DOI: 10.1007/s10924-016-0865-5

Jabeen, N., & Atif, M. (2024). Polysaccharides based biopolymers for biomedical applications: A review. *Polymers for Advanced Technologies*, *35*(1), e6203. DOI: 10.1002/pat.6203

Jain, K., Avsar, P., Patton, D., Moore, Z., & Murray, B. (2025). What specific challenges do patients with chronic wounds encounter when attending medical appointments related to wound care? A systematic review. *Journal of Tissue Viability*, *100865*(2), 100865. Advance online publication. DOI: 10.1016/j.jtv.2025.100865 PMID: 39978175

Jang, M. J., Bae, S., Jung, Y.-S., Kim, J. C., Park, S. K., Suh, J. S., Yi, S. J., Ahn, S. H., & Lim, J. O. (2021). Enhanced wound healing using a 3D printed VEGF-mimicking peptide incorporated hydrogel patch in a pig model. *Biomedical Materials (Bristol, England)*, *16*(4), 045013. DOI: 10.1088/1748-605X/abf1a8 PMID: 33761488

Jara, C. P., Catarino, C. M., Lei, Y., Velloso, L. A., Karande, P., Velander, W. H., & de Araujo, E. P. (2020). Demonstration of re-epithelialization in a bioprinted human skin equivalent wound model. *Bioprinting (Amsterdam, Netherlands)*, *24*, e00102. DOI: 10.1016/j.bprint.2020.e00102

Jayakumar, R., Prabaharan, M., Kumar, P. S., Nair, S. V., & Tamura, H. J. B. A. (2011). Biomaterials based on chitin and chitosan in wound dressing applications. *Biotechnology Advances*, *29*(3), 322–337. DOI: 10.1016/j.biotechadv.2011.01.005 PMID: 21262336

Jee, C.-H., Eom, N.-Y., Jang, H.-M., Jung, H.-W., Choi, E.-S., Won, J.-H., Hong, I.-H., Kang, B.-T., Jeong, D. W., & Jung, D. I. (2016). Effect of autologous platelet-rich plasma application on cutaneous wound healing in dogs. *Journal of Veterinary Science (Suwon-si, Korea)*, *17*(1), 79–87. DOI: 10.4142/jvs.2016.17.1.79 PMID: 27051343

Jeong, Y. G., Yoo, J. J., Lee, S. J., & Kim, M. S. (2024). 3D digital light process bioprinting: Cutting-edge platforms for resolution of organ fabrication. *Materials Today. Bio*, *101284*, 101284. Advance online publication. DOI: 10.1016/j.mtbio.2024.101284 PMID: 39430572

Jiang, Y., Li, R., Han, C., & Huang, L. (2021). Extracellular matrix grafts: From preparation to application. *International Journal of Molecular Medicine*, *47*(2), 463–474. DOI: 10.3892/ijmm.2020.4818 PMID: 33416123

Johnson, R., & Wang, Y. (2015). Drug delivery systems for wound healing. *Current Pharmaceutical Biotechnology*, *16*(7), 621–629. DOI: 10.2174/138920101666615 0206113720 PMID: 25658378

Jung, J. A., Yoon, Y. D., Lee, H. W., Kang, S. R., & Han, S. K. (2018). Comparison of human umbilical cord blood-derived mesenchymal stem cells with healthy fibroblasts on wound-healing activity of diabetic fibroblasts. *International Wound Journal, 15*(1), 133–139. DOI: 10.1111/iwj.12849 PMID: 29115054

Kelly, B. E., Bhattacharya, I., Heidari, H., Shusteff, M., Spadaccini, C. M., & Taylor, H. K. (2019). Volumetric additive manufacturing via tomographic reconstruction. *Science, 363*(6431), 1075–1079. DOI: 10.1126/science.aau7114 PMID: 30705152

Kennedy, J. F., Knill, C. J., & Thorley, M. (2001). Natural polymers for healing wounds. In *Recent advances in environmentally compatible polymers* (pp. 97–104). Woodhead Publishing., DOI: 10.1533/9781845693749.2.97

Kølle, S. T., Fischer-Nielsen, A., Mathiasen, A. B., Elberg, J. J., Oliveri, R. S., Glovinski, P. V., Kastrup, J., Kirchhoff, M., Rasmussen, B. S., Talman, M. M., Thomsen, C., Dickmeiss, E., & Drzewiecki, K. T. (2013). Enrichment of autologous fat grafts with ex-vivo expanded adipose tissue-derived stem cells for graft survival: A randomised placebo-controlled trial. *Lancet, 382*(9898), 1113–1120. DOI: 10.1016/S0140-6736(13)61410-5 PMID: 24075051

Koshy, J., & Sangeetha, D. (2024). Recent progress and treatment strategy of pectin polysaccharide based tissue engineering scaffolds in cancer therapy, wound healing and cartilage regeneration. *International Journal of Biological Macromolecules, 257*, 128594. DOI: 10.1016/j.ijbiomac.2023.128594 PMID: 38056744

Kubinová, Š., & Syková, E. (2010). Nanotechnologies in regenerative medicine. *Minimally Invasive Therapy & Allied Technologies, 19*(3), 144–156. DOI: 10.3109/13645706.2010.481398 PMID: 20497067

Kusindarta, D. L., & Wihadmadyatami, H. (2018). The role of extracellular matrix in tissue regeneration. *Tissue Regeneration, 65*. Advance online publication. DOI: 10.5772/intechopen.75728

Lacci, K. M., & Dardik, A. (2010). Platelet-rich plasma: Support for its use in wound healing. *The Yale Journal of Biology and Medicine, 83*, 1–9. PMID: 20351977

Lai, J., & Wang, M. (2023). Developments of additive manufacturing and 5D printing in tissue engineering. *Journal of Materials Research, 38*(21), 4692–4725. DOI: 10.1557/s43578-023-01193-5

Laidmäe, I., Ērglis, K., Cēbers, A., Janmey, P. A., & Uibo, R. (2018). Salmon fibrinogen and chitosan scaffold for tissue engineering: In vitro and in vivo evaluation. *Journal of Materials Science. Materials in Medicine, 29*(12), 1–12. DOI: 10.1007/s10856-018-6192-8 PMID: 30506370

Lehmann, T., Vaughn, A. E., Seal, S., Liechty, K. W., & Zgheib, C. (2022). Silk fibroin-based therapeutics for impaired wound healing. *Pharmaceutics*, *14*(3), 651. DOI: 10.3390/pharmaceutics14030651 PMID: 35336024

Li, S., Zhang, H., Sun, L., Zhang, X., Guo, M., Liu, J., Wang, W., & Zhao, N. (2024). 4D printing of biological macromolecules employing handheld bioprinters for in situ wound healing applications. *International Journal of Biological Macromolecules*, *280*(3), 135999. DOI: 10.1016/j.ijbiomac.2024.135999 PMID: 39326614

Liu, X., Michael, S., Bharti, K., Ferrer, M., & Song, M. J. (2020). A biofabricated vascularized skin model of atopic dermatitis for preclinical studies. *Biofabrication*, *12*(3), 035002. DOI: 10.1088/1758-5090/ab76a1 PMID: 32059197

Lopez-Vidal, L., Juskaite, K., Ramöller, I. K., Real, D. A., McKenna, P. E., Priotti, J., Donnelly, R. F., & Paredes, A. J. (2024). Advanced drug delivery systems for the management of local conditions. *Therapeutic Delivery*, *16*(3), 285–303. DOI: 10.1080/20415990.2024.2437978 PMID: 40020739

Majtan, J & Jesenak, M. (2018). β-Glucans: Multi-Functional Modulator of Wound Healing. *Molecules*. Apr 1;23:806. DOI: 10.3390/molecules23040806

Masri, S., & Fauzi, M. (2021). Current Insight of Printability Quality Improvement Strategies in Natural-Based Bioinks for Skin Regeneration and Wound Healing. *Polymers*, *13*(7), 1011. DOI: 10.3390/polym13071011 PMID: 33805995

Masri, S., Zawani, M., Zulkiflee, I., Salleh, A., Fadilah, N. I., Maarof, M., Wen, A. P. Y., Duman, F., Tabata, Y., Aziz, I. A., Bt Hj Idrus, R. B. H., & Fauzi, M. B. (2022). Cellular Interaction of Human Skin Cells towards Natural Bioink via 3D-Bioprinting Technologies for Chronic Wound: A Comprehensive Review. *International Journal of Molecular Sciences*, *23*(1), 476. DOI: 10.3390/ijms23010476 PMID: 35008902

Matai, I., Kaur, G., Seyedsalehi, A., McClinton, A., & Laurencin, C. T. (2020). Progress in 3D bioprinting technology for tissue/organ regenerative engineering. *Biomaterials*, *226*, 119536. DOI: 10.1016/j.biomaterials.2019.119536 PMID: 31648135

Mathew-Steiner, S. S., Roy, S., & Sen, C. K. (2021). Collagen in wound healing. *Bioengineering (Basel, Switzerland)*, *8*(5), 63. DOI: 10.3390/bioengineering8050063 PMID: 34064689

Mayet, N., Choonara, Y. E., Kumar, P., Tomar, L. K., Tyagi, C., Du Toit, L. C., & Pillay, V. (2014). A comprehensive review of advanced biopolymeric wound healing systems. *Journal of Pharmaceutical Sciences*, *103*(8), 2211–2230. DOI: 10.1002/jps.24068 PMID: 24985412

Mazini, L., Rochette, L., Admou, B., Amal, S., & Malka, G. (2020). Hopes and Limits of Adipose-Derived Stem Cells (ADSCs) and Mesenchymal Stem Cells (MSCs) in Wound Healing. *International Journal of Molecular Sciences*, *21*(4), 1306. DOI: 10.3390/ijms21041306 PMID: 32075181

Melrose, J. (2016). Glycosaminoglycans in wound healing. *Bone and Tissue Regeneration Insights*, *7*, BTRI.S38670. Advance online publication. DOI: 10.4137/BTRI.S38670

Milan, P. B., Pazouki, A., Joghataei, M. T., Mozafari, M., Amini, N., Kargozar, S., Amoupour, M., Latifi, N., & Samadikuchaksaraei, A. (2020). Decellularization and preservation of human skin: A platform for tissue engineering and reconstructive surgery. *Methods (San Diego, Calif.)*, *171*, 62–67. DOI: 10.1016/j.ymeth.2019.07.005 PMID: 31302179

Miri, Z., Farè, S., Ma, Q., & Haugen, H. J. (2023). Updates on polyurethane and its multifunctional applications in biomedical engineering. *Progress in Biomedical Engineering (Bristol, England)*, *5*(4), 042001. DOI: 10.1088/2516-1091/acef84

Mogoşanu, G. D., & Grumezescu, A. M. (2014). Natural and synthetic polymers for wounds and burns dressing. *International Journal of Pharmaceutics*, *463*(2), 127–136. DOI: 10.1016/j.ijpharm.2013.12.015 PMID: 24368109

Mogoşanu, G. D., Popescu, F. C., Busuioc, C. J., Pârvănescu, H., & Lascăr, I. (2012). Natural products locally modulators of the cellular response: Therapeutic perspectives in skin burns. *Romanian Journal of Morphology and Embryology = Revue Roumaine de Morphologie et Embryologie*, *53*, 249–262. PMID: 22732793

Murphy, S. V., & Atala, A. (2014). 3D bioprinting of tissues and organs. *Nature Biotechnology*, *32*(8), 773–785. DOI: 10.1038/nbt.2958 PMID: 25093879

Naomi, R., Bahari, H., Ridzuan, P. M., & Othman, F. (2021). Natural-based biomaterial for skin wound healing (Gelatin vs. collagen): Expert review. *Polymers*, *13*(14), 2319. DOI: 10.3390/polym13142319 PMID: 34301076

Neuman, M. G., Nanau, R. M., Oruña-Sanchez, L., & Coto, G. (2015). Hyaluronic acid and wound healing. *Journal of Pharmacy & Pharmaceutical Sciences*, *18*(1), 53–60. DOI: 10.18433/J3K89D PMID: 25877441

Nor-Azlan, A. Y. H., Katas, H., Habideen, N. H., & Mh Busra, M. F. (2020). Dual-action of thermoresponsive gels containing DsiRNA-loaded gold nanoparticles for diabetic wound therapy: Characterization, in vitro safety and healing efficacy. *Saudi Pharmaceutical Journal : SPJ : the Official Publication of the Saudi Pharmaceutical Society*, *28*(11), 1420–1430. DOI: 10.1016/j.jsps.2020.09.007 PMID: 33250649

Nosrati, H., Khouy, R. A., Nosrati, A., Khodaei, M., Banitalebi-Dehkordi, M., Ashrafi-Dehkordi, K., Sanami, S., & Alizadeh, Z. (2021). Nanocomposite scaffolds for accelerating chronic wound healing by enhancing angiogenesis. *Journal of Nanobiotechnology*, *19*(1), 1. Advance online publication. DOI: 10.1186/s12951-020-00755-7 PMID: 33397416

Ovington, L. G. (2007). Advances in wound dressings. *Clinics in Dermatology*, *25*(1), 33–38. DOI: 10.1016/j.clindermatol.2006.09.003 PMID: 17276199

Pallua, N., Wolter, T., & Markowicz, M. (2010). Platelet-rich plasma in burns. *Burns*, *36*(1), 4–8. DOI: 10.1016/j.burns.2009.05.002 PMID: 19541423

Pang, C., Fan, K. S., Wei, L., & Kolar, M. K. (2021). Gene therapy in wound healing using nanotechnology. *Wound Repair and Regeneration*, *29*(2), 225–239. DOI: 10.1111/wrr.12881 PMID: 33377593

Petrie, K., Cox,C.T, Becker,B.C, MacKay, B. J. (2022). Clinical applications of acellular dermal matrices: A review. *Scars Burn Heal*. 19. . Pivec, T., Smole, M. S., Gašparič, P., & Kleinschek, K. S. (2017). Polyurethanes for Medical Use. *Tekstilec*, 60 . https://doi.org/DOI: 10.1177/20595131211038313

Pollini, M., & Paladini, F. (2020). Bioinspired materials for wound healing application:the potential of silk fibroin. *Materials (Basel)*, *13*(15), 3361. DOI: 10.3390/ma13153361 PMID: 32751205

Qu, W., Wang, Z., Hunt, C., Morrow, A. S., Urtecho, M., Amin, M., Shah, S., Hasan, B., Abd-Rabu, R., & Ashmore, Z. (2021). Mayo Clinic Proceedings. Elsevier; Amsterdam, The Netherlands. The Effectiveness and Safety of Platelet-Rich Plasma for Chronic Wounds: A Systematic Review and Meta-analysis; pp. 2407–2417. DOI: 10.3390/biomedicines12010007

Rasouli, M., Rahimi, A., Soleimani, M., & keshel, S. H. (2021). The interplay between extracellular matrix and progenitor/stem cells during wound healing: Opportunities and future directions. *Acta Histochemica*, *123*(7), 151785. DOI: 10.1016/j.acthis.2021.151785 PMID: 34500185

Rimondo, S., Perale, G., & Rossi, F. (2019). Polysaccharide-based scaffold for tissue-regeneration. In Functional polysaccharides for biomedical applications, pp. 189-212 DOI: 10.1016/B978-0-08-102555-0.00006-6

Robin, A., Nandakumar, K., & Sabu, T. (2017). Microbial barrier property and blood compatibility studies of electrospun Poly- -caprolactone/zinc oxide nanocomposite scaffolds. *Journal of Siberian Federal University.Biology (Basel)*, *10*, 226–236.

Saghazadeh, S., Rinoldi, C., Schot, M., Kashaf, S. S., Sharifi, F., Jalilian, E., Nuutila, K., Giatsidis, G., Mostafalu, P., Derakhshandeh, H., Yue, K., Swieszkowski, W., Memic, A., Tamayol, A., & Khademhosseini, A. (2018). Drug delivery systems and materials for wound healing applications. *Advanced Drug Delivery Reviews, 127*, 138–166. DOI: 10.1016/j.addr.2018.04.008 PMID: 29626550

Sala, D. F., Longobardo, G., Fabozzi, A., di Gennaro, M., & Borzacchiello, A. (2022). Hyaluronic acid-based wound dressing with antimicrobial properties for wound healing application. *Applied Sciences (Basel, Switzerland), 12*(6), 3091. DOI: 10.3390/app12063091

Sarheed, O., Ahmed, A., Shouqair, D., & Boateng, J. (2016). Antimicrobial dressings for improving wound healing. *Wound Healing-Nnew Insights into Ancient Challenges*, 374-398.

Shaabani, E., Sharifiaghdam, M., Faridi-Majidi, R., De Smedt, S. C., Braeckmans, K., & Fraire, J. C. (2022). Gene therapy to enhance angiogenesis in chronic wounds. *Molecular Therapy. Nucleic Acids, 29*, 871–899. DOI: 10.1016/j.omtn.2022.08.020 PMID: 36159590

Sharda, D., Attri, K., & Choudhury, D. (2024). Greener healing: Sustainable nanotechnology for advanced wound care. *Discover Nano, 19*(1), 127. DOI: 10.1186/s11671-024-04061-1 PMID: 39136798

Shenoy, Sandhya R., Manasi J. Wagdarikar, and Namita D. Desai. (2024). Polymers in medical devices and pharmaceutical packaging. *Polymers for Pharmaceutical and biomedical Applications*,333-382. DOI: 10.1016/B978-0-323-95496-9.00009-0

Shi, S., Ou, X., Long, J., Lu, X., Xu, S., & Zhang, L. (2024). Nanoparticle-based therapeutics for enhanced burn wound healing: A comprehensive review. *International Journal of Nanomedicine, 19*, 11213–11233. DOI: 10.2147/IJN.S490027 PMID: 39513089

Sierpinski, P., Garrett, J., Ma, J., Apel, P., Klorig, D., Smith, T., Koman, L. A., Atala, A., & Van Dyke, M. (2007). The use of keratin biomaterials derived from human hair for the promotion of rapid regeneration of peripheral nerves. *Biomaterials, 29*(1), 118–128. DOI: 10.1016/j.biomaterials.2007.08.023 PMID: 17919720

Singh, R., Shitiz, K., & Singh, A. (2017). Chitin and chitosan: Biopolymers for wound management. *International Wound Journal, 14*(6), 1276–1289. DOI: 10.1111/iwj.12797 PMID: 28799228

Sivamaruthi, B. S., Nallasamy, P., Suganthy, N., Kesika, P., & Chaiyasut, C. (2022). Pharmaceutical and biomedical applications of starch-based drug delivery system: A review. *Journal of Drug Delivery Science and Technology*, *77*, 103890. DOI: 10.1016/j.jddst.2022.103890

Skylar-Scott, M. A., Mueller, J., Visser, C. W., & Lewis, J. A. (2019). Voxelated soft matter via multimaterial multinozzle 3D printing. *Nature*, *575*(7782), 330–335. DOI: 10.1038/s41586-019-1736-8 PMID: 31723289

Srivastava, A., Yadav, T., Sharma, S., Nayak, A., Kumari, A. A., & Mishra, N. (2015). Polymers in drug delivery. *Journal of Biosciences and Medicines*, *4*(1), 69–84. DOI: 10.4236/jbm.2016.41009

Su, L., Zheng, J., Wang, Y., Zhang, W., & Hu, D. (2019). Emerging progress on the mechanism and technology in wound repair. *Biomedicine and Pharmacotherapy*, *117*, 109191. DOI: 10.1016/j.biopha.2019.109191 PMID: 31387187

Sulaeva, I., Henniges, U., Rosenau, T., & Potthast, A. (2015). Bacterial cellulose as a material for wound treatment: Properties and modifications. A review. *Biotechnology Advances*, *33*(8), 1547–1571. DOI: 10.1016/j.biotechadv.2015.07.009 PMID: 26253857

Suri, S. S., Fenniri, H., & Singh, B. (2007). Nanotechnology-based drug delivery systems. *Journal of Occupational Medicine and Toxicology (London, England)*, *2*(1), 1–6. DOI: 10.1186/1745-6673-2-16 PMID: 18053152

Sutcliffe, J. E., Thrasivoulou, C., Serena, T. E., Madden, L., Richards, T., Phillips, A. R., & Becker, D. L. (2017). Changes in the extracellular matrix surrounding human chronic wounds revealed by 2-photon imaging. *International Wound Journal*, *14*(6), 1225–1236. DOI: 10.1111/iwj.12789 PMID: 28730726

Suthar, M., Gupta, S., Bukhari, S., & Ponemone, V. (2017). Treatment of chronic non-healing ulcers using autologous platelet rich plasma: A case series. *Journal of Biomedical Science*, *24*(1), 16. DOI: 10.1186/s12929-017-0324-1 PMID: 28241824

Tocco, I., Zavan, B., Bassetto, F., & Vindigni, V. (2012). Nanotechnology-based therapies for skin wound regeneration. *Journal of Nanomaterials*, *714134*(1), 1–11. DOI: 10.1155/2012/714134

Tumbleston, J. R., Shirvanyants, D., Ermoshkin, N., Janusziewicz, R., Johnson, A. R., Kelly, D., Chen, K., Pinschmidt, R., Rolland, J. P., Ermoshkin, A., Samulski, E. T., & DeSimone, J. M. (2015). Continuous liquid interface production of 3D objects. *Science*, *347*(6228), 1349–1352. DOI: 10.1126/science.aaa2397 PMID: 25780246

Turner, N. J. (2021). Application of extracellular matrix in regenerative medicine. *Applied Sciences (Basel, Switzerland), 11*(7), 3262. DOI: 10.3390/app11073262

Uddin, F., Rudin, C. M., & Sen, T. (2020). CRISPR gene therapy: Applications, limitations, and implications for the future. *Frontiers in Oncology, 10*, 1387. DOI: 10.3389/fonc.2020.01387 PMID: 32850447

Vasconcelos, A., & Cavaco-Paulo, A. (2011). Wound dressings for a proteolytic-rich environment. *Applied Microbiology and Biotechnology, 90*(2), 445–460. DOI: 10.1007/s00253-011-3135-4 PMID: 21360151

Velasco, D., Quílez, C., Garcia, M., Del Cañizo, J.F., Jorcano, J.L. (2018). 3D human skin bioprinting: A view from the bio side. Journal of 3D Printing in Medicine, 2, 141–162.

Wallace, E. R., Yue, Z., Dottori, M., Wood, F. M., Fear, M., Wallace, G. G., & Beirne, S. (2023). Point of care approaches to 3D bioprinting for wound healing applications. *Progress in Biomedical Engineering (Bristol, England), 5*(2), 023002. DOI: 10.1088/2516-1091/acceeb

Weiliang, Z., & Lili, G. (2021). Research advances in the application of adipose-derived stem cells derived exosomes in cutaneous wound healing. *Annals of Dermatology, 33*(4), 309. DOI: 10.5021/ad.2021.33.4.309

Wu, S. C., Marston, W., & Armstrong, D. G. (2010). Wound care: The role of advanced wound-healing technologies. *Journal of the American Podiatric Medical Association, 100*(5), 385–394. DOI: 10.7547/1000385

Ye, K. Y., Sullivan, K. E., & Black, L. D. (2011). Encapsulation of cardiomyocytes in a fibrin hydrogel for cardiac tissue engineering. *Journal of Visualized Experiments, 19*(55), 3251. DOI: 10.3791/3251-v

Zhang, X., Shu, W., Yu, Q., Qu, W., Wang, Y., & Li, R. (2020). Functional biomaterials for treatment of chronic wounds. *Frontiers in Bioengineering and Biotechnology, 8*, 516. DOI: 10.3389/fbioe.2020.00516

Zhang, X., Yang, J., Li, Y., Liu, S., Long, K., Zhao, Q., Zhang, Y., Deng, Z., & Jin, Y. (2011). Functional neovascularization in tissue engineering with porcine acellular dermal matrix and human umbilical vein endothelial cells. *Tissue Engineering. Part C, Methods, 17*(4), 423–433. DOI: 10.1089/ten.tec.2010.0466

Zhong, W., Xing, M. M., & Maibach, H. I. (2010). Nanofibrous materials for wound care. *Cutaneous and Ocular Toxicology, 29*(3), 143–152. DOI: 10.3109/15569527.2010.489307

Chapter 9
Regenerative Medicine and Tissue Engineering: Transforming Healthcare

Vivek Pazhamalai
https://orcid.org/0000-0003-2088-7545
Vels Institute of Science, Technology and Advanced Studies, Chennai, India

S. Ivo Romauld
https://orcid.org/0000-0003-0610-0646
Vels Institute of Science, Technology and Advanced Studies, Chennai, India

P. Dharshika
https://orcid.org/0009-0009-7342-297X
Vels Institute of Science, Technology and Advanced Studies, Chennai, India

S. S. Meenambiga
https://orcid.org/0000-0002-5445-525X
Vels Institute of Science, Technology and Advanced Studies, Chennai, India

Kosireddy Vanitha
https://orcid.org/0009-0008-7348-1235
Vels Institute of Science, Technology and Advanced Studies, Chennai, India

K. Rajakumari
https://orcid.org/0000-0002-8102-9512
Vels Institute of Science, Technology and Advanced Studies, Chennai, India

V. T. Thanush
https://orcid.org/0009-0009-6895-3442
Vels Institute of Science, Technology and Advanced Studies, Chennai, India

ABSTRACT

Tissue engineering, stem cells, and cloning are just a few of the technological fields that falls under regenerative medicine. Tissue engineering techniques utilize the cellular matrices, which rely on the body's inherent capacity for regeneration to ensure that new tissue growth is properly oriented and directed, and the use of matrices containing cells. Biomaterials give cells a three-dimensional environment in which to develop into new tissues with the right structure and function. They can

DOI: 10.4018/979-8-3373-1305-4.ch009

also facilitate the distribution of cells and the right bioactive substances, such as growth factors and cell adhesion peptides, to the body's intended locations. Current regulations and ethical considerations advise that before a novel tissue engineering and regenerative medicine technique or instrument is implemented into standard clinical practice and used by numerous patients, controlled randomized clinical trials must be carried out. Clinical studies involving regeneration treatments have revealed some restrictions, difficulties, and unknowns.

1. INTRODUCTION TO TISSUE ENGINEERING AND REGENERATIVE MEDICINE

Living cells, biocompatible materials, appropriate biochemical (like growth factors), physical (like cyclic mechanical stress) components, and their combinations are used in the relatively young subject of tissue engineering to produce structures that resemble tissue. Placing these tissue constructs into the body to fix damage or replace a failing organ's function is usually the end objective. Bone and cartilage are examples of structural components; skin and blood arteries are examples of barrier and transport components; and the liver and pancreas are examples of biochemical and secretory components. The two main types of tissue engineering techniques are the use of acellular matrices, which rely on the body's inherent capacity for regeneration to ensure that new tissue growth is properly oriented and directed, and the use of matrices containing cells, (Atala, 2004). To advance and develop innovative and sophisticated strategies, such as bio-inspired modeling of human diseases, novel drug screening tools, micro-tissue engineering, and biomarker identification with predictive and therapeutic action, tissue engineering has been branching out into new and exciting areas of biomedicine, combining its inherent multidisciplinary nature with technological advancements, (Gomes et al., 2017). Most tissue engineering techniques now in use rely on a sample of autologous cells taken from the host's damaged organ. However, a tissue biopsy may not produce enough normal cells for growth and transplantation in many patients with significant end-stage organ failure, (Atala, 2006). Tissue engineering, stem cells, and cloning are just a few of the technological fields that fall under the umbrella of regenerative medicine. One of the key subfields of regenerative medicine, tissue engineering, applies materials science, engineering, and cell transplantation concepts to create biological replacements that can preserve and restore normal function. Acellular scaffolds, which rely on the body's inherent capacity for regeneration to ensure the correct orientation and direction of new tissue formation, and scaffolds seeded with cells are the two main types of tissue engineering techniques, (Olson, Atala, & Yoo, 2011). Tissue Engineering and Regenerative Medicine (TERM) takes a multidisciplinary approach to creating and using novel therapeutic techniques and products to treat and repair tissue defects and modulate illness. Significant advancements have been made in this sector since the end of the previous century, and the TERM scientists' results in recent years have been particularly remarkable, (Cancedda, Murphy, & Van Griensven, 2023). Since most human tissues do not regenerate independently, "regenerative medicine engineering" is one of the most promising alternative therapies available today. The idea is straightforward: cells are gathered and inserted into damaged tissue, either with or without changes to their biological characteristics, or they are preserved in a porous three-dimensional medium where their mechanical and physicochemical characteristics are maintained, once these tissues or cells are fully developed, they can be grafted, heart failure, blood vessels, diabetes, osteoarthritis, liver disease, bladder, skin, etc. may be one of the main therapeutic uses for the middle term, (Stoltz *et al.*, 20120. Tissue engineering and regenerative medicine (TERM) are cutting-edge fields that, by providing innovative approaches to the regeneration and restoration of damaged organs and tissues, have the potential to substantially alter healthcare. By combining the concepts of cellular biology, material science, and engineering, TERM addresses significant problems like tissue defects and organ failure, providing hope for a range of medical conditions. Micro-tissue engineering, bio-inspired modeling, and biomaterial design are recent examples of how rapidly the field is evolving. Even though issues like obtaining enough cells for transplantation still exist, TERM's multidisciplinary approach and ongoing research are making it a crucial part of future medical innovation and are leading to the development of revolutionary treatments.

2. PRINCIPLES OF TISSUE ENGINEERING

Using advanced material science, stem cell science, physics, developmental biology, and clinical translation to regenerate complex tissues and organ systems. Regenerative engineering is a development of tissue engineering, which aims to promote the integration of engineering science and medicine. Its goal is to establish an interdisciplinary team of scientists, engineers, physicists, and clinicians for integrated approaches to treating different diseases. This has led to recent developments in the field of tissue engineering based on biomaterials. New techniques for producing induced pluripotent stem cells have also been made possible by a better understanding of adult and embryonic stem (ES) cells, (Esdialle, Washington, & Laurencin, 2021). The majority of tissue engineering uses living cells, therefore getting enough cells is a crucial problem. Usually, cells come from either (a) stem or progenitor cells or (b) donor tissue, which is frequently quite scarce. The two main characteristics of stem cells—their great proliferative potential and their pluripotency, or capacity to develop into cells of numerous lineages—make them appealing for the extraction of vast amounts of cells. Controlled delivery methods can also be employed to extend the initial soluble factor load's life. Among the techniques used include chemical conjugation to the scaffold material itself, encapsulation in tiny biodegradable particles, and the expression and release of the factors via transfected cells. After identifying the cells, scaffolds, and environmental requirements, one must think about suitable assembly methods. There were many significant mistakes in the early studies in this field, which simply combined all the components at random before implantation, (Berthiaume, Maguire, & Yarmush, 2011).

2.1 Scaffold Design and Fabrication

To create mechanically strong structures with controlled rates of degradation and porosity for the passage of nutrients, gases, and regulatory factors, TERM has primarily used 3D porous scaffolds and hydrogels. Some of the traditional technological techniques that have been employed for scaffold manufacturing and have shown cheap costs and ideal physicochemical qualities structures are the foam replica method, particulate-leaching, freeze-drying, gas foaming, and phase separation. Supercritical fluid technologies, microfluidics, and advanced manufacturing techniques like 3D printing and robocasting have recently been used to create complex structures for faulty tissue regeneration. These structures are superior to traditional ones in several ways, including enhanced cellular adhesion, structural and mechanical qualities, and porosity, (Pina *et al.,* 2019). Despite the complexity of scaffold functional requirements, these design goals can be quantitatively defined using particular tissue constitutive models. Numerous factors can impact tissue regeneration both separately and in combination, such as mass transport problems, controlled growth factor release, and cell-matrix interaction, making it even more difficult to determine quantitative design targets for improving tissue regeneration. In the early 1990s, Robert Langer and associates established two essential scaffold-design requirements: the need to satisfy cellular metabolic demands through scaffold diffusivity and the enhancement of tissue regeneration through regulation of cell–scaffold interaction, (Hollister, 2009). There are two types of scaffolds: natural and manmade. There are benefits and disadvantages to both kinds of materials. Donor tissues, such as donor trachea, are used to create natural scaffolds, which are then decellularized to eliminate any immunogenic cellular components. Enzymatic, physical, or chemical methods can all be used to accomplish decellularization. Removing every cellular component while maintaining the extracellular matrix composition and angiogenic factors is the goal of the optimal decellularization process. Regretfully, there is currently no consensus regarding the best decellularization technique for tracheal tissue. Furthermore, there is ongoing discussion regarding a variety of decellularization-related topics, including the quantity of cycles and the "grade" of decellularization. Good biocompatibility and the existence of an extracellular matrix (ECM) with the same original tissue composition, microarchitecture, microvasculature, and signaling components are two benefits of a natural scaffold. However, after being implanted, decellularized tissues will unavoidably experience resorption and degradation; additionally, the decellularization procedure and post-implantation tissue degradation mean that the scaffold's stiffness is frequently insufficient to preserve a patent airway lumen. Finally, a natural scaffold necessitates a variable duration for the decellularization process, which typically takes weeks to months, and an animal donor source, which may be scarce. Finally, a scaffold may consist of several layers, known as hybrid scaffolds, in which natural and synthetic tissues are mixed to overcome their drawbacks. Ghorbani et al.'s study serves as an example. They created a scaffold with an inner layer made of decellularized aorta and an exterior layer made of electrospun nanofibers made of a combination of collagen and polycaprolactone (PCL), (Mammana et al., 2024). Tissue engineering is one possible strategy to drastically reduce the demand for tissues and organs. Significant challenges still need to be overcome to guarantee the viability of tissue engineering, even if current research has focused on producing functional tissues. Current concerns that still plague tissue engineering include creating materials for cell transplantation, preventing tissue and cell rejection, maintaining tissues and cells for long-term preservation, and promoting blood vessel and neuron growth. Understanding the fundamentals of tissue engineering and how to modify each component to satisfy the intended requirements of tissue regeneration is crucial in attempts to address these problems. Cells, scaffolds, and growth factors are essential components and instruments for successful tissue engineering, (Do et al., 2018).

Representation of basic characteristics of tumor tissue engineered (TTE) scaffolds in combination with varied nanostructured materials, regulatory and growth factors and cell types are all illustrated in Figure 1.

Figure 1 Representation of basic characteristics of tumor tissue engineered (TTE) scaffolds in combination with varied nanostructured materials, regulatory and growth factors and cell types

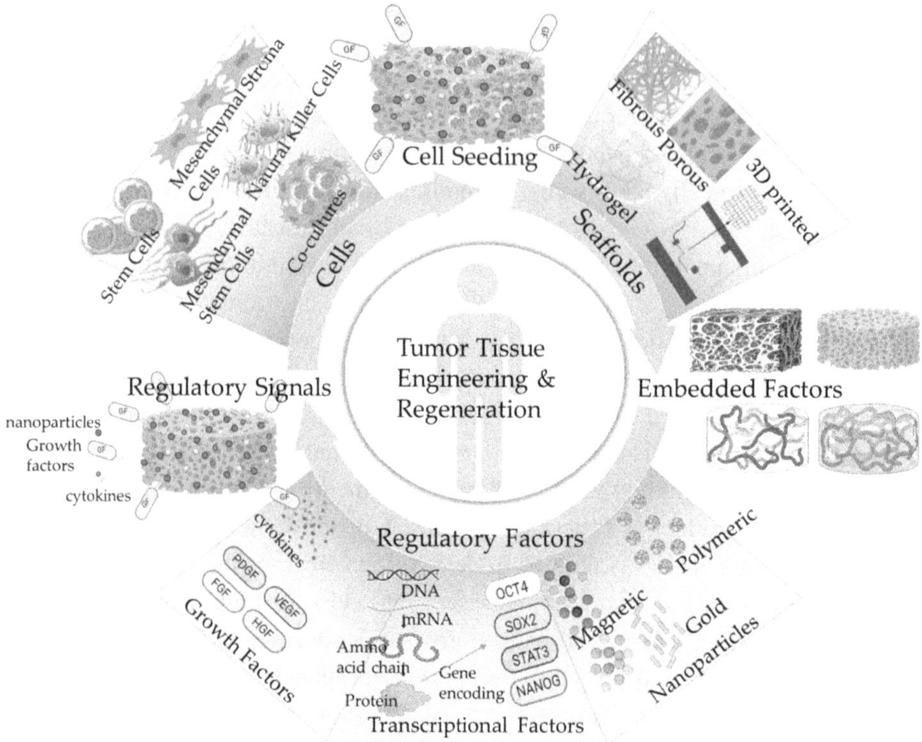

3. BIOMATERIALS FOR TISSUE ENGINEERING

Biomaterials, cells, and bioactive chemicals are typically used in some combination in tissue engineering (TE), which blends biology and engineering concepts. The application in question, the tissue replacement plan, and patient characteristics like age and co-morbidities, among others, determine each factor's proper contribution. Both in-vitro and in-vivo procedures can be used in TE tactics, and as stem cell biology, biomaterial science, and bioreactor technology progress, the best strategy for each clinical application will continue to change. The need for the engineered tissue to grow and adapt to the surrounding tissue presents another challenge for TE in the pediatric population because patients are still developing. In the field of TE, biomaterials are crucial, if not vital. Although biomaterials have been utilized for millennia for procedures like dental fillings and intraocular lens replacement, developments in cell and molecular biology, chemistry, materials science, and engineering have opened up a wide range of clinical application options. The perfect biomaterial has seen significant modification over the past 50 years and will differ depending on the application. The objective of early biomaterial design was to produce a level of functional output that closely matched natural tissue while avoiding tissue damage or a harmful host response, as well as to match mechanical and material qualities, (Keane & Badylak, 2014). The word "biomaterial" has several meanings in the legal and scientific domains. "Any instrument, apparatus, implant, machine, appliance, in vitro reagent or calibrator, software, material, or other similar or related articles, intended by the manufacturer to be used, alone or in combination, for human beings for one or more of the specific purposes of diagnosing, preventing, monitoring, treating, investigating, supporting or sustaining life, controlling conception, and disinfecting medical devices" is the legal meaning of a medical device. Biomaterials are essential to the creation of tissue constructions because they serve as a three-dimensional support environment and artificial extracellular matrix for cells that migrate from the host tissue in vivo or are entrained in vitro to regenerate a wound site. Polymers, ceramics, composites, and even metals—whether synthetic or natural—can all be used as biomaterials in tissue engineering. With the exception of orthopedics, polymers are the most widely used biomaterials in tissue engineering because of their mechanical adaptability and resemblance to the structural properties of tissue. Biodegradable polymers have emerged as the standard for the majority of medical and related applications because they also show little long-term inflammation or problems linked to repeated surgical procedures. Thermoplastic polyesters like poly(lactic acid) (PLA), poly(glycolic acid) (PGA), and polycaprolactone (PCL), as well as their mixes or copolymers, currently dominate the market for polymeric biomaterials, (Chen, Liang, & Thouas, 2013). The goal of tissue engineering is to use various techniques to regenerate and repair damaged tissues. Any substance, structure, or surface that interacts with biological processes is referred to as a biomaterial. It is utilized for partial or complete tissue replacement and can be produced synthetically or from natural sources, (Eldeeb, Salah, & Elkasabgy, 2022). Because of their many benefits, including biocompatibility, ease of manufacture, renewability, cheap cost, availability, and Non immunogenicity, biomaterials derived from natural sources are currently the subject of considerable study. Four major categories can be used to classify biomaterials that come from natural sources: materials derived from proteins, polysaccharides, glycosaminoglycans, and extracellular matrix. Natural biomaterials are typically employed for (i) replacing or repairing damaged tissue or organs, (ii) encouraging tissue regeneration, (iii) delivering drugs, and (iv) creating bone scaffolds, (Chelu & Musuc, 2023).

3.1 Advances in 3D Printing and Bio-Inks

The bio-ink and bioprinter are essential components for creating 3D bioprinted structures. The fabrication process affects crucial elements including strength, resolution, and shape. Originally developed in the early 2000s, droplet-based bioprinting (DBB) is a quick and easy method for precisely and carefully depositing biologics. Without the nozzle coming into contact with the substrate, picoliter droplets are piled on top of it. Because it can print inks with low viscosities (3.5–12 mPa s−1), is compatible with a wide range of biological materials, and allows for fast speed and high resolution, DBB is incredibly flexible. For DBB, inkjet bioprinting is the most used method. It encompasses electrodynamic inkjet bioprinting, drop-on-demand inkjet, and continuous inkjet. Because of the Rayleigh-Plateau instability, the bio-ink solution in the chamber is extruded through a nozzle during continuous inkjet bioprinting, causing the stream to fragment into droplets. Bio-inks are essential parts of bioprinting since they are biomaterial solutions that contain living cells. The biomaterial solution's constituents must shield the cells from stresses during the printing process. Hydrogels, microcarriers, cell aggregates, and decellularized matrix components are the four primary categories of bio-ink materials. In DBB, bioink droplets should produce accurate deposition and shield the cells from stresses. Droplet integrity is a crucial property for this, and it can be changed by the bio-inks material components, (Donderwinkel, Van Hest, & Cameron, 2017). In conclusion, droplet-based bioprinting (DBB) represents a versatile and precise method for creating 3D bioprinted structures. Its ability to handle low-viscosity bio-inks, achieve high resolution, and support a wide range of biological materials makes it a powerful tool in tissue engineering and regenerative medicine. DBB's efficacy, however, is largely dependent on the characteristics of the bio-ink, which must maintain droplet integrity and cell viability while reducing printing stress. Continued advancements in bio-ink formulations and printing techniques are essential to overcome current limitations, paving the way for future more complex and functional printed structures.

4. STEM CELLS IN REGENERATIVE MEDICINE

4.1 Types of Stem Cells

Stem cells can regenerate themself. In the early phases of life and development, it can change into different kinds of cells in the body. There are numerous types of stem cells, including nonembryonic/somatic stem cells, induced pluripotent stem cells, and pluripotent stem cells, which can be embryonic stem cells. Pluripotent stem cells tend to be able to differentiate into all the cells in the body. The stem cells present in the tissue and organ can be differentiated into different specialized cell types.

4.1.1 Pluripotent Stem Cells

The inner cell mass and trophectoderm cells are two of the cell types found in the blastocyst of early embryos. While the inner cell mass would also grow into specialized cell types, tissues, and organs, the trophectoderm cells are found in the placenta. Some matured human adult cells can be regenerated into an embryonic stem cell. These stem cells are known to be induced pluripotent stem cells (iPSCs). Pluripotent stem cells are said to be undifferentiated as they do not possess tissue-specific characteristics like morphology to perform specialized functions.

4.1.2 Adult Stem Cells

The Adult stem cells contribute as an internal repair system that helps in the replacement of cells that have been lost through cell tears, injury, or some disease. Adult stem cells are found in tissues and organs. Adult stem cells may also stay undivided for a long period until they stay activated for more cells by default which helps to sustain tissue repairs, (Mahla, 2016).

4.1.3 Embryonic Stem Cells

Embryonic stem cells (ESC) are the most likely to differentiate into different tissues, which require the reconstruction of human embryos. In a recent study by Harvard University, they fused human embryonic stem cells to human fibroblast cells, resulting in stable tetraploid DNA content, which is the hybrid cells that represent the source of the therapeutic approach, (Cowan et al., 2005). The ESC can proliferate in a pluripotent state yet to be undifferentiated and can transform into differentiated cell types. The ESC is taken from the embryo's inner cell mass in the blastocyte.

Human ESC has differentiated in vitro cells from the embryonic germ layers. The skin, neurons contribute to ectodermal differentiation. Blood, cells of cardiac, cartilage, endothelial tissue, and muscle cells differentiate from the mesodermal tissue, and the pancreatic cells have contributed to endodermal distinction.

4.2 Regenerative Medicine

Regenerative medicine is the most unfold branch of medical field, that revolves with restoring function of tissues and organs of patients those who were suffering from severe injuries or chronic disease conditions, where the body's regenerative responses are sufficient, (Mason & Dunnill, 2008). Stem cells are used for all tissues and organ systems in the body, and they play a diversified role in the progression, development, and tissue repair processes. Based on regenerative medicine applications stem cells can be classified as ESCs, tissue-specific progenitor stem cells, mesenchymal stem cells, umbilical cord stem cells, bone marrow stem cells, and iPSCs. Stem cells show major histocompatibility complex receptors less and they secret chemokine that recruits the endothelial and immune cells for enables the tissue tolerance at the graft site.

Stem cells, such as the ESC, secrete vasculogenic and neurogenic factors, which support tissue in spinal cord-associated diseases. Regenerating this spinal tissue would improve balance. In cardiovascular diseases, stem cells are applied in ESC-derived CMs. Cardiomyocytes show GCaMP3, and Tbox3 distinct ESCs. In the MSCs, in case of dental problems, the mode of action of stem cells occurs in transplants of the EMSCs as biopolymer tissue. IPSCs have derived NPCs transplantation. TSPSCs in regenerative medicine involve the tissue-specific stem cells and the progenitor cells which can differentiate into various cells of the tissue. MSCs includes $CD73^+$, $CD34^-$, $CD45^-$, $CD14^-$, $CD19^-$, and $CD79a^-$ cells, known to be stromal cells. These MSCs do not involve in the bone marrow.

BMSCs and UCSCs are vital components in the regenerative medicine, each offering unique benefits and applications. BMSCs are derived from the spongy bone marrow tissue and comprise a variety of cell types, including mesenchymal, stromal, and hematopoietic stem cells. These cells, which can differentiate into a variety of cell types and are crucial for the production of blood, are especially useful for bone regeneration and the repair of tissues damaged by illnesses like heart conditions. On the other hand, UCSCs—which come from umbilical cord tissue offer a convenient alternative for individualized medical care. By restoring tissue balance in cases of neuroblastoma and regenerating myelin in patients with Krabbe's disease, they have shown great promise in the treatment of neurodegenerative diseases. Additionally, UCSCs can be injected intravenously to treat a variety of illnesses, such as diabetes, Hodgkin's lymphoma, systemic lupus erythematosus, and long-term dialysis-related complications like peritoneal fibrosis. When combined, BMSCs and UCSCs offer hope for novel treatments for a range of illnesses, representing a promising new area in regenerative medicine, (Mahla, 2016).

Stem cell types and their therapeutic applications are listed in Table 1.

4.2.1 ESCs

ESCs are known to be pluripotent, which can give rise to more than 150 cell types that promise to give various types of treatment to any kind of disease, (Thomson, 1998). The transcription factors OCT4 and SOX2 control the rate of pluripotency of the ESCs. In connection with the retinal ganglion cells, medicines are being generated from CRISPR-Cas9, where the gene BRN3B is specifically expressed in RGSs and can be used to specific and purify the other generated RGSs from the other cells, (Sluch et al., 2015). To restore heart functions and increase the rate of survival of heart patients, the regeneration of cardiac tissue is done using cardiomyocyte transplantation. Cardiovascular progenitor-ECSs derived, and bone marrow-derived mononuclear cells are the mature cardiomyocytes would have tissue healing activity which suppresses the heart arrhythmias, proving without involving any of the tumorigenic associated effects, (Shiba et al., 2012) (Fernandes et al., 2015).

Table 1. Different stem cell types and their therapeutic applications

Stem Cell Type	Applications	Mechanisms/Key Insights
ESCs (Embryonic Stem Cells)	Treats ARMD, spinal cord injuries, diabetes, osteoarthritis, cardiovascular diseases, etc.	Differentiates into >200 cell types. CRISPR-Cas9 enhances retinal ganglion cell generation. Forskolin boosts axonal growth.
Retinal Ganglion Cells	ARMD and glaucoma therapy	CRISPR-Cas9 targets BRN3B gene. Incorporation into biomaterial scaffolds improves axonal differentiation.
Cardiomyocytes	Cardiovascular therapy, reduces arrhythmias, supports electrical repair of the heart	Derived from ESCs and progenitors. Integrates with heart tissues for mechanical and electrical repair.
Hepatocytes	Liver injury treatment, drug screening	ESCs stimulated by VitK12 and lithocholic acid differentiate into hepatocytes producing albumin and apolipoprotein B100.
Pancreatic Cells	**β**-Diabetes treatment (T2DM)	ESCs transdifferentiated into insulin-secreting β-cells via PDX1 epigenetic reprogramming.
Chondrocytes	Osteoarthritis treatment	ESC-derived cells embedded in fibrin gel regenerate cartilage in joint injuries.
Pacemaker Cells	Biological pacemaker for heart rhythm regulation	ESCs with TBox3 expression generate pacemaker-like cells.
TSPSCs (Tissue-Specific Progenitor Stem Cells)	Diverse tissue regeneration (intestinal, dental, corneal, etc.)	Multipotent; retains tissue specificity. Can differentiate into neurons, goblet cells, cochlear hair cells, and more.
PPCs (Pancreatic Progenitor Cells)	Diabetes treatment; produces β-cells	Grows in 3D scaffolds to form insulin-producing cell clusters.
DPSCs (Dental Pulp Stem Cells)	Neurodental therapies and nerve regeneration	Differentiates into neuronal cells responsive to neurotransmitters (e.g., acetylcholine, GABA).
IESCs (Inner Ear Stem Cells)	Deafness treatment	Notch signaling inhibition via LY411575 promotes cochlear hair cell regeneration.

continued on following page

Table 1. Continued

Stem Cell Type	Applications	Mechanisms/Key Insights
IPCs (Intestinal Progenitor Cells)	Treatment of intestinal injuries (e.g., necrotizing enterocolitis)	Combines progenitors with immune and connective tissue cells in 3D biomaterials to regenerate intestinal mucosa.
LPSCs (Limbal Progenitor Stem Cells)	Corneal regeneration	Transplanted cells regrow into functional human corneal tissue.
Mesoangioblasts (MABs)	Muscle regeneration for Duchenne muscular dystrophy (DMD)	Coaxing MABs in PEG-fibrinogen hydrogel supports muscle fiber formation.
AdSCs (Adipose-Derived Stem Cells)	Retinal vascular repair, heart regeneration	Produces vasoprotective factors; differentiates into endothelial cells, vascular smooth muscle cells, and cardiomyocytes.
SKPs (Skin-Derived Precursors)	Wound healing and angiogenesis	Derived from dermal papilla; gives rise to neurons, Schwann cells, chondrocytes, and vascular smooth muscle cells.
Fallopian Tube Stem Cells	Fertility restoration, ovarian cancer research	Differentiates into fallopian tube organoids under active Wnt and Notch signaling.
CA-AdSCs (Cardiac Adipose-Derived Stem Cells)	Myocardial ischemia therapy	Differentiates into heart tissue and improves cardiac function.

4.2.2 TSPSCs

TSPSCs is a well-known stem cell that helps in sustaining the homeostasis of tissue by the progression of continuous cell division. The TSPSCs contribute to maintaining the plasticity and differentiation of the stem cells, which also give rise to new types of cells. It contributes to the therapeutic application on progenitor cells (PPCs), dental pulp stem cells (DPSCs), intestinal progenitor cells (IPCs), skin-derived precursors (SKPs), epithelial progenitor stem cells (EPSCs), and adipose-derived stem cells (ADSCs).

The PPCs differentiation to change into the -cells is regulated by insulin negatively, (Ye et al., 2016). So, the PPCs require notch signalling to grow faster rather than a single population for renewing itself and differentiation. The transplantation of the cornea stem cells of mice to fully regrown functional human cornea is made efficient through the blood-eye barrier, which is used for the treatment of various types of eye diseases and is vital for the regenerating corneal tissue that is essential for the restoration of the vision, (Ksander et al., 2014).

4.2.3 MSCs

The MSCs are the stromal cells, which are multi stem cells that can differentiate into the tissue of the mesodermal origin only, which is categorized into tendons, bone, cartilages, ligaments, muscles, and neurons. Bone marrow-derived MSCs (BMDMSCs) are employed to regenerate bladder tissue and share morphological and phenotypic similarities with bladder stem cells, (Mahla, 2016). Stem cell therapies are mostly in the experimental stage. However, there is hope for the future as researchers work on new compounds that can activate tissue-specific stem cells. This activation could help these stem cells move to areas of tissue injury and transform into the specific cells needed for repair. Advances in using stem cells to treat conditions like muscle damage, cancer, autoimmune diseases, and spinal cord injuries could lead to significant benefits for patients facing a variety of health challenges. As this field continues to evolve, it holds great promise for improving patient outcomes across many different diseases.

5. GROWTH FACTORS AND TISSUE ENGINEERING

The growth factors support the tissues' cellular development, multiplication, and differentiation. Following a wound, transforming growth factor-β1 (TGF-β1) and platelet-derived growth factor (PDGF) are two of the growth factors that will be present in the case of natural regeneration as soon as the blood vessels are damaged. During the healing process, this growth consists of endothelial cells, fibroblasts, and macrophages. Growth factors support wound closure by preserving the integrity of the tissue in question.

Together with TGF-β1 and FGF-2, BMPs are known to be essential osteogenic factors in the context of bone regeneration, supporting the differentiation of mesenchymal stem cells into osteoblasts. employing polymer scaffolds that have the ability to release growth factors, which improves these progenitor cells' recruitment and differentiation. Additionally, adding growth factors to scaffold materials has proven successful in encouraging chondrocyte differentiation and guaranteeing appropriate tissue integration.

Hepatocyte function and survival are enhanced by growth factors like EGF and HGF, which are also advantageous for hepatic tissue engineering. For transplanted cells to survive, there must be sufficient vascularization at the transplantation site. In skin tissue engineering, growth factors such as TGF-β and PDGF are used to effectively treat chronic wounds. Scaffolds infused with vascular endothelial growth factor (VEGF) aid in cardiac tissue engineering's cardiac repair procedures. Tissue engineering applications in a variety of biological systems depend on the effective fusion of cells, scaffolds, and growth factors, (Hassanzadeh, 2012).

5.1 Growth Factor Interaction With GAGs

Growth factors are immobilized by glycosaminoglycans (GAGs), particularly heparan sulfate-GAGs (HS-GAGs), which are an essential part of the extracellular matrix (ECM). The process by which these GAGs interact non-covalently with different growth factors, referred to as "heparin-binding," includes vascular endothelial growth factor (VEGF), platelet-derived growth factor, and basic fibroblast growth factor. Positively charged amino acids in the growth factors attach to the negatively charged sulfate and carboxyl groups present in HS-GAGs through ionic and van der Waals forces. To stabilize growth factors and increase their biological activity by encouraging receptor activation and starting downstream signaling pathways, such binding is necessary for their sequestration within the extracellular matrix. Consequently, these growth factors are stored in the extracellular matrix (ECM), making them easily accessible for critical cellular functions such as tissue repair, differentiation, and proliferation. In conclusion, preserving cellular processes and promoting tissue health depend heavily on the interaction between growth factors and GAGs, (Mitchell *et al.,* 2016).

5.2 Growth Factors and Biomaterials

To help damaged tissues regenerate, tissue engineering uses a variety of biomaterials, with solid synthetics and hydrogel-type materials being especially common. Matrigel, an extracellular matrix comprising essential elements such as laminin, fibronectin, and proteoglycans, is one prominent example. In addition to promoting cell division, matrigel preserves the structural characteristics of Schwann and olfactory ensheathing cells. Its ability to promote axonal regeneration with vascular endothelial growth factor (VEGF) has been demonstrated through its successful use as a scaffold for delivering Schwann cells in spinal cord injuries. Fibronectin mats, which are derived from plasma fibronectin and contain components like neurotrophin-3 and brain-derived neurotrophic factor, are another crucial substance that has demonstrated promise in fostering nerve regeneration. A biocompatible polysaccharide called alginate works well as a scaffold for neutrosphere cell transplantation and improves spinal cord injury recovery. Polyethylene glycol (PEG) has also been used to improve growth factor pharmacokinetics and seal cell membrane breaches, making it easier for growth factors to pass through the blood-brain barrier.

Because of their biocompatibility and ability to mimic the effects of cell scaffold constructs—which are sometimes improved with basic fibroblast growth factor (bFGF) to promote nerve extension—fibrin-based scaffolds are gaining popularity. Growth factor-loaded poly (2-hydroxyethyl methacrylate-co-methyl methacrylate) (PHEMA) hydrogels have also demonstrated promise in supporting nerve regeneration. Collagen gels are being researched for the localized delivery of therapeutic medicines following spinal cord injury because they may encourage axonal regrowth. Poly[N-(2-hydroxypropyl) methacrylamide] (PHPMA) hydrogels are recent innovations that promote axonal regrowth following brain damage. Although side effects have complicated clinical trials, ciliary neurotrophic factor (CNTF) has shown promise as a treatment for degenerative motoneuron disorders such as amyotrophic lateral sclerosis (ALS).

To improve CNTF's stability and delivery while reducing systemic effects, researchers are looking into microencapsulation techniques. All things considered, the advancement of tissue engineering techniques meant to successfully repair and regenerate damaged tissues depends on the combination of different biomaterials and growth factors, (Hassanzadeh, 2012).

5.3 Delivery Systems in Tissue Engineering

In tissue engineering, creating delivery systems is crucial for releasing drugs and bioactive proteins over extended periods. These systems can be made from a variety of natural or synthetic polymers, which may be either degradable or non-degradable. Recently, particle-based delivery systems have become increasingly popular due to their ability to enhance the solubility of poorly water-soluble compounds, extend the half-life of therapeutic agents in the bloodstream, and allow for targeted drug delivery that minimizes side effects. To improve drug delivery to the central nervous system (CNS), researchers have developed non-invasive techniques using nano systems and colloidal carriers, which are often lipid- or polymer-based. Among these, polymeric nanoparticles stand out as promising candidates because they can encapsulate drugs, protecting them from metabolism and enabling their transport across the blood-brain barrier without causing damage. Various polymers, such as polylactide-co-glycolide (PLGA), chitosan, poly (butyl cyanoacrylate) (PBCA), and poly (cyanoacrylate-co-hexadecyl cyanoacrylate) (PHDCA), have been used to create these nanoparticles. Additionally, strategies like using blood-brain barrier permeabilizers, genetically engineered cells, and biodegradable or non-biodegradable polymeric devices have been explored to ensure a continuous supply of neuroactive agents. Overall, advancements in these delivery systems are essential for improving the effectiveness of drug therapies in tissue engineering, especially when targeting the complex environment of the CNS.

6. STEM CELL THERAPY

Stem cell treatment replaces or overrides defective cells to indirectly erase or make up for the genetic weakness. Although there are specific difficulties with each technique (as each method depends on the type and source of cells), stem cell therapy is recognized to show potential in the treatment of numerous human diseases. These difficulties include problems with immunity, rejection of graft vs host, teratoma or cancer hazards, purification, growth, upkeep, cost, and reproducibility. Many businesses tried to advance embryonic stem cells (ESC) technology in the early to mid-2000s, but most of them gave up on the technology due to ethical and technical difficulties and turned their focus to more conventional pharmaceuticals like small molecule compounds.

Because of the simplicity of CRISPR-Cas gene editing, other stem cell methods, such that of induced pluripotent stem cells (iPSCs), are probably going to see a comeback in the therapeutic field. Certain of the epigenetic issues may be addressed by researchers using CRISPR-Cas technologies difficulties that iPSCs have previously been linked to. Eventually, rekindled interest in iPSC therapies will compete with other, more well-established stem cell therapies like Mesenchymal Stem Cell (MSC) medications like Alofisel a TiGenix (Leuven, Belgium) and Takeda Pharmaceutical Company's (Osaka, Osaka Prefecture, Japan) recently approved European product. In general, a wave of innovation is expected to sweep over the stem cell sector in the years ahead, (Malcolm, Mitchell, & Muni, 2020).

7. IMMUNOLOGICAL CHALLENGES AND SOLUTIONS

7.1 Immunological Challenges for Protein Thiol Oxidation State

Click PEGylation is an innovative method used to analyze the redox state of protein thiols by attaching polyethylene glycol (PEG) to specific sites on proteins. However, this technique encounters several significant challenges that can hinder its effectiveness in immunological applications. Steric hindrance is a major issue; the PEG polymer can prevent antibodies from attaching to the protein's epitope, which could lead to a partial or total loss of signal in assays. PEGylation of multiple thiols exacerbates this problem because it reduces the possibility of antibody binding, especially with polyclonal antibodies.

Furthermore, PEGylation-induced mass shift makes it more difficult to transfer and detect proteins on membranes, which could result in an underestimation of signals for mass-shifted proteins. It can be challenging to correctly interpret results when sodium dodecyl sulfate (SDS) is present because it can further distort the bands of PEGylated proteins during electrophoresis. Reversible oxidation processes also add complexity because oxidized thiols can contaminate reduced thiol bands, making selective reduction techniques necessary to successfully distinguish between different oxidation states. Finally, exposure to dioxygen during cell lysis can result in the artificial oxidation of thiols via free radical mechanisms, which are influenced by various factors like the availability of metal ions. Improving Click PEGylation's dependability and suitability for researching protein thiol redox states requires addressing these issues, (Cobley & Husi, 2020).

7.2 Immunological Solutions for Protein Thiol Oxidation State

The proposed solutions to enhance Click PEGylation for assessing protein thiol redox states focus on implementing an "antibody first" immunocapture workflow. This involves labeling the primary antibody with dibenzocyclooctyne (DBCO) functionalized N-hydroxysuccinimide to form stable bonds with primary amines. The labeled antibody is then incubated with the sample and captured using an azide-functionalized resin through strain-promoted azide-alkyne cycloaddition (SPAAC). The antibody-target complex, which can be eluted even in the absence of the antibody, can be isolated with high stringency using this technique. Tz-PEG5 is added after elution to start the IEDDA reaction, which allows mass changes in the gel to be seen using Coomassie or silver staining. For large proteins like ryanodine receptor 1 (RYR1), which has numerous solvent-exposed thiols, substituting Tz-PEG5 with a fluorescently labeled compound such as Tz-Cy5 can facilitate quantification of thiol exposure. Additionally, anti-PEG antibodies can be utilized to assess various reversible thiol oxidation types using a single antibody, streamlining the screening process. To address the reactivity of alkylating agents with sulfenic acid (SOH), researchers suggest using Dyn-2, a reagent that selectively labels SOH. This could enhance the specificity of Click PEGylation workflows. Collectively, these strategies aim to improve the reliability and applicability of Click PEGylation in studying protein thiol redox states while overcoming existing challenges, (Cobley & Husi, 2020).

8. SCAFFOLDS IN CLINICAL APPLICATIONS

In order to successfully infiltrate and attach with the right bioactive molecules to support cell division and growth the scaffold requires to be biocompatible mechanically and structurally stable be biodegradable and provide temporary support to repair injured cartilage a variety of natural biomaterials have been produced including gelatin hyaluronan fibrin adhesive sodium alginate hydrogel or chitosan and additionally artificial materials such polylactic acid 23 due primarily to the potential of immunoreaction and disease transmission these materials are now only used in limited clinical settings, (Iwasa et al., 2009).

Depending on the application or disease modeling, a number of tissue engineering techniques can be used, including selecting the appropriate cell source, creating organoids using natural or composite scaffolds, and adding bioreactor tools, as shown in Figure 2.

Figure 2. The development of organoids with natural or composite scaffold support, the careful selection of GI cell sources, and bioreactor technologies are current GI efforts to construct tissue-engineered intestines.

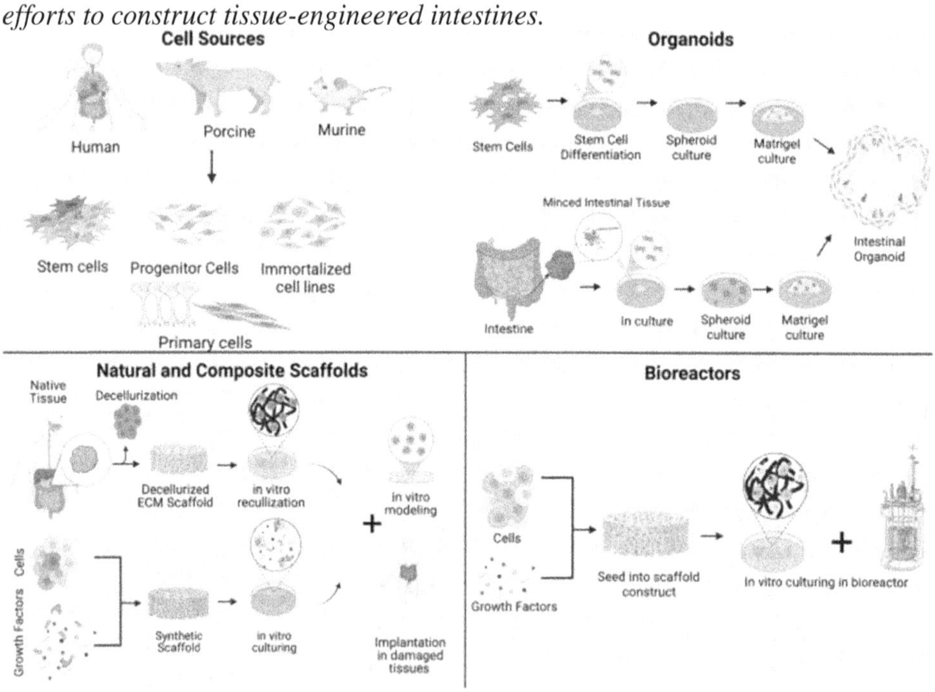

9. CLINICAL TRAILS

during the years 2000 and 2002 the USAs share of labor force fell from 80 to 54 20 tissue-engineered goods were commencing research studies with the food and drug administration fda by the close of 2002 though four have been authorized not one of them have become financial success as of yet six additional requests have either dropped or did not acquire approval of the product there remained ten products in clinical studies the most of those that were in phase iphase ii and some of which had been funded by investigators despite spending over 45 billion on research and development as a whole this sector is yet to create a viable product it is clear that tissue engineering is finding it difficult to achieve the shift from an experimental stage to one with a profitable product line, (Lysaght & Hazlehurst, 2004).

10. BARRIERS TO CLINICAL TRANSLATION

Since they are easier to reach and have more tissue available, the bone marrow & fatty tissues have historically been the best tissue sources for MSC extraction. In addition to producing better chondrogenic differentiation than bone marrow-derived MSCs, adipose-derived MSCs have been demonstrated to isolate more MSCs per tissue volume than bone-derived MSCs. The two adipose tissue harvest sites most frequently utilized for MSC isolation are the infrapatellar fat pad (IFP) and abdominal subcutaneous tissue. IFP tissue has been demonstrated to have a higher chondrogenic potential despite the fact that abdominal fat underneath the skin is more prevalent, (Francis *et al.,* 2018).

11. CHALLENGES AND FUTURE PERSPECTIVE

The goal of "prevascularization" techniques is to create neo-organs that have an existing channel structure in order to make it easier to create a functional vascular network. This can be done by either pre-seeding endothelial lineage cells into the channels or by recruiting them in vivo via biochemical cues that the scaffold releases or embeds. The challenge remains, though, of how to design channels so that the body will perceive them as its own vascular network. Decellularized tissue could be used as the scaffold as a solution, (Olson, Atala, & Yoo, 2011).

although autologous vascular tissue has been effectively used to treat a variety of cardiovascular disorders cvds such as atherosclerosis it is frequently insufficient for transplantation 12 consequently the goal of tissue-engineered vascular graft tevg development is to offer substitutes for autologous tissue even though numerous research have been published on the development of tevgs utilizing various materials and techniques some of the drawbacks of traditional grafts like the potential for blood clots still exist in this study we examined the findings from recent publications in the area of developing tevgs for use in human and animal models, (Kitsuka et al., 2022).

In a way, the most advanced "smart" biomaterials are created when cells are included through electrospinning or printing. Biomaterials that exhibit interactive activity, capable of responding to and modulating cellular activities and the surrounding environment, can be created even in the absence of cells. At the molecular level, several teams have investigated the creation of biomaterials that combi2e the biological properties of proteins with the benefits of synthetic polymers. The term "smart polymers" was first used to describe materials that change their structure significantly according to environmental cues like slight variations in pH, temperature, or ionic strength. Polymer crosslinking can be triggered by light stimulation. DNA uptake can be aided by ultrasound, which can also cause nanobubble creation, (Furth & Atala, 2014).

12. CONCLUSION

The rapidly developing fields of tissue engineering and regenerative medicine have enormous potential to revolutionize healthcare by providing creative ways to regenerate and repair damaged tissues and organs. This multidisciplinary approach creates biological replacements that can return to normal function by combining concepts from biology, materials science, and engineering. Fundamentally, it makes use of living cells, biocompatible materials, and biochemical variables to create tissue constructs that can be inserted into the body to treat a range of illnesses, such as tissue defects and organ failure. As a result of the developments, new methods like micro-tissue engineering and 3D printing are being investigated, which improve the functionality and appearance of scaffolds used in tissue regeneration. These scaffolds, which can be constructed from natural or synthetic materials and offer different benefits and difficulties, offer a supportive environment for cell growth. For example, natural scaffolds frequently have problems with availability and degradation, even though they closely resemble the structure of human tissues. However, while synthetic scaffolds can be designed to have particular characteristics, they might not have all of the biological cues present in natural tissues. Even though this field has made great strides, there are still obstacles to overcome, especially in obtaining enough cells for transplantation and guaranteeing successful integration with host tissues.

REFERENCES

Atala, A. (2004). Tissue engineering and regenerative medicine: Concepts for clinical application. *Rejuvenation Research*, *7*(1), 15–31. DOI: 10.1089/154916804323105053 PMID: 15256042

Atala, A. (2006). Recent developments in tissue engineering and regenerative medicine. *Current Opinion in Pediatrics*, *18*(2), 167–171. DOI: 10.1097/01.mop.0000193294.94646.be PMID: 16601497

Berthiaume, F., Maguire, T. J., & Yarmush, M. L. (2011). Tissue engineering and regenerative medicine: History, progress, and challenges. *Annual Review of Chemical and Biomolecular Engineering*, *2*(1), 403–430. DOI: 10.1146/annurev-chembioeng-061010-114257 PMID: 22432625

Cancedda, R., Murphy, J. M., & Van Griensven, M. (2023). Insights in tissue engineering and regenerative medicine 2021: Novel developments, current challenges, and future perspectives. *Frontiers in Bioengineering and Biotechnology*, *10*, 1125027. DOI: 10.3389/fbioe.2022.1125027 PMID: 36714627

Chelu, M., & Musuc, A. M. (2023). Advanced biomedical applications of multifunctional natural and synthetic biomaterials. *Processes (Basel, Switzerland)*, *11*(9), 2696. DOI: 10.3390/pr11092696

Chen, Q., Liang, S., & Thouas, G. A. (2013). Elastomeric biomaterials for tissue engineering. *Progress in Polymer Science*, *38*(3-4), 584–671. DOI: 10.1016/j.progpolymsci.2012.05.003

Cobley, J. N., & Husi, H. (2020). Immunological techniques to assess protein thiol redox state: Opportunities, challenges and solutions. *Antioxidants*, *9*(4), 315. DOI: 10.3390/antiox9040315 PMID: 32326525

Cowan, C. A., Atienza, J., Melton, D. A., & Eggan, K. (2005). Nuclear reprogramming of somatic cells after fusion with human embryonic stem cells. *Science*, *309*(5739), 1369–1373. DOI: 10.1126/science.1116447 PMID: 16123299

Do, A. V., Smith, R., Acri, T. M., Geary, S. M., & Salem, A. K. (2018). 3D printing technologies for 3D scaffold engineering. In *Functional 3D tissue engineering scaffolds* (pp. 203–234). Woodhead Publishing. DOI: 10.1016/B978-0-08-100979-6.00009-4

Donderwinkel, I., Van Hest, J. C., & Cameron, N. R. (2017). Bio-inks for 3D bioprinting: Recent advances and future prospects. *Polymer Chemistry*, *8*(31), 4451–4471. DOI: 10.1039/C7PY00826K

Eldeeb, A. E., Salah, S., & Elkasabgy, N. A. (2022). Biomaterials for tissue engineering applications and current updates in the field: A comprehensive review. *AAPS PharmSciTech*, *23*(7), 267. DOI: 10.1208/s12249-022-02419-1 PMID: 36163568

Esdaille, C. J., Washington, K. S., & Laurencin, C. T. (2021). Regenerative engineering: A review of recent advances and future directions. *Regenerative Medicine*, *16*(5), 495–512. DOI: 10.2217/rme-2021-0016 PMID: 34030463

Fernandes, S., Chong, J. J. H., Paige, S. L., Iwata, M., Torok-Storb, B., Keller, G., Reinecke, H., & Murry, C. E. (2015). Comparison of human embryonic stem cell-derived cardiomyocytes, cardiovascular progenitors, and bone marrow mononuclear cells for cardiac repair. *Stem Cell Reports*, *5*(5), 753–762. DOI: 10.1016/j.stemcr.2015.09.011 PMID: 26607951

Francis, S. L., Di Bella, C., Wallace, G. G., & Choong, P. F. (2018). Cartilage tissue engineering using stem cells and bioprinting technology—Barriers to clinical translation. *Frontiers in Surgery*, *5*, 70. DOI: 10.3389/fsurg.2018.00070 PMID: 30547034

Furth, M. E., & Atala, A. (2014). Tissue engineering: future perspectives. In *Principles of tissue engineering* (pp. 83–123). Academic Press. DOI: 10.1016/B978-0-12-398358-9.00006-9

Gomes, M. E., Rodrigues, M. T., Domingues, R. M., & Reis, R. L. (2017). Tissue engineering and regenerative medicine: New trends and directions—a year in review. *Tissue Engineering. Part B, Reviews*, *23*(3), 211–224. DOI: 10.1089/ten.teb.2017.0081 PMID: 28457175

Hassanzadeh, P. (2012). Tissue engineering and growth factors: Updated evidence. *Biomedical Reviews*, *23*(0), 19–35. DOI: 10.14748/bmr.v23.26

Hollister, S. J. (2009). Scaffold design and manufacturing: From concept to clinic. *Advanced Materials*, *21*(32-33), 3330–3342. DOI: 10.1002/adma.200802977 PMID: 20882500

Iwasa, J., Engebretsen, L., Shima, Y., & Ochi, M. (2009). Clinical application of scaffolds for cartilage tissue engineering. *Knee Surgery, Sports Traumatology, Arthroscopy : Official Journal of the ESSKA*, *17*(6), 561–577. DOI: 10.1007/s00167-008-0663-2 PMID: 19020862

Keane, T. J., & Badylak, S. F. (2014, June). Biomaterials for tissue engineering applications. [). WB Saunders.]. *Seminars in Pediatric Surgery*, *23*(3), 112–118. DOI: 10.1053/j.sempedsurg.2014.06.010 PMID: 24994524

Kitsuka, T., Hama, R., Ulziibayar, A., Matsuzaki, Y., Kelly, J., & Shinoka, T. (2022). Clinical Application for Tissue Engineering Focused on Materials. *Biomedicines, 10*(6), 1439. DOI: 10.3390/biomedicines10061439 PMID: 35740460

Ksander, B. R., Kolovou, P. E., Wilson, B. J., Saab, K. R., Guo, Q., Ma, J., McGuire, S. P., Gregory, M. S., Vincent, W. J. B., Perez, V. L., Cruz-Guilloty, F., Kao, W. W. Y., Call, M. K., Tucker, B. A., Zhan, Q., Murphy, G. F., Lathrop, K. L., Alt, C., Mortensen, L. J., & Frank, N. Y. (2014). ABCB5 is a limbal stem cell gene required for corneal development and repair. *Nature, 511*(7509), 353–357. DOI: 10.1038/nature13426 PMID: 25030174

Lysaght, M. J., & Hazlehurst, A. L. (2004). Tissue engineering: The end of the beginning. *Tissue Engineering, 10*(1-2), 309–320. DOI: 10.1089/107632704322791943 PMID: 15009955

Mahla, R. S. (2016). Stem cells applications in regenerative medicine and disease therapeutics. *International Journal of Cell Biology, 2016*(1), 6940283. DOI: 10.1155/2016/6940283 PMID: 27516776

Malcolm, T., Mitchell, D. A., & Muni, N. (2020). Second Generation Genome Editing Technologies in Drug Discovery. In *Second Generation Cell and Gene-based Therapies* (pp. 213–242). Academic Press. DOI: 10.1016/B978-0-12-812034-7.00008-X

Mammana, M., Bonis, A., Verzeletti, V., Dell'Amore, A., & Rea, F. (2024). Tracheal Tissue Engineering: Principles and State of the Art. *Bioengineering (Basel, Switzerland), 11*(2), 198. DOI: 10.3390/bioengineering11020198 PMID: 38391684

Mason, C., & Dunnill, P. (2008). A brief definition of regenerative medicine. *Regenerative Medicine, 3*(1), 1–5. DOI: 10.2217/17460751.3.1.1 PMID: 18154457

Mitchell, A. C., Briquez, P. S., Hubbell, J. A., & Cochran, J. R. (2016). Engineering growth factors for regenerative medicine applications. *Acta Biomaterialia, 30*, 1–12. DOI: 10.1016/j.actbio.2015.11.007 PMID: 26555377

Olson, J. L., Atala, A., & Yoo, J. J. (2011). Tissue engineering: Current strategies and future directions. *Chonnam Medical Journal, 47*(1), 1–13. DOI: 10.4068/cmj.2011.47.1.1 PMID: 22111050

Olson, J. L., Atala, A., & Yoo, J. J. (2011). Tissue engineering: Current strategies and future directions. *Chonnam Medical Journal, 47*(1), 1–13. DOI: 10.4068/cmj.2011.47.1.1 PMID: 22111050

Pina, S., Ribeiro, V. P., Marques, C. F., Maia, F. R., Silva, T. H., Reis, R. L., & Oliveira, J. M. (2019). Scaffolding strategies for tissue engineering and regenerative medicine applications. *Materials (Basel)*, *12*(11), 1824. DOI: 10.3390/ma12111824 PMID: 31195642

Shiba, Y., Fernandes, S., Zhu, W.-Z., Filice, D., Muskheli, V., Kim, J., Palpant, N. J., Gantz, J., Moyes, K. W., Reinecke, H., Van Biber, B., Dardas, T., Mignone, J. L., Izawa, A., Hanna, R., Viswanathan, M., Gold, J. D., Kotlikoff, M. I., Sarvazyan, N., & Laflamme, M. A. (2012). Human ES-cell-derived cardiomyocytes electrically couple and suppress arrhythmias in injured hearts. *Nature*, *489*(7415), 322–325. DOI: 10.1038/nature11317 PMID: 22864415

Sluch, V. M., Davis, C.-H. O., Ranganathan, V., Kerr, J. M., Krick, K., Martin, R., Berlinicke, C. A., Marsh-Armstrong, N., Diamond, J. S., Mao, H.-Q., & Zack, D. J. (2015). Differentiation of human ESCs to retinal ganglion cells using a CRISPR engineered reporter cell line. *Scientific Reports*, *5*(1), 16595. Advance online publication. DOI: 10.1038/srep16595 PMID: 26563826

Stoltz, J. F., Zhou, Y. F., He, X. H., Chen, Y., Stoltz, J. F., Decot, V., & Bensoussan, D. (2012). Introduction to regenerative medicine and tissue engineering. *Bio-Medical Materials and Engineering*, *22*(1-3), 3–16. DOI: 10.3233/BME-2012-0684 PMID: 22766697

Thomson, J. A., Itskovitz-Eldor, J., Shapiro, S. S., Waknitz, M. A., Swiergiel, J. J., Marshall, V. S., & Jones, J. M. (1998). Embryonic stem cell lines derived from human blastocysts. *Science*, *282*(5391), 1145–1147. DOI: 10.1126/science.282.5391.1145 PMID: 9804556

Ye, L., Robertson, M. A., Mastracci, T. L., & Anderson, R. M. (2016). An insulin signaling feedback loop regulates pancreas progenitor cell differentiation during islet development and regeneration. *Developmental Biology*, *409*(2), 354–369. DOI: 10.1016/j.ydbio.2015.12.003 PMID: 26658317

Chapter 10
Scaffold for Tissue Engineering Design Fabrication and Applications

Nida Iqbal
https://orcid.org/0000-0002-8502-4954
University of Engineering and Technology Lahore, Pakistan

Muhammad Asad Ullah
University of Engineering and Technology, Lahore, Pakistan

Muhammad Zaeem Khalid
https://orcid.org/0009-0007-3517-0746
University of Engineering and Technology, Lahore, Pakistan

Syed Tasawar Hussain
University of Engineering and Technology, Lahore, Pakistan

ABSTRACT

Recently, Tissue engineering (TE) has been rapidly growing field in biomedical field, it provides the solutions to the problem such as immunological rejection and a shortage of available donors. TE scaffolds encourage cell adhesion, proliferation, and differentiation by simulating the extracellular matrix with three-dimensional matrices. Current, advancements in artificial intelligence (AI) and nanotechnology have improved the design, pore size, mechanical properties. However, scaffolds lack the ability of vascularization, immune compatibility, and scalability. In order to address this issue, scaffolds surface-functionalized with anti-inflammatory cyto-

DOI: 10.4018/979-8-3373-1305-4.ch010

kines such as IL-10 that can increase the integration, less rejection, and long-term performance. Therefore, it is considered that the combination of nanotechnology and AI scaffold design will enhance bioactivity, mechanical strength, and cellular behavior modeling. Regenerative medicine is poised for a revolution due to significant advancements in scaffold-based TE.

INTRODUCTION

Many conditions and illnesses could have severe consequences on the body, including organ failure and, in some cases, even possible death; other conditions can only be well controlled. Although current methods, such as autografting, which is the procedure of transplanting an organ or tissue from the same organism, and allografting, which is transplanting of an organ or tissue from one member of the same species to another, also come to replace or repair damaged tissues or organs but it is not readily accessible. There is a risk of producing an immune response in a patient and spreading infectious diseases. Tissue engineering holds great promise in regenerative healthcare, particularly in developing biomimetic scaffolds that can significantly mitigate the environmental impact on various aspects of medical research (Tajurahim et al., 2025).

The historical development of scaffold-based tissue engineering and Bioprinting is the key to the development of regenerative medicine. Autografts and natural biomaterials were the primary reliance in the initial years of tissue engineering but were not scalable and not highly biocompatible. Synthetic scaffolds, bioactive composites, and sophisticated polymeric matrices have, over time, transformed tissue engineering with better control over mechanical properties and degradation rates. The development of 3D Bioprinting in the early 2000s brought unprecedented precision in scaffold production, enabling the production of patient-specific tissue architecture. Volumetric Bioprinting, light-based printing, and artificial intelligence-based scaffold design are revolutionizing regenerative medicine. Incorporating nanotechnology, innovative biomaterials, and bioinformatics, the latest bioprinting technologies now allow real-time tissue growth modeling and organ regeneration, a breakthrough in healthcare (Gharibshahian et al., 2024). These techniques provide the solution to address the shortcomings of the existing scaffold materials and tissue engineering. Scaffolds, which are biomaterials used to assist with the development of tissue repair, augmentation, and maintenance, are part of tissue engineering. Other functions of these cells include working as the template for repairing and regenerating the damaged tissue and delivering the best possible way for different elements to ensure their cell is still alive, experiencing proliferation, and finally, differentiation (Suamte et al., 2023). In recent advancements, porous scaffold biomaterials are combined with cells to facilitate the regeneration of damaged tissues. If the replacing, regenerating, and repairing are the kind of treatment for disease or trauma-induced tissue degeneration or injury, then the treatment in the case is. Success is made possible by life-saving and innovative techniques, such as autograft or allograft. Unfortunately, these are prone to many more serious problems, such as tissue rejection.

Improvements in tissue engineering and regenerative medicine can overcome such limitations by replacing biological tissues with biological replacements that allow tissue function. A component of tissue engineering is the application of biological science and engineering concepts. A significant function of the porous three-dimensional (3D) scaffolds used as a template is to provide a suitable environment for tissue regeneration.

Recently, nano-scaffolds have been utilized in tissue engineering applications because of their nanoscale architecture mimicking the extracellular matrix in nature. Biomedical use of nanofibrous scaffolds was discussed and exemplified based on their potential in bone, cardiovascular, and neural regeneration. In addition, research on using Nano topographies in bone tissue engineering reveals nano-scaffolds' capacity to modulate the immune system and osteogenic differentiation. Evidence depicts the relevance of nano-scaffolds in enhancing scaffold functionality for tissue regeneration (Omidian & Gill, 2024).

Scaffolds are prepared by seeding growth factors and viable cells and directly translated into the body for transplantation or in vitro tissue generation. Different types of biomaterials are used to construct scaffolds, such as bioceramics (hydroxyapatite, bioglasses), natural and synthetic polymers, polymers (polylactic acid (PLLA), poly dl lactic acid (PLGA), polystyrene, and polyglycolic acid (PGA)). Biomaterials can perform functions in the biological environment, such as assessing, treating, and replacing any tissue or organ in the body. An advantage of these polymers is that the change may vary degrading characteristics in the composition of the polymer. Despite this, they would suffer a rejection risk due to decreased bioactivity. Natural material scaffolds have superior cell adhesion and biological activity. Collagen, alginate-based scaffolds, chitosan, and proteoglycans are the most commonly used natural materials. They are biodegradable and do not prevent host cells from forming the extracellular matrix (ECM) (Koyyada & Orsu, 2021).

Therefore, tissue engineering has emerged as a promising field that can situate itself in solving the problems of classical grafting techniques by using scaffolds in tissue regeneration. Scaffolds have three-dimensional (3D) structures to support cell adhesion, proliferation, and differentiation and guide the new growth of functional tissues.

Nano-scaffolds address many of the fundamental issues of tissue engineering with improved mechanical stability, bioactivity, and cell response. Experiments have demonstrated that incorporating nanoparticles into scaffolding structures improves vascularization, reduces inflammation, and controls drug delivery for regenerative medicine. Functionalizing the nanostructure surface enhances cell adhesion, growth, and differentiation, improving tissue integration and survival.

The field of scaffold-based tissue engineering has experienced incredible development in recent decades. Scaffolds were initially derived from natural biomaterials such as collagen, alginate, chitosan, and fibrin, and these demonstrated fair biocompatibility and bioactivity.

Metallic nanoparticles like silver (Ag), zinc oxide (ZnO), and titanium dioxide (TiO_2) have been added to scaffolds for their improved mechanical strength, antimicrobial properties, and biocompatibility. The work with scaffolds based on nanoparticles revealed immense potential for healing and preventing infection from bacteria. Thus, they are highly beneficial to tissue engineering applications. Adding metallic nanoparticles improves mechanical strength but can also be used for drug delivery and controlled degradation, making their performance in regenerative medicine superior.

Their mechanical properties and degradation patterns were difficult to manage, and they were restricted to application in load-bearing tissues to some extent. Due to such shortcomings, researchers shifted towards synthetic polymers such as polylactic acid (PLA), Polycaprolactone (PCL) and polyglycolic acid (PGA) were characterized by controlled degradation rates and mechanical properties. These polymers possessed better structural strength and were suitable for orthopedic, dental, and soft tissue engineering applications. Synthetic polymers are often deficient in high bioactivity and, therefore, are less than optimal. Hence, to improve biological performance, various tyeps of bioactive ceramics (hydroxyapatite and bioactive glass) or functionalizing with biomolecules are thus essential to enhance cellular response and tissue integration(*WIREs Nanomed Nanobiotechnol - 2023 - Rahmani Del Bakhshayesh - Recent Advances in Nano-scaffolds for Tissue Engineering.Pdf*, n.d.). With computational modeling and artificial intelligence (AI) development, scaffold design has become a precision engineering task. Previously, scaffolding manufacturing was performed through trial-and-error techniques, which were costly and time-consuming. Recent developments have integrated machine learning algorithms and computational simulations to tailor scaffold porosity, mechanical properties, and degradation rates before physical manufacturing. AI-aided approaches, such as generative design and topology optimization, enable scientists to predict the behavior of scaffolds in biological environments, thereby maximizing nutrient diffusion, vascularization, and cell attachment(Mukasheva et al., 2024). In addition, bioprinting and electrospinning technologies are combined with AI to print hierarchical architecture scaffolds that replicate the extracellular matrix (ECM) at the nanoscale. Patient-specific scaffolds designed in line with a patient's anatomy, innovative biomaterials that can detect physiological stimuli, and nanotechnology-based modifications (e.g., nanoparticle coatings for drug targeting) are future trends from 2023 to 2025. These advances represent a milestone shift from static scaffolds to dynamic, bioactive systems with the potential to drive regeneration, reduce immune rejection, and improve long-term clinical outcomes (Cheng et al., 2024).

Figure 1. Key components of tissue engineering

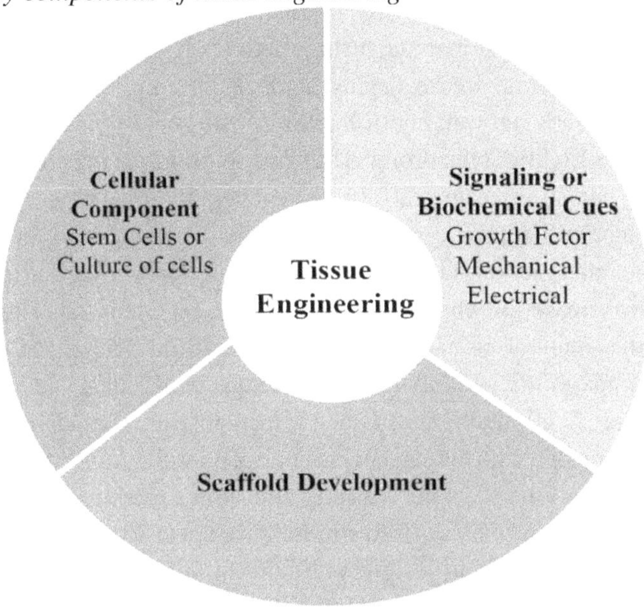

Tissue engineering uses interactions between cells, signaling molecules (like growth factors), and an underlying scaffold structure. However, according to the diagram above, the two opposites must simultaneously achieve the best tissue regeneration. Hence, scaffolds provide temporary extracellular matrix (ECM) substitutes that allow the cells to migrate, attach, secrete their own ECM, and form functional tissues (Collins et al., 2021). Current treatment methods fail due to the lack of availability of autografts, the risk of immune rejection with allografts, and ethical issues associated with xenografts, where scaffolds are needed (Y. Chen et al., 2022a). It is essential to choose the material of the scaffold to be regenerated successfully. Based on its potential use, scaffolds have been developed from different materials such as natural and synthetic polymers, ceramics, and composites (Kanwar & Vijayavenkataraman, 2021). Collagen, chitosan, and other natural polymers of similar structural framework to native ECM can promote bioactivity in cell attachment and proliferation. On the other hand, synthetic polymers such as polycaprolactone (PCL), polylactic acid (PLA), and poly(lactic-co-glycolic acid) (PLGA) have tunable degradation rates and mechanical properties that are suitable for various types of tissues (Cinici et al., 2024),(Top et al., 2021). Owing to osteoconductive properties and facilitating mineralization, extensive use of ceramics, such as hydroxyapatite (Mehmandoost et al., 2024), and bioactive glass (X. Zhang et al., 2021),(Andrea et al., 2025), has been made for bone tissue engineering. A combination of various materials, such as bioceramics and polymers, called composite materials, can improve both biocompatibility and mechanical properties (Jin et al., 2021).

The recent advancements in scaffold fabrication transformed tissue engineering. Various traditional scaffold manufacturing methods have been used increasingly, including solvent casting, freeze drying, and gas foaming. However, control of scaffold architecture is not well controllable.

Recent studies highlight the promise of nano-scaffolds to transform tissue engineering. Using nanocomposite scaffolds in regenerative medicine highlights their ability to enhance cell adhesion, proliferation, and differentiation. In addition, the development of nanogel-based scaffolds with high water-retention capacity and controlled drug release for wound healing and bone regeneration. These advances demonstrate that integrating nanotechnology in scaffold design can significantly improve biocompatibility and functionality (Cengiz et al., 2022).

Integrating artificial intelligence (AI) and computational modeling has revolutionized scaffold design with the capacity to control pore size, mechanical properties, and bioactivity precisely. Machine learning algorithms read through vast volumes of data to predict the optimal scaffold structure for specific tissue types. Artificial intelligence transforms scaffold design by utilizing high-performance computational modeling and real-time optimization. Harvard's Wyss Institute researchers use AI-based computational models to forecast scaffold degradation rates and facilitate optimized tissue regeneration. Scientists at Stanford University have created an AI-augmented scaffold printing system that controls material deposition in real time based on live imaging feedback, enhancing accuracy and reproducibility. However, ETH Zurich uses deep learning algorithms to analyze the biomechanical characteristics of scaffolds and forecast long-term integration with biological tissues.

Though it has come a long way, AI in scaffold technology has problems. One such problem is the lack of standardized datasets since AI models require enormous amounts of good-quality data to train on, and scaffold research lacks such data. Computational problems also occur since scaffolds designed at high-resolution demand huge computational power, thus making real-time applications not so easy to implement. Finally, regulatory problems persist since AI-based scaffold design has to contend with bureaucratic FDA and EMA regulations, thus making its universal application in clinics difficult.

Artificial Intelligence has revolutionized scaffold-based tissue engineering by enabling predictive modeling, real-time monitoring, and optimizing Bio-Printed constructs (X. Wang et al., 2024). AI-based deep learning models hold the potential to:

- Predict Cell Behavior & Differentiation – Computer simulations based on AI study stem cell behavior in scaffolds, optimizing growth conditions before implantation.
- Improve Bioprinting Accuracy – Machine learning controls change print settings in real time to minimize scaffold topology and mechanics discrepancies.
- Real-time monitoring during Scaffold Fabrication – Computer vision and image analytics with AI identify defects in deposition layers to increase reproducibility.
- Overcome AI Limitations – Despite its advantages, AI is not without its limitations, such as the lack of standard data sets, enormous computational resources, and regulatory issues.

AI-based techniques, such as machine learning and neural networks, also assist in the real-time monitoring of 3D printing and bioprinting processes, which provides superb reproducibility and reduces fabrication defects. The future of scaffold design will likely be in the form of self-adapting materials that can change their properties based on biological signals. With the advancement of emerging fabrication techniques, including electrospinning, 3D printing, and computer-aided design (CAD), fabrication in the broader aspect of scaffold structure and more porosity, mechanical properties, and spatial organization has become possible (Radhakrishnan et al., 2021),(Y. Chen et al., 2022b),(Serrano-Aroca et al., 2022). In particular, nanofiber-based scaffolds were made from electron spinning with the mimicked architecture of the ECM at the nanoscale level to improve cell scaffold interactions (Q. Yang et al., 2022). However, due to 3D printing, they have manufactured patient-specific scaffolds with drug-releasable, specific geometry, controlled biodegradation, and regenerative medicine (Fu et al., 2022).

Another critical aspect of scaffold design is the interaction of scaffolds with cells and biological systems. Cell behavior is influenced by scaffold architecture, including porosity, surface topography, and mechanical properties (C. Wang & Zhou, 2024). A recent development in biomedical engineering, tissue engineering (TE), replaces or regenerates different types of biological tissues by combining cells, materials, and biochemical elements. Making biopolymeric scaffolds with the proper porosity structure is crucial for replicating the complex architecture of native tissues and directing three-dimensional cell development. Several techniques, starting with polymer melts or solutions, are used to treat and convert natural and synthetic biomaterials into porous scaffolds (Capuana et al., 2021).

High porosity and interconnectivity facilitate nutrient diffusion and cell migration, while surface modifications, such as bioactive coatings and functionalization with growth factors, enhance cellular responses (P. Xu et al., 2024). Porous materials have gained significant attention because of their applications in gas storage, drug encapsulation and release, cell scaffolds, separation membranes, and numerous others. Scaffolds with interconnected pore networks accommodate nutrient exchange, release proteins, and allow gas exchange. In addition, porosity affects the mechanical properties of the scaffold (Jurczak et al., 2025).

Nano-scaffolds have benefits over traditional scaffolds, including enhanced mechanical properties, controllable biodegradation, and increased bioactivity. A recent study shows that nanofibrous scaffolds improve cellular interaction in a biomimetic environment, enhancing differentiation and tissue growth. Moreover, nano-coatings in scaffolds improved osteointegration and angiogenesis, enhancing clinical efficacy in bone and soft tissue engineering.

Scaffold porosity is a crucial factor in simulating the complex in vivo microenvironment. It has a direct impact on vascularization, migration, nutrient transport, cell-cell interactions, and the formation of functional tissue. Several factors, including composition, shape, mechanical stability, and cellular compatibility, determine a scaffold's design to guarantee optimal tissue creation. For tissues of different kinds, specific pore size ranges enhance scaffold performance: tiny pores (~1-2 μm) encourage skin regeneration by promoting epidermal cell adhesion, moderate pores (~2-12 μm) permit dermal migration, and broader pores (~40-100 μm) allow for vascular structures. For bone, the ideal scaffolds are multi-layered with tiny holes (50–100 μm). Tissue engineering of cell adhesion and the use of broader (200–400 μm) pores to allow for angiogenesis and transport of nutrients. Intermediary pore diameters (~25 – 60 μm) are required to address cell integration and nutrient production needs in lung and cardiovascular tissues (Mukasheva et al., 2024).

Cellular responses such as proliferation and tissue cell migration directly influence tissue vascularization and, eventually, form the new tissue. In addition, tissue formation should dictate scaffold degradation, which should occur in a way that releases scaffold within the tissue without causing mechanical instability at any point (Tamo et al., 2024).

This chapter discusses the application of scaffold design, fabrication methods, and tissue engineering applications in detail. It focuses on various materials used in scaffold fabrication and the critical properties required for umbilical tissue regeneration. It also describes scaffold-cell interaction, essential for tissue formation and integration.

Scaffold Design

Types of Scaffold Design

I. One-Dimensional (1D) Scaffolds:

The template structures for tissue development are the 1D scaffolds, fibers, nanotubes, and nanowires, all linear structures. Critical to navigation of axon growth for regenerating cerebral tissue, engineering of blood vessels, and muscle fiber alignment in the regeneration of muscle tissue. Materials used for 1D scaffolds include natural polymers, polymer of poly (lactic acid) (PLA), poly (glycolic acid) (PGA), and their copolymers. These carbon nanotubes are used to improve the electrical and mechanical properties.

The fabrication of 1D channel scaffolds is therefore done by 1) electrospinning to make nanofiber scaffolds, 2) template-assisted synthesis by removing the sacrificial templates, and 3) self-assembly methods. Characterized by fiber diameter, alignment, mechanical properties, cell attachment, and the downloads associated with the scaffold. Proliferation (Patil et al., 2024).

II. Two-Dimensional (2D) Scaffolds:

2D Scaffolds are planar structures that provide surfaces usable for cell adhesion, proliferation, and differentiation. For their intended function, these scaffolds must be load-bearing, biodegradable, and biocompatible. Factors that affect cell viability and proliferation, such as porosity, median pore size, and pore shape, were found to determine optimization(Patil et al., 2024).

Conventional methods of 2D scaffold fabrication (thermally induced phase separation, emulsion freeze drying, solvent casting, gas foaming, and electrospinning) exist. Recently, 3D printing technologies have been used to improve scaffold architecture for bone tissue engineering.

III. Three-Dimensional (3D) Scaffolds:

3D integration of cells or growth factors necessary for tissue repair or replacement. Cells need to exchange nutrients, oxygen should move through them, and waste should exit them; the porous, networked network that makes this possible is called tissue. Different fabrication methods (conventional or rapid prototyping techniques) can control pore sizes or porosity.

3D scaffold design is one of the most essential aspects, being the one in which graded porosity, mimicking in vivo environments with varying degrees of exposed cells to different levels of characteristics, is very important. 3D scaffold creates mechanical stability, diffusion of nutrients, and cell infiltration, improving tissue integration.

Various techniques, such as 3D Bioprinting, hydrogels, and nanofibers, are used to achieve complex 3D structures. Material selection, pore structure, and degradation rates need to be controlled to balance mechanical strength and biological functionality(Patil et al., 2024).

Figure 2. Dimensionally visualization of scaffold

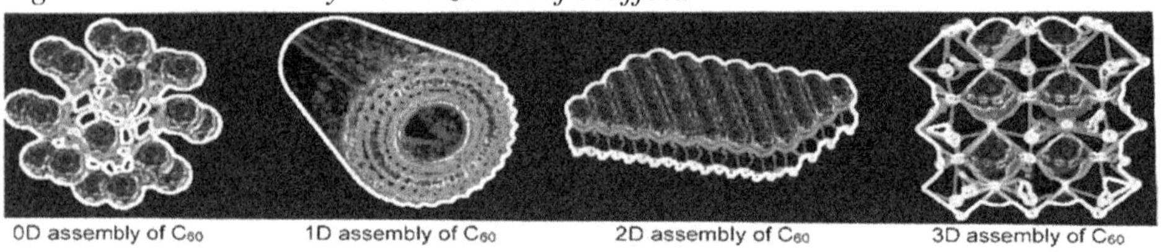

Materials for Scaffold Design

A tissue engineering scaffold material's biocompatibility, mechanical integrity, and degradation behavior are critical. Commonly used materials include:

- **Biopolymers:** The widely used natural polymers (collagen, chitosan, alginate, and hyaluronic acid) are biocompatible or bioactive, mimicking the native ECM. Wound healing and soft tissue (Serrano-Aroca et al., 2022),(Q. Yang et al., 2022).
- **Ceramics:** Hydroxyapatites and bioactive glass materials tend to be high-strength materials well suited to bone tissue engineering. The osteoconductive augments bone generation and is excellent for orthopedic use applications (Fu et al., 2022).
- **Composites**: This is due to hybrid materials made up of biopolymers mixed with ceramics, which makes them biocompatible and more durable in a compromise between these two properties. These materials have particular utility since they apply to the coexistence of both flexibility and strength, such as cartilage repair (C. Wang & Zhou, 2024).
- **Synthetic Polymers:** PLA, PCL, and PLGA enable tunable mechanical and degradation properties and are appropriate for tissue engineering applica-

tions. They are easy to process and scale to large sizes, making them desirable for scaffold production (P. Xu et al., 2024).

NEXT-GENERATION BIOINKS FOR NEXT-GENERATION SCAFFOLD FABRICATION

Bio-inks' evolution has significantly improved the function, mechanical properties, and biocompatibility of bio-printed scaffolds. Recent advances in bio-ink materials include:

- **Hybrid Hydrogels- Combinations** of natural polymers (e.g., gelatin, alginate, collagen) with synthetic biomaterials (e.g., PEGDA, PCL) to improve mechanical stability and bioactivity.
- **Decellularized ECM (dECM) Bioinks-**
  These bio-inks are derived from tissue and maintain biochemical cues for cell differentiation and tissue regeneration.
- **Bio printable Synthetic Polymers-** Synthetic polymers like PLGA, PEGDA, and PCL have their degradation rates adjusted and are employed in bone, cartilage, and vascularized tissue engineering.

These second-generation bioinks improve patient-specific scaffold fabrication by replicating the extracellular matrix (ECM) and offering the best cell adhesion, proliferation, and differentiation (Dzobo et al., 2019),(Cao et al., 2021).

PROPERTIES OF SCAFFOLDS

The following are the key properties for a successful scaffold design.:

Porosity and Pore Interconnectivity: Migration of cells, diffusion of nutrients, and waste removal play critical roles in cell survival and tissue generation, and the high porosity and interconnected pores allow such phenomenon to occur. For example, optimal scaffolds of bone type require porosity above, whereas optimal scaffolds of adipose type require porosity below 50% (Serrano-Aroca et al., 2022).

Mechanical Strength: The scaffold must provide adequate mechanical support, e.g., bone scaffolds must have high compressive strength, and soft tissue scaffolds must be flexible. Materials such as bioactive glass and polymer ceramic composites use to enhance mechanical integrity (Zenobi et al., 2023).

Biocompatibility: The material should not provoke an adverse immune response, fungal adhesion, and proliferation. A further surface modification to improve cellular interactions is coating with bioactive molecules (Collins et al., 2021).

Degradation Rate: Regeneration scaffolds should destruct at a speed consistent with new tissue formation, at the same time as structural integrity during the regeneration. PLGA can be engineered to degrade at different timescales as polymers to meet particular application needs (Y. Chen et al., 2022b).

Figure 3. Properties of bone tissue engineering (BTE)

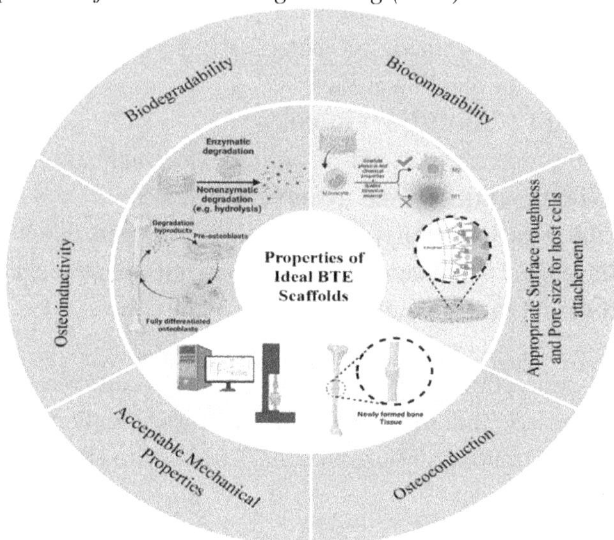

Biomechanical Properties & Degradation of Scaffolds for Tissue Engineering

Scaffold biomechanical properties are essential in tissue growth, regeneration, and attachment. The strength must be similar to the target tissue, with elastic and flexible ability. The main biomechanical parameters are:

Mechanical Strength & Elasticity – Scaffolds should be able to bear cell growth under physiological loads.

Porosity & Pore Size – Critical for oxygen and nutrient diffusion, deciding cell viability.

Hydration & Swelling Behavior – Hydrogels and polymer scaffolds absorb water, affecting biomechanical stability.

SCAFFOLD DEGRADATION AND ITS INFLUENCE ON TISSUE REGENERATION

Scaffold degradation is a critical factor in tissue regeneration, as it determines how the scaffold is degraded in a natural tissue environment. The degradation rate must match the tissue formation speed to avoid premature scaffold collapse or residual material accumulation. Polymer scaffolds (e.g., PLA, PGA) are hydrolyzed, and natural biomaterials are degraded enzymatically. Mechanical strength is reduced with degradation, which compromises tissue integrity.

SURFACE FUNCTIONALIZATION

Chemical modification of tissue-engineered scaffolds with bioactive molecules, growth factors, or antimicrobial agents may increase cellular interactions, essential for stopping infection. The authors explored functionalization techniques (surface coatings and nanopatterning) to improve the performance of the scaffold.

CELL-SCAFFOLD INTERACTIONS

The interaction between scaffolds and cells dictates the success of tissue engineering applications. Attaching to the scaffold is possible, and the scaffold surface is adhered to through the integrin receptors, mediating adhesion, signaling, and differentiation to the scaffold. Surface modifications of the scaffolds, such as functionalization with bioactive molecules and Nano-structuring, will enhance cellular response (Amnieh et al., 2024). In addition, cell behavior is scaffold-dependent, and cells align and migrate depending on scaffold architecture. Several studies have shown that nano-topographical features can induce stem cell differentiation and tissue integration.

Finally, the degradation behavior of scaffolds also depends on cell response and tissue development. However, ideally, a scaffold should degrade preferably in a controlled manner according to the rate of new tissue formation. Degradation products are nontoxic and quickly metabolized or excreted from the body.

Moreover, scaffold stiffness and elasticity influence cell differentiation, as a soft scaffold tends to be favored by neural differentiation, while a stiffer scaffold is associated with osteogenesis. Mechanical properties were also tunable, directing stem cell fate and tissue regeneration outcomes.

Figure 4. Interaction of bone and scaffold in BTE (Dixon & Gomillion, 2022)

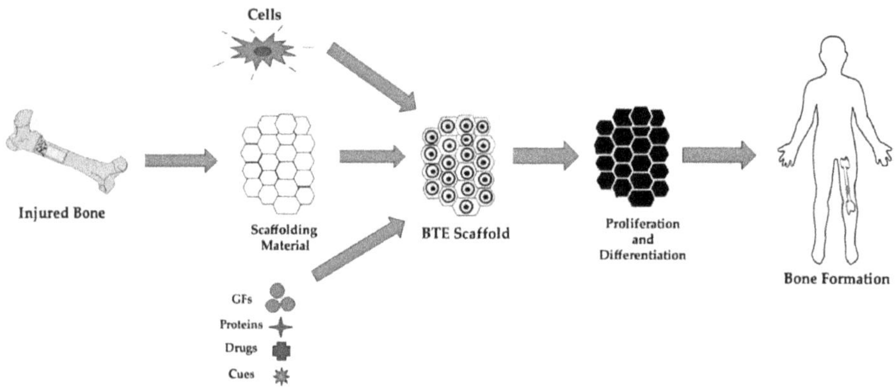

FABRICATION TECHNIQUES

In tissue engineering, scaffold construction is essential because it directly impacts tissue regeneration, cell adhesion, and proliferation. Tissue engineering is a multidisciplinary field that links genetic engineering, biotechnology, clinical medicine, mechanical engineering, and biomedical engineering. The combination of computational modeling and artificial intelligence (AI) has revolutionarily changed scaffold design by allowing for exact control of essential parameters like pore size, mechanical strength, and bioactivity. The conventional scaffold fabrication techniques like solvent casting, gas foaming, and freeze-drying are not reproducible or accurate. AI-based approaches avoid the time-consuming trial-and-error process of scaffold design through predictive algorithms operating on vast biological databases to design optimized scaffold structures that are tissue-type specific. Perhaps the most significant of the advantages of AI in tissue engineering is its ability to enhance 3D printing and bioprinting protocols. AI image analysis and deep learning capabilities allow real-time monitoring of printed scaffold architecture with high reproducibility and less likelihood of fabrication flaws such as inconsistent porosity or mechanical vulnerability. AI can also read patient-specific data, such as CT scans and MRI, to develop tailored scaffolds that precisely match a patient's anatomy, with higher clinical success.

Furthermore, machine learning algorithms are used to model cell-scaffold interactions and predict cell behavior in different scaffold geometries. The algorithms are used to refine scaffold parameters such as biodegradation rates, surface roughness, and Bio-functional coatings to enhance tissue integration and regeneration. Shortly, AI will be instrumental in developing self-adjusting scaffolds that adjust their properties dynamically per biological signals like pH, enzymatic activity, or mechanical stress. These future scaffolds will facilitate innovative tissue engineering solutions in which the scaffold form and function will adapt to the healing tissue, offering a better biomimetic and effective regenerative platform (Omigbodun & Oladapo, 2025). The application of AI in scaffold design is growing in popularity as a way to increase accuracy and efficiency. Later in this chapter, a thorough explanation of its uses is given. Machine learning algorithms read through vast volumes of data to predict the optimal scaffold structure for specific tissue types. AI-based techniques such as machine learning and neural networks also assist in the real-time monitoring of 3D printing and bioprinting processes, which provides superb reproducibility and reduces fabrication defects. The future of scaffold design will likely be in the form of self-adapting materials that can change their properties based on biological signals. Tissue regeneration is a complicated process that depends on several variables, including surface characteristics, porosity, mechanical stability, solubility, degradability, and the preservation of cell-cell connections. The bones, cartilage, and tissues are seriously damaged by diseases and accidents such as osteomyelitis, arthritis, anemia, malignancies, hereditary multiple exostoses, and hereditary bone marrow failure syndromes. The worldwide market is anticipated to reach a value of 11.5 billion US dollars by the end of 2025 due to the rise in demand for bone grafts in organ transplantation and substitution surgery (Kumar & Jacob, 2022). Creating porous scaffolds to create an environment conducive to tissue growth and regeneration for complicated organs is known as tissue engineering.

Three-dimensional scaffolds are made of permeable, fibrous, and porous biomaterials. It facilitates the movement of bodily fluids and encourages cell-to-cell communication, extracellular matrix deposition, and survivability against a range of pathogens with low inflammatory response and toxicity rates. Chemical components used in 3D scaffolding production include metals and non-metals, composites, hydrogels, natural and synthetic polymers, ceramics, and non-ceramics (Kirallah & Hussein, 2025). The primary components of human bone, a bio-composite, are organic collagen and inorganic minerals. In the hierarchical structure of bone, hydroxyapatite (Ca10(PO4)6(OH)2) nanocrystals are deposited on collagen fibrils. The outside architecture is complex, compact bone (~10%) because of the high mineral content. In contrast, the inner architecture is composed of cancellous or spongy bone (~80–90%), which is highly vascularized and has an interconnected porous structure (Bhushan et al., 2022). They are responsible for the synthesis and secretion of the osteoid, the organic bone matrix. Ribosomes, Golgi apparatuses, endoplasmic Reticulum, and mitochondria are abundant. The matrix envelops active osteoblasts to create osteocytes, which comprise several cytoplasmic organelles and a small number of endoplasmic Reticulum. The interaction between osteoblasts and osteocytes aids in controlling the movement of mineral ions between the bone's extracellular space and matrix (Bhushan et al., 2022).

The methods employed fall into two general categories:

- Conventional approaches.
- Current ways.

CONVENTIONAL APPROACH

I. Sol-Gel Technique:

A popular wet-chemical method for creating bioactive scaffolds is the sol-gel procedure. It provides reasonable control over porosity, composition, and structure at low processing temperatures. Bioinks generated from sol-gel are used in the 3D printing process called "robocasting" to create scaffolds.

In the sol-gel process, metal alkoxides or inorganic salts are hydrolyzed and condensed to create a stable sol that gels into a porous network. in order to improve the mechanical properties, the gel is heat-treated at 675°C and 700°C for 1 hour after being aged at 60°C for 7 days and dried. While drawbacks include long processing time and fragility, benefits include controlled porosity, uniform composition, and low processing temperature. In bone tissue engineering, the procedure works best with bioactive glass scaffolds (Deliormanlı, 2025).

Figure 5. Scaffold fabrication via sol-gel technique

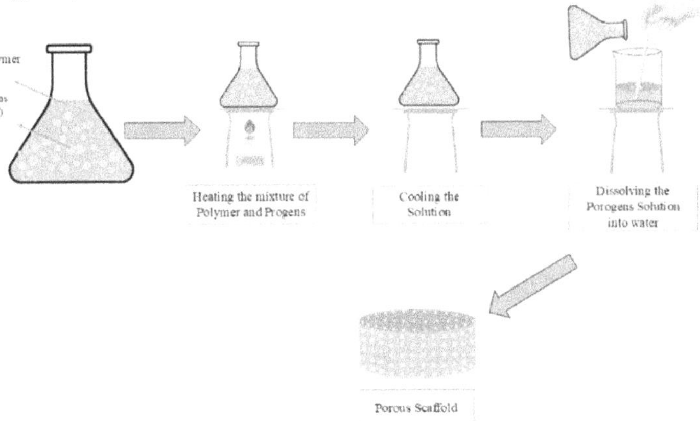

The procedure provides biocompatibility and homogeneity, making it suitable for tissue engineering. The characteristics of scaffolds for bone and soft tissue regeneration are improved when sol-gel and robocasting are combined (Ishikawa et al., 2020).

II. Freeze Drying:

Figure 6. Scaffold fabrication via freeze drying

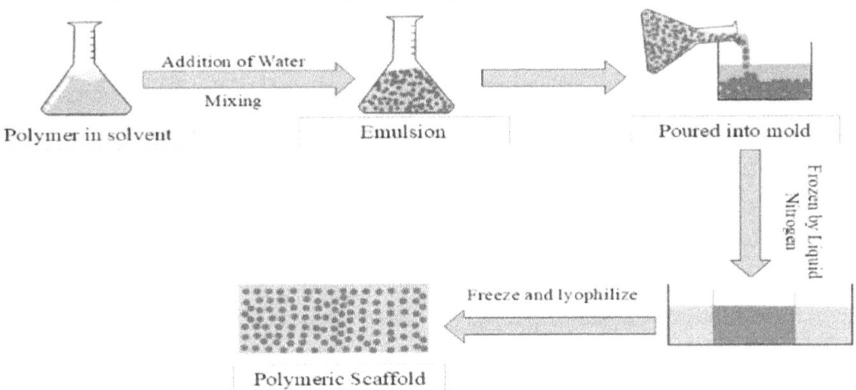

One intriguing method for creating scaffolds in tissue engineering is freeze-drying or lyophilization. The three primary processes are preparing the solution, casting or molding, freezing, and low-pressure drying. When the polymeric solution freezes, ice crystals are formed, providing a porous structure. A highly porous and interconnected scaffold with porosities of up to around 90% is retained after the ice sublimes and any leftover unfrozen water is desorbed. By altering the freezing rate, polymer concentration, and processing temperature, the pore size—typically between 20 and 200 μm—can be changed (Collins et al., 2021). The approach preserves the bioactivity of temperature-sensitive biomolecules and is best suited for creating scaffolds from polymers, ceramics, and composite materials. The main benefit of freeze-drying is its capacity to produce highly porous, interconnected structures for nutrient transport and cell penetration. However, freeze-drying requires specialized equipment and a strong vacuum for the best moisture removal. Despite these drawbacks, freeze-dried scaffolds have many uses in soft tissue engineering and bone and cartilage regeneration, where regulated porosity and biocompatibility are crucial for appropriate tissue integration.

III. Solvent Casting:

One such inexpensive method of making porous scaffolds is solvent casting. The first step occurs by dissolving a biodegradable polymer in a suitable solvent to produce a homogeneous solution. Then, the solution is poured into a mold or onto a Porogen, such as dispersed sugar particles or salt crystals, to provide the structure with pores. It proceeds through carefully controlled conditions, and then the polymer solidifies (under solvent) to make a shaped scaffold with a network of pores, leaving the solvent to evaporate slowly. Finally, Porogen is leached away to obtain a very porous structure. The injection of a Porogen with a different pore size or distribution can be accomplished by varying the type of Porogen and determining how much or what %age of the Porogen is used.

It is achieved using polymer scaffolds like poly (lactic-co-glycolic acid (PLGA), polycaprolactone (PCL), and polylactic acid (PLA) to fabricate these porous structures with attachment and proliferation of cells (Suhaimin et al., 2025).

The technique's main disadvantage is that the dripping solvents are very toxic, and the leftover solvents can potentially be not biocompatible after post-processing. It also lacks substantial control of pore size and interconnectivity compared to other, more mature fabrication methods. While these limitations may restrict the use of the technique, it is very popular as a means of scaffolding soft tissue—engineering and bone tissue regeneration.

Figure 7. Scaffold fabrication via solvent casting

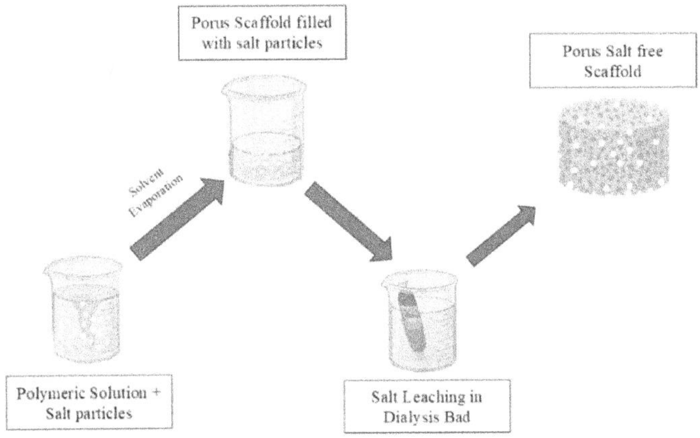

MODERN AND CURRENT WAYS

I.3-D Printing:

3D printing is a recent state-of-the-art scaffold production method used for tissue engineering due to its ability to superimpose exactly layer by layer of biomaterials, resulting in high customizability of the structures. Unlike conventional methods such as solvent casting or electrospinning, 3D printing can produce anisotropic architectures resembling the extracellular matrix, thereby providing better cellular adhesion and subsequent cellular growth and differentiation (Profile, 2025). The particular use for patient-specific applications, where structural integrity and accurate bone scaffold porosity are essential, is beneficial. It makes it a viable method for creating functioning tissue structures in regenerative medicine, particularly in the healing of bone and cartilage (Prakoso et al., 2025).

Figure 8. Scaffold fabrication via 3D printing

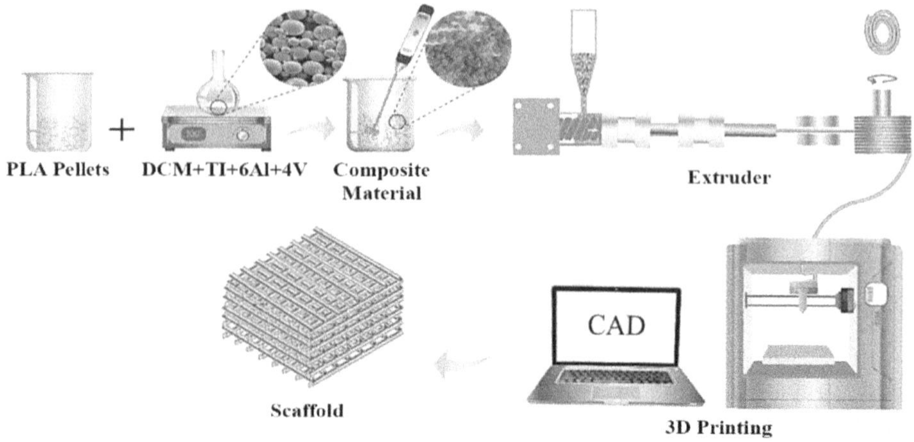

II. Electrospinning:

Electrospinning is a widely adopted method for producing nanofibrous scaffolds with ECM features, whereby a polymer solution is ejected through a high-voltage electric field. Materials such as collagen, gelatin, polycaprolactone (PCL), polylactic acid (PLA), poly(lactic-co-glycolic acid) (PLGA), polysulfide, and polycaprolactone (PCL) are dissolved in solvents (dimethylformamide (DMF) or trifluoroethanol (TFE)). During the process, parameters of polymer concentration 5–30% w/v, applied voltage 5–30 kV, flow rate 0.1–5 mL/h, and tip-to-collector distance 5–10 cm are affected; environmental factors (temperature 20–40 °C; humidity 20–60%) (S. Chen et al., 2025).

They have a very high surface area for cell adhesion, are biodegradable and biomimetic, and have adjustable fiber diameter. Despite these drawbacks, such as poor control of fiber alignment, limited penetration or cell contact, need for organic solvents, and batch-to-batch variations, these include, however. There are difficulties when using electrospinning in skin tissue engineering, cartilage tissue engineering, wound healing, neuron regeneration, and drug delivery systems.

Electrospun scaffolds also have the advantage of the biomimetic nanofibrous structure as the extracellular matrix, the high surface area for cell adhesion, adjustable fiber diameter, and degradation. They have the disadvantages of batch-to-batch irregularities, poor ability to introduce live cells, poor fiber alignment control, and hazardous chemical solvents. Nevertheless, electrospinning has been employed in neurological regeneration, wound healing, skin, cartilage tissue engineering, and delivery systems.

Figure 9. Scaffold fabrication via electrospinning

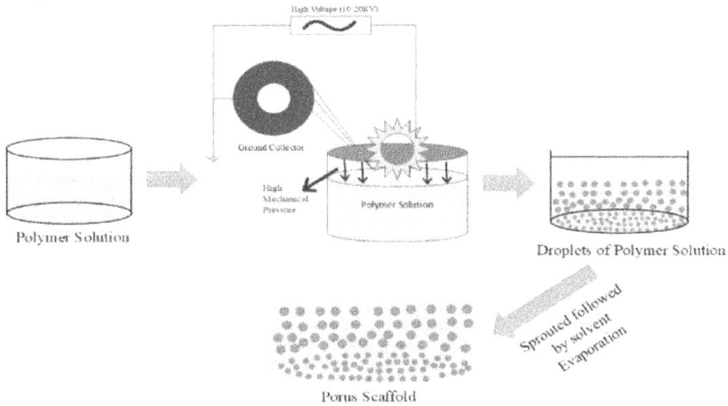

III. Bio-Printing:

Bioprinting is a complex tissue engineering method that utilizes the bio-inks containing living cells to construct structures with cells implanted in them. Materials used: alginate, gelatin, collagen, fibrin, and hyaluronic acid are used in depositing. Hydrogel-based bio-inks, cells, and growth factors layer by layer. Nozzle diameter (100–500 μm), extrusion pressure (1–200 kPa), temperature (4–37°C), and cross-linking time (seconds to minutes) are essential printing parameters to maintain cell viability and structural integrity. Bioprinting offers other benefits, such as making intricate tissue structures, boosting cell division and proliferation, and better functional tissue regeneration (Kasturi et al., 2024). Therefore, there are different ways in which Bioprinting is hindered, such as the need for specific bioinks, exorbitant costs, technological difficulty, and ongoing research. Despite these apparent challenges, Bioprinting can be used in wound healing, vascular grafts, cartilage, organ tissue engineering, and custom-made regenerative medicine.

Figure 10. Scaffold fabrication via bioprinting, (a). schematic illustration of bioprinting of hydrogel scaffolds for bone and cartilage defect repair (Z. Yang et al., 2022). (b). A simple step-by-step process for bioprinting from bio-ink in tissue engineering

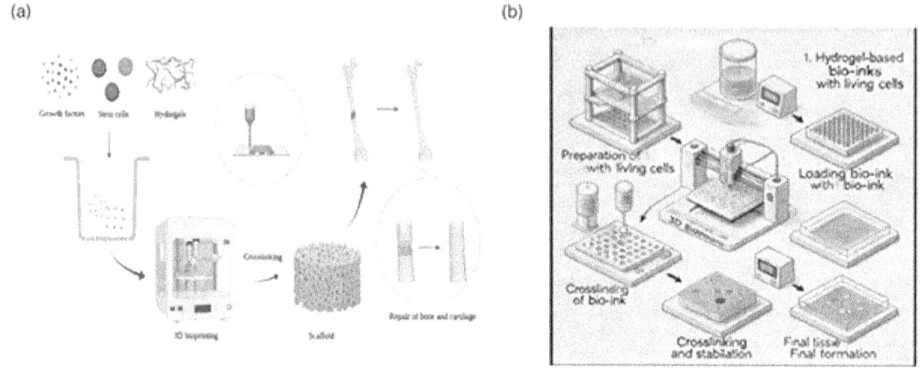

CLASSIFICATION OF BIOPRINTING TECHNOLOGIES IN TISSUE ENGINEERING

Tissue engineering has been transformed by contemporary bioprinting methods, which provide accurate scaffold creation tailored to each patient. Currently, regenerative medicine uses four main categories of bioprinting technologies:

1. <u>Extrusion-Based Bioprinting:</u>

   Extrusion-based Bioprinting utilizes mechanical stress to extrude bio-inks from a nozzle and cause continuous layer-by-layer deposition. It is extensively used to regenerate cartilage and bone tissue but can potentially lead to cell destruction by shear stress.
2. <u>Inkjet-Based Bioprinting:</u>

   Inkjet-based Bioprinting can print tiny bio-ink droplets on a substrate through controlled ejection. It possesses high accuracy and economical printing but is ideal for low-viscosity materials.
3. <u>Laser-Assisted Bioprinting:</u>

   Laser-assisted Bioprinting utilizes laser pulses to deposit bioink on the surface of a scaffold. It has high patterning accuracy and cell viability and can be used for vascularized tissue engineering. It is costly and scalable.
4. <u>Volumetric & Light-Based Bioprinting:</u>

Emerging technologies use holographic projection of light to print scaffolds in seconds. These technologies can enable speedy bio-fabrication but require more effort for regulatory clearance.

All of these approaches to Bioprinting are tissue-specific, and experimentation is now optimizing print resolution, bio-ink composition, and scale-up (Mirshafiei et al., 2024).

Table 1. Comparison table of fabrication methods

Fabrication Method	Advantages	Disadvantages
Solvent Casting	Simple, cost-effective	Poor pore connectivity, residual solvents
Freeze-Drying	High porosity, biocompatible	Long processing time, brittle structures
3D Printing	High precision, customizable	Expensive, requires specialized equipment
Electrospinning	Mimics ECM, high surface area	Poor cell penetration, limited mechanical strength
Bioprinting	Integrates live cells, controlled architecture	High cost, limited Bio-ink options

CHALLENGES AND FUTURE DIRECTIONS

The biggest challenge is that an engineered tissue has to maintain or establish a healthy blood supply to prosper and support integration with the host tissue. Nanotechnology also significantly contributes to scaffold development, with improved mechanical properties and biological interactions. Electrospun nanofiber scaffolds have been developed at MIT, which enhance cell attachment and mechanical strength for improved tissue integration. Johns Hopkins University uses nanoparticle-laden scaffolds to improve targeted drug release, wound healing, and complication reduction. Graphene-based bio-scaffolds have been reported at Imperial College London and have found tremendous potential to enhance neuronal regeneration, especially in spinal cord injury.

Practical applications of nanotechnology in scaffolds (nanofiber scaffolds, nanoparticle-based drug delivery, graphene-based scaffolds) and future challenges. Examples of AI applied to scaffold design (Harvard, Stanford, ETH Zurich) and limitations (non-availability of standard datasets, computational complexity, regulatory barriers). Vascularization remains the overarching limiting factor in scaffold-based tissue engineering. Without a functional vascular network, tissue-engineered constructs are prone to cell necrosis and restricted integration. In response to this challenge, many vascularization strategies have been conceived, such as:

- Microfluidic-Based Bioprinting: able to mimic capillary networks by creating microchannel-embedded scaffolds to permit oxygen and nutrient diffusion.
- Endothelial Co-Culture Techniques- Employ a co-culture of endothelial cells (ECs) and mesenchymal stem cells (MSCs) to cause spontaneous vessel formation in scaffolds.
- Growth Factor Integration- Vascular endothelial growth factor (VEGF) supplementation enhances angiogenesis, resulting in the formation of blood vessels at a high rate.
- Scaffold Pre-Vascularization- Pre-vascularized constructs are pre-made and can be implanted in the patient, seamlessly integrating with host blood vessels.

The restricted vascularization of larger scaffolds causes cell necrosis in the central region. (Mukasheva et al., 2024), (Chae et al., 2023). The body's immune response impairs the effectiveness of the scaffold in regeneration by an immune response that will reject the scaffold or by inflammation. They also have to overcome additional hurdles in scaffolds that approximate the mechanical properties of native tissue and maintain structural integrity over time while being able to define adequate cell shape and connectivity to the scaffold substrate. Another issue is that most scaffold manufacturing techniques are relatively expensive and require particular conditions, so mass production for other medical applications is quite costly and not feasible.

Here, AI and nanotechnologies are used to design scaffolds to overcome the above challenges. Although there are excellent advances in scaffold engineering, clinical translation is restricted due to cost and regulatory factors. The FDA (Food Drug Administration) and EMA (European Medicines Agencies) place strict demands on biomaterial-derived scaffolds, necessitating extensive preclinical work before approval. The literature suggests that the absence of standardization in scaffold production and quality control is a significant bottleneck for commercialization. The cost of producing intricate, patient-specific scaffolds also remains prohibitive, restricting the widespread use of regenerative medicine. Future studies must overcome scalability, cost issues, and long-term in vivo behavior to close the gap between lab and clinic (Malkani et al., 2024). AI and nanotechnologies enhance productivity and personalization because AI models already process vast amounts of data to build the AI process, predict cellular behavior, and improve the scaffold architecture. Machine learning systems can also choose the best biomaterials and production parameters for tissue engineering applications. At this time, nanotechnology makes it possible to construct nanoengineered scaffolds for improving mechanical strength, facilitating adherence of cells, and increasing the bioactivity of the contents of nanofibers, nanoparticles, and surface functionalization. For example, coatings of nanoparticles can be used to release growth factors to control cell regeneration and reduce immunological rejection.

The innovative scaffolds with biosensors and responsive materials can dynamically engage with cells in real-time in response to environmental cues.

Scaffold-based approaches have made revolutionary strides in clinical applications, revolutionizing regenerative medicine. Bioactive scaffolds have successfully regenerated bone in orthopedic patients with extensive fractures, promoting faster healing and structural integrity. A landmark 2024 clinical trial confirmed that 3D-printed polycaprolactone (PCL) scaffolds, in combination with stem cell therapy, significantly accelerated cartilage regeneration in knee injuries, offering a promising alternative to traditional grafts. Further, hydrogel-based scaffolds have emerged as a game-changer in wound healing, with impressive efficacy in treating chronic ulcers by accelerating tissue repair and reducing complications. These advances demonstrate the vast potential of scaffolds in personalized medicine, where patient-specific designs and bioengineered solutions can lead to more effective, targeted, and long-term regenerative therapies (N. Xu et al., 2023),(W. Zhang et al., 2023),(Cao et al., 2021).

CONCLUSION

Scaffold-based tissue engineering has revolutionized regenerative medicine with novel organ regeneration and tissue repair strategies. With the integration of advanced fabrication techniques such as Bioprinting and electrospinning, scientists have achieved unprecedented accuracy in scaffold design. The use of biocompatible polymers, bioactive ceramics, and hybrid hydrogels has led to improved mechanical strength, controlled degradation, and improved cellular response. AI-based scaffold modeling and machine learning algorithms enable predictive optimization to ensure patient-specific scaffold designs with improved clinical outcomes.

Although there has been such advancement, particular key challenges exist, including vascularization limitations, immune rejection, and scalability in bulk manufacturing. Future research would need to target the development of pre-vascularized scaffolds, bioactive surface coatings, and innovative scaffolds with the ability to perceive physiological signals. Integrating AI, nanotechnology, and bioinformatics will play a central role in breaking through the constraints, with the next-generation scaffolds providing real-time tissue monitoring, improved biocompatibility, and improved healing rates.

With further development, scaffold-based tissue engineering can be one of the cornerstones of personalized medicine, enabling tailored regenerative therapies to enhance treatment outcomes and define the future of biomedical science and medicine.

REFERENCES

Amnieh, Y. A., Karbasi, S., Dehkordi, S. H., Shadkhast, M., & Basiri, A. (2024). Evaluation of the Effects of Decellularized Wharton Jelly Nanoparticles on Poly-hydroxy Butyrate-Chitosan Electrospun Scaffolds for Cartilage Tissue Engineering Applications. *Journal of Polymers and the Environment*, *33*(1), 545–569. DOI: 10.1007/s10924-024-03385-4

Andrea, L. D., Gabrieli, R., Milano, L., Magagnin, L., De, A., Alidoost, D., Schwentenwein, M., Verné, E., Baino, F., & Vena, P. (2025). Acta Materialia Elastic and failure characterization of hydroxyapatite TPMS scaffolds using a combined approach of ultrasound, compression tests and micro-CT based numerical models. *Acta Materialia, 287*(September 2024), 120776. DOI: 10.1016/j.actamat.2025.120776

Bhushan, S., Singh, S., Maiti, T. K., Sharma, C., Dutt, D., Sharma, S., Li, C., & Tag Eldin, E. M. (2022). Scaffold Fabrication Techniques of Biomaterials for Bone Tissue Engineering. *Critical Reviews in Bioengineering*, *9*(12), 728. Advance online publication. DOI: 10.3390/bioengineering9120728 PMID: 36550933

Cao, Y., Cheng, P., Sang, S., Xiang, C., An, Y., Wei, X., Yan, Y., & Li, P. (2021). 3D printed PCL/GelMA biphasic scaffold boosts cartilage regeneration using co-culture of mesenchymal stem cells and chondrocytes: In vivo study. *Materials & Design*, *210*, 110065. DOI: 10.1016/j.matdes.2021.110065

Capuana, E., Lopresti, F., Carfì Pavia, F., Brucato, V., & La Carrubba, V. (2021). Solution-based processing for scaffold fabrication in tissue engineering applications: A brief review. *Polymers*, *13*(13), 2041. Advance online publication. DOI: 10.3390/polym13132041 PMID: 34206515

Cengiz, I. F., Reis, R. L., & Oliveira, J. M. (2022). Engineering scaffolds for tissue engineering and regenerative medicine. *Advances in Biomedical Polymers and Composites: Materials and Applications*, *5*(1), 109–130. DOI: 10.1016/B978-0-323-88524-9.00030-9

Chae, S., Ha, D. H., & Lee, H. (2023). 3D bioprinting strategy for engineering vascularized tissue models. *International Journal of Bioprinting*, *9*(5), 748. Advance online publication. DOI: 10.18063/ijb.748 PMID: 37502273

Chen, S., Xie, C., Long, X., Wang, X., Li, X., Liu, P., Liu, J., & Wang, Z. (2025). Development of Electrospinning Setup for Vascular Tissue-Engineering Application with Thick-Hierarchical Fiber Alignment. *Tissue Engineering and Regenerative Medicine*, *22*(2), 195–210. DOI: 10.1007/s13770-024-00691-9 PMID: 39825992

Chen, Y., Dong, X., Shafiq, M., Myles, G., Radacsi, N., & Mo, X. (2022a). Recent Advancements on Three-Dimensional Electrospun Nanofiber Scaffolds for Tissue Engineering. *Advanced Fiber Materials, 4*(5), 959–986. DOI: 10.1007/s42765-022-00170-7

Chen, Y., Dong, X., Shafiq, M., Myles, G., Radacsi, N., & Mo, X. (2022b). Recent Advancements on Three-Dimensional Electrospun Nanofiber Scaffolds for Tissue Engineering. *Advanced Fiber Materials, 4*(5), 959–986. DOI: 10.1007/s42765-022-00170-7

Cheng, F., Song, D., Li, H., Ravi, S. K., & Tan, S. C. (2024). Recent Progress in Biomedical Scaffold Fabricated via Electrospinning: Design, Fabrication and Tissue Engineering Application. *Advanced Functional Materials, 2406950*, 1–28. DOI: 10.1002/adfm.202406950

Cinici, B., Yaba, S., Kurt, M., Yalcin, H. C., Duta, L., & Gunduz, O. (2024). Fabrication Strategies for Bioceramic Scaffolds in Bone Tissue Engineering with Generative Design Applications. *Biomimetics, 9*(7), 409. Advance online publication. DOI: 10.3390/biomimetics9070409 PMID: 39056850

Collins, M. N., Ren, G., Young, K., Pina, S., Reis, R. L., & Oliveira, J. M. (2021). Scaffold Fabrication Technologies and Structure/Function Properties in Bone Tissue Engineering. *Advanced Functional Materials, 31*(21), 2010609. Advance online publication. DOI: 10.1002/adfm.202010609

Deliormanlı, A. M. (2025). Novel Sol - Gel Inks for the Direct Writing of SiO 2 - Based Bioactive Glass Scaffolds for Tissue Engineering Applications. *Silicon, 0123456789*(4), 775–787. Advance online publication. DOI: 10.1007/s12633-025-03224-8

Dixon, D. T., & Gomillion, C. T. (2022). Conductive scaffolds for bone tissue engineering: Current state and future outlook. *Journal of Functional Biomaterials, 13*(1), 1. Advance online publication. DOI: 10.3390/jfb13010001 PMID: 35076518

Dzobo, K., Motaung, K. S. C. M., & Adesida, A. (2019). Recent trends in decellularized extracellular matrix bioinks for 3D printing: An updated review. *International Journal of Molecular Sciences, 20*(18), 4628. Advance online publication. DOI: 10.3390/ijms20184628 PMID: 31540457

Fu, J. N., Wang, X., Yang, M., Chen, Y. R., Zhang, J. Y., Deng, R. H., Zhang, Z. N., Yu, J. K., & Yuan, F. Z. (2022). Scaffold-Based Tissue Engineering Strategies for Osteochondral Repair. *Frontiers in Bioengineering and Biotechnology, 9*(January), 1–21. DOI: 10.3389/fbioe.2021.812383 PMID: 35087809

Gharibshahian, M., Torkashvand, M., Bavisi, M., Aldaghi, N., & Alizadeh, A. (2024). Recent advances in artificial intelligent strategies for tissue engineering and regenerative medicine. *Skin Research and Technology : Official Journal of International Society for Bioengineering and the Skin (ISBS) and International Society for Digital Imaging of Skin (ISDIS) and International Society for Skin Imaging (ISSI), 30*(9), 1–15. DOI: 10.1111/srt.70016 PMID: 39189880

Ishikawa, K., Garskaite, E., & Kareiva, A. (2020). Sol–gel synthesis of calcium phosphate-based biomaterials—A review of environmentally benign, simple, and effective synthesis routes. *Journal of Sol-Gel Science and Technology, 94*(3), 551–572. DOI: 10.1007/s10971-020-05245-8

Jin, Y., Xie, C., Gao, Q., Zhou, X., Li, G., Du, J., & He, Y. (2021). Fabrication of multi-scale and tunable auxetic scaffolds for tissue engineering. *Materials & Design, 197*, 109277. DOI: 10.1016/j.matdes.2020.109277

Jurczak, K. M., Zhang, R., Hinrichs, W. L. J., Grijpma, D. W., Schuurmann, R. C. L., de Vries, J. P. P. M., & van Rijn, P. (2025). Porous polytrimethylenecarbonate scaffolds: Design considerations and porosity modulation techniques. *Materials and Design, 250*(September 2024). DOI: 10.1016/j.matdes.2025.113588

Kanwar, S., & Vijayavenkataraman, S. (2021). Design of 3D printed scaffolds for bone tissue engineering: A review. *Bioprinting (Amsterdam, Netherlands), 24*(August), e00167. DOI: 10.1016/j.bprint.2021.e00167

Kasturi, M., Mathur, V., Gadre, M., Srinivasan, V., & Vasanthan, K. S. (2024). Three Dimensional Bioprinting for Hepatic Tissue Engineering: From In Vitro Models to Clinical Applications. *Tissue Engineering and Regenerative Medicine, 21*(1), 21–52. DOI: 10.1007/s13770-023-00576-3 PMID: 37882981

Kirallah, A. A., & Hussein, B. F. (2025). Assessment of Sheep Omentum for Soft-tissue Engineering Scaffolds. *Egyptian Journal of Veterinary Science(Egypt), 56*(1), 101–108. DOI: 10.21608/ejvs.2024.269178.1842

Koyyada, A., & Orsu, P. (2021). Recent Advancements and Associated Challenges of Scaffold Fabrication Techniques in Tissue Engineering Applications. *Regenerative Engineering and Translational Medicine, 7*(2), 147–159. DOI: 10.1007/s40883-020-00166-y

Kumar, A., & Jacob, A. (2022). Techniques in scaffold fabrication process for tissue engineering applications: A review. *Journal of Applied Biology and Biotechnology, 10*(3), 163–176. DOI: 10.7324/JABB.2022.100321

Malkani, S., Prado, O., & Stevens, K. R. (2024). Sacrificial Templating for Accelerating Clinical Translation of Engineered Organs. *ACS Biomaterials Science & Engineering*. Advance online publication. DOI: 10.1021/acsbiomaterials.4c01824 PMID: 39701582

Mehmandoost, M., Oveisi, H., & Meshkini, A. (2024). *Comparative study on physicochemical properties of macroporous hydroxyapatite coatings on 316L stainless steel implants using sol-gel and inverse opal templating*. Materials Science and Technology., DOI: 10.1177/02670836241249250

Mirshafiei, M., Rashedi, H., Yazdian, F., Rahdar, A., & Baino, F. (2024). Advancements in tissue and organ 3D bioprinting: Current techniques, applications, and future perspectives. *Materials and Design, 240*(October 2023), 112853. DOI: 10.1016/j.matdes.2024.112853

Mukasheva, F., Adilova, L., Dyussenbinov, A., Yernaimanova, B., Abilev, M., & Akilbekova, D. (2024). Optimizing scaffold pore size for tissue engineering: Insights across various tissue types. *Frontiers in Bioengineering and Biotechnology, 12*(November), 1–21. DOI: 10.3389/fbioe.2024.1444986 PMID: 39600888

Omidian, H., & Gill, E. J. (2024). Nanofibrous Scaffolds in Biomedicine. *Journal of Composites Science*, *8*(7), 269. Advance online publication. DOI: 10.3390/jcs8070269

Omigbodun, F. T., & Oladapo, B. I. (2025). AI-Optimized Lattice Structures for Biomechanics Scaffold Design. *Biomimetics*, *10*(2), 1–19. DOI: 10.3390/biomimetics10020088 PMID: 39997111

Patil, S. J., Thorat, V. M., Koparde, A. A., Bhosale, R. R., Bhinge, S. D., Chavan, D. D., & Tiwari, D. D. (2024). Theranostic Applications of Scaffolds in Current Biomedical Research. *Cureus*, *16*(10). Advance online publication. DOI: 10.7759/cureus.71694 PMID: 39559663

Prakoso, A. T., Syahrom, A., Arifin, A., & Basri, H. (2025). Mechanical Characterisation of 3D-Printed Porous PLA Scaffolds with Complex Microarchitectures for Bone Tissue Engineering Applications. *Journal of Advanced Research in Applied Sciences and Engineering Technology*, *47*(1), 39–55. DOI: 10.37934/araset.47.1.3955

Profile, S. E. E. (2025). *Applications and Advances in 3D Scaffolds for Tissue Regeneration Applications and Advances in 3D Scaffolds for Tissue Regeneration. January*.

Radhakrishnan, S., Nagarajan, S., Belaid, H., Farha, C., Iatsunskyi, I., Coy, E., Soussan, L., Huon, V., Bares, J., Belkacemi, K., Teyssier, C., Balme, S., Miele, P., Cornu, D., Kalkura, N., Cavaillès, V., & Bechelany, M. (2021). Fabrication of 3D printed antimicrobial polycaprolactone scaffolds for tissue engineering applications. *Materials Science and Engineering C, 118*(August 2020), 111525. DOI: 10.1016/j.msec.2020.111525

Serrano-Aroca, Á., Cano-Vicent, A., Sabater i Serra, R., El-Tanani, M., Aljabali, A. A., Tambuwala, M. M., & Mishra, Y. K. (2022). Scaffolds in the microbial resistant era: Fabrication, materials, properties and tissue engineering applications. *Materials Today. Bio*, *16*(August), 100412. Advance online publication. DOI: 10.1016/j.mtbio.2022.100412 PMID: 36097597

Suamte, L., Tirkey, A., Barman, J., & Jayasekhar Babu, P. (2023). Various manufacturing methods and ideal properties of scaffolds for tissue engineering applications. *Smart Materials in Manufacturing, 1*(June 2022), 100011. DOI: 10.1016/j.smmf.2022.100011

Suhaimin, I. S., Abu Kassim, S., Ahmad Zubir, S., & Abdullah, T. K. (2025). Effect of bioactive glass on the properties of glass/polymer composite scaffold fabricated by solvent casting/particulate leaching technique. *Journal of Thermoplastic Composite Materials*, *0*(0), 1–19. DOI: 10.1177/08927057251314420

Tajurahim, N. A. N., Mahmood, S., Ngadiman, N. H. A., & Sing, S. L. (2025). Biomaterials for tissue engineering scaffolds: Balancing efficiency and eco-friendliness through life cycle assessment. *Cleaner Environmental Systems, 16*(March 2024), 100253. DOI: 10.1016/j.cesys.2024.100253

Tamo, A. K., Djouonkep, L. D. W., & Selabi, N. B. S. (2024). 3D printing of polysaccharide-based hydrogel scaffolds for tissue engineering applications: A review. *International Journal of Biological Macromolecules*, *270*(P2), 132123. DOI: 10.1016/j.ijbiomac.2024.132123 PMID: 38761909

Top, N., Şahin, İ., Gökçe, H., & Gökçe, H. (2021). Computer-aided design and additive manufacturing of bone scaffolds for tissue engineering: State of the art. *Journal of Materials Research, 36*(19), 3725–3745. DOI: 10.1557/s43578-021-00156-y

Wang, C., & Zhou, Y. (2024). Sacrificial biomaterials in 3D fabrication of scaffolds for tissue engineering applications. *Journal of Biomedical Materials Research. Part B, Applied Biomaterials*, *112*(1), e35312. Advance online publication. DOI: 10.1002/jbm.b.35312 PMID: 37572033

Wang, X., Zhang, D., Pratap Singh, Y., Yeo, M., Deng, G., Lai, J., Chen, F., Ozbolat, I. T., & Yu, Y. (2024). Progress in Organ Bioprinting for Regenerative Medicine—Article. *Engineering (Beijing)*, *42*, 121–142. DOI: 10.1016/j.eng.2024.04.023

WIREs Nanomed Nanobiotechnol - 2023 - Rahmani Del Bakhshayesh - Recent advances in nano-scaffolds for tissue engineering.pdf. (n.d.).

Xu, N., Lu, D., Qiang, L., Liu, Y., Yin, D., Wang, Z., Luo, Y., Yang, C., Ma, Z., Ma, H., & Wang, J. (2023). 3D-Printed Composite Bioceramic Scaffolds for Bone and Cartilage Integrated Regeneration. *ACS Omega*, *8*(41), 37918–37926. DOI: 10.1021/acsomega.3c03284 PMID: 37867636

Xu, P., Kankala, R. K., Wang, S., & Chen, A. (2024). Decellularized extracellular matrix-based composite scaffolds for tissue engineering and regenerative medicine. *Regenerative Biomaterials, 11*(September 2023). DOI: 10.1093/rb/rbad107

Yang, Q., Peng, J., Xiao, H., Xu, X., & Qian, Z. (2022). Polysaccharide hydrogels: Functionalization, construction and served as scaffold for tissue engineering. *Carbohydrate Polymers, 278*(September 2021), 118952. DOI: 10.1016/j.carbpol.2021.118952

Yang, Z., Yi, P., Liu, Z., Zhang, W., Mei, L., Feng, C., Tu, C., & Li, Z. (2022). Stem Cell-Laden Hydrogel-Based 3D Bioprinting for Bone and Cartilage Tissue Engineering. *Frontiers in Bioengineering and Biotechnology*, *10*(May), 865770. Advance online publication. DOI: 10.3389/fbioe.2022.865770 PMID: 35656197

Zenobi, E., Merco, M., Mochi, F., Ruspi, J., Pecci, R., Marchese, R., Convertino, A., Lisi, A., Del Gaudio, C., & Ledda, M. (2023). Tailoring the Microarchitectures of 3D Printed Bone-like Scaffolds for Tissue Engineering Applications. *Bioengineering (Basel, Switzerland)*, *10*(5), 567. Advance online publication. DOI: 10.3390/bioengineering10050567 PMID: 37237637

Zhang, W., Liu, L., Cheng, H., Zhu, J., Li, X., Ye, S., & Li, X. (2023). Hydrogel-based dressings designed to facilitate wound healing. *Materials Advances*, *5*(4), 1364–1394. DOI: 10.1039/D3MA00682D

Zhang, X., Li, Z., Yang, P., Duan, G., Liu, X., Gu, Z., & Li, Y. (2021). Polyphenol scaffolds in tissue engineering. *Materials Horizons*, *8*(1), 145–167. DOI: 10.1039/D0MH01317J PMID: 34821294

Chapter 11
Role of Biomaterials in Promoting Wound Healing

Saeedeh Zare Jalise
Department of Tissue Engineering and Applied Cell Sciences, School of Medicine, Qom University of Medical Sciences, Qom, Iran

Mohsen Sheykhhasan
https://orcid.org/0000-0002-4610-2278
Cellular and Molecular Research Center, Qom University of Medical Sciences, Qom, Iran

ABSTRACT

Because biomaterials can improve tissue repair and regeneration, their use in wound healing has drawn much attention. Biomaterials facilitate cellular connections, create favorable microenvironments, and offer mechanical support, making them vital for promoting wound healing. These materials fall into three categories: natural, synthetic, and hybrid. Natural polymers such as collagen, alginate, and chitosan mimic the extracellular matrix and offer biocompatibility, while synthetic polymers like PLGA provide adjustable qualities such as mechanical strength and degradation rates. Advanced biomaterials like hydrogels, nanoparticles, and electrospun fibers enhance moisture retention, control drug release, and reduce infection. They can release bioactive chemicals like growth factors and antimicrobial peptides, promoting healing and preventing chronic wounds. This chapter examines various biomaterials used in wound healing, their therapeutic uses, and modes of action, as well as future developments and challenges in design, biocompatibility, and scalability.

DOI: 10.4018/979-8-3373-1305-4.ch011

1. INTRODUCTION: ROLE OF BIOMATERIALS IN WOUND HEALING

Biomaterials play a pivotal role in enhancing wound healing by modulating various biological processes and providing structural support. These materials, ranging from natural polymers to advanced nanomaterials, are designed to address the complexities of wound healing, which involves stages of inflammation, proliferation, and remodeling. For example, macrophages are crucial in regulating these stages, and biomaterials can modulate their behavior to promote healing (Li et al., 2024). Bacterial nanocelluloses (BNCs) have emerged as promising materials because of their mechanical strength, biocompatibility, and ability to deliver antimicrobial compounds, making them suitable for various types of wounds, including burns and diabetic wounds (Zarepour et al., 2024). Hydrogels, particularly those integrated with cell-conditioned media, offer biocompatibility and biodegradability, enhancing cellular activities such as proliferation and angiogenesis, which are critical for tissue regeneration (Nifontova et al., 2024). Bioceramics, known for their ion-releasing capabilities, support cellular metabolism and exhibit antibacterial properties, facilitating both hard and soft tissue repair without the side effects associated with conventional medications (Al-Naymi et al., 2024). Protein- and lipid-based biomaterials are also significant because of their biodegradability and biocompatibility, which help reduce inflammation and accelerate healing (Abeysinghe & Bandara, 2024). Chitosan and hyaluronic acid-based materials are known for their antimicrobial and anti-inflammatory properties, further enhancing their utility in wound care (Alkabli, 2024). The integration of nanomaterials in wound dressings has shown potential in improving the wound microenvironment by promoting hemostasis, immune regulation, and tissue proliferation, thus accelerating wound closure (Rani et al., 2025). Despite these advancements, challenges such as stability, toxicity, and the need for smart biomaterials that can surpass synthetic products remain. Future research is directed toward optimizing these materials for better clinical outcomes, including the development of intelligent wound dressings that can detect and treat infections synergistically (Cao et al., 2024; Zhong et al., 2024). Biomaterials offer a multifaceted approach to wound healing, combining structural support with biological modulation to improve patient outcomes and reduce healthcare burdens.

2. TYPES OF BIOMATERIALS IN WOUND HEALING

2.1. Natural Polymers

Natural polymers have emerged as promising materials in the field of wound healing because of their biocompatibility, biodegradability, and ability to mimic the extracellular matrix, which is crucial for tissue regeneration. For example, aloe vera-based hydrogels have been developed to enhance wound healing by improving mechanical strength and adhesion properties, promoting fibroblast proliferation, and modulating macrophage activity to reduce inflammation and enhance healing processes (X. Wang et al., 2024). Similarly, the integration of natural polymers such as aloe vera and calendula with polycaprolactone (PCL) in wound dressings has been shown to enhance antimicrobial properties and maintain hydration, which are essential for effective wound healing (Al-Hasani & Al-Hassani, 2024). Other natural polymers, such as chitosan, alginate, and hyaluronic acid, have been extensively studied for their regenerative capabilities, with innovations focused on their chemical composition and cross-linking mechanisms to improve their mechanical and biological performance (Chelu et al., 2024). The use of cellulose and chitosan in suture materials, which are enhanced with graphene oxide nanoparticles, has also been explored to improve biocompatibility and antibacterial activity, further supporting wound healing (Gayathri et al., 2024). Moreover, biodegradable polymers, both natural and synthetic, have been utilized to control the release of bioactive molecules, thereby increasing cell proliferation and angiogenesis, which are critical for wound repair (Halder et al., 2024). The incorporation of biosensors into wound dressings, which use natural polymers such as alginate and chitosan, has led to the development of smart bandages that can respond to physiological changes, offering a more dynamic approach to wound management (Basu et al., 2024). Honey hydrogels combined with natural polymers such as chitosan and gelatin have been highlighted for their potential in treating chronic wounds, although challenges remain in improving their mechanical strength (Chin et al., 2024). The development of self-healing nanomaterials based on natural polymers has also been noted for their ability to autonomously repair damage, reducing the need for frequent dressing changes and enhancing wound care efficiency (Anand et al., 2024). Despite promising advancements, challenges such as scaling up production and ensuring the sterility and stability of these materials persist, necessitating further research and investment in innovative wound care solutions (Cai et al., 2024). Additionally, marine-derived polysaccharides have shown potential in managing diabetic wounds because of their hemostatic and antimicrobial properties, although further research is needed to fully understand their mechanisms and optimize their use (Sudhakaran, 2024). The integration of natural polymers in wound healing applications has significant potential for improving patient outcomes and advancing the field of regenerative medicine.

Patient-Centric Considerations

Natural polymer dressings typically offer comfort and familiarity to patients due to their gentle texture and ease of application. These materials often align well with cultural preferences for natural or plant-derived remedies, increasing patient acceptance. However, ensuring consistency in sensory characteristics, such as odor and texture, and meeting diverse cultural expectations remains critical in broader patient populations.

In the use of natural polymers for wound healing focus on enhancing the healing process while ensuring safety, comfort, and efficacy. Natural polymers such as chitosan, alginate, collagen, and hyaluronic acid are favored due to their biocompatibility, biodegradability, and structural similarity to the extracellular matrix, which supports tissue regeneration and reduces the risk of adverse reactions (Mehvari et al., 2024). These materials are particularly beneficial in managing complex wounds, such as those associated with diabetes, where they help modulate the wound environment, promote cell proliferation, and provide antimicrobial properties to prevent infections (Bhardwaj et al., 2023). The versatility of natural polymers allows for the development of advanced wound dressings that can be tailored to specific patient needs, offering features like moisture regulation, breathability, and the ability to deliver therapeutic agents directly to the wound site (Shahzadi et al., 2022). Innovations such as self-healing materials and stimuli-responsive dressings further enhance patient care by reducing the frequency of dressing changes and adapting to the wound's healing stage (Anand et al., 2024). Moreover, the integration of natural polymers with modern fabrication techniques, including 3D bioprinting, holds promise for creating personalized wound care solutions that align with individual patient profiles (Ho et al., 2024). Despite these advancements, challenges remain, such as ensuring consistent quality and mechanical strength, which are critical for patient safety and the effectiveness of wound dressings (Ho et al., 2024). The patient-centric approach in utilizing natural polymers for wound healing emphasizes the need for materials that not only accelerate healing but also enhance the overall patient experience by being safe, effective, and adaptable to various wound types and conditions (Sharma et al., 2022).

2.2. Synthetic Polymers

Synthetic polymers have emerged as pivotal components in the field of wound healing, offering a range of applications from drug delivery systems to structural scaffolds that mimic the extracellular matrix (ECM). These polymers, such as polyurethane, polyethylene glycol, polylactic acid, and polycaprolactone, are favored for their biocompatibility, biodegradability, and mechanical properties, which are crucial for effective wound management (Halder et al., 2024; Quadir et al., 2024). The integration of synthetic polymers into hydrogels and electrospun scaffolds has been particularly noteworthy. Hydrogels, which are composed of a polymer network and water, provide a moist environment conducive to healing and can be engineered to release bioactive factors that promote cell growth and angiogenesis (Manjit & Mishra, 2024). On the other hand, electrospun scaffolds offer a nanoarchitecture that supports cell adhesion and proliferation, which are essential for tissue regeneration (Gill et al., 2023). The versatility of synthetic polymers allows for the incorporation of biosensors and nanoparticles, enhancing their functionality by enabling targeted drug delivery and antibacterial properties (M. Kumar et al., 2024). Moreover, the development of smart dressings that respond to physiological changes, such as pH or glucose levels, exemplifies the innovative use of synthetic polymers in creating adaptive wound care solutions (M. Kumar et al., 2024). Despite these advancements, challenges such as ensuring in vivo biocompatibility and long-term stability remain, necessitating ongoing research to optimize these materials for clinical applications (Manjit & Mishra, 2024). The future of synthetic polymers in wound healing looks promising, with potential for further customization and integration with advanced technologies such as 3D printing to create more effective and personalized wound care solutions (Gill et al., 2023; Xu et al., 2023).

Patient-Centric Considerations

Synthetic biomaterials offer advantages in durability and reliability, but their clinical acceptance often depends on comfort, ease of use, and appearance. Materials that minimize discomfort during dressing changes and reduce dressing frequency are preferred by patients. Smart dressings designed with discreet sensors enhance user autonomy and confidence in wound management, but they must also address patient concerns regarding privacy, aesthetics, and ease of interpretation.

In the use of synthetic polymers for wound healing are multifaceted, focusing on the customization of wound dressings to meet specific patient needs and wound types. Synthetic polymers offer significant advantages due to their customizable properties, which allow for the creation of dressings that can be tailored to the unique requirements of different wounds, thereby deviating from a 'one size fits all' approach (Mir et al., 2018). Electrospun scaffolds, for instance, are highly valued for their ability to mimic the natural extracellular matrix, providing a conducive environment for cell proliferation and differentiation, which is crucial for effective wound healing (Gill et al., 2023). The mechanical and thermal properties of synthetic polymers, such as polylactic acid (PLA) and polycaprolactone (PCL), make them suitable for creating durable and effective wound dressings that can be tailored to specific healing needs (Xu et al., 2023). Moreover, the integration of biodegradable and biocompatible synthetic polymers addresses the limitations of natural polymers, offering enhanced mechanical properties and controlled degradation rates, which are essential for patient comfort and effective healing (Halder et al., 2024). The use of bioresorbable polymers, which degrade naturally in the body, eliminates the need for surgical removal, thus reducing patient discomfort and the risk of infection (Quadir et al., 2024). Additionally, the incorporation of antimicrobial agents, such as metal/metal oxide nanoparticles, into synthetic polymer matrices enhances the antimicrobial properties of wound dressings, providing an added layer of protection against infections (Gobi et al., 2021). The development of stimuli-responsive and drug-delivery systems within synthetic polymer dressings further enhances their functionality, allowing for targeted and controlled release of therapeutic agents, which can be crucial for managing chronic wounds (Chen et al., 2024). The patient-centric approach in the development of synthetic polymer-based wound dressings emphasizes the importance of customization, biocompatibility, and functionality to improve healing outcomes and patient satisfaction (Prete et al., 2023).

2.3. Hybrid Materials

Hybrid materials have emerged as promising candidates in the field of wound healing because of their multifunctional properties, which can be tailored to address various aspects of the healing process. These materials often combine biocompatible polymers with bioactive agents to increase their therapeutic efficacy. For example, graphene oxide and silver oxide integrated with polyvinyl alcohol (PVA) and chitosan have been shown to mimic natural body compositions and provide electrical stimulation to promote cell migration and proliferation, thus enhancing wound healing capabilities (Unnikrishnan et al., 2024). Similarly, chitosan and hyaluronic acid-based hybrids are noted for their biocompatibility, biodegradability, and inherent biological activities, such as antimicrobial and anti-inflammatory properties, making them suitable for skin protection and regeneration (Alkabli, 2024). The incorporation of reduced graphene oxide (rGO) into collagen-based hydrogels has led to improved conductivity and stability, which are crucial for effective wound closure (He et al., 2024). Additionally, the use of essential oils in polymer-based dressings has been explored for their antimicrobial properties, which are attributed to compounds such as eugenol and cinnamaldehyde, further enhancing the healing process (Buriti et al., 2024). Advanced composites, such as those made from human placenta and sodium alginate, have shown promising results in promoting angiogenesis and tissue formation, which are crucial for deep wound healing (Alizadeh et al., 2024). Sepiolite-based hydrogels with CuxO nanoparticles have been developed for their self-healing and antibacterial properties, effectively aiding in hemostasis and wound healing (Jiang et al., 2024). Moreover, polysaccharide-based hydrogels with interpenetrating networks have been designed to offer robust mechanical properties and effective drug delivery, ensuring comprehensive wound repair (He et al., 2024). Innovative approaches also include the use of biomimetic hydrogels that modulate immune responses to expedite healing in infection-related wounds (Bao et al., 2024). Furthermore, hybrid hydrogels combining polyacrylamide and photodynamic nanoparticles have been developed to address chronic wound infections without antibiotics (Kang et al., 2024). Chitosan/Bi2Se3 nanocomposites have shown enhanced antibacterial activity and biocompatibility, promoting cell proliferation and wound healing in vitro (Swaminathan et al., 2024). These studies underscore the potential of hybrid materials in creating advanced wound dressings that offer multiple benefits, including antimicrobial activity, enhanced mechanical properties, and improved healing outcomes (**Figure 1**).

Patient-Centric Considerations

Hybrid materials are promising due to their multifunctionality and potential to reduce treatment duration and complexity. However, acceptance can be influenced by patient perceptions regarding the safety and origins of hybrid or nanoparticle-based components. Clear communication regarding the safety, efficacy, and benefits of these materials, alongside addressing any patient anxieties regarding novel technologies, is essential for successful clinical adoption.

In the development of hybrid materials for wound healing focus on enhancing the healing process while minimizing adverse effects and improving patient comfort. Hybrid materials, such as those incorporating essential oils, graphene, polycaprolactone (PCL), and other bioactive compounds, offer promising solutions by mimicking the extracellular matrix and providing antimicrobial properties, which are crucial for preventing infections and promoting faster healing (Zhao et al., 2019). For instance, the integration of essential oils like eugenol and cinnamaldehyde in polymer-based dressings has shown potential in reducing inflammation and accelerating wound closure due to their antimicrobial properties (Buriti et al., 2024). Similarly, graphene oxide (GO) combined with PCL in hybrid patches has demonstrated efficacy in protecting cells from bacterial infections, thus facilitating wound healing in complex cases such as open abdomen and intestinal fistula wounds (Zhao et al., 2019). The use of natural oils, such as andiroba oil in PCL films, has been shown to enhance the thermal stability and cell viability of the dressing, making it a suitable candidate for biomedical applications (Silva et al., 2021). Moreover, hybrid hydrogels incorporating self-assembling peptides and nanoparticles have been developed to address infected chronic wounds, offering strong tissue adhesion and self-healing properties without the need for antibiotics (Kang et al., 2024). These materials not only promote rapid wound closure but also ensure a controlled inflammatory response, which is crucial for effective healing, as demonstrated by the use of hybrid biomaterials that modulate neutrophil activity to resolve inflammation and promote tissue regeneration (Liu et al., 2022). Additionally, the incorporation of nanotechnology and smart materials, such as electroactive polymers, into wound dressings has enhanced their mechanical strength and drug release capabilities, further supporting patient-centric therapeutic interventions (Nasra et al., 2024). These advancements highlight the importance of integrating bioactive compounds and innovative technologies in hybrid materials to improve wound healing outcomes while prioritizing patient safety and comfort.

2.4. Integrative Perspective

Each biomaterial type plays a complementary role in wound healing, and their selection often depends on wound severity, type, and healing stage. **Natural polymers** are ideal for early-stage healing and chronic wounds due to their biological affinity, while **synthetic polymers** serve well in structural and smart applications requiring durability. **Hybrid materials** are best suited for complex or infected wounds, where multifunctional performance is required. Integrating these approaches through combination dressings or staged application strategies can optimize healing outcomes and patient care.

The integration of various biomaterial types in wound healing is a multifaceted approach that leverages the unique properties of both natural and synthetic materials to address the complex requirements of wound care. Biomaterials such as hydrogels, films, foams, and membranes are commonly employed due to their ability to create an optimal healing environment by maintaining hydration, providing structural support, and facilitating gas exchange (Moreira et al., 2024). Natural biomaterials, including polysaccharides and proteins, are favored for their biomimicry of the extracellular matrix (ECM) and their role in native wound healing processes, although they often require enhancement through combination with synthetic materials to overcome limitations like low mechanical strength (Ansari & Darvishi, 2024). Synthetic polymers, such as polylactic acid and polycaprolactone, offer customizable properties that can be tailored to specific wound types, enhancing their utility in wound dressings (Mir et al., 2018). Advanced composite materials, such as multipolymeric systems and nanofibrous structures, aim to fulfill multiple wound dressing requirements, including anti-infective properties and controlled biodegradation, although a single material meeting all these criteria remains elusive (Pillay et al., 2015). The development of trilayered constructs, which mimic the full thickness of skin, represents a promising approach for chronic wound healing by providing a dense superficial layer, a bioactive middle layer, and a porous lower layer to support cell proliferation and tissue regeneration (Ijaola et al., 2022). Smart biomaterials, capable of responding to environmental stimuli, offer precise control over the wound healing process, enhancing the effectiveness of treatment across different healing stages (Liu et al., 2023). The integration of drug delivery systems and nanotechnologies further augments the functionality of biomaterials, enabling targeted delivery of therapeutic agents and enhancing the overall healing process (Piraino & Selimović, 2015). Despite the advancements, challenges such as cost, scalability, and processing difficulties persist, necessitating ongoing research to optimize the synthesis and application of these biomaterials in clinical settings (Das et al., 2023).

Ultimately, integrating patient perspectives—such as comfort, cultural appropriateness, usability, aesthetics, and clear patient education—is vital. Addressing these factors ensures successful clinical translation, adherence, and broader community acceptance of biomaterial-based wound care technologies.

Figure 1. Schematic representation of biomaterials used in wound healing applications

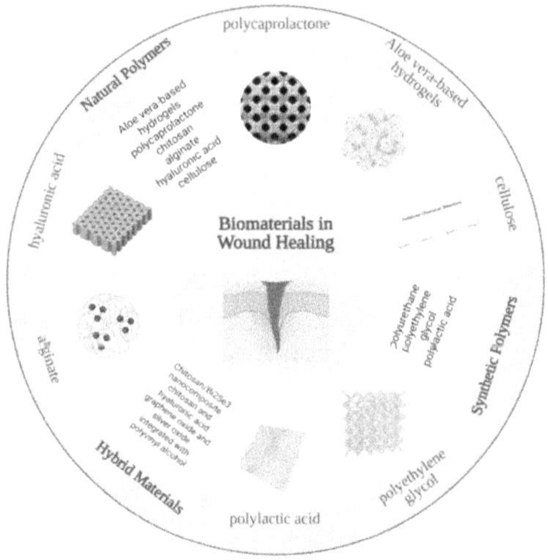

The materials are categorized into three main groups: natural polymers (e.g., aloe vera-based hydrogels, polycaprolactone, chitosan, alginate, hyaluronic acid, and cellulose), synthetic polymers (e.g., polyurethane, polyethylene glycol, and polylactic acid), and hybrid materials (e.g., chitosan/Bi2Se3 nanocomposites, chitosan, hyaluronic acid, graphene oxide, and silver oxide integrated with polyvinyl alcohol). Each category is illustrated with representative images and structures, highlighting their role in wound healing.

Table 1. Comparative overview of biomaterials for wound healing

Biomaterial Type	Representative Materials	Advantages	Disadvantages	Clinical Applications
Natural Polymers	Chitosan, Alginate, Hyaluronic acid, Aloe vera	Biocompatible, biodegradable, mimics ECM, bioactive	Mechanical weakness, batch variability, scalability issues	Chronic wounds, diabetic ulcers, burn dressings
Synthetic Polymers	Polycaprolactone (PCL), Polyurethane, PEG, PLA	Tunable mechanical properties, reproducibility, integration with sensors	Biodegradation products may be inflammatory, less bioactive	Drug delivery scaffolds, smart dressings, tissue engineering
Hybrid Materials	Chitosan/PVA + silver/graphene oxide, Collagen-rGO hydrogels	Combine bioactivity and mechanical strength, multifunctional, tailored responses	Complex fabrication, regulatory challenges	Antimicrobial dressings, chronic/infected wound treatment, electroactive scaffolds

3. MECHANISMS OF BIOMATERIAL ACTION IN WOUND REPAIR

3.1. Cellular Interaction

Cellular interaction biomaterials play crucial roles in wound repair by modulating the wound microenvironment and influencing the cellular behaviors essential for healing. The interaction between biomaterials and cells, such as macrophages, fibroblasts, and mast cells, is pivotal in determining the healing outcome. For example, the crosslinking density of hydrogels can significantly affect macrophage and fibroblast behavior, with lightly crosslinked hydrogels promoting better cellular infiltration and smaller scars than heavily crosslinked hydrogels do, which increases inflammation and profibrotic activity (Butenko et al., 2024). Similarly, the composition of wound dressings, such as Atrauman and Melolin, can influence the retention or absorption of key cell types such as M2 macrophages, impacting the healing trajectory (Saberianpour et al., 2024). Biomaterials can also be engineered to provide biochemical cues that guide cellular responses, such as peptide therapy and collagen matrices, which are crucial for advanced wound repair (Singh et al., 2022). Moreover, bioactive materials can modulate the wound microenvironment at the molecular level, promoting hemostasis, anti-inflammatory effects, tissue regeneration, and matrix remodeling (Li et al., 2022). The role of the immune system is particularly significant, as biomaterials can interact with immune cells to reduce scarring and enhance regeneration, with some studies showing the potential for complete tissue regeneration through immune modulation (Butenko et al., 2023). Additionally, the use of acellular biomaterials combined with bone marrow-derived stem cells has shown promise in improving wound healing through paracrine effects, enhancing collagen production and reducing inflammatory cytokines (de Souza et al., 2023). The interaction of human dermal fibroblasts with bacterial nanocellulose composite hydrogels further exemplifies how biomaterials can support cell viability and influence gene expression related to wound healing (Xi Loh et al., 2018).

3.2. Release of Bioactive Molecules

Biomaterials that release bioactive molecules play crucial roles in wound repair by modulating the wound microenvironment and promoting healing through various mechanisms. Granular biomaterials, such as jammed microgels, have been developed to sequester and release signaling molecules such as interleukin 6 (IL-6) and vascular endothelial growth factor A (VEGF-A), thereby tailoring the local concentrations of pro- and anti-inflammatory factors to enhance wound healing (Emiroglu et al., 2024). Bioactive materials, including those derived from natural compounds such as polyphenols, have shown promise in modulating cell behaviors and the wound microenvironment, facilitating processes such as angiogenesis, fibroblast migration, and inflammation control (Zhao et al., 2023). Nanomaterials, particularly those encapsulating natural bioactive agents, offer advantages such as improved solubility, improved stability, and controlled release, which are essential for the prolonged and effective treatment of wounds (Kant et al., 2021). Stimuli-responsive biomaterials have been designed to provide spatiotemporal control over the delivery of therapeutics, addressing the complexity of wound healing by enabling localized and timely release of bioactive molecules (Oliva & Almquist, 2020). Surfactants and biosurfactants, with their anti-inflammatory and antibacterial properties, also contribute to wound healing by maintaining a balanced wound environment (Ohadi et al., 2023). Furthermore, innovative approaches such as the use of silk fibroin and gold nanorods in nanomaterial dressings have been shown to stimulate immune responses and enhance tissue repair processes, particularly in challenging conditions such as diabetic wounds (Ghosh et al., 2024). The integration of bioactive molecules into biomaterials offers a multifaceted approach to wound healing, addressing both the biological and mechanical aspects of tissue repair and regeneration (Chen et al., 2019).

4. ADVANCED BIOMATERIALS FOR ENHANCED WOUND HEALING

4.1. Nanomaterials and Nanotechnology

Nanomaterials and nanotechnology have significantly advanced the field of wound healing by offering innovative solutions that address the complexities of wound management. Titanium dioxide nanoparticles (TiO2 NPs) have been highlighted for their antioxidant, anti-inflammatory, and antimicrobial properties, which are crucial for accelerating wound healing and enhancing tissue regeneration when incorporated into scaffolds and dressings (Nosrati & Heydari, 2025). The integration of various nanomaterials, such as nanoparticles, nanofibers, and nanocomposites, into wounds has facilitated controlled drug delivery, improved mechanical strength, and provided a conducive environment for cellular processes, thereby promoting tissue regeneration and reducing chronic inflammation (Goyal et al., 2024). Nanotechnology has also enabled the development of smart dressings and regenerative scaffolds that mimic the extracellular matrix, promoting cell proliferation and tissue regeneration, particularly in hard-to-heal wounds such as diabetic ulcers and severe burns (Alencar et al., 2024). Furthermore, gas-releasing nanomaterials have emerged as a novel strategy, offering broad-spectrum antibacterial properties without inducing bacterial resistance, thus proving effective in treating chronic nonhealing wounds (Duan et al.). The use of bioactive nanoparticles in wound dressings has been shown to enhance the healing of prolonged wounds and burns by creating a microenvironment that mimics physiological tissue regeneration processes (Mittal et al., 2024). Additionally, the combination of nanopolymers with plant extracts in hydrogels has accelerated healing and improved tissue regeneration because of their antioxidant, anti-inflammatory, and antimicrobial properties (Jessy Mercy et al., 2024). Despite these advancements, challenges such as the high cost of nanotechnological products and the need for more large-scale clinical trials remain, highlighting the necessity for further research and improved accessibility to ensure the broad adoption of these technologies in wound care (Alencar et al., 2024). Overall, the integration of nanotechnology into wound management represents a paradigm shift, offering promising avenues for addressing longstanding challenges in cellular and tissue repair (R. Kumar et al., 2024; Nameeta, 2024).

For instance, clinical trials utilizing silver nanoparticles incorporated into dressings have demonstrated accelerated healing rates in chronic diabetic wounds compared to conventional dressings, significantly reducing infection rates and hospital stays (Alencar et al., 2024). Gas-releasing nanomaterials, known for their broad-spectrum antibacterial properties without inducing resistance, have been successfully used in treating antibiotic-resistant infections in chronic nonhealing wounds (Duan et al., 2025). Additionally, plant-derived nanopolymer hydrogels have demonstrated clinical effectiveness in accelerating wound closure and minimizing inflammation in burn patients, highlighting their practical advantages (Jessy Mercy et al., 2024). The use of nanomaterials in wound dressings, such as hydrogel/nano silver-based dressings and copper oxide-infused dressings, has been particularly beneficial in treating diabetic foot wounds and difficult-to-treat wounds, respectively (Prabhu et al., 2023). Despite these advancements, challenges such as reproducibility, stability, toxicity, and histocompatibility remain, necessitating further research to ensure successful clinical translation (Rani et al., 2025). Moreover, the high cost of some nanotechnological products poses a barrier to widespread implementation, especially in resource-limited settings (Alencar et al., 2024). Nonetheless, the ongoing research and development in this field continue to pave the way for improved patient outcomes and reduced healthcare burdens, with future prospects including intelligent wound dressings that can detect and treat infections synergistically (Wang et al., 2021). Nanotechnology holds tremendous promise for revolutionizing wound care, offering advanced therapeutic interventions that can significantly enhance wound healing outcomes (Naskar & Kim, 2020).

4.2. Hydrogels and Moisture Retention

Owing to their unique properties, such as high water retention, biocompatibility, and ability to create a moist environment conducive to tissue regeneration, hydrogels have emerged as promising solutions for enhancing wound healing. These hydrophilic polymer networks mimic natural tissue environments, which increase cell viability and function, making them ideal for wound dressings and tissue engineering applications (Kaur et al., 2024; McKenzie et al., 2015). The moisture retention capability of hydrogels is particularly beneficial, as it promotes cell migration and proliferation, reduces inflammation, and prevents infection, thereby accelerating the healing process (Olteanu et al., 2024). Hydrogels can be engineered to deliver bioactive agents and antibiotics directly to the wound site, further enhancing their therapeutic efficacy (Kaur et al., 2024). Various types of hydrogels, including those based on natural polymers such as chitosan and hyaluronic acid, have been developed to improve wound healing outcomes. For example, quaternized chitosan hydrogels offer enhanced antibacterial properties and solubility across a range of pH values, making them effective in wound regeneration (Mottaghitalab et al., 2024). Similarly, hyaluronic acid-based self-healing hydrogels are particularly effective for diabetic wounds, as they can maintain a moist environment and repair themselves when damaged, thus providing a customized therapeutic approach (Chhillar & Jaiswal, 2025). The integration of fibroblast-derived extracellular vesicles into hydrogels has also been shown to significantly accelerate wound healing by promoting cell migration, differentiation, and angiogenesis (Galbiati et al., 2025). Moreover, the development of bioadhesive and self-healing hydrogels addresses the need for dressings that can withstand mechanical stress and adhere well to tissue, which is crucial for managing chronic wounds (Nezhad-Mokhtari et al., 2024). Despite these advancements, challenges remain in optimizing the mechanical strength, adhesion, and scalability of hydrogel-based wound dressings, indicating a need for continued research and development in this field. Overall, the versatility and adaptability of hydrogels make them valuable tools in modern wound care, offering potential for improved patient outcomes across various clinical scenarios (Olteanu et al., 2024).

Clinical studies have demonstrated that hydrogels incorporating bioactive compounds, such as quaternized chitosan or hyaluronic acid, significantly enhance wound healing outcomes in diabetic foot ulcers and pressure injuries by maintaining an optimal healing environment (Chhillar & Jaiswal, 2025; Mottaghitalab et al., 2024). In one illustrative clinical case, self-healing hyaluronic acid hydrogels achieved approximately 20% faster healing times compared to conventional dressings in diabetic ulcers, improving patient comfort and reducing dressing-change frequency (Chhillar & Jaiswal, 2025). Additionally, hydrogels enriched with fibroblast-derived extracellular vesicles have shown remarkable efficacy in treating chronic wounds, accelerating angiogenesis and tissue regeneration, thus demonstrating significant potential for clinical translation (Galbiati et al., 2025). Clinical trials have also highlighted the superiority of specific hydrogels, such as the Olea europaea leaf extract hydrogel, which significantly accelerated wound healing compared to traditional amorphous hydrogels in a randomized controlled trial involving various ulcer types (Verdú-Soriano et al., 2022). Additionally, hydrogels like the M-CMCS/O-HES have shown promising results in rat models by providing excellent water retention, biocompatibility, and biodegradability, leading to faster wound closure and improved tissue regeneration (Li et al., 2020). Systematic reviews have consistently reported that hydrogel dressings significantly shorten healing times and alleviate pain in various wound types, including diabetic foot ulcers and burns, without severe adverse reactions (Satti et al., 2023). Furthermore, smart hydrogels with responsiveness to external stimuli, such as pH and temperature, have been developed to enhance wound healing by modulating inflammation and promoting angiogenesis

(Tehrany et al., 2023). The incorporation of antibacterial agents, such as tobramycin, into hydrogels has also been shown to combat bacterial infections effectively, further optimizing the wound healing process (Xiao et al., 2024). The integration of hydrogels in wound management represents a significant advancement, offering multifunctional capabilities that address the diverse challenges of wound healing (Kuddushi et al., 2023).

4.3. Electrospun Fibers

Electrospun fibers have emerged as a promising technology for enhancing wound healing because of their unique properties and versatility in incorporating various therapeutic agents. These fibers, produced through electrospinning, mimic the extracellular matrix (ECM) of the skin, providing a conducive environment for cell proliferation and tissue regeneration, which is crucial for effective wound healing (Dai et al., 2024; Lu et al., 2024). The incorporation of natural polymers and bioactive compounds, such as chitosan, gelatin, curcumin, and rutin, enhances the antimicrobial, anti-inflammatory, and antioxidant properties of the fibers, promoting faster wound closure and reduced scarring (Liu et al., 2024; P. D. Yadav et al., 2024). Multifunctional electrospun nanofiber films, such as those incorporating rhamnose and therapeutic agents such as fluticasone and mupirocin, have shown significant potential in treating infected burn wounds by offering antimicrobial and regenerative properties, achieving up to 30% faster healing than controls do (Ijaz & Khan, 2025). The high porosity and surface area of electrospun fibers facilitate the absorption of wound exudate and the controlled release of therapeutic agents, which are essential for managing chronic wounds and minimizing scarring (Shariatzadeh et al., 2024). Additionally, the integration of advanced materials such as silver nanocrystals and graphene oxide into electrospun fibers enhances their mechanical strength and antimicrobial efficacy, making them suitable for chronic and burn-related wounds (Reyes-Guzmán et al., 2024). With their biomimetic structure and ability to incorporate smart features such as stimuli-responsive components, electrospun hydrogel fibers further advance wound care by providing real-time monitoring and tailored therapeutic delivery (P. Yadav et al., 2024). Despite these advancements, challenges remain in optimizing the synthesis process and ensuring consistent clinical performance, necessitating further research to fully realize the clinical potential of electrospun nanofiber dressings (Lu et al., 2024; P. D. Yadav et al., 2024). Electrospun fibers represent a significant advancement in wound healing technologies, offering a multifaceted approach to accelerate healing and improve outcomes (**Figure 2**).

Clinically, electrospun dressings containing therapeutic agents such as fluticasone and mupirocin have proven highly effective for infected burns, achieving wound closure up to 30% faster than conventional gauze dressings, with significantly reduced infection rates (Ijaz & Khan, 2025). Electrospun fibers embedded with silver nanocrystals or graphene oxide have similarly demonstrated clinical success in treating chronic and burn wounds by providing sustained antimicrobial protection and mechanical support, facilitating improved healing outcomes in difficult-to-treat wounds (Reyes-Guzmán et al., 2024). Additionally, electrospun hydrogel fibers with stimuli-responsive features enable real-time wound monitoring and personalized therapeutic responses, showing clinical promise in managing chronic and non-healing wounds (J. P. Yadav et al., 2024).

Clinical trials have demonstrated the efficacy of electrospun fiber matrices in treating chronic wounds, such as diabetic foot ulcers, where they have shown superior results compared to standard care, achieving higher rates of complete wound re-epithelialization and faster healing times (Husain et al., 2024). The incorporation of antimicrobial agents and growth factors into these fibers further enhances their wound healing capabilities by reducing infection and inflammation, as evidenced by studies using fibers loaded with drugs like enrofloxacin and flunixin meglumine, which showed significant antibacterial activity and accelerated healing in animal models (Li et al., 2021). Additionally, innovative approaches such as self-powered electrospun fibers that provide electrical stimulation have been developed, offering multifunctional benefits including enhanced antibacterial properties and improved hemostasis, which are crucial for chronic wound management (Zhang et al., 2024). The versatility of electrospun fibers allows for the integration of various therapeutic agents, enabling tailored treatments for different wound types, including infected burn wounds and pressure ulcers (Ijaz & Khan, 2025). Despite these advancements, challenges remain in optimizing the synthesis processes and ensuring consistent clinical performance, necessitating further research to fully realize the potential of electrospun fibers in wound healing (P. Yadav et al., 2024). The clinical application of electrospun fibers represents a significant advancement in wound care, offering a promising alternative to conventional dressings with their ability to enhance healing through biomimetic structures and multifunctional capabilities (Liu et al., 2017).

Figure 2. Overview of advanced biomaterials for enhanced wound healing

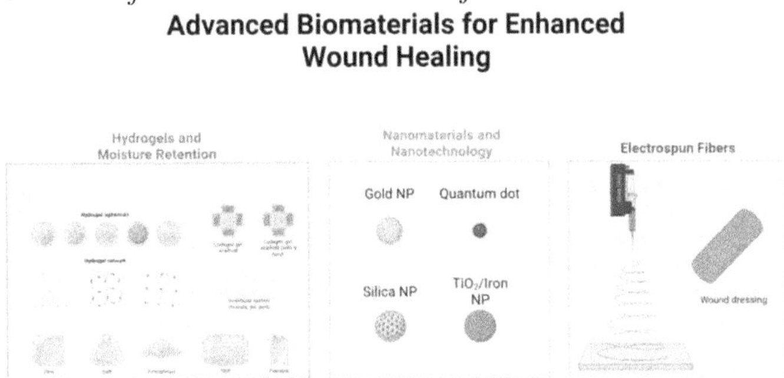

The overview is categorized into three main approaches: hydrogels and moisture retention, nanomaterials and nanotechnology, and electrospinning fibers. Hydrogels provide moisture retention and structural support through different forms, such as spherical hydrogels, hydrogel networks, and collagen gel scaffolds. Nanomaterials, including gold nanoparticles (NPs), silica NPs, quantum dots, and TiO_2/Iron NPs, enhance wound healing through antimicrobial, anti-inflammatory, and regenerative properties. Electrospun fibers, shown in the form of wound dressings, offer a nanofiber-based scaffold for improved healing and tissue regeneration.

5. CLINICAL APPLICATIONS OF BIOMATERIALS IN WOUND HEALING

Biomaterials have emerged as pivotal tools in the clinical management of wound healing, offering innovative solutions to enhance tissue repair and regeneration. Biomaterial-based scaffolds, such as those discussed by Sindhi et al., provide a three-dimensional framework that supports cellular processes and facilitates the delivery of cells, medications, and genes, thereby promoting skin tissue regeneration (Sindhi et al., 2025). In the context of chronic wounds, biomaterials address the challenges posed by slow healing and frequent infections, with a focus on improving biocompatibility and integrating drug delivery systems to enhance therapeutic outcomes (Barbu et al., 2025). Green synthesized biomaterials, including chitosan, collagen, and alginate, are known for their biocompatibility and ability to maintain moisture at the wound site, which accelerates healing (Farasati Far et al., 2025). Bacterial nanocelluloses (BNCs) are highlighted for their mechanical strength, biodegradability, and ability to serve as carriers for antimicrobial compounds, making them suitable for various types of wounds, including diabetic and ischemic wounds (Zarepour et al., 2024). The integration of hydrogels with cell-conditioned media and extracellular vesicles has shown promise in modulating cellular activities crucial for wound healing, such as proliferation and angiogenesis, while providing a moist environment conducive to tissue regeneration (Nifontova et al., 2024). Furthermore, the modulation of macrophage function through biomaterials is crucial, as macrophages play a significant role in the inflammatory and tissue repair phases of wound healing (Li et al., 2024). Novel biomaterials, including nanofibers and composite hydrogels, are being developed to enhance wound healing and tissue regeneration, with a focus on maintaining internal homeostasis (Zhong et al., 2024). Bioceramics, known for their ability to release inorganic ions, contribute to cellular metabolism and exhibit bactericidal activity, offering a cost-effective and efficient alternative for wound repair (Al-Naymi et al., 2024). These advancements underscore the transformative potential of biomaterials in wound healing, emphasizing their role in improving therapeutic efficacy and patient outcomes across various clinical scenarios.

Despite these promising developments, the transition of biomaterial-based wound healing products from the laboratory to clinical practice is often hindered by complex regulatory and approval processes. Historically, regulatory agencies such as the United States Food and Drug Administration (FDA) and the European Medicines Agency (EMA) have played critical roles in shaping the clinical introduction of new biomaterials. Early regulations focused primarily on safety and basic biocompatibility; however, as biomaterials became more sophisticated (e.g., incorporating cells, genes, and bioactive molecules), guidelines evolved to address issues such as immunogenicity, long-term stability, and environmental impact (Khanna et al., 2025).

To meet regulatory expectations, manufacturers must demonstrate robust quality control measures through standardized testing protocols. These include physicochemical characterization, sterilization validation, and batch-to-batch reproducibility to ensure product consistency and patient safety. Recent changes in policies also emphasize post-market surveillance, requiring ongoing monitoring of device performance and adverse events once biomaterials have entered clinical use (Vinchurkar et al., 2025). In tandem, the International Organization for Standardization (ISO) has issued standards outlining requirements for design, risk management, and performance evaluation of medical devices, thereby promoting harmonized global practices.

From a historical standpoint, many early biomaterials (such as first-generation synthetic polymers) were subject to relatively minimal oversight, as regulatory bodies primarily concentrated on drug products rather than combination products or advanced tissue engineering strategies. Over the last two decades, increasing complexity in tissue engineering has prompted a shift toward more stringent assessments. For instance, the FDA introduced the Breakthrough Devices Program to expedite the review of innovative products with potential to address life-threatening conditions, which includes certain biomaterial-based wound dressings. Similarly, the EMA has launched adaptive licensing pathways that encourage early collaboration between developers and regulators, aiming to balance patient safety with timely access to novel therapies (Jones & Patel, 2018).

These evolving frameworks highlight the importance of close collaboration among researchers, manufacturers, clinicians, and regulatory authorities. By understanding both the technological innovations and the regulatory landscape, stakeholders can navigate clinical translation more efficiently. Continuous updates to policies—spurred by advances in biomaterial science—demand proactive engagement with the latest guidelines and standardization measures. As such, incorporating regulatory strategies into product development cycles from the outset is now viewed as essential for the successful clinical implementation of biomaterials in wound healing.

5.1. Acute and Chronic Wounds

Biomaterials have emerged as pivotal tools in the clinical management of both acute and chronic wounds, offering innovative solutions to enhance wound healing and tissue regeneration. Biomaterial-based scaffolds, particularly those incorporating nanotechnology, have shown promise in skin tissue regeneration because they provide structural support and facilitate the cellular processes essential for healing (Sindhi et al., 2025). Natural biomaterials, such as polysaccharides and proteins, are increasingly favored for their biomimetic properties and ability to integrate with the body's native healing processes, although they often require enhancement with synthetic materials to improve their mechanical properties (Ansari & Darvishi, 2024). Hydrogels, a type of biomaterial, are particularly effective in wound healing because of their ability to maintain a moist environment, deliver bioactive substances, and prevent infections, thereby accelerating the healing process (P. Wang et al., 2024). Collagen-based scaffolds have been specifically highlighted for their efficacy in treating chronic wounds, such as diabetic ulcers, by promoting tissue regeneration and addressing the underlying pathophysiological issues that impede healing (La Monica et al., 2024). The integration of nanomaterials into wound dressings has further advanced the field by offering antimicrobial, anti-inflammatory, and angiogenic benefits, which are crucial for managing complex wound environments (Rani et al., 2025). Moreover, the modulation of the immune system through biomaterials and nanomedicine has been recognized as a critical strategy in chronic wound healing, emphasizing the role of immune cells in the repair process (Las Heras et al., 2024). Oxygen-releasing biomaterials represent another innovative approach, addressing hypoxia in chronic wounds and facilitating improved healing outcomes through enhanced oxygen delivery (He et al., 2023). Collectively, these advancements underscore the diverse applications of biomaterials in wound care, highlighting their potential to revolutionize treatment strategies and improve patient outcomes across various wound types (Moreira et al., 2024).

5.2. Burns and Surgical Wounds

Biomaterials have emerged as pivotal tools in the clinical management of burns and surgical wounds, offering innovative solutions to enhance healing and tissue regeneration. These materials, including scaffolds, hydrogels, and chitosan, are integral to the tissue engineering triad, which combines cells, scaffolds, and growth-stimulating signals to promote re-epithelialization and limit scar formation in burn injuries (Vishali et al.). Scaffolds, particularly those based on biomaterials, provide structural support and a conducive environment for cell adhesion, proliferation, and differentiation, which are crucial for skin tissue regeneration (Vishali et al.). The incorporation of micro/nanostructures in biomaterials has been shown to influence cell behavior, promote angiogenesis, and regulate immune responses, thereby enhancing wound healing and reducing scar areas (Tao et al., 2023). Both natural and synthetic polymers are extensively used in wound healing applications, with their success rates varying on the basis of the severity of the wound and the properties of the biomaterial (Das et al., 2023). Advanced biomaterials, developed through interdisciplinary approaches, offer multifunctional capabilities that accelerate wound repair and improve tissue regeneration quality (Luo & Zhou, 2024). These materials are designed to address the complex pathophysiological processes of wound healing, which include coagulation, inflammation, proliferation, and tissue remodeling (Dias-Ferreira et al., 2023). In the context of burn injuries, biomaterials serve as scaffolds or dressings that mimic the extracellular matrix, providing mechanical support and facilitating the release of bioactive molecules to enhance healing (Bhar & Das, 2024). The development of smart biomaterials that can control wound healing temporally and spatially further underscores their potential in personalized wound therapy (Liu et al., 2023). Despite promising advancements, challenges such as the scarcity of certain biomaterials, high costs, and processing difficulties remain, necessitating ongoing research to optimize their clinical applicability (Das et al., 2023). The integration of biomaterials in wound healing strategies represents a significant advancement in medical science, offering new avenues for the effective treatment of burns and surgical wounds.

6. CHALLENGES IN BIOMATERIAL DESIGN AND CLINICAL TRANSLATION

The design and clinical translation of biomaterials face numerous challenges, as highlighted across various studies. One significant hurdle is the regulatory landscape, which is often complex and lacks international harmonization, posing barriers to the clinical implementation of advanced biomaterials such as nanomaterial-enabled biosensors and 3D-printed scaffolds (Talreja et al., 2024). Safety and toxicity concerns, particularly with nanomaterials and liquid metals, further complicate their clinical adoption owing to potential immune rejection and long-term biological safety issues (Xu et al., 2024). Additionally, there is a notable gap between the optimism of scientists and the cautious approach of clinicians, particularly in the context of bone defect treatments, which underscores the need for interdisciplinary collaboration to align clinical needs with research outcomes (Laubach et al., 2024). Manufacturing challenges, including scalability and maintaining the structural integrity of complex delivery systems, are also prevalent, especially in the context of protein delivery and adoptive cell therapies (Gorantla et al., 2024). Ethical considerations are increasingly critical as biomaterials become more complex, necessitating updated ethical guidelines and training to ensure responsible scientific inquiry (Hunckler & Levine, 2022). Moreover, the economic constraints and hesitancy in adopting new technologies further impede the translation of innovative biomaterials into clinical practice (Talreja et al., 2024). Despite these challenges, the potential of biomaterials in regenerative medicine, diagnostics, and therapeutic applications remains vast, with ongoing research focusing on overcoming these barriers through improved design, regulatory clarity, and interdisciplinary collaboration (Capella-Monsonís et al., 2024; Q. Zhu et al., 2024). The integration of biomaterials into clinical settings requires a concerted effort to address these multifaceted challenges, ensuring that innovations can effectively transition from the bench to the bedside (**Figure 3**) (Bayon et al., 2024).

Real-world applications illustrate both the promise and pitfalls of biomaterial research. For example, hydroxyapatite-based bone graft substitutes have achieved clinical success by promoting osteointegration in certain orthopedic procedures, yet broader adoption has been slowed by variability in patient responses and cost considerations (Kauke-Navarro et al., 2024). Conversely, metal-on-metal hip implants initially showed promise due to their durability but were later associated with significant wear-particle generation, adverse local tissue reactions, and increased regulatory scrutiny, demonstrating how unanticipated outcomes can impede clinical uptake (Stoops et al., 2025). These contrasting scenarios underscore the importance of robust preclinical testing, long-term surveillance, and responsive regulatory frameworks to facilitate responsible innovation.

An evolving trend that significantly influences biomaterial design is the shift toward personalized medicine. Advancements in genomics, proteomics, and tissue engineering techniques enable the tailoring of biomaterial-based implants and drug delivery systems to match individual patient profiles. Such personalization can optimize therapeutic effectiveness and minimize adverse events by taking into account patient-specific factors—ranging from genetic markers to lifestyle and environmental exposures (Raheem et al., 2025). For instance, 3D-bioprinted scaffolds designed with patient-derived stem cells are increasingly explored in regenerative therapies, allowing for more precise healing outcomes while reducing immunogenicity and graft failure rates. However, implementing personalized biomaterials at scale requires rethinking manufacturing processes, regulatory guidelines, and reimbursement models, underscoring the need for ongoing dialogue among industry stakeholders, clinicians, and policymakers.

Despite these challenges, the potential of biomaterials in regenerative medicine, diagnostics, and therapeutic applications remains vast, with ongoing research focusing on overcoming barriers through improved design, regulatory clarity, and interdisciplinary collaboration (Capella-Monsonís et al., 2024; L. Zhu et al., 2024). The integration of biomaterials into clinical settings requires a concerted effort to address these multifaceted issues, ensuring that innovations can effectively transition from the bench to the bedside (Figure 3) (Brassesco et al., 2024).

6.1. Biocompatibility and Safety

Biocompatibility and safety challenges in biomaterial design and clinical translation are multifaceted and involve a complex interplay of biological, regulatory, and ethical considerations. Biocompatibility is a critical factor, as biomaterials must interact safely with biological systems without provoking adverse reactions. This ability is assessed through a combination of in vitro, in vivo, and clinical assays, as outlined by the ISO 10993 standard, which evaluates aspects such as cytotoxicity, genotoxicity, and immunotoxicology (Nasiri et al., 2025). Nanomaterials, for example, require careful consideration of properties such as surface chemistry and size, which significantly influence biological responses and pose challenges in ensuring safe clinical applications. Regulatory frameworks, such as the EU Medical Device Regulation, aim to ensure patient safety but can also slow the translation of innovative biomaterials due to complex approval processes (Ke et al., 2022). The development of ECM-based biomaterials and protein delivery systems further highlights the need for advanced manufacturing techniques and regulatory navigation to ensure biocompatibility and efficacy (Gorantla et al., 2024). Despite their promising properties, liquid metal biomaterials face challenges related to biosafety and material stability, which hinder their widespread clinical translation (Xu et al.,

2024). The biological response to biomaterials is influenced by their structural and physio-chemical properties, necessitating precise engineering to optimize interactions with biological systems (Anderson, 2001). Ethical considerations also play a crucial role, as the rapid advancement of biomaterials science demands proactive measures to address potential ethical dilemmas, ensuring responsible research and development practices (Hunckler & Levine, 2022). The successful clinical translation of biomaterials requires a comprehensive approach that integrates biocompatibility testing, regulatory compliance, and ethical considerations to overcome the inherent challenges in this dynamic field.

6.2. Scalability and Manufacturing

Scalability and manufacturing challenges in biomaterial design and clinical translation are multifaceted and involve technical, regulatory, and economic considerations. A significant challenge is the scalability of production processes, which is crucial for commercial success and clinical application. For example, stem cell culture methods and tissue engineering approaches often lack scalability, necessitating innovations such as bioreactors to improve production efficiency and quality (Wall et al., 2016). The integration of advanced fabrication techniques, such as 3D and 4D printing, offers potential solutions but also introduces challenges related to regulatory compliance and material standardization (Murphy et al., 2020). The complexity of manufacturing is further compounded by the need for biocompatibility and stability, as seen in the development of protein-delivering biomaterials and liquid metal biomaterials, which face hurdles in maintaining structural integrity and ensuring long-term safety (Xu et al., 2024). Additionally, the translation of extracellular matrix (ECM) biomaterials and other regenerative materials is hindered by the need for manageable regulatory pathways and cost-effective manufacturing processes (Capella-Monsonís et al., 2024). The role of high-throughput screening and machine learning in biomaterialomics is emerging as a promising approach to address these challenges by enabling rapid characterization and optimization of biomaterials (Yi et al., 2024). However, the successful clinical translation of these innovations requires robust academic–industry partnerships and the establishment of consistent regulatory guidelines to ensure quality and efficacy (Chandra et al., 2015). Furthermore, the integration of image-based design with 3D printing within a regulatory framework is essential for developing patient-specific devices, highlighting the need for a multidisciplinary approach to overcome these translational barriers (Hollister et al., 2016). Addressing these challenges requires a concerted effort across scientific, industrial, and regulatory domains to realize the full potential of biomaterials in clinical settings.

6.3. Sustainability and Environmental Impact

Biomaterials used in wound healing have varying environmental impacts during their production, use, and disposal, which are influenced by their composition and the processes involved. The production of traditional synthetic materials, such as petroleum-based ointments and plastic films, often results in significant environmental harm due to their non-biodegradable nature and the pollution associated with their manufacturing processes (Elfawy et al., 2023). In contrast, the development of green biomaterials, such as collagen, cellulose, and chitosan, offers a more sustainable alternative. These materials are not only biocompatible and biodegradable but also reduce environmental impact due to their eco-friendly production methods (Farasati Far et al., 2025). The use of natural biomaterials, like those derived from marine resources, further exemplifies this trend, as they are sourced sustainably and possess properties that enhance wound healing while minimizing ecological footprints (Coman et al., 2024). During their use, biomaterials such as hydrogels and nanofibrous structures provide an optimal healing environment by maintaining moisture and promoting cell proliferation, which can accelerate the healing process and reduce the need for frequent dressing changes, thereby minimizing waste (Ijaola et al., 2022). However, challenges remain, such as the need for improved mechanical properties and cost-effective extraction methods for natural biomaterials, which can limit their widespread adoption (Ansari & Darvishi, 2024). Disposal of biomaterials also poses environmental concerns, particularly for synthetic polymers that are not biodegradable. Advances in biodegradable polymers and eco-friendly nanoparticles aim to address these issues by ensuring that biomaterials break down without leaving harmful residues (Saxena et al., 2024). While significant progress has been made in developing environmentally sustainable biomaterials for wound healing, ongoing research is essential to enhance their efficacy and reduce their environmental impact throughout their lifecycle (Farasati Far et al., 2025).

To quantify the environmental costs associated with biomaterial synthesis, usage, and end-of-life processing in wound healing, a comprehensive methodological approach is required that integrates life cycle assessment (LCA) and sustainable synthesis strategies. The environmental impact of biomaterials begins with their sourcing, where the use of renewable and non-polluting feedstocks, such as agricultural residues, is crucial to minimize ecological footprints and avoid competition with food production (Stathatou et al., 2023). The synthesis of biomaterials, particularly those involving nanoparticles, often involves significant energy consumption and environmental releases, as seen in the production of nanosilver-enabled bandages, where upstream electricity production and mining wastes contribute heavily to environmental impacts (Pourzahedi & Eckelman, 2015). Green synthesis methods, which utilize non-toxic solvents and minimize waste, offer a more sustainable alternative, reducing the environmental hazards associated with conventional nanoparticle synthesis (Ma'aruf et al., 2024). During the usage phase, biomaterials like biopolymers and placental-derived materials provide biocompatibility and biodegradability, essential for reducing long-term environmental impacts (Verma et al., 2024). The end-of-life processing of biomaterials, including recycling and composting, is critical for sustainability. However, challenges such as contamination and degradation during recycling need to be addressed to enhance resource efficiency and reduce pollution (Wiśniewska et al., 2023). Furthermore, the integration of antioxidant properties in biomaterials can enhance their therapeutic efficacy while potentially reducing oxidative stress-related environmental impacts (Fadilah et al., 2023). A holistic approach that combines LCA, sustainable sourcing, green synthesis, and effective end-of-life strategies is essential to accurately quantify and mitigate the environmental costs of biomaterials in wound healing applications.

Integrating eco-friendly materials and processes in wound healing is a burgeoning field that aims to minimize environmental footprints while enhancing clinical efficacy. The use of renewable resources for wound dressings is a foundational step in reducing environmental impact, as highlighted by the sourcing of materials from natural and biodegradable polymers such as chitin, which offers good biocompatibility and antibacterial properties when combined with nanosilver for enhanced wound healing rates (Zhou et al., 2017). The application of green chemistry principles, such as using enzymes instead of chemical crosslinkers and employing process intensification strategies like microwave radiation, further supports sustainable production methods (Gupta et al., 2025). Advanced biomaterials, including biodegradable polymers and eco-friendly nanoparticles, are being developed to promote green recovery and minimize environmental impact, with hydrogel dressings and electrospun biopolymer nanofibers being notable examples (El-Sherbiny & Ali, 2015). The eco-friendly synthesis of silver nanoparticles using plant extracts, such as Nitrosalsola vermiculata, demonstrates a novel approach to wound healing, offering substantial reductions in wound size and improvements in tissue regeneration (Abdellatif et al., 2023). Additionally, the development of polyvinyl alcohol/carboxymethyl cellulose dressings using natural agents and physical crosslinking techniques exemplifies a low-cost, environmentally friendly method that accelerates wound healing without cytotoxicity (Mariello et al., 2024). The incorporation of reduced graphene oxide synthesized via eco-friendly methods, along with collagen and fibrinogen from waste sources, into bio sheets for dressings further underscores the potential of sustainable materials in wound care technologies (Preethy et al., 2024). Electrospun nanofibrous materials, derived from biodegradable polymers, mimic the extracellular matrix and support tissue growth, offering a promising avenue for advanced wound dressings that align with environmental sustainability goals (Azimi et al., 2020). These innovations collectively highlight the intersection of scientific efficacy and environmental sustainability in the development of wound healing solutions.

Figure 3. Clinical applications of biomaterials in wound healing

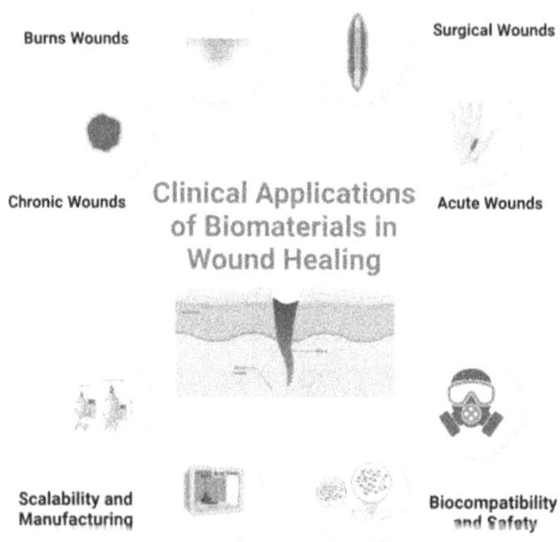

The applications highlight their role in treating different wound types and addressing key challenges. Biomaterials are utilized for burn wounds, chronic wounds, surgical wounds, and acute wounds, providing structural support and promoting tissue regeneration. Additionally, considerations such as scalability and manufacturing (e.g., bioprinting and industrial production) and biocompatibility and safety (e.g., ensuring nontoxicity and regulatory compliance) are crucial for the successful implementation of biomaterials in wound care.

7. CONCLUSION AND FUTURE DIRECTIONS

This comprehensive review of biomaterials used in wound healing highlights the transformative impact these materials have had on regenerative medicine. Biomaterials, ranging from natural and synthetic polymers to innovative hybrid systems, have demonstrated significant potential in modulating the wound microenvironment, supporting cellular functions, and promoting tissue regeneration. The intricate interplay between material properties and biological responses—whether through cellular interactions or the controlled release of bioactive molecules—has paved the way for advanced wound care strategies that effectively address both acute and chronic conditions. Clinical applications have underscored the value of these materials in treating diverse types of wounds, including burns and surgical wounds, where they not only expedite healing but also reduce scarring and infection risks. Despite these advancements, the field continues to face challenges in biocompatibility, regulatory approval, scalability, and manufacturing, which must be addressed to fully transition these innovations from the laboratory to routine clinical practice.

Future directions in biomaterials for wound healing include the development of smart, responsive systems that integrate biosensors for real-time monitoring and adaptive therapeutic delivery, as well as the advancement of personalized wound care through technologies such as 3D and 4D printing to create patient-specific scaffolds and dressings. Researchers are also focusing on improving biocompatibility and safety by refining the chemical and physical properties of these materials to minimize adverse reactions, whereas interdisciplinary collaborations among material scientists, clinicians, and regulatory experts aim to streamline the transition of innovations from the laboratory to clinical practice. Additionally, advancements in manufacturing techniques, including high-throughput screening and machine learning, are expected to increase scalability and cost-effectiveness, ultimately ensuring that next-generation biomaterials provide more effective and tailored solutions for diverse wound healing challenges.

REFERENCES

Abdellatif, A. A., Rugaie, O. A., Alhumaydhi, F. A., Tolba, N. S., & Mousa, A. M. (2023). Eco-Friendly Synthesis of Silver Nanoparticles by Nitrosalsola vermiculata to Promote Skin Wound Healing. *Applied Sciences (Basel, Switzerland)*, *13*(12), 6912. DOI: 10.3390/app13126912

Abeysinghe, N., & Bandara, N. (2024). Protein-and Lipid-based Wound-healing Materials.

Al-Hasani, F. J., & Al-Hassani, E. S. (2024). Preparation and Characterization of Anti-Microbial Wound Healing Materials from Natural Origins. Journal of Physics: Conference Series, Al-Naymi, H. A. S., Al-Musawi, M. H., Mirhaj, M., Valizadeh, H., Pajooh, A. M. D., Shahriari-Khalaji, M., Sharifianjazi, F., Tavamaishvili, K., Kazemi, N., & Salehi, S. (2024). Exploring nanobioceramics in wound healing as effective and economical alternatives. *Heliyon*.

Alencar, M. S. F., Silva, G. H. C., da Silva, A. A., de Azevedo, A. K. R., Pereira, M. A., do Nascimento, J. C. C., dos Santos, P. S., da Silva Campos, J., Bernardes, M. S. V., & de Deus Caparroz, D. P. P. (2024). Evidence-based practices on nanotechnology in wound treatment. *Caderno Pedagógico*, *21*(12), e10234–e10234. DOI: 10.54033/cadpedv21n12-037

Alizadeh, S., Nasiri, M., Saraei, M., Zahiri, M., Khosrowpour, Z., Sineh Sepehr, K., Nouri, M., Zarrabi, M., Kalantari, N., Shafikhani, S. H., & Gholipourmalekabadi, M. (2024). Optimization of an Affordable and Efficient Skin Allograft Composite with Excellent Biomechanical and Biological Properties Suitable for the Regeneration of Deep Skin Wounds: A Preclinical Study. *ACS Applied Bio Materials*, *7*(11), 7378–7390. DOI: 10.1021/acsabm.4c01016 PMID: 39475164

Alkabli, J. (2024). Recent advances in the development of chitosan/hyaluronic acid-based hybrid materials for skin protection, regeneration, and healing: A review. *International Journal of Biological Macromolecules*, *279*, 135357. DOI: 10.1016/j.ijbiomac.2024.135357 PMID: 39245118

Anand, K., Sharma, R., & Sharma, N. (2024). Recent advancements in natural polymers-based self-healing nano-materials for wound dressing. *Journal of Biomedical Materials Research. Part B, Applied Biomaterials*, *112*(6), e35435. DOI: 10.1002/jbm.b.35435 PMID: 38864664

Anderson, J. M. (2001). Biological responses to materials. *Annual Review of Materials Research*, *31*(1), 81–110. DOI: 10.1146/annurev.matsci.31.1.81

Ansari, M., & Darvishi, A. (2024). A review of the current state of natural biomaterials in wound healing applications. *Frontiers in Bioengineering and Biotechnology*, *12*, 1309541. DOI: 10.3389/fbioe.2024.1309541 PMID: 38600945

Azimi, B., Maleki, H., Zavagna, L., De la Ossa, J. G., Linari, S., Lazzeri, A., & Danti, S. (2020). Bio-based electrospun fibers for wound healing. *Journal of Functional Biomaterials*, *11*(3), 67. DOI: 10.3390/jfb11030067 PMID: 32971968

Bao, X., Huo, S., Wang, Z., Yang, S., Dou, L., Liu, Y., Huang, J., Cai, C., Fang, B., & Xu, G. (2024). Multifunctional biomimetic hydrogel dressing provides anti-infection treatment and improves immunotherapy by reprogramming the infection-related wound microenvironment. *Journal of Nanobiotechnology*, *22*(1), 80. DOI: 10.1186/s12951-024-02337-3 PMID: 38418972

Barbu, V.-S., Gaboreanu, M.-D., Marinas, I. C., Paun, A.-M., Ionel, I. P., & Avram, S. (2025). Implications of Biomaterials for Chronic Wounds. *Mini-Reviews in Medicinal Chemistry*. PMID: 39781714

Basu, P., Banerjee, A., Okoro, P. D., Masoumi, A., Kanjilal, B., Akbari, M., Martins-Green, M., Armstrong, D. G., & Noshadi, I. (2024). Integration of Functional Polymers and Biosensors to Enhance Wound Healing. *Advanced Healthcare Materials*, *13*(29), 2401461. DOI: 10.1002/adhm.202401461 PMID: 39235365

Bayon, Y., Bureau, C., Perreira, M. J., Aubert, F., Caillibotte, M., Vestberg, R., & Letourneur, D. (2024). Journey of medical device development from the bench to the bedside—Four real-life examples of commercial biomaterials development. *Exploration of Biomat-X*, *1*(1), 23–33. DOI: 10.37349/ebmx.2024.00004

Bhar, A., & Das, S. (2024). From scars to solutions: Exploring biomaterials for skin graft and tissue engineering in response to burn injury.

Bhardwaj, H., Khute, S., & Jangde, R. K. (2023). Biopolymeric Materials in the Management of Diabetic Wound Healing: A Comprehensive Review. *Journal of Ravishankar University*, *36*(2), 94–108. DOI: 10.52228/JRUB.2023-36-2-7

Brassesco, M. E., Cortez, J., Triacca, V., Payen, J., & Bayon, Y. (2024). Translating Ideas into Commercial Biomaterial Devices: A Path to Improving Healthcare. *ACS Biomaterials Science & Engineering*, *10*(4), 1910–1920. DOI: 10.1021/acsbiomaterials.3c01441 PMID: 38452343

Buriti, B. M. A. B., Figueiredo, P. L. B., Passos, M. F., & da Silva, J. K. R. (2024). Polymer-based wound dressings loaded with essential oil for the treatment of wounds: A review. *Pharmaceuticals (Basel, Switzerland)*, *17*(7), 897. DOI: 10.3390/ph17070897 PMID: 39065747

Butenko, S., Miwa, H., Liu, Y., Plikus, M. V., Scumpia, P. O., & Liu, W. F. (2023). Engineering immunomodulatory biomaterials to drive skin wounds toward regenerative healing. *Cold Spring Harbor Perspectives in Biology*, *15*(5), a041242. DOI: 10.1101/cshperspect.a041242 PMID: 36123029

Butenko, S., Nagalla, R. R., Guerrero-Juarez, C. F., Palomba, F., David, L.-M., Nguyen, R. Q., Gay, D., Almet, A. A., Digman, M. A., Nie, Q., Scumpia, P. O., Plikus, M. V., & Liu, W. F. (2024). Hydrogel crosslinking modulates macrophages, fibroblasts, and their communication, during wound healing. *Nature Communications*, *15*(1), 6820. DOI: 10.1038/s41467-024-50072-y PMID: 39122702

Cai, C., Li, W., Zhang, X., Cheng, B., Chen, S., & Zhang, Y. (2024). Natural Polymer–Based Hydrogel Dressings for Wound Healing. *Advances in Wound Care*, wound.2024.0024. DOI: 10.1089/wound.2024.0024 PMID: 38623809

Cao, Y., Sun, J., Qin, S., Zhou, Z., Xu, Y., & Liu, C. (2024). Advances and Challenges in Immune-Modulatory Biomaterials for Wound Healing Applications. *Pharmaceutics*, *16*(8), 990. DOI: 10.3390/pharmaceutics16080990 PMID: 39204335

Capella-Monsonís, H., Crum, R. J., Hussey, G. S., & Badylak, S. F. (2024). Advances, challenges, and future directions in the clinical translation of ECM biomaterials for regenerative medicine applications. *Advanced Drug Delivery Reviews*, *211*, 115347. DOI: 10.1016/j.addr.2024.115347 PMID: 38844005

Chandra, P., Yoo, J. J., & Lee, S. J. (2015). Biomaterials in regenerative medicine: Challenges in technology transfer from science to process development. In *Translational Regenerative Medicine* (pp. 151–167). Elsevier. DOI: 10.1016/B978-0-12-410396-2.00013-X

Chelu, M., Calderon Moreno, J. M., Musuc, A. M., & Popa, M. (2024). Natural regenerative hydrogels for wound healing. *Gels (Basel, Switzerland)*, *10*(9), 547. DOI: 10.3390/gels10090547 PMID: 39330149

Chen, D., Hou, Q., Zhong, L., Zhao, Y., Li, M., & Fu, X. (2019). Bioactive molecules for skin repair and regeneration: Progress and perspectives. *Stem Cells International*, *2019*(1), 6789823. DOI: 10.1155/2019/6789823 PMID: 32082386

Chen, Y., Chai, M., Xuan, C., Lin, J., Yang, H., Li, C., Xie, M., Ostrovidov, S., Shi, X., & Mao, C. (2024). Tuning the properties of surgical polymeric materials for improved soft-tissue wound closure and healing. *Progress in Materials Science*, *143*, 101249. DOI: 10.1016/j.pmatsci.2024.101249

Chhillar, A., & Jaiswal, A. (2025). Hyaluronic Acid-Based Self-Healing Hydrogels for Diabetic Wound Healing. *Advanced Healthcare Materials*, *14*(4), 2404255. DOI: 10.1002/adhm.202404255 PMID: 39722163

Chin, S. W., Azman, A. S., & Tan, J. W. (2024). Incorporation of natural and synthetic polymers into honey hydrogel for wound healing: A review. *Health Science Reports*, *7*(7), e2251. DOI: 10.1002/hsr2.2251 PMID: 39015423

Coman, A. E., Marin, M. M., Ro ca, A. M., Albu Kaya, M. G., Constantinescu, R. R., & Titorencu, I. (2024). Marine Resources Gels as Main Ingredient for Wound Healing Biomaterials: Obtaining and Characterization. *Gels (Basel, Switzerland)*, *10*(11), 729. DOI: 10.3390/gels10110729 PMID: 39590085

Dai, X., Nie, W., Shen, H., Machens, H.-G., Böker, K., Taheri, S., Lehmann, W., Shen, Y., & Schilling, A. F. (2024). Electrospinning based biomaterials for biomimetic fabrication, bioactive protein delivery and wound regenerative repair. *Regenerative Biomaterials*, •••, rbae139. PMID: 39803356

Das, P., Manna, S., Roy, S., Nandi, S. K., & Basak, P. (2023). Polymeric biomaterials-based tissue engineering for wound healing: A systemic review. *Burns and Trauma*, *11*, tkac058. DOI: 10.1093/burnst/tkac058 PMID: 36761088

de Souza, I. C., Takejima, A. L., Simeoni, R. B., Gamba, L. K., Ribeiro, V. S. T., Foltz, K. M., de Noronha, L., de Almeida, M. B., Neto, J. R. F., de Carvalho, K. A. T., da Silveira, P. C. L., Pinho, R. A., Francisco, J. C., & Guarita-Souza, L. C. (2023). Acellular biomaterials associated with autologous bone marrow-derived mononuclear stem cells improve wound healing through paracrine effects. *Biomedicines*, *11*(4), 1003. DOI: 10.3390/biomedicines11041003 PMID: 37189621

Dias-Ferreira, J., Teixeira, M., Severino, P., Boonme, P., Jovanovic, J., Zielińska, A., & Souto, E. B. (2023). Applications of biomaterials in wound healing management: from fundamental physiology to advanced technology. In *Nanotechnology and Regenerative Medicine* (pp. 349–369). Elsevier. DOI: 10.1016/B978-0-323-90471-1.00020-7

Duan, Y., Li, L., Hu, J., Zheng, B., & He, K. (2025). Engineering Gas-Releasing Nanomaterials for Efficient Wound Healing. *ChemBioChem*, *26*(4), e202400790. DOI: 10.1002/cbic.202400790 PMID: 39592412

Duan, Y., Li, L., Hu, J., Zheng, B., & He, K. Engineering Gas-Releasing Nanomaterials for Efficient Wound Healing. *ChemBioChem*, e202400790.

El-Sherbiny, I. M., & Ali, I. H. (2015). Eco-friendly electrospun polymeric nanofibers-based nanocomposites for wound healing and tissue engineering. *Eco-friendly Polymer Nanocomposites: Processing and Properties*, 399-431.

Elfawy, L. A., Ng, C. Y., Amirrah, I. N., Mazlan, Z., Wen, A. P. Y., Fadilah, N. I. M., Maarof, M., Lokanathan, Y., & Fauzi, M. B. (2023). Sustainable approach of functional biomaterials–tissue engineering for skin burn treatment: A comprehensive review. *Pharmaceuticals (Basel, Switzerland)*, *16*(5), 701. DOI: 10.3390/ph16050701 PMID: 37242483

Emiroglu, D. B., Singh, A., Marco-Dufort, B., Speck, N., Rivano, P. G., Oakey, J. S., Nakatsuka, N., deMello, A. J., Labouesse, C., & Tibbitt, M. W. (2024). Granular Biomaterials as Bioactive Sponges for the Sequestration and Release of Signaling Molecules. *Advanced Healthcare Materials*, •••, 2400800. DOI: 10.1002/adhm.202400800 PMID: 38808536

Fadilah, N. I. M., Phang, S. J., Kamaruzaman, N., Salleh, A., Zawani, M., Sanyal, A., Maarof, M., & Fauzi, M. B. (2023). Antioxidant biomaterials in cutaneous wound healing and tissue regeneration: A critical review. *Antioxidants*, *12*(4), 787. DOI: 10.3390/antiox12040787 PMID: 37107164

Farasati Far, B., Jameie, L., Taromi, P., Nahavndi, R., & Jamshidi, E. (2025). Dermal and Oral Wound Healing. In *Green Biomaterials in Tissue Engineering* (pp. 297–329). ACS Publications. DOI: 10.1021/bk-2025-1497.ch009

Galbiati, M., Maiullari, F., Ceraolo, M. G., Bousselmi, S., Fratini, N., Gega, K., Recchia, S., Ferretti, A. M., Scala, G., Costantini, M., Sciarra, T., Rizzi, R., & Bearzi, C. (2025). Bioactive hydrogel supplemented with stromal cell-derived extracellular vesicles enhance wound healing. *Pharmaceutics*, *17*(2), 162. DOI: 10.3390/pharmaceutics17020162 PMID: 40006529

Gayathri, R., ArulJothi, K., Raj, K. H., & Gnanavel, S. (2024). NEXT-GENERATION SUTURES: COMBINING NATURAL POLYMERS AND GRAPHENE FOR OPTIMAL WOUND HEALING. *Results in Surfaces and Interfaces*, 100287.

Ghosh, D., Yaron, J. R., Abedin, M. R., Godeshala, S., Kumar, S., Kilbourne, J., Berthiaume, F., & Rege, K. (2024). Bioactive nanomaterials kickstart early repair processes and potentiate temporally modulated healing of healthy and diabetic wounds. *Biomaterials*, *306*, 122496. DOI: 10.1016/j.biomaterials.2024.122496 PMID: 38373363

Gill, A. S., Sood, M., Deol, P. K., & Kaur, I. P. (2023). Synthetic polymer based electrospun scaffolds for wound healing applications. *Journal of Drug Delivery Science and Technology*, *89*, 105054. DOI: 10.1016/j.jddst.2023.105054

Gobi, R., Ravichandiran, P., Babu, R. S., & Yoo, D. J. (2021). Biopolymer and synthetic polymer-based nanocomposites in wound dressing applications: A review. *Polymers*, *13*(12), 1962. DOI: 10.3390/polym13121962 PMID: 34199209

Gorantla, A., Hall, J. T., Troidle, A., & Janjic, J. M. (2024). Biomaterials for protein delivery: Opportunities and challenges to clinical translation. *Micromachines*, *15*(4), 533. DOI: 10.3390/mi15040533 PMID: 38675344

Goyal, K., Ahalwat, S., & Jogpal, V. (2024). Transforming Wound Management: Advancement in Nanomaterials-based Therapeutics. *Recent Advances in Inflammation & Allergy Drug Discovery*, *19*. Advance online publication. DOI: 10.2174/0127722708314632241117192456

Gupta, M. N., Rangaraju, A., & Ambre, P. (2025). Sustainable dressings for wound healing. *Biotechnology for Sustainable Materials*, *2*(1), 1. DOI: 10.1186/s44316-024-00023-w

Halder, T., Barot, H., Kumar, B., Kaushik, V., Patel, H., Bhut, H., Saha, B., Poddar, S., & Acharya, N. (2024). An Insight into Biodegradable Polymers and their Biomedical Applications for Wound Healing. *Current Pharmaceutical Design*, *30*(31), 2425–2444. DOI: 10.2174/0113816128295935240425101509 PMID: 38982925

He, Q., Gao, X., Wu, Z., Zhu, J., Chen, H., Liu, X., & Zhang, X. (2024). Robust, superabsorbent and antibacterial polysaccharide-based hybrid-network hydrogels for wound repair. *International Journal of Biological Macromolecules*, *279*, 134626. DOI: 10.1016/j.ijbiomac.2024.134626 PMID: 39128759

He, Y., Chang, Q., & Lu, F. (2023). Oxygen-releasing biomaterials for chronic wounds breathing: From theoretical mechanism to application prospect. *Materials Today. Bio*, *20*, 100687. DOI: 10.1016/j.mtbio.2023.100687 PMID: 37334187

Ho, T. T. P., Tran, H. A., Doan, V. K., Maitz, J., Li, Z., Wise, S. G., Lim, K. S., & Rnjak-Kovacina, J. (2024). Natural Polymer-Based Materials for Wound Healing Applications. *Advanced NanoBiomed Research*, *4*(5), 2300131. DOI: 10.1002/anbr.202300131

Hollister, S. J., Flanagan, C. L., Morrison, R. J., Patel, J. J., Wheeler, M. B., Edwards, S. P., & Green, G. E. (2016). Integrating image-based design and 3D biomaterial printing to create patient specific devices within a design control framework for clinical translation. *ACS Biomaterials Science & Engineering*, *2*(10), 1827–1836. DOI: 10.1021/acsbiomaterials.6b00332 PMID: 31231678

Hunckler, M. D., & Levine, A. D. (2022). Navigating ethical challenges in the development and translation of biomaterials research. *Frontiers in Bioengineering and Biotechnology*, *10*, 949280. DOI: 10.3389/fbioe.2022.949280 PMID: 36204464

Husain, K., Malik, A., Kirchens, J., & Choi, G. (2024). A prospective, blinded, randomized controlled clinical trial evaluating the effect of the synthetic electrospun fiber matrix in the treatment of chronic diabetic foot ulcers. *Foot & Ankle Surgery: Techniques. Foot & Ankle Surgery (New York, N.Y.)*, *4*(1), 100362. DOI: 10.1016/j.fastrc.2024.100362

Ijaola, A. O., Akamo, D. O., Damiri, F., Akisin, C. J., Bamidele, E. A., Ajiboye, E. G., Berrada, M., Onyenokwe, V. O., Yang, S.-Y., & Asmatulu, E. (2022). Polymeric biomaterials for wound healing applications: A comprehensive review. *Journal of Biomaterials Science. Polymer Edition*, *33*(15), 1998–2050. DOI: 10.1080/09205063.2022.2088528 PMID: 35695023

Ijaz, M., & Khan, M. (2025). Multifunctional electrospun nanofiber films of polyacrylonitrile and polyvinyl alcohol incorporating rhamnose and therapeutic agents for enhanced healing of infected burn wounds. *Journal of Biomaterials Science. Polymer Edition*, •••, 1–33. DOI: 10.1080/09205063.2024.2449297 PMID: 39799519

Jessy Mercy, D., Thirumalai, A., Udayakumar, S., Deepika, B., Janani, G., Girigoswami, A., & Girigoswami, K. (2024). Enhancing Wound Healing with Nanohydrogel-Entrapped Plant Extracts and Nanosilver: An In Vitro Investigation. *Molecules (Basel, Switzerland)*, *29*(21), 5004. DOI: 10.3390/molecules29215004 PMID: 39519646

Jiang, Y., Wang, L., Qi, W., Yin, P., Liao, X., Luo, Y., & Ding, Y. (2024). Antibacterial and self-healing sepiolite-based hybrid hydrogel for hemostasis and wound healing. *Biomaterials Advances*, *159*, 213838. DOI: 10.1016/j.bioadv.2024.213838 PMID: 38531257

Jones, D. P., & Patel, J. (2018). Therapeutic approaches targeting inflammation in cardiovascular disorders. *Biology (Basel)*, *7*(4), 49. DOI: 10.3390/biology7040049 PMID: 30453474

Kang, T., Guo, Z., Lu, Y., Cun, J., Gao, W., Pu, Y., & He, B. (2024). Hybrid Hydrogels of Polyacrylamide and Self-assembly Photodynamic Nanoparticles with Diverse Adhesion for Infected Chronic Wound Healing. *Biomacromolecules*, *25*(11), 7475–7484. DOI: 10.1021/acs.biomac.4c01162 PMID: 39428619

Kant, V., Kumari, P., Jitendra, D. K., Ahuja, M., & Kumar, V. (2021). Nanomaterials of natural bioactive compounds for wound healing: Novel drug delivery approach. *Current Drug Delivery*, *18*(10), 1406–1425. DOI: 10.2174/1567201818666210729103712 PMID: 34325636

Kauke-Navarro, M., Knoedler, L., Knoedler, S., & Safi, A. F. (2024). Advancements in facial implantology: A review of hydroxyapatite applications and outcomes. *Frontiers in Surgery*, *11*, 1409733. DOI: 10.3389/fsurg.2024.1409733 PMID: 39092153

Kaur, H., Gogoi, B., Sharma, I., Das, D. K., Azad, M. A., Pramanik, D. D., & Pramanik, A. (2024). Hydrogels as a potential biomaterial for multimodal therapeutic applications. *Molecular Pharmaceutics*, *21*(10), 4827–4848. DOI: 10.1021/acs.molpharmaceut.4c00595 PMID: 39290162

Ke, D., Niu, C., & Yang, X. (2022). Evolution of 3D bioprinting-from the perspectives of bioprinting companies. *Bioprinting (Amsterdam, Netherlands)*, *25*, e00193. DOI: 10.1016/j.bprint.2022.e00193

Khanna, D., Gemechu, E., Mahbub, N., Joy, J., & Kumar, A. (2025). Assessment of life cycle environmental impacts of materials, driving pattern, and climatic conditions on battery electric and hydrogen fuel cell vehicles in a cold region. *Environmental Impact Assessment Review*, *110*, 107680. DOI: 10.1016/j.eiar.2024.107680

Kuddushi, M., Shah, A. A., Ayranci, C., & Zhang, X. (2023). Recent advances in novel materials and techniques for developing transparent wound dressings. *Journal of Materials Chemistry. B*, *11*(27), 6201–6224. DOI: 10.1039/D3TB00639E PMID: 37306212

Kumar, M., Mahmood, S., Chopra, S., & Bhatia, A. (2024). Biopolymer based nanoparticles and their therapeutic potential in wound healing–A review. *International Journal of Biological Macromolecules*, *267*, 131335. DOI: 10.1016/j.ijbiomac.2024.131335 PMID: 38604431

Kumar, R., Igwegbe, C. A., & Khandel, S. K. (2024). Nanotherapeutic and Nano–Bio Interface for Regeneration and Healing. *Biomedicines*, *12*(12), 2927. DOI: 10.3390/biomedicines12122927 PMID: 39767834

La Monica, F., Campora, S., & Ghersi, G. (2024). Collagen-based scaffolds for chronic skin wound treatment. *Gels (Basel, Switzerland)*, *10*(2), 137. DOI: 10.3390/gels10020137 PMID: 38391467

Las Heras, K., Garcia-Orue, I., Rancan, F., Igartua, M., Santos-Vizcaino, E., & Hernandez, R. M. (2024). Modulating the immune system towards a functional chronic wound healing: A biomaterials and Nanomedicine perspective. *Advanced Drug Delivery Reviews*, *210*, 115342. DOI: 10.1016/j.addr.2024.115342 PMID: 38797316

Laubach, M., Whyte, S., Chan, H. F., Frankenbach-Désor, T., Mayer-Wagner, S., Hildebrand, F., Holzapfel, B. M., Kneser, U., Dulleck, U., & Hutmacher, D. W. (2024). Lost in translation: The lack of agreement between surgeons and scientists regarding biomaterials research and innovation for treating bone defects. *BMC Medicine*, *22*(1), 517. DOI: 10.1186/s12916-024-03734-z PMID: 39506708

Li, C., Chen, C., Zhao, J., Tan, M., Zhai, S., Wei, Y., Wang, L., & Dai, T. (2021). Electrospun fibrous membrane containing a cyclodextrin covalent organic framework with antibacterial properties for accelerating wound healing. *ACS Biomaterials Science & Engineering*, *7*(8), 3898–3907. DOI: 10.1021/acsbiomaterials.1c00648 PMID: 34279078

Li, J., Xie, J., Wang, Y., Li, X., Yang, L., Zhao, M., & Chen, C. (2024). Development of Biomaterials to Modulate the Function of Macrophages in Wound Healing. *Bioengineering (Basel, Switzerland)*, *11*(10), 1017. DOI: 10.3390/bioengineering11101017 PMID: 39451393

Li, J., Yu, F., Chen, G., Liu, J., Li, X.-L., Cheng, B., Mo, X.-M., Chen, C., & Pan, J.-F. (2020). Moist-retaining, self-recoverable, bioadhesive, and transparent in situ forming hydrogels to accelerate wound healing. *ACS Applied Materials & Interfaces*, *12*(2), 2023–2038. DOI: 10.1021/acsami.9b17180 PMID: 31895528

Li, R., Liu, K., Huang, X., Li, D., Ding, J., Liu, B., & Chen, X. (2022). Bioactive materials promote wound healing through modulation of cell behaviors. *Advancement of Science*, *9*(10), 2105152. DOI: 10.1002/advs.202105152 PMID: 35138042

Liu, M., Duan, X.-P., Li, Y.-M., Yang, D.-P., & Long, Y.-Z. (2017). Electrospun nanofibers for wound healing. *Materials Science and Engineering C*, *76*, 1413–1423. DOI: 10.1016/j.msec.2017.03.034 PMID: 28482508

Liu, Q., Luo, S., Peng, J., & Chang, R. (2024). Electrospun Nanofibers from Plant Natural Products: A New Approach Toward Efficient Wound Healing. *International Journal of Nanomedicine*, *19*, 13973–13990. DOI: 10.2147/IJN.S501970 PMID: 39742091

Liu, W., Zu, L., Wang, S., Li, J., Fei, X., Geng, M., Zhu, C., & Shi, H. (2023). Tailored biomedical materials for wound healing. *Burns and Trauma*, *11*, tkad040. DOI: 10.1093/burnst/tkad040 PMID: 37899884

Liu, X., Dou, G., Li, Z., Wang, X., Jin, R., Liu, Y., Kuang, H., Huang, X., Yang, X., Yang, X., Liu, S., Wu, M., Guo, H., Ding, F., Xu, H., Liu, S., Jin, Y., & Xuan, K. (2022). Hybrid biomaterial initiates refractory wound healing via inducing transiently heightened inflammatory responses. *Advancement of Science*, *9*(21), 2105650. DOI: 10.1002/advs.202105650 PMID: 35603963

Lu, X., Zhou, L., & Song, W. (2024). Recent Progress of Electrospun Nanofiber Dressing in the Promotion of Wound Healing. *Polymers, 16*(18), 2596. DOI: 10.3390/polym16182596 PMID: 39339060

Luo, G., & Zhou, X. (2024). Application of advanced biomaterials in wound repair. *Zhonghua Shao Shang Yu Chuang Mian Xiu Fu Za Zhi, 40*(1), 26–32. PMID: 38296234

Ma'aruf, M., Mustapha, S., & Giriraj, T. (2024). Sustainable synthesis strategies: Biofabrication's impact on metal and metal oxide nanoparticles. *African Journal of Environment and Natural Science Research, 7*(2), 229–252. DOI: 10.52589/AJENSR-JTFPYHUK

Manjit, M., & Mishra, B. (2024). Synthetic Polymer-Based Hydrogels for Tissue Engineering. In *Biomaterial-based Hydrogels: Therapeutics Carrier and Tissue Regeneration* (pp. 357-385). Springer. DOI: 10.1007/978-981-99-8826-6_13

Mariello, M., Binetti, E., Todaro, M. T., Qualtieri, A., Brunetti, V., Siciliano, P., De Vittorio, M., & Blasi, L. (2024). Eco-Friendly Production of Polyvinyl Alcohol/Carboxymethyl Cellulose Wound Healing Dressing Containing Sericin. *Gels (Basel, Switzerland), 10*(6), 412. DOI: 10.3390/gels10060412 PMID: 38920958

McKenzie, M., Betts, D., Suh, A., Bui, K., Kim, L. D., & Cho, H. (2015). Hydrogel-based drug delivery systems for poorly water-soluble drugs. *Molecules (Basel, Switzerland), 20*(11), 20397–20408. DOI: 10.3390/molecules201119705 PMID: 26580588

Mehvari, F., Ramezanzade, V., An, J., Kim, J., Dinari, M., & Kim, J. S. (2024). Biopolymer-based hydrogels for biomedical applications: Bioactivity and wound healing properties. *Coordination Chemistry Reviews, 518*, 216093. DOI: 10.1016/j.ccr.2024.216093

Mir, M., Ali, M. N., Barakullah, A., Gulzar, A., Arshad, M., Fatima, S., & Asad, M. (2018). Synthetic polymeric biomaterials for wound healing: A review. *Progress in Biomaterials, 7*(1), 1–21. DOI: 10.1007/s40204-018-0083-4 PMID: 29446015

Mittal, P., Rana, P., Goyal, C., Kapoor, R., Soni, M. L., & Gautam, R. K. (2024). Bionanomaterials in Wound Dressings. In *Bionanomaterials for Industrial Applications* (pp. 301–309). CRC Press. DOI: 10.1201/9781003432791-20

Moreira, T. D., Martins, V. B., da Silva Júnior, A. H., Sayer, C., de Araújo, P. H. H., & Immich, A. P. S. (2024). New insights into biomaterials for wound dressings and care: Challenges and trends. *Progress in Organic Coatings, 187*, 108118. DOI: 10.1016/j.porgcoat.2023.108118

Mottaghitalab, F., Yazdi, M. K., Saeb, M. R., Bączek, T., & Farokhi, M. (2024). Green and sustainable hydrogels based on quaternized chitosan to enhance wound healing. *Chemical Engineering Journal*, *492*, 152288. DOI: 10.1016/j.cej.2024.152288

Murphy, S. V., De Coppi, P., & Atala, A. (2020). Opportunities and challenges of translational 3D bioprinting. *Nature Biomedical Engineering*, *4*(4), 370–380. DOI: 10.1038/s41551-019-0471-7 PMID: 31695178

Nameeta, J. M. (2024). Whispers of Healing: Navigation of Nanomaterials for Wound Restoration and Inflammation Control. *Materials Research Foundations, 171.*

Nasiri, S. N., Aghajanloo, B., Nasiri, N., & Nazarnezhad, S. (2025). Cytotoxicity and Biocompatibility of Green Biomaterials. In *Green Biomaterials in Tissue Engineering* (pp. 175–205). ACS Publications. DOI: 10.1021/bk-2025-1497.ch005

Naskar, A., & Kim, K. (2020). Recent advances in nanomaterial-based wound-healing therapeutics. *Pharmaceutics*, *12*(6), 499. DOI: 10.3390/pharmaceutics12060499 PMID: 32486142

Nasra, S., Pramanik, S., Oza, V., Kansara, K., & Kumar, A. (2024). Advancements in wound management: Integrating nanotechnology and smart materials for enhanced therapeutic interventions. *Discover Nano*, *19*(1), 159. DOI: 10.1186/s11671-024-04116-3 PMID: 39354172

Nezhad-Mokhtari, P., Hasany, M., Kohestanian, M., Dolatshahi-Pirouz, A., Milani, M., & Mehrali, M. (2024). Recent advancements in bioadhesive self-healing hydrogels for effective chronic wound care. *Advances in Colloid and Interface Science*, *334*, 103306. DOI: 10.1016/j.cis.2024.103306 PMID: 39423587

Nifontova, G., Safaryan, S., Khristidis, Y., Smirnova, O., Vosough, M., Shpichka, A., & Timashev, P. (2024). Advancing wound healing by hydrogel-based dressings loaded with cell-conditioned medium: A systematic review. *Stem Cell Research & Therapy*, *15*(1), 371. DOI: 10.1186/s13287-024-03976-x PMID: 39420416

Nosrati, H., & Heydari, M. (2025). Titanium dioxide nanoparticles: A promising candidate for wound healing applications. *Burns and Trauma*, *13*, tkae069. DOI: 10.1093/burnst/tkae069 PMID: 39759542

Ohadi, M., Forootanfar, H., Dehghannoudeh, N., Banat, I. M., & Dehghannoudeh, G. (2023). The role of surfactants and biosurfactants in the wound healing process: a review. *Journal of Wound care, 32*(Sup4a), xxxix-xlvi.

Oliva, N., & Almquist, B. D. (2020). Spatiotemporal delivery of bioactive molecules for wound healing using stimuli-responsive biomaterials. *Advanced Drug Delivery Reviews*, *161*, 22–41. DOI: 10.1016/j.addr.2020.07.021 PMID: 32745497

Olteanu, G., Neac u, S. M., Joi a, F. A., Musuc, A. M., Lupu, E. C., Ioni ă-Mîndrican, C.-B., Lupuliasa, D., & Mititelu, M. (2024). Advancements in regenerative hydrogels in skin wound treatment: A comprehensive review. *International Journal of Molecular Sciences*, *25*(7), 3849. DOI: 10.3390/ijms25073849 PMID: 38612660

Pillay, V., Kumar, P., & Choonara, Y. E. (2015). Integrated biomaterial composites for accelerated wound healing. *Biomaterials in Regenerative Medicine and the Immune System*, 209-223.

Piraino, F., & Selimović, Š. (2015). A current view of functional biomaterials for wound care, molecular and cellular therapies. *BioMed Research International*, *2015*(1), 403801. DOI: 10.1155/2015/403801 PMID: 26509154

Pourzahedi, L., & Eckelman, M. J. (2015). Environmental life cycle assessment of nanosilver-enabled bandages. *Environmental Science & Technology*, *49*(1), 361–368. DOI: 10.1021/es504655y PMID: 25489789

Prabhu, A., Baliga, V., Bhat, S., Thenkondar, S. T., Nayak, Y., & Nayak, U. Y. (2023). Transforming wound management: Nanomaterials and their clinical impact. *Pharmaceutics*, *15*(5), 1560. DOI: 10.3390/pharmaceutics15051560 PMID: 37242802

Preethy, K., Petrecia, P. D., & Chamundeeswari, M. (2024). Development of bio sheet using nanoparticles and the confederation of protein for casting wound. *International Journal of Biological Macromolecules*, *274*, 133178. DOI: 10.1016/j.ijbiomac.2024.133178 PMID: 38906355

Prete, S., Dattilo, M., Patitucci, F., Pezzi, G., Parisi, O. I., & Puoci, F. (2023). Natural and synthetic polymeric biomaterials for application in wound management. *Journal of Functional Biomaterials*, *14*(9), 455. DOI: 10.3390/jfb14090455 PMID: 37754869

Quadir, S. S., Puri, D., Joshi, G., Choudhary, D., Kumar, S., Singh, M., & Sawhney, S. K. (2024). Bioresorbable polymers for wound healing. In *Bioresorbable Polymers and their Composites* (pp. 353–383). Elsevier. DOI: 10.1016/B978-0-443-18915-9.00003-3

Raheem, A., Mandal, K., Biswas, S., Ahari, A., Hassani Najafabadi, A., Farhadi, N., Zehtabi, F., Gangrade, A., Mecwan, M., Maity, S., Sharma, S., Arputharaj, J. N., Khan, P. A., Udduttula, A., Kouchehbaghi, N. H., Khorsandi, D., Vasita, R., Haghniaz, R., Herculano, R. D., & Manivasagam, G. (2025). Smart biomaterials in healthcare: Breakthroughs in tissue engineering, immunomodulation, patient-specific therapies, and biosensor applications. *Applied Physics Reviews*, *12*(1), 011333. DOI: 10.1063/5.0238817

Rani, K., Singh, G., Narwal, S., Chopra, B., & Dhingra, A. K. (2025). Nanomaterials in Wound Healing: Mechanisms, Applications, and Future Prospects. *Current Nanomedicine*, *15*(1), 50–69. DOI: 10.2174/0124681873294822240517073406

Reyes-Guzmán, V. L., Villarreal-Gómez, L. J., Vázquez-Mora, R., Méndez-Ramírez, Y. I., Paz-González, J. A., Zizumbo-López, A., Borbón, H., Lizarraga-Medina, E. G., Cornejo-Bravo, J. M., Pérez-González, G. L., Ontiveros-Zepeda, A. S., Pérez-Sánchez, A., Chavira-Martínez, E., Huirache-Acuña, R., & Estévez-Martínez, Y. (2024). Integrating an antimicrobial nanocomposite to bioactive electrospun fibers for improved wound dressing materials. *Scientific Reports*, *14*(1), 25118. DOI: 10.1038/s41598-024-75814-2 PMID: 39443526

Saberianpour, S., Melotto, G., Redhead, L., Terrazzini, N., Forss, J. R., & Santin, M. (2024). Harnessing the interactions of wound exudate cells with dressings biomaterials for the control and prognosis of healing pathways. *Pharmaceuticals (Basel, Switzerland)*, *17*(9), 1111. DOI: 10.3390/ph17091111 PMID: 39338276

Satti, M. K., Humayun, S., Sajid, M., Asdaq, K. N., Ashraf, T., & Aftab, M. (2023). Hydrogels for wound dressing applications-A systematic review. *Pakistan Journal of Medical & Health Sciences*, *17*(03), 2–2. DOI: 10.53350/pjmhs20231732

Saxena, A., Anandhi, R., Rashmi, K., Singh, N., Yadav, D. K., & Zabibah, R. S. (2024). Biomedical Materials for Sustainable Wound Care: A Review of Environmental Impact and Clinical Efficacy. E3S Web of Conferences, Shahzadi, M., Hassan, T., & Saeed, S. (2022). Application of Natural Polymers in Wound Dressings. *Pakistan Journal of Medical & Health Sciences*, *16*(10), 1–1.

Shariatzadeh, F. J., Currie, S., Logsetty, S., Spiwak, R., & Liu, S. (2024). Enhancing wound healing and minimizing scarring: A comprehensive review of nanofiber technology in wound dressings. *Progress in Materials Science*, •••, 101350.

Sharma, S., Sharma, B., Shekhar, S., & Jain, P. (2022). Natural polymer-based composite wound dressings. *Polymeric and Natural Composites: Materials, Manufacturing and Biomedical Applications*, 401-423.

Silva, D. F., Lima, K. T., Bastos, G. N., Oliveira, J. A. R., do Nascimento, L. A. S., Costa, C. E. F., Filho, G. N., Concha, V. O., & Passos, M. F. (2021). PCL/andiroba oil (Carapa guianensis Aubl.) hybrid film for wound healing applications. *Polymers*, *13*(10), 1591. DOI: 10.3390/polym13101591 PMID: 34069314

Sindhi, K., Pingili, R. B., Beldar, V., Bhattacharya, S., Rahaman, J., & Mukherjee, D. (2025). The role of biomaterials-based scaffolds in advancing skin tissue construct. *Journal of Tissue Viability*, *34*(2), 100858. DOI: 10.1016/j.jtv.2025.100858 PMID: 39827732

Singh, V., Marimuthu, T., Makatini, M. M., & Choonara, Y. E. (2022). Biopolymer-based wound dressings with biochemical cues for cell-instructive wound repair. *Polymers, 14*(24), 5371. DOI: 10.3390/polym14245371 PMID: 36559739

Stathatou, P. M., Corbin, L., Meredith, J. C., & Garmulewicz, A. (2023). Biomaterials and regenerative agriculture: A methodological framework to enable circular transitions. *Sustainability (Basel), 15*(19), 14306. DOI: 10.3390/su151914306

Stoops, T. K., Layuno-Matos, J. G., Simon, P., Gustke, K. A., & Bernasek, T. L. (2025). Metal-on-Metal Total Hip Arthroplasties: Why Do They Fail? *Arthroplasty Today, 33*, 101662. DOI: 10.1016/j.artd.2025.101662 PMID: 40207181

Sudhakaran, G. (2024). Blue healing: Marine biopolymers' dual role in diabetic wounds and palliative care. *Natural Product Research,* •••, 1–3. DOI: 10.1080/14786419.2024.2358523 PMID: 38780166

Swaminathan, U., Marimuthu, K., Kasinathan, K., Choi, H. K., Sivakumar, P., Krishnasamy, R., & Palanisamy, R. (2024). Synthesis of novel liquid phase exfoliation of chitosan/Bi2Se3 hybrid nanocomposites for in-vitro wound healing. *International Journal of Biological Macromolecules, 255*, 128257. DOI: 10.1016/j.ijbiomac.2023.128257 PMID: 37984575

Talreja, R. K., Sable, H., Chaudhary, V., Kadian, S., Singh, M., Kumar, M., Kishore, J., Chaudhary, V., & Khosla, A. (2024). Challenges in Lab-to-Clinic Translation of 5th/6th Generation Intelligent Nanomaterial-enabled Biosensors. *ECS Sensors Plus, 3*(4), 041602. DOI: 10.1149/2754-2726/ad9f7e

Tao, Y., Shi, K., & Xiao, J. (2023). Research progress of biomaterials with ordered micro-nano structure in wound repair. *Zhonghua Shao Shang za zhi= Zhonghua Shaoshang Zazhi= Chinese Journal of Burns, 39*(9), 896-900.

Tehrany, P. M., Rahmanian, P., Rezaee, A., Ranjbarpazuki, G., Fard, F. S., Zandieh, M. A., Ranjbarpazuki, A., Asghari, S., Javani, N., & Nabavi, N. (2023). Multifunctional and theranostic hydrogels for wound healing acceleration: An emphasis on diabetic-related chronic wounds. *Environmental Research, 238*, 117087. DOI: 10.1016/j.envres.2023.117087 PMID: 37716390

Unnikrishnan, G., Muthuswamy, S., Kolanthai, E., Megha, M., Thomas, J., Haris, M., Gopinath, G., Varghese, R., & Ayyasamy, S. (2024). Synthesis and analysis of multifunctional graphene oxide/Ag2O-PVA/chitosan hybrid polymeric composite for wound healing applications. *International Journal of Biological Macromolecules, 277*, 134301. DOI: 10.1016/j.ijbiomac.2024.134301 PMID: 39094875

Verdú-Soriano, J., de Cristino-Espinar, M., Luna-Morales, S., Dios-Guerra, C., Caballero-Villarraso, J., Moreno-Moreno, P., Casado-Díaz, A., Berenguer-Pérez, M., Guler-Caamaño, I., Laosa-Zafra, O., Rodríguez-Mañas, L., & Lázaro-Martínez, J. L. (2022). Superiority of a novel multifunctional amorphous hydrogel containing olea europaea leaf extract (EHO-85) for the treatment of skin ulcers: A randomized, active-controlled clinical trial. *Journal of Clinical Medicine*, *11*(5), 1260. DOI: 10.3390/jcm11051260 PMID: 35268352

Verma, D., Okhawilai, M., Nangan, S., Thakur, V. K., Gopi, S., Kuppusamy, K., Sharma, M., & Uyama, H. (2024). A sustainable and green approach towards the utilization of biopolymers for effective wound dressing applications: A detailed review. *Nano-Structures & Nano-Objects*, *37*, 101086. DOI: 10.1016/j.nanoso.2023.101086

Vinchurkar, K., Bukke, S. P. N., Jain, P., Bhadoria, J., Likhariya, M., Mane, S., Suryawanshi, M., Veerabhadrappa, K. V., Eftekhari, Z., & Onohuean, H. (2025). Advances in sustainable biomaterials: Characterizations, and applications in medicine. *Discover Polymers*, *2*(1), 2. DOI: 10.1007/s44347-025-00014-8

Vishali, J. K., Sharma, P., Jassal, R., Singh, B., Sayam, M., & Kajla, V. Transformative Biomaterials in Burn Care: Utilizing Scaffolds, Hydrogels, And Chitosan for Optimized Healing and Scar Reduction.

Wall, I., de Silva Thompson, D., Peticone, C., & Perez, R. (2016). Industrial translation requirements for manufacture of stem cell–derived and tissue-engineered products. *Tissue Engineering and Regeneration in Dentistry: Current Strategies*, 110-123.

Wang, M., Huang, X., Zheng, H., Tang, Y., Zeng, K., Shao, L., & Li, L. (2021). Nanomaterials applied in wound healing: Mechanisms, limitations and perspectives. *Journal of Controlled Release*, *337*, 236–247. DOI: 10.1016/j.jconrel.2021.07.017 PMID: 34273419

Wang, P., Cai, F., Li, Y., Yang, X., Feng, R., Lu, H., Bai, X., & Han, J. (2024). Emerging trends in the application of hydrogel-based biomaterials for enhanced wound healing: A literature review. *International Journal of Biological Macromolecules*, *261*, 129300. DOI: 10.1016/j.ijbiomac.2024.129300 PMID: 38216016

Wang, X., Yang, J., Zhao, Q., Xie, X., Deng, F., Wang, Z., Jiang, K., Li, X., Liu, H., Shi, Z., Zhu, X., Chen, L., & Lv, D. (2024). A tissue-adhesive, mechanically enhanced, natural Aloe Vera-based injectable hydrogel for wound healing: Macrophage mediation and collagen proliferation. *International Journal of Biological Macromolecules*, *283*, 137452. DOI: 10.1016/j.ijbiomac.2024.137452 PMID: 39522911

Wiśniewska, P., Saeb, M. R., & Bencherif, S. A. (2023). Biomaterials recycling: A promising pathway to sustainability. *Frontiers in Biomaterials Science*, *2*, 1260402. DOI: 10.3389/fbiom.2023.1260402 PMID: 38550558

Xi Loh, E. Y., Fauzi, M. B., Ng, M. H., Ng, P. Y., Ng, S. F., Ariffin, H., & Mohd Amin, M. C. I. (2018). Cellular and molecular interaction of human dermal fibroblasts with bacterial nanocellulose composite hydrogel for tissue regeneration. *ACS Applied Materials & Interfaces*, *10*(46), 39532–39543. DOI: 10.1021/acsami.8b16645 PMID: 30372014

Xiao, J., Liang, Y., Sun, T., Liu, M., & He, X. (2024). A functional dual responsive CMC/OHA/SA/TOB hydrogel as wound dressing to enhance wound healing. *Scientific Reports*, *14*(1), 26854. DOI: 10.1038/s41598-024-78044-8 PMID: 39501050

Xu, H., Lu, J., Xi, Y., Wang, X., & Liu, J. (2024). Liquid metal biomaterials: Translational medicines, challenges and perspectives. *National Science Review*, *11*(2), nwad302. DOI: 10.1093/nsr/nwad302 PMID: 38213519

Xu, R., Fang, Y., Zhang, Z., Cao, Y., Yan, Y., Gan, L., Xu, J., & Zhou, G. (2023). Recent advances in biodegradable and biocompatible synthetic polymers used in skin wound healing. *Materials (Basel)*, *16*(15), 5459. DOI: 10.3390/ma16155459 PMID: 37570163

Yadav, J. P., Singh, A. K., Grishina, M., Pathak, P., Verma, A., Kumar, V., Kumar, P., & Patel, D. K. (2024). Insights into the mechanisms of diabetic wounds: Pathophysiology, molecular targets, and treatment strategies through conventional and alternative therapies. *Inflammopharmacology*, *32*(1), 149–228. DOI: 10.1007/s10787-023-01407-6 PMID: 38212535

Yadav, P., Gupta, M., Singh, S. P., & Parashar, P. (2024). Biocompatible Electrospun Hydrogel Fibers for Advanced Wound Healing Therapies. *Current Pharmaceutical Design*, *30*(41), 3240–3254. DOI: 10.2174/0113816128322485240826065135 PMID: 39279109

Yadav, P. D., Londhe, P. V., Chavan, S. S., Mohite, D. D., Firame, G. B., Kadam, S. S., Patil, M. J., & Ansari, M. (2024). Electrospun composite nanofibers for wound healing: Synthesis, characterization, and clinical potential of biopolymer-based materials. *Discover Materials*, *4*(1), 1–21. DOI: 10.1007/s43939-024-00173-8

Yi, Y., An, H. W., & Wang, H. (2024). Intelligent biomaterialomics: Molecular design, manufacturing, and biomedical applications. *Advanced Materials*, *36*(22), 2305099. DOI: 10.1002/adma.202305099 PMID: 37490938

Zarepour, A., Gok, B., Kılıç, Y. B., Khosravi, A., Iravani, S., & Zarrabi, A. (2024). Bacterial nanocelluloses as sustainable biomaterials for advanced wound healing and dressings. *Journal of Materials Chemistry. B*, *12*(48), 12489–12507. DOI: 10.1039/D4TB01024H PMID: 39533945

Zhang, J., Wang, M., Yuan, H., Zeng, X.-F., Wang, J.-X., & Le, Y. (2024). Accelerated Wound Healing by Electrospun Multifunctional Fibers with Self-Powered Performance. *Langmuir*, *40*(17), 9134–9143. DOI: 10.1021/acs.langmuir.4c00545 PMID: 38636482

Zhao, C., Wu, X., Huang, J., Chen, C., Yu, J., Fang, M., Wang, G., & Ren, J. (2019). Hybrid material for open abdomen: Saving the wound from intestinal fistula. *Journal of Materials Science. Materials in Medicine*, *30*(9), 1–10. DOI: 10.1007/s10856-019-6311-1 PMID: 31535210

Zhao, S., Han, L., Yan, L., & Lu, X. (2023). The recent research progress of polyphenol-derived biomaterials in wound repair. *Biosurface and Biotribology*, *9*(4), 114–128. DOI: 10.1049/bsb2.12074

Zhong, Y., Wei, E., Wu, L., Wang, Y., Lin, Q., Wu, N., Chen, H., & Tang, N. (2024). Novel Biomaterials for Wound Healing and Tissue Regeneration. *ACS Omega*, *9*(30), 32268–32286. DOI: 10.1021/acsomega.4c02775 PMID: 39100297

Zhou, D., Yang, T., & Luo, G. (2017). Nanosilver coated Chitin derived membrane as an Eco-friendly Dressing and Its Effect on Wound Healing.

Zhu, L., Yu, Z.-L., Li, S., Xu, C.-Z., Hou, Y.-J., Liao, L.-X., Xu, Y.-L., Zhang, J.-T., Wei, B.-M., Wen, W., & Wang, H.-B. (2024). Recent advances on collagen biomaterial: From extraction, cross-linking to tissue regeneration. *Polymer Reviews (Philadelphia, Pa.)*, *64*(4), 1031–1059. DOI: 10.1080/15583724.2024.2382128

Zhu, Q., Sun, E., Sun, Y., Cao, X., & Wang, N. (2024). Biomaterial Promotes Triboelectric Nanogenerator for Health Diagnostics and Clinical Application. *Nanomaterials (Basel, Switzerland)*, *14*(23), 1885. DOI: 10.3390/nano14231885 PMID: 39683273

KEY TERMS AND DEFINITIONS

Biomaterials: Substances engineered to interact with biological systems for a medical purpose—either therapeutic (treat, augment, repair, or replace tissue function) or diagnostic.

Wound Healing: A complex biological process involving multiple stages—hemostasis, inflammation, proliferation, and remodeling—aimed at tissue repair and regeneration after injury.

Hydrogels: Hydrophilic polymer networks capable of retaining large amounts of water, often used in wound dressings to maintain a moist healing environment and deliver bioactive compounds.

Natural Polymers: Biopolymers derived from natural sources (e.g., chitosan, alginate, hyaluronic acid) that mimic components of the extracellular matrix and are typically biodegradable and biocompatible.

Synthetic Polymers: Man-made polymers (e.g., polycaprolactone, polylactic acid) engineered for controlled mechanical properties and degradation rates, used in advanced wound dressings and scaffolds.

Hybrid Materials: Composites that combine natural and synthetic components or integrate nanoparticles, essential oils, or other functional additives to provide multifunctionality (e.g., antimicrobial, self-healing, conductive).

Macrophage Modulation: The influence of biomaterials on macrophage polarization (e.g., promoting M2 anti-inflammatory phenotype), which plays a pivotal role in regulating inflammation and tissue repair.

Electrospinning: A fabrication technique that produces nanofibers mimicking the extracellular matrix, often used to create scaffolds that support cell attachment and tissue regeneration.

Nanomaterials: Engineered materials at the nanoscale (1–100 nm) used in wound care for their enhanced properties such as antimicrobial activity, bioactive molecule delivery, and cellular modulation.

Smart Dressings: Advanced wound dressings that incorporate sensors or stimuli-responsive systems to monitor wound conditions or release therapeutic agents based on environmental cues.

Biocompatibility: The ability of a material to perform its desired function without eliciting adverse local or systemic effects in the host.

Angiogenesis: The formation of new blood vessels, a crucial component in the proliferation stage of wound healing, often promoted by bioactive materials.

Extracellular Matrix (ECM): A complex network of proteins and polysaccharides surrounding cells, providing structural support and signaling cues; often mimicked in biomaterial design.

Stimuli-Responsive Materials: Materials that change their properties or behavior in response to external stimuli (e.g., pH, temperature, glucose), used to create adaptive wound care systems.

Bacterial Nanocellulose (BNC): A naturally derived nanomaterial known for its strength, purity, and moisture retention capabilities, increasingly used in wound dressings.

Self-Healing Materials: Biomaterials capable of repairing their structure autonomously after damage, thereby reducing dressing changes and enhancing durability.

Regenerative Medicine: A field focused on restoring or establishing normal function in damaged tissues and organs, with biomaterials often playing a critical support role.

Scaffolds: 3D structures made from biomaterials designed to support cell growth, tissue regeneration, and vascularization in wound healing applications.

Angiogenic Factors: Molecules like VEGF (vascular endothelial growth factor) that promote the development of blood vessels, often incorporated into biomaterials to enhance healing.

Biodegradability: The capability of a material to be broken down by biological systems, an important feature for temporary implants or dressings that should not remain permanently in the body.

Chapter 12

Nano-Engineered Therapies for Breast Cancer: A New Paradigm to Overcome Multidrug Resistance

Banashree Bondhopadhyay
https://orcid.org/0000-0002-6679-7791
Amity University, Noida, India

Tanmay J. Urs
Amity University, Noida, India

Shreya Gupta
https://orcid.org/0009-0003-0795-6881
Amity University, Noida, India

Ruchika Ruchika
https://orcid.org/0009-0003-6685-4359
Amity University, Ghaziabad, India

ABSTRACT

The effectiveness of the conventional treatment strategies is falling, as tumors are gradually becoming chemoresistant. Breast cancer cells are persistently overexposed to therapeutic agents, leading them to develop multidrug resistance. Molecular mechanisms causing Multidrug Resistance (MDR) include the overexpression of drug efflux transporters, evasion of apoptosis, activation of NF-κB and other signaling pathways supporting tumor proliferation, dysregulation of DNA repair

DOI: 10.4018/979-8-3373-1305-4.ch012

mechanisms, epigenetic modulations and tumor-supportive microenvironment. This present study explores the biomedical applications of nanoparticles to combat multidrug resistance (MDR) in breast cancer. We focus on nanoparticles that can bypass drug efflux pumps, deliver agents precisely, co-deliver siRNA/miRNA for DNA repair, and release drugs responsively. Looking ahead, we identify future research opportunities in multi-targeting pathways, hypoxia/enzyme-triggered drug release, genetic/epigenetic modulation, personalized medicines, and AI-driven optimization of nanoparticle properties.

1. INTRODUCTION

The aggressive and resistant breast cancers can survive and proliferate despite extensive exposure to various chemotherapeutic agents. Multidrug resistance (MDR) presents a significant clinical challenge. It reduces the effectiveness of conventional treatments, leading to disease progression, treatment failure, and poor outcomes for patients (Wind & Holen, 2011). MDR in breast cancer is driven by multiple molecular and microenvironmental mechanisms. The key factors include the overexpression of ATP-binding cassette (ABC) transporters, regulation of pro- and anti-apoptotic proteins, DNA repair mechanisms, interactions within the tumour microenvironment (TME), and epigenetic modifications. These factors contribute to the complication of treatment strategies (Kinnel et al., 2023). The existing conventional treatment modalities, such as chemotherapy and combination therapy, primarily target the underlying mechanisms. The strategies to overcome drug efflux involve, verapamil and tariquidar, to block P-gp, BRCP and MRP1 activity. However, these inhibitors often exhibit poor specificity, causing off-target effects and systemic toxicities. The efflux pump inhibitors upregulate alternative efflux mechanisms, along with unfavourable pharmacokinetics and drug interactions (Xue & Liang, 2012).

Targeting DNA repair pathways with PARP inhibitors Olaparib and Talazoparib, has shown effectiveness in BRCA-mutated breast cancers by inducing synthetic lethality. However, resistance can develop through secondary BRCA mutations or the upregulation of DNA damage response proteins like RAD51 (Hobbs et al., 2021). Therapies targeting anti-apoptotic proteins, such as venetoclax, a BCL-2 inhibitor are used to restore apoptosis. However, resistance persistently arise from MCL-1 overexpression and mutations in pro-apoptotic proteins like BAX, limiting long-term efficacy (H. Wang et al., 2021).

Additionally, DNA methyltransferase inhibitors, azacytadine and decitabine and histone deacetylase inhibitors, vorinostat and entinostat, reactivate tumour suppressor genes silenced by hypermethylation and hyperacetylation (Emran et al., 2022).

However, their low bioavailability, off-target toxicity, and negative effects on gene expression pose significant challenges (Brown et al., 2022).

In addition to specific challenges, traditional modalities are limited by poor bioavailability, transient effects and off-target toxicities, despite their potential to reverse resistance. Moreover, tumour heterogeneity, redundancy in resistance mechanisms, gaps in clinical translation and adaptability of breast cancer cells further complicate treatment outcomes. It necessitates the exploration of approaches to enhance drug delivery, increase specificity, and simultaneously target multiple resistance pathways.

Nanoparticle based strategies are in boom in the recent years, particularly for the treatment of MDR in multi-dimensional diseases like breast cancer (Martinelli & Biglietti, 2020a). Nanoparticles are ultra fine particles ideally ranging from 1-100nm in dimensions (Mba & Nweze, 2021). Owing to their small size, they possess unique physicochemical properties. The characteristics include a high surface area-to-volume ratio, good reactivity and penetration of complex biological barriers (Lan et al., 2023). The underlying physical, chemical and biological properties make NPs the ideal option for drug delivery applications in cancer therapy. The versatile nature of NPs allows for their mechanical engineering, to perform desired functions. NPs passively target through the enhanced permeability and retention (EPR) effect and actively bind to overexpressed receptors on tumor cells through specific ligands, incorporated on the surface (Attia et al., 2019).

The nano-based systems are produced from a variety of biomaterial sources. Lipid based such as liposomes (Hamad et al., 2024), PLGA and PEG based polymeric NPs (Salari et al., 2022), metallic NPs (Hheidari et al., 2024) such gold, silver and platinum, magnetic NPs such as iron oxide and super paramagnetic iron oxide NPs (Meng et al., 2024), solid-lipid NPs (Mo et al., 2023), dendrimer and micelle-based NPs (Alven & Aderibigbe, 2020) have been developed and widely utilized for performing selective or multifaceted treatment role.

Nanotechnology and nano-based platforms have evolved significantly over the time. Early formulations were primarily designed for the purpose of passive drug delivery. Early NPs include liposomes and polymeric NPs (Dastidar et al., 2022). The primitive NPs now stand as the foundation for the development of novel systems. Advancements in nanotechnology led to the creation of current multifunctional nanoparticles with versatile and multifaceted roles in different stages of breast cancer treatment (Li et al., 2024). The latest platforms can deliver multiple therapeutic agents simultaneously without off-target payloads. The systems additionally offer real-time monitoring of the incorporated agent through imaging techniques. Current biomedical applications have reached to targeted delivery of chemotherapeutics, gene and immunotherapy, achieving stimuli-triggered sustained release (Raheem et al., 2023).

Nanoparticles have significant potential as alternatives to conventional drug delivery systems. These advanced strategies have improved the poor solubility and bioavailability issues of traditional means. Nanoparticle formulations can encapsulate hydrophobic drugs such as paclitaxel and doxorubicin for controlled release and better therapeutic efficacy (Yadav et al., 2022). This capability is particularly crucial in the context of multidrug resistance (MDR), where cancer cells often eject out agents before they can even employ their therapeutic effects. Employing NPs that inhibit efflux transporters like P-glycoprotein (P-gp) or delivering combination therapies that simultaneously target multiple pathways, address the mechanisms that contribute to drug resistance (Gao et al., 2024a).

The multifunctionality of nanoparticles allow the co-delivery of chemotherapeutic agents synergistically with efflux-pump inhibitors and gene-silencer molecules (Bhattacharjee, 2022). The novel strategies can be engineered to respond to specific acidic TME mediated stimuli and trigger a sustained drug release. These stimuli include pH, temperature, light, redox, elevated ROS levels and hypoxia, improving bioavailability and pharmacokinetics beneficial for counteracting MDR in breast cancer (Zhou et al., 2018a) **(Table 1)**.

Table 1. A comparative analysis of conventional and nano-based strategies in breast cancer treatment

Features	Conventional strategies	Nano-based strategies	References
Drug resistance	Drug resistance due to DNA repair, efflux pumps and tumour.	Overcoming drug resistance thought blocking drug efflux.	(Gote et al., 2021b; Guan et al., 2024)(Gote et al., 2021b; Guan et al., 2024)
Toxicity	High toxicity due to off targeting.	Tumor specific accumulation reduces systemic toxicity.	(Ombredane et al., 2021) (Ombredane et al., 2021)
Therapeutic agents	Mainly chemotherapy and immunotherapy.	Gene therapy and PTT agents	(Ovejero-Paredes et al., 2022)
Targeting mechanism	Non-specific drug delivery, which also harms healthy tissue.	Passive targeting and active targeting	(Nabil et al., 2021)(Nabil et al., 2021)
Drug delivery	Poor drug delivery due to limited solubility and short circulation half-life.	Enhanced drug delivery through increased solubility, controlled drug release and prolonged circulation	(Ashrafizadeh et al., 2023) (Ashrafizadeh et al., 2023)

2. BACKGROUND (MULTIDRUG RESISTANCE IN BREAST CANCER)

MDR is intrinsic among several cancerous cells, allowing them to survive and proliferate regardless of the persistent exposure to various anti-cancer drugs. The phenomenon is present or acquired from the onset of treatment, developing substantially over time as a response to therapy. MDR is characterized to resist multiple influence of therapeutic drugs, often resulting in failed treatment strategies and progression of the disease. It has been a major contributing factor of mortality among aggressive subtypes of breast cancer, particularly $HER2^+$ and TNBC.

Several molecular mechanisms harmfully drive the development of MDR in the breast tumor microenvironment (TME). Elevated expression of drug efflux transporters belonging to the ATP-binding cassette (ABC) superfamily has a major influence on MDR (Gote et al., 2021). Key transporters include P-glycoprotein (P-gp), multidrug resistance protein 1 (MRP1), and breast cancer resistance protein (BCRP). The transporters actively pump and eject out chemotherapeutic agents like doxorubicin (DOX) and paclitaxel (PTX) from cancer cells. P-gp is the most well-characterized among these, often linked to decrease drug accumulation in breast cancer (Mechanism of Multidrug Resistance to Chemotherapy Mediated by P-glycoprotein (Review), n.d.). MRP1 and BCRP facilitate the efflux of various other anticancer drugs (Xue & Liang, n.d.).

The deregulation and evasion of apoptosis, a hallmark of cancer, is another primary reason for MDR. Tumors gradually develop strategies such as overexpression of anti-apoptotic proteins, downregulation of pro-apoptotic proteins and disruption of signalling pathways to control cell death (Neophytou et al., 2021). The activation of nuclear factor-kappa B (NF-κB) signaling promotes cell survival, proliferation and resistance to apoptosis. NF-κB upregulates anti-apoptotic proteins such as BCL-2 and inhibits pro-apoptotic pathways, allowing cancer cells to withstand chemotherapy-induced stress and develop MDR (Pavitra et al., 2023).

3. ADDITIONALLY, DYSREGULATED DNA REPAIR MECHANISMS DRIVE MDR

Defected pathways such as homologous recombination or non-homologous end joining, allows cancerous cells to persist DNA damage caused by chemotherapeutic agents (Gao et al., 2024b). Epigenetic modifications such as DNA methylation and histone acetylation, alter the expression of genes involved in drug metabolism, cell cycle regulation and apoptosis. Moreover, TME creates a protective niche for cancer cells. Hypoxia, acidosis and interactions with stromal cells enhance drug resistance by promoting angiogenesis, immune evasion, and the survival of cancer stem cells (CSCs), which are inherently resistant to therapy (Aravindan et al., 2024)

Classification of nanoparticles for breast cancer treatment

Nanoparticles for breast cancer treatment is a significant area of research and development. They are classified into three major categories organic, inorganic and carbon-based nanomaterial. Nanomaterial offers unique therapeutic benefits that are used to improve treatment outcomes for breast cancer patients (Eynde et al., 2024).

Organic nanomaterials are known for their biocompatibility and biodegradability, which makes them excellent candidates for targeted drug delivery system. liposomes are spherical vesicles that can encapsulate chemotherapeutic drug like doxorubicin. This encapsulation not only improves the solubility of the drug but also significantly decreases systematic toxicity, thereby limiting side effects associated. Moreover, polymeric nanoparticle, can be engineered from various biodegradable polymers, allow for controlled release of drugs in response to specific stimuli. Dendrimers, with their highly branched structures and surface modifications, facilitate precise drug loading and delivery, ensuring that therapeutic agents are effectively transported to cancer cells (Ovejero-Paredes et al., 2022).

Inorganic nanomaterial is known for their stability and multifunctional properties, making them suitable for a various of applications in cancer therapy. metal nanoparticles, like gold nanoparticles, have exceptional photothermal conversion efficiency. They can be used in photothermal therapy to selectively destruct cancer cells by converting light into heat when exposed to near infrared radiation (Sargazi et al., 2022). Silver nanoparticle exhibits intrinsic anticancer activity and also serve as carriers for phytochemical that enhance therapeutic efficacy. Moreover, metal oxide nanoparticles like manganese dioxide, combined with polydopamine creates a hybrid system that provides both PTT and chemotherapy. Mesoporous silica nanoparticles are class of inorganic materials known for their high drug loading capacity and controlled release properties, which can be finely tuned to match the needs of specific therapies (Cheraghi et al., 2023; Rani et al., 2023).

Carbon based nanoparticles are significant in breast cancer treatment due to their unique and mechanical properties. Graphene oxide is one such material that has been utilised in photothermal ablation and drug delivery applications. It interacts with light which makes it an excellent candidate for PTT, while its surface allows for the attachment of various therapeutic agents. Carbon nanotubes have emerged as diverse platform that act both as biosensors and drug carrier, improving tumour imaging capabilities while allowing targeted delivery of chemotherapeutics. Furthermore, carbon dots specially, lipid coated carbon dots enable fluorescence guided PTT, enhancing the precision of treatment delivery (Hosseini et al., 2023).

4. BIOMEDICAL APPLICATIONS OF NPS FOR THE CHALLENGES OF MULTI DRUG-RESISTANT BREAST CANCER

NPs employ a variety of mechanisms to target and mitigate MDR in breast cancer. NPs accumulate in the tumor tissues, owing to the leaky vasculature and poor lymphatic drainage. The passive targeting approach bypasses the need for specific molecular recognition which make them effective in drug resistant tumors. NPs deliver chemotherapeutic agents directly to the tumor site through the enhanced permeability and retention (EPR) effect (C. Duan et al., 2023). On the other hand, NPs are functionalized with ligands such as aptamers and antibodies. The ligand-coated NPs bind to the overexpressed receptors such as HER2, EGFR, or CD44 on drug-resistant tumors. The system ensures cellular uptake and precise drug delivery (Ganesan et al., 2021a).

Multifunctional nanoparticles integrate therapeutic agents with MDR-reversing strategies such as efflux pump inhibitors and gene-silencing tools. The system exploits synergistic effects to downregulate drug efflux pumps, inhibit survival pathways and induce apoptosis in resistant cells lines of breast cancer. Stimuli-responsive NPs release their payload in response to specific TME triggers and conditions. They include hypoxia, pH, redox potential or enzymatic activity (Chang et al., 2021).

4.1 Nanoparticles to Bypass Drug Efflux Pumps

A study developed chitosan-based polymeric NPs to encapsulate and promote controlled release of both CUR and DOX. *In vitro* studies on human breast cancer models demonstrated effective downregulation of ABC transporters and NF-κB activity. The system enhanced intracellular drug retention and promoted apoptosis in resistant cancer cells (J. Duan et al., 2012).

DOX and resveratrol (RES) were co-encapsulated in a poly(lactic-co-glycolic acid) (PLGA) modified polymeric NPs by (Y. Zhao et al., 2016). The DOX/RES-loaded NPs delivered the compounds into the nucleus of MDA-MB-231/ADR and MCF-7/ADR cell lines. The dual delivery resulted in significant cytotoxicity, and it overcame drug resistance by inhibiting the expression of P-gp, MRP-1 and BCRP. Additionally, the NPs down-regulated NF-κB and BCL-2 expression and induced apoptosis. *In vivo* studies, DOX/RES-loaded NPs primarily targeted tumor tissue and reduced tumor growth compared to free DOX.

A study by (Lai et al., 2025), developed a macrophage membrane camouflaged liposome (DOX-Tet NPs). This was designed to reverse DOX resistance in MCF-7/ADR cells. The core of the liposome was loaded with DOX and tetrandrine (Tet). The macrophage membrane served as the outer shell. The combination of DOX and Tet allowed effective binding to P-glycoprotein (P-gp) and blocked the drug efflux. The blockage increased the accumulation of DOX at the tumor sites. *In vitro* assays reduced the resistance index for MCF-7/ADR cells, when treated with these particles compared to free DOX or DOX-Tet solutions. The macrophage membrane functionalization simultaneously improved cellular uptake due to α4-integrin binding to VCAM-1, facilitating immune evasion.

A different CAM/DOX PEGylated liposome showed the inhibition of P-gp in a study. The nanoparticles were capable of high encapsulation of both DOX and CAM. The study reported a notable decrease in P-gp levels with the PEGylated liposomes, reversing MDR with improved drug penetration in MCF-7/ADR cell line. Furthermore, CAM along with the inhibition of P-gp, disrupted autophagy and sensitized tumor cells to DOX drug (Alfreahat et al., 2025).

A study investigated the Ex@MTX-CQDs, exosomes were designed to encapsulate carbon quantum dots (CQDs) derived from Folic Acid and methotrexate (MTX). The exosomes had excellent drug-loading efficiency and pH-sensitive release properties. Exosomes facilitated endocytosis through EPR effect in MCF-7/ADR cell line, allowing to bypass P-gp efflux pumps. Additionally, specific targeting of folic acid enabled to bind to cancer cells which overexpressed folate receptors, enhancing internalization and cytotoxicity. Cellular studies showed significant apoptosis induction in MCF-7 breast cancer cells compared to free MTX, indicating the effectiveness of this nanocarrier in overcoming drug resistance (Kazeminava et al., 2024).

Figure 1. The multifunctional nanoparticles, responsive to pH, redox and enzymatic conditions in the tumor microenvironment. The nanoparticles encapsulate the drug, releases the drug upon exposure to acidic pH, high glutathione levels and MMP enzyme (This picture was created using Canva.com on 1st Feb 2025)

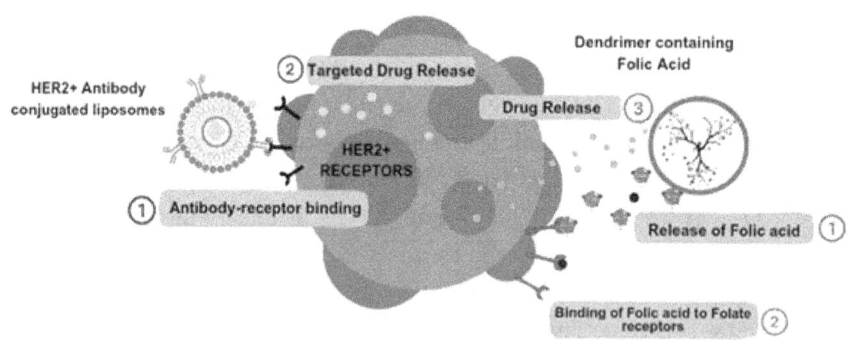

Another study focused the successful development of mixed micelle NPs loaded with docetaxel (DTX) and CUR for co-delivery against MCF-7/ADR cells. *in vitro* release profiles of the combination showed sustained drug release through EPR effect. Mixed micelles had a better cellular uptake, cytotoxicity, apoptosis rates and reactive oxygen species (ROS) levels. Along with the improved bioavailability, the duration of the drug concentrations in the plasma were prolonged (Dian et al., 2024).

HA-MIL-125 nanoparticles were used in a study to co-encapsulate a pH-sensitive DOX prodrug (DV) and an autophagy inhibitor 3-methyladenine (3-MA). HA-MIL -125@DVMA nanoparticles were created with desirable size and pH-sensitive release properties. Notably, the release of DOX from these nanoparticles was enhanced in the acidic TME. HA-MIL-125@DVMA nanoparticles improved drug accumulation in MCF-7/ADR cells through receptor-mediated endocytosis, effectively killing tumor cells and reversing MDR.

The development of DOX-resistant tumors was inhibited *in vivo,* reducing harmful effects associated with DOX. Compared to free DOX therapy, the inhibition rate of HA-MIL-125@DVMA was increased for more than 3.5 times in resistant tumors. 3-MA inhibited autophagy, while the HA modification actively targeted CD44 receptors on the MCF-7/ADR cells, to prevent the P-gp efflux pump and enhance DOX accumulation (Q. Guo et al., 2023).

In a different study, CUR, a water insoluble agent was loaded into solid lipid nanoparticles (SLNs) with a size range of 175-190 nm. The chitosan-coated SLNs (CURC-CS-SLN) had a better hydrophilicity. This improved their biocompatibility and prevented immune clearance. CURC-CS-SLN resensitized doxorubicin-resistant triple-negative breast cancer (TNBC) cells at 5-10 times lower concentrations than free CURC. The NPs targeted cells with elevated ROS levels, inhibited the NF-κB signaling pathway and downregulated P-gp. Superior chemotherapeutic efficiency was observed without any significant toxicity or cardiac damage *in vivo* (Abd-Ellatef et al., 2020).

Polymeric lipid hybrid nanoparticles (E-PLNs) were encapsulated emodin (EMO), natural active ingredient alongside DOX to address MDR in MCF-7/ADR cells. Exogenous interleukin-6 (IL-6) and inhibitors of the JAK2/STAT3 signaling pathway were employed. *In vitro* results showed inhibited IL-6-induced overactivation of the JAK2/STAT3 pathway, by EMO and E-PLNs in combination with DOX. This was followed by decreased cell proliferation, reduction of EMT, lower invasion rates and reversal of DOX resistance in MCF-7/ADR cells (Gu et al., 2024).

4.2 Targeted Delivery by NPs for MDR Reversal

A study developed an immunoliposome-based delivery system. It was engineered with HER2 antibodies to specifically bind with HER2-expressing tumor in HER2$^+$ BC. The formulation delivered doxorubicin (DOX) and bevacizumab in combination. The system triggered positively charged electrostatic interactions with the negatively charged tumor membrane. Both DOX and bevacizumab were successfully encapsulated within the liposomes, to provide controlled release and sustained drug action at the tumor site.

Preferred bioaccumulation of the administered liposomes was facilitated in the tumor tissues. The system reduced drug efflux problems through EPR effect, exploiting the leaky vasculature. In vitro studies assessed increased DOX concentrations by immunoliposomes, compared to free release in tumor cells. The combination of bevacizumab and DOX inhibited tumor growth and improved survival rates *in vivo* models that were both HER2$^+$ and MDR$^+$ (Y. Tang et al., 2017).

A similar study synthesized anti-EGFR immunoliposomes (anti-EGFR-ILs) for the same targeted delivery of DOX to EGFR overexpressed cells in advanced TNBC. The anti-EGFR antibody fragments were integrated into PEGylated liposome membranes for specific binding to the MDA-MB-231 cells. The engineered anti-EGFR-ILs showed better payload and delivery of DOX, as desired, compared to the traditional antibody-drug conjugates.

In vitro results confirmed the increase in DOX concentrations and increased cytotoxicity in MDA-MB-231 cell lines. However, questions have raised regarding the suitability of EGFR as a target molecule for advanced TNBCs, despite acceptable safety profiles from phase II trials (Mamot et al., 2023).

In a different study, Trastuzumab engineered nylon NPs were loaded with sorafenib, a multi-kinase inhibitor with anti-angiogenic properties and nutlin-3a, an MDM2 inhibitor reactivating p53 pathway. The complex system was characterised for pH-sensitive therapeutic delivery profiles in acidic environments of HER2$^+$ SK-BR-3 cells.

Along with their therapeutic interventions, the system was also capable of tumor imaging and remodelling, detection and localization. The platform showed clear spectral discrimination, upon conjugation with near-infrared (NIR) dyes. Their uniform and optimum photoacoustic spectrum enabled precise PA imaging of biological environments *in vitro* (Şen et al., 2024).

Researchers from another study developed DOX loaded copper oxide NPs coated with biocompatible chitosan (Cs-CuO NPs). This nano formulation had high drug loading capacity and pH-dependent drug release in MCF-7/MDR cells. The approach induced apoptosis by causing oxidative stress and a loss of mitochondrial membrane potential (Khursheed et al., 2022).

Another prospect was the development of PTX/MNPs/QDs@Biotin–PEG–PCDA for dual-modal targeting approach to overcome MDR. This integrated PTX, MNPs and QDs within a biotin-based polymeric carrier for therapy and imaging. The MNPs facilitated magnetic targeting, under the influence of an external magnetic field for precise localization. The conjugate had a better cellular uptake *in vitro* MCF-7/ADR cell.

QDs provided sensitive fluorescence tracking. This allowed real-time monitoring of the biodistribution and cellular internalization of the drug *in vitro*. The combination of these modalities showed effective GSH triggered release of PTX and CUR within the TME. CUR downregulated the drug efflux transporters P-gp, often upregulated in MDR cell lines, increasing PTX accumulation (J. Wang et al., 2016).

4.3 Co-Delivery of Agents by Nanoparticles to Counter MDR

The targeted/pH/reduction-sensitive polymer micelles were developed to co-deliver DOX and 10-hydroxycamptothecin (HCPT) in MCF-7/ADR breast cancer cells. Each chemotherapeutic agent was synchronously encapsulated through π-π stacking within a single micelle. The complex bypassed from the recognition by drug efflux pumps such as P-gp and BCRP. The dual-drug formulation evaded all the cellular repair mechanisms, through synergistic effects between DOX and HCPT.

A light-responsive polysaccharide NP was co-loaded with DOX and an ATP-binding cassette transporter inhibitor, APA. The irradiation of light disassembled the nanoparticle, releasing both DOX and APA simultaneously. APA thoroughly inhibited P-gp activity and restored DOX sensitivity in resistant cells. Similarly, lapatinib (LPA), a tyrosine kinase inhibitor (TKI), was incorporated into micelles with DOX to reverse MDR by suppressing P-gp activity (Wei et al., 2021a).

In a study, NV@CaP-RGD NP was incorporated with a drug efflux inhibitor Verapamil (VRP), and a chemotherapeutic agent novantrone (NVT). In this approach, a PS-PEG core encapsulated NVT and a CaP shell adsorbed VRP. RGD peptide was functionalized as a targeted ligand to navigate the nanoparticles to breast cancer cells. NV@CaP-RGD significantly enhanced the concentration of NVT in MDR tumor cells through drug internalization. The action inhibited the efflux of these agents and prevented lysosomal escape. This led to increased apoptosis via activated mitochondrial pathway and the suppression of the ERK signalling transduction pathway *in vitro* (Dong et al., 2019).

One more study developed mesoporous silica nanoparticles (MSNPs) to co-load DOX and P-gp siRNA. This strategy was employed to eradicate DOX resistance in a MDR BC xenograft model. The NPs were further functionalized with a polyethyleneimine-PEG (PEI-PEG) copolymer for protective delivery of stable DOX and P-gp siRNA to the tumor site. In vivo studies proved that co-delivery system achieved greater tumor growth inhibition compared to free DOX or nanoparticles loaded with either DOX or siRNA alone (Xiao et al., 2016).

Self-assembled polycurcumin NPs integrate CUR into an intracellular cleavable polymer. The complex facilitates specific degradation and drug co-release at elevated levels of intracellular GSH. The design allows for simultaneous release of CUR and encapsulated DOX against MCF-7/ADR cells. The hydrophilic outer shell composing biotin-PEG provides a stealth shielding from recognition by the reticuloendothelial system. It reversed DOX resistance by suppressing the expression of P-gp and ATP activity (S. Guo et al., 2016).

Liposomes co-deliver DOX alongside a Ras-related nuclear protein, Ran-GTP. The inhibitory peptide targets faulty DNA repair mechanisms, which are driven by Ran-GTP, thereby implicating drug resistance. By inhibiting this protein, the Ran-GTP inhibitory peptide effectively reversed MDR. The complex sensitized the MCF-7/ADR cell to DOX drug (Wei et al., 2021b).

4.4 Nanoparticles for siRNA and miRNA delivery for DNA Repair Mechanisms

A hyperbranched polymeric (HBP) NP was utilized by a study to develop a theranostic system. The system efficiently delivered both therapeutic agents and gene silencing tools. Bispecific antibodies were incorporated for the targeted delivery of DOX alongside siRNA. More than 80% of available sites were conjugated with siRNA for strong gene silencing, to restore drug sensitivity in MDR cancer cells. The HBP/DOX/siRNA/BsAb formulation inhibited tumor cell growth more efficiently compared to control groups. Additionally, the system inhibited mitochondrial respiration and glycolytic activity targeting the metabolic pathways of MDR cells (Y. Zhao et al., 2022)(Y. Zhao et al., 2022)(Y. Zhao et al., 2022).

Figure 2. The nanoparticles are engineered for controlled drug release, tumor specific targeting and enhanced therapeutic effects. Encapsulating the therapeutic siRNA gene for silencing of ABCB1 gene. Hence, reducing P-gp transporter expression and increasing intracellular drug retention (This picture was created using Canva.com on 1st Feb 2025)

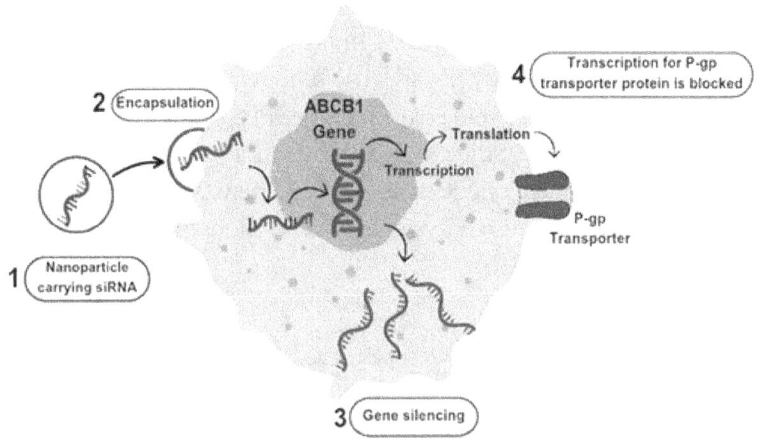

The siRNA gene is utilized to target and silence the MDR1. The siRNA is implicated in MDR to restore their sensitivity to therapy. However, the instability of siRNA inside the body and its susceptibility to nuclease degradation pose significant challenges for its clinical applications. To overcome these issues, human serum albumin (HSA) NPs are developed. Owing to their excellent biocompatibility, low immunogenicity, and natural affinity for drugs. HSA nanoparticles are modified with specific ligands, such as cetuximab, an antibody targeting the EGFR. The modification enhanced tumor-specific targeting by allowing selective binding of NPs to EGFR. The cetuximab-HSA system was loaded with DOX and siMDR1. In vitro studies indicated that it significantly enhanced cellular uptake of DOX and improved siMDR1 transfection efficiency in MCF-7/ADR cells. Furthermore, treatment with these nanoparticles resulted in a notable decrease in MDR1 mRNA levels and P-gp protein expression and restored the sensitivity of the cells to chemotherapy (Evers et al., 2022).

4.5 Stimuli Responsive NPs for Controlled Drug Release

A dual-responsive nano carrying system (HPPDC) was developed, capable of responding to pH and redox conditions. The system was characterized to promote the synergistic effects of DOX and celecoxib (CXB) in drug-resistant breast cancers. The HPPDC system demonstrated good stability *in vitro* and facilitated accelerated drug release in acidic and redox environments. In drug-resistant human breast cancer MCF-7/ADR cells, HPPDC NPs improved the cellular uptake of DOX through endocytosis, mediated by the specific binding of CD44 to hyaluronic acid. It simultaneously downregulated the expression of P-gp via COX-2 inhibition. The combination notably increased the cytotoxic as well as apoptotic effects of DOX. In MCF-7/ADR tumor-bearing nude mice, HPPDC nanoparticles exhibited tumor-targeting, enhanced chemosensitivity and reduced the expression of COX-2 and P-gp *in vivo* (Zhang et al., 2019).

Figure 3. The figure illustrates the nanoparticles developed for selective drug delivery to tumor cells overexpressing the folate receptors and HER2 receptors. The surface characteristics of nanoparticles are modified with anti-HER2 antibodies and folic acids for enhanced targeting and drug release (This picture was created using Canva.com on 1st Feb 2025)

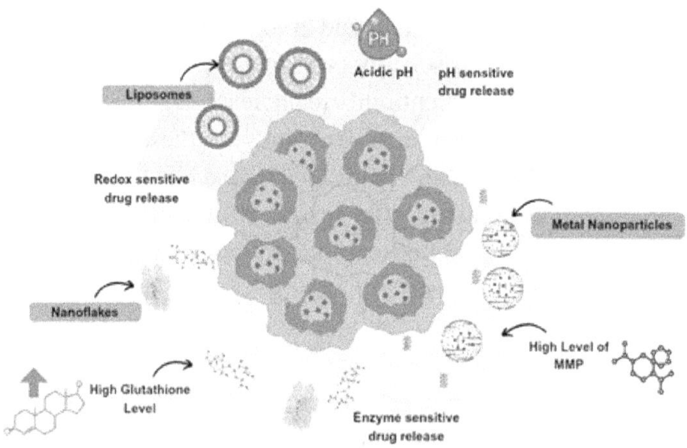

Zhou et al., 2018b study, highlighted the development of acidity-triggered ligand-presenting (ATLP) NPs to expose iRGD ligands for enhanced cellular uptake in MCF-7/ADR cells. This system dissociates in acidic microenvironments and facilitate the release of P85 and DOX through matrix metalloproteinase-2 cleavage. It inhibited P-gp and promoted tumor cell death. Additionally, NIR laser irradiation generated reactive oxygen species (ROS)in presence of Ce6 to alter gene expression and tackle drug resistance.

Han et al., 2015 designed a pH/redox-sensitive nano delivery system. They used multi-layered nanocomplexes for the sequential release of siRNA and DOX in MCF-7/ADR cell line. The outer layer encapsulated siRNA via disulfide bonds. The mesoporous silica NPs were loaded with DOX to form the core. Glutathione (GSH) triggered siRNA release in the cytoplasm, simultaneously TAT peptide recognition facilitated DOX delivery into the nucleus.

Table 2. Summarised list of nanoparticles and their mechanistic action to eliminate MDR in breast cancer using different formulations

Serial No	Nanoparticles	Delivered Drugs	Mechanism of Action	References
1.	Chitosan based polymeric nanoparticles	Curcumin + Doxorubicin	Down regulation of ABC transporters	(J. Duan et al., 2012)(J. Duan et al., 2012)(J. Duan et al., 2012)
2.	PLGA based nanoparticles	Doxorubicin+ Resveratrol	Downregulation of NF-kB and P-gp inhibition	(M. X. Zhao & Zhu, 2016) (M. X. Zhao & Zhu, 2016) (M. X. Zhao & Zhu, 2016)
3.	Liposomes	Doxorubicin + Bevacizumab	Controlled drug release	(X. Tang et al., 2017)(X. Tang et al., 2017)(X. Tang et al., 2017)
4.	Anti-EGFR	Doxorubicin	EGFR targeted uptake and retention of drug	(Mamot et al., 2023) (Mamot et al., 2023) (Mamot et al., 2023)
5.	Trastuzumab Nylon nanoparticles	Sorafenib + Nutlin-3a	pH sensitive drug delivery	(Şen et al., 2024)
6.	Biotin-PEG Polymeric nanoparticles	PTX+ MNPs+ Quantum dots	Magnetic Targeting, GSH triggered drug release	(J. Wang et al., 2016)
7.	HSA Nanoparticles	Doxorubicin + SIMDR1	EGFR targeted delivery and silences MDR1	(Evers et al., 2022)
8.	Hyperbranched polymeric nanoparticles	Doxorubicin + siRNA	Gene silencing and inhibition of metabolism	(Y. Zhao et al., 2022)

5. LIMITATIONS

Compatibility issues arise due to the complex interaction between nanoparticles, drug payloads, and the biological systems. These interactions alter the drug release kinetics, compromising therapeutic outcomes by either prematurely releasing the drug into action sites or limiting its availability (Martinelli & Biglietti, 2020b).

The nanoparticles accumulate in non-target tissues, causing off-target effects and systemic toxicities. This accumulation may trigger inflammatory responses or damage vital organs, making biocompatibility assessments essential before clinical use (Kawish et al., 2024). The scalability of manufacturing processes is challenging. Producing nanoparticles consistently at a large scale while maintaining uniform size and surface characteristics is complex. Variability in nanoparticle properties can lead to inconsistent therapeutic effects, complicating clinical applications (Hua et al., 2018).

Patient outcomes vary due to tumor heterogeneity and inter-patient variability in drug response. These differences can affect the effectiveness of nanoparticle-mediated therapies, as patients may respond differently based on genetic and phenotypic traits in their tumors (Ganesan et al., 2021b).

There is also a lack of long-term safety and efficacy data for nano-based therapies. The absence of comprehensive studies on delayed adverse effects raises concerns about potential toxicities that may not appear until after extended treatment periods (Desai, 2012; *Nanoparticle-Based Drug Delivery Systems: Advances and Challenges in Nanomedicine – Traditional Medicine*, n.d.). Research must focus to optimize nanoparticle design, improve targeting strategies, and address these challenges before widespread clinical adopt

6. FUTURE PERSPECTIVES

Nanoparticles have substantially grown as the solution for ever-evolving breast cancer disease. However, nanotechnology is constantly evolving to meet the multi-dimensional challenges of the breast cancer hazard. Future advancements in the use of NPs to overcome MDR involve the exploration of innovative strategies and systems. These systems should aim to improve the efficacy, specificity and clinical applicability of NPs.

A key area in the development of the targeting strategies is the administration of dual or multi-targeting approaches. While current NPs utilize single targeting ligands, this will allow the advanced systems to address tumor heterogeneity and improve specificity. NPs can be engineered with ligands for both HER2 and EGFR, for targeting multiple pathways simultaneously.

Current research has shown the efficacy of NPs to allow stimuli-responsive controlled release of the therapeutic payload. The exploration and better understanding of the Tumor Microenvironment (TME) will allow the exploitation of hypoxia, overexpressed enzyme-triggered drug release, specifically in MDR cell lines. This will ensure precise and accurate drug release minimizing off-target unloading.

Integrating genetic and epigenetic modulations with NP-based therapies will enable the repair of defective DNA mechanisms. Future NPs can incorporate CRISPR/Cas9 and similar systems to eliminate MDR-related challenges. Research should focus on the potential delivery of epigenetic modulators, such as HDAC inhibitors or DNA methyltransferase inhibitors. This can possibly allow the reversal of epigenetic changes related to drug resistance. The future holds potential for personalized nanoparticle-based medicines. NPs can potentially be tailored to individual patient profiles. It can be based on tumor genetics, biomarker expression and specific drug resistance mechanisms.

Research can potentially focus on the combination of immune checkpoint inhibitors with NPs, particularly for multi drug-resistant breast cancers. Nano vaccines that deliver tumor-specific antigens to trigger immune response can be developed. NPs can be engineered to modulate TME and enhance the activity of immune cells and overcome evasion in MDR tumors. The application of artificial intelligence (AI) can optimize the design and architecture of NPs. AI tools can be utilized to assess the optimal properties such as size, charge and drug release profiles of NPs for MDR mechanisms.

7. CONCLUSION

Drug efflux, active DNA repair mechanisms, impaired apoptosis and tumor-supportive signaling pathways are some of the multifaceted mechanisms of MDR in BC. Nanoparticles have flexible designs and drug loading for targeted drug delivery, prolonged circulation of the drugs *in vitro* and *in vivo*. The systems employ a variety of strategies to evade the molecular mechanisms driving multidrug resistance. One of the primary approaches is bypassing drug efflux pumps, such as P-glycoprotein (P-gp), MRP-1, and BCRP, which are overexpressed in resistant cancer cells. NPs like chitosan-based polymeric nanoparticles and PLGA-modified NPs encapsulate both chemotherapeutic agents DOX, CUR and efflux pump inhibitors such as resveratrol, tetrandrine. They NPs favoured controlled drug release and increased intracellular drug retention. These systems downregulated ABC transporters and inhibit NF-κB signaling, to block drug efflux and develop apoptosis in resistant cells.

NPs are functionalized with ligands such HER2 antibodies, EGFR-targeting fragments to bind to the overexpressed receptors on cancer cells. The NPs precisely delivered the drug and improved cellular uptake, as seen by immunoliposomes and anti-EGFR-ILs. Targeted NPs passively target by exploiting the EPR effect, to accumulate in tumor tissues. MSNPs and polymeric micelles were characterized with co-delivery of agents. The NPs efficiently co-encapsulated DOX, PTX with MDR-reversing agents P-gp siRNA and autophagy inhibitors. The synergy inhibited drug efflux, downregulated survival pathways and induced apoptosis among breast tumor cell lines.

Stimuli-responsive NPs reversed MDR by releasing therapeutic payloads in response to TME based triggers such as redox potential, acidic pH, or enzymatic activity. Systems like HA-MIL-125@DVMA NPs released drugs in acidic TME. Likewise, light-responsive NPs disassembled upon irradiation for controlled and targeted drug release. Several NPs facilitate gene and miRNA delivery for the silencing of MDR-related genes such as MDR1 and restore drug sensitivity. HAS NPs and hyperbranched polymeric NPs deliver siRNA synergistically with chemotherapeutics to downregulate P-gp and enhance intracellular drug accumulation.

REFERENCES

Abd-Ellatef, G. E. F., Gazzano, E., Chirio, D., Hamed, A. R., Belisario, D. C., Zuddas, C., Peira, E., Rolando, B., Kopecka, J., Marie, M. A. S., Sapino, S., Fahmy, S. R., Gallarate, M., Abdel-Hamid, A. H. Z., & Riganti, C. (2020). Curcumin-Loaded Solid Lipid Nanoparticles Bypass P-Glycoprotein Mediated Doxorubicin Resistance in Triple Negative Breast Cancer Cells. *Pharmaceutics 2020, Vol. 12, Page 96, 12*(2), 96. DOI: 10.3390/pharmaceutics12020096

Alfreahat, I., Nsairat, H., Aldeeb, I. D., Al-Samydai, A., & Alshaer, W. (2025). In Vitro Potentiation of Doxorubicin Cytotoxicity Utilizing Clarithromycin Loaded-PEGylated Liposomes. *Technology in Cancer Research & Treatment, 24*, 15330338241312560. DOI: 10.1177/15330338241312561 PMID: 39865928

Alven, S., & Aderibigbe, B. A. (2020). The Therapeutic Efficacy of Dendrimer and Micelle Formulations for Breast Cancer Treatment. *Pharmaceutics, 12*(12), 1212. DOI: 10.3390/pharmaceutics12121212 PMID: 33333778

Aravindan, A., Gupta, A., Moorkoth, S., & Dhas, N. (2024). Implications of nanotherapeutic advancements to leverage multi-drug resistant breast cancer: The state-of-the-art review. *Journal of Drug Delivery Science and Technology, 100*, 106007. DOI: 10.1016/j.jddst.2024.106007

Attia, M. F., Anton, N., Wallyn, J., Omran, Z., & Vandamme, T. F. (2019). An overview of active and passive targeting strategies to improve the nanocarriers efficiency to tumour sites. *The Journal of Pharmacy and Pharmacology, 71*(8), 1185–1198. DOI: 10.1111/jphp.13098 PMID: 31049986

Bhattacharjee, S. (2022). Craft of Co-encapsulation in Nanomedicine: A Struggle To Achieve Synergy through Reciprocity. *ACS Pharmacology & Translational Science, 5*(5), 278–298. DOI: 10.1021/acsptsci.2c00033 PMID: 35592431

Brown, L. J., Achinger-Kawecka, J., Portman, N., Clark, S., Stirzaker, C., & Lim, E. (2022). Epigenetic Therapies and Biomarkers in Breast Cancer. *Cancers (Basel), 14*(3), 474. DOI: 10.3390/cancers14030474 PMID: 35158742

Chang, D., Ma, Y., Xu, X., Xie, J., & Ju, S. (2021). Stimuli-Responsive Polymeric Nanoplatforms for Cancer Therapy. *Frontiers in Bioengineering and Biotechnology, 9*, 707319. DOI: 10.3389/fbioe.2021.707319 PMID: 34249894

Dastidar, D. G., Ghosh, D., & Das, A. (2022). Recent developments in nanocarriers for cancer chemotherapy. *OpenNano, 8*, 100080. DOI: 10.1016/j.onano.2022.100080

Desai, N. (2012). Challenges in Development of Nanoparticle-Based Therapeutics. *The AAPS Journal*, *14*(2), 282–295. DOI: 10.1208/s12248-012-9339-4 PMID: 22407288

Dian, C., Qian, Z., Ran, M., Yan, X., & Dian, L. (2024). Co-Delivery of Docetaxel and Curcumin Functionalized Mixed Micelles for the Treatment of Drug-Resistant Breast Cancer by Oral Administration. *International Journal of Nanomedicine*, *19*, 8603–8620. DOI: 10.2147/IJN.S472445 PMID: 39188859

Dong, Y., Liao, H., Yu, J., Fu, H., Zhao, D., Gong, K., Wang, Q., & Duan, Y. (2019). Incorporation of drug efflux inhibitor and chemotherapeutic agent into an inorganic/organic platform for the effective treatment of multidrug resistant breast cancer. *Journal of Nanobiotechnology*, *17*(1), 1–15. DOI: 10.1186/s12951-019-0559-y PMID: 31870362

Duan, C., Yu, M., Xu, J., Li, B. Y., Zhao, Y., & Kankala, R. K. (2023). Overcoming Cancer Multi-drug Resistance (MDR): Reasons, mechanisms, nanotherapeutic solutions, and challenges. *Biomedicine and Pharmacotherapy*, *162*, 114643. DOI: 10.1016/j.biopha.2023.114643 PMID: 37031496

Duan, J., Mansour, H. M., Zhang, Y., Deng, X., Chen, Y., Wang, J., Pan, Y., & Zhao, J. (2012). Reversion of multidrug resistance by co-encapsulation of doxorubicin and curcumin in chitosan/poly(butyl cyanoacrylate) nanoparticles. *International Journal of Pharmaceutics*, *426*(1–2), 193–201. DOI: 10.1016/j.ijpharm.2012.01.020 PMID: 22274587

Emran, T., Shahriar, A., Mahmud, A. R., Rahman, T., Abir, M. H., Siddiquee, M. F.-R., Ahmed, H., Rahman, N., Nainu, F., Wahyudin, E., Mitra, S., Dhama, K., Habiballah, M. M., Haque, S., Islam, A., & Hassan, M. M. (2022). Multidrug Resistance in Cancer: Understanding Molecular Mechanisms, Immunoprevention and Therapeutic Approaches. *Frontiers in Oncology*, *12*, 891652. DOI: 10.3389/fonc.2022.891652 PMID: 35814435

Evers, M. J. W., van de Wakker, S. I., de Groot, E. M., de Jong, O. G., Gitz-François, J. J. J., Seinen, C. S., Sluijter, J. P. G., Schiffelers, R. M., & Vader, P. (2022). Functional siRNA Delivery by Extracellular Vesicle-Liposome Hybrid Nanoparticles. *Advanced Healthcare Materials*, *11*(5), 2101202. Advance online publication. DOI: 10.1002/adhm.202101202 PMID: 34382360

Ganesan, K., Wang, Y., Gao, F., Liu, Q., Zhang, C., Li, P., Zhang, J., & Chen, J. (2021a). Targeting Engineered Nanoparticles for Breast Cancer Therapy. *Pharmaceutics*, *13*(11), 1829. DOI: 10.3390/pharmaceutics13111829 PMID: 34834243

Ganesan, K., Wang, Y., Gao, F., Liu, Q., Zhang, C., Li, P., Zhang, J., & Chen, J. (2021b). Targeting Engineered Nanoparticles for Breast Cancer Therapy. *Pharmaceutics, 13*(11), 1829. DOI: 10.3390/pharmaceutics13111829 PMID: 34834243

Gao, L., Meng, F., Yang, Z., Lafuente-Merchan, M., Fernández, L. M., Cao, Y., Kusamori, K., Nishikawa, M., Itakura, S., Chen, J., Huang, X., Ouyang, D., Riester, O., Deigner, H. P., Lai, H., Pedraz, J. L., Ramalingam, M., & Cai, Y. (2024a). Nano-drug delivery system for the treatment of multidrug-resistant breast cancer: Current status and future perspectives. *Biomedicine and Pharmacotherapy, 179*, 117327. DOI: 10.1016/j.biopha.2024.117327 PMID: 39216449

Gao, L., Meng, F., Yang, Z., Lafuente-Merchan, M., Fernández, L. M., Cao, Y., Kusamori, K., Nishikawa, M., Itakura, S., Chen, J., Huang, X., Ouyang, D., Riester, O., Deigner, H. P., Lai, H., Pedraz, J. L., Ramalingam, M., & Cai, Y. (2024b). Nano-drug delivery system for the treatment of multidrug-resistant breast cancer: Current status and future perspectives. *Biomedicine and Pharmacotherapy, 179*, 117327. DOI: 10.1016/j.biopha.2024.117327 PMID: 39216449

Gote, V., Nookala, A. R., Bolla, P. K., & Pal, D. (2021). Drug Resistance in Metastatic Breast Cancer: Tumor Targeted Nanomedicine to the Rescue. *International Journal of Molecular Sciences 2021, Vol. 22, Page 4673, 22*(9), 4673. DOI: 10.3390/ijms22094673

Gu, H., Meng, F., Sun, H., Yang, L., Li, Q., Chen, Z., Cai, T., Yang, Z., & Cai, Y. (2024). Polymer lipid hybrid nanoparticles encapsulated with Emodin combined with DOX reverse multidrug resistance of breast cancer via IL-6/JAK2/STAT3 signaling pathway. *Cancer Nanotechnology, 15*(1), 1–21. DOI: 10.1186/s12645-023-00237-z

Guo, Q., Li, J., Mao, J., Chen, W., Yang, M., Yang, Y., Hua, Y., & Qiu, L. (2023). Hollow MIL-125 Nanoparticles Loading Doxorubicin Prodrug and 3-Methyladenine for Reversal of Tumor Multidrug Resistance. *Journal of Functional Biomaterials 2023, Vol. 14, Page 546, 14*(11), 546. DOI: 10.3390/jfb14110546

Guo, S., Lv, L., Shen, Y., Hu, Z., He, Q., & Chen, X. (2016). A nanoparticulate pre-chemosensitizer for efficacious chemotherapy of multidrug resistant breast cancer. *Scientific Reports 2016 6:1, 6*(1), 1–11. DOI: 10.1038/srep21459

Hamad, I., Harb, A. A., & Bustanji, Y. (2024). Liposome-Based Drug Delivery Systems in Cancer Research: An Analysis of Global Landscape Efforts and Achievements. *Pharmaceutics 2024, Vol. 16, Page 400, 16*(3), 400. DOI: 10.3390/pharmaceutics16030400

Han, L., Tang, C., & Yin, C. (2015). Dual-targeting and pH/redox-responsive multi-layered nanocomplexes for smart co-delivery of doxorubicin and siRNA. *Biomaterials*, *60*, 42–52. DOI: 10.1016/j.biomaterials.2015.05.001 PMID: 25982552

Hheidari, A., Mohammadi, J., Ghodousi, M., Mahmoodi, M., Ebrahimi, S., Pishbin, E., & Rahdar, A. (2024). Metal-based nanoparticle in cancer treatment: Lessons learned and challenges. *Frontiers in Bioengineering and Biotechnology*, *12*, 1436297. DOI: 10.3389/fbioe.2024.1436297 PMID: 39055339

Hobbs, E. A., Litton, J. K., & Yap, T. A. (2021). Development of the PARP inhibitor talazoparib for the treatment of advanced BRCA1 and BRCA2 mutated breast cancer. *Expert Opinion on Pharmacotherapy*, *22*(14), 1825–1837. DOI: 10.1080/14656566.2021.1952181 PMID: 34309473

Hua, S., de Matos, M. B. C., Metselaar, J. M., & Storm, G. (2018). Current trends and challenges in the clinical translation of nanoparticulate nanomedicines: Pathways for translational development and commercialization. *Frontiers in Pharmacology*, *9*(JUL), 403086. DOI: 10.3389/fphar.2018.00790 PMID: 30065653

Kawish, S. M., Sharma, S., Gupta, P., Ahmad, F. J., Iqbal, M., Alshabrmi, F. M., Anwer, M. K., Fathi-karkan, S., Rahdar, A., & Aboudzadeh, M. A. (2024). Nanoparticle-Based Drug Delivery Platform for Simultaneous Administration of Phytochemicals and Chemotherapeutics: Emerging Trends in Cancer Management. *Particle & Particle Systems Characterization*, *41*(12), 2400049. DOI: 10.1002/ppsc.202400049

Kazeminava, F., Javanbakht, S., Latifi, Z., Rasoulzadehzali, M., Abbaszadeh, M., Alimohammadzadeh, B., Mahdipour, M., Fattahi, A., Hamishehkar, H., Adibag, Z., & Nouri, M. (2024). Ultrasound-assisted encapsulating folic acid-based carbon quantum dots within breast cancer cell-derived exosomes as a co-receptors-mediated anticancer nanocarrier for enhanced breast cancer therapy. *Scientific Reports 2024 14:1*, *14*(1), 1–12. DOI: 10.1038/s41598-024-67934-6

Khursheed, R., Dua, K., Vishwas, S., Gulati, M., Jha, N. K., Aldhafeeri, G. M., Alanazi, F. G., Goh, B. H., Gupta, G., Paudel, K. R., Hansbro, P. M., Chellappan, D. K., & Singh, S. K. (2022). Biomedical applications of metallic nanoparticles in cancer: Current status and future perspectives. *Biomedicine and Pharmacotherapy*, *150*, 112951. DOI: 10.1016/j.biopha.2022.112951 PMID: 35447546

Kinnel, B., Singh, S. K., Oprea-Ilies, G., & Singh, R. (2023). Targeted Therapy and Mechanisms of Drug Resistance in Breast Cancer. *Cancers (Basel)*, *15*(4), 1320. DOI: 10.3390/cancers15041320 PMID: 36831661

Lai, Y., Pang, S., Li, C., Song, J., Wang, M., Chen, M., & Ren, X. (2025). Breast cancer-targeted therapy and doxorubicin multidrug resistance are reversed via macrophage membrane-camouflaged liposomes. *Colloids and Surfaces. B, Biointerfaces, 245*, 114310. DOI: 10.1016/j.colsurfb.2024.114310 PMID: 39405948

Lan, H., Jamil, M., Ke, G., & Dong, N. (2023). The role of nanoparticles and nanomaterials in cancer diagnosis and treatment: A comprehensive review. *American Journal of Cancer Research, 13*(12), 5751. https://pmc.ncbi.nlm.nih.gov/articles/PMC10767363/ PMID: 38187049

Li, X., Peng, X., Zoulikha, M., Boafo, G. F., Magar, K. T., Ju, Y., & He, W. (2024). Multifunctional nanoparticle-mediated combining therapy for human diseases. *Signal Transduction and Targeted Therapy 2023 9:1, 9*(1), 1–33. DOI: 10.1038/s41392-023-01668-1

Mamot, C., Wicki, A., Hasler-Strub, U., Riniker, S., Li, Q., Holer, L., Bärtschi, D., Zaman, K., von Moos, R., Dedes, K. J., Boos, L. A., Novak, U., Bodmer, A., Ritschard, R., Obermann, E. C., Tzankov, A., Ackermann, C., Membrez-Antonioli, V., Zürrer-Härdi, U., … Rochlitz, C. (2023). A multicenter phase II trial of anti-EGFR-immunoliposomes loaded with doxorubicin in patients with advanced triple negative breast cancer. *Scientific Reports 2023 13:1, 13*(1), 1–9. DOI: 10.1038/s41598-023-30950-z

Martinelli, C., & Biglietti, M. (2020a). Nanotechnological approaches for counteracting multidrug resistance in cancer. *Cancer Drug Resistance (Alhambra, Calif.), 3*(4), 1003. DOI: 10.20517/cdr.2020.47 PMID: 35582219

Martinelli, C., & Biglietti, M. (2020b). Nanotechnological approaches for counteracting multidrug resistance in cancer. *Cancer Drug Resistance (Alhambra, Calif.), 3*(4), 1003. DOI: 10.20517/cdr.2020.47 PMID: 35582219

Mba, I. E., & Nweze, E. I. (2021). Nanoparticles as therapeutic options for treating multidrug-resistant bacteria: Research progress, challenges, and prospects. *World Journal of Microbiology & Biotechnology, 37*(6), 1–30. DOI: 10.1007/s11274-021-03070-x PMID: 34046779

Mechanism of multidrug resistance to chemotherapy mediated by P-glycoprotein (Review). (n.d.). Retrieved February 1, 2025, from https://www.spandidos-publications.com/10.3892/ijo.2023.5567

Meng, Y. Q., Shi, Y. N., Zhu, Y. P., Liu, Y. Q., Gu, L. W., Liu, D. D., Ma, A., Xia, F., Guo, Q. Y., Xu, C. C., Zhang, J. Z., Qiu, C., & Wang, J. G. (2024). Recent trends in preparation and biomedical applications of iron oxide nanoparticles. *Journal of Nanobiotechnology, 22*(1), 24. DOI: 10.1186/s12951-023-02235-0 PMID: 38191388

Mo, K., Kim, A., Choe, S., Shin, M., & Yoon, H. (2023). Overview of Solid Lipid Nanoparticles in Breast Cancer Therapy. *Pharmaceutics, 15*(8), 2065. DOI: 10.3390/pharmaceutics15082065 PMID: 37631279

Nanoparticle-Based Drug Delivery Systems: Advances and Challenges in Nanomedicine – Traditional medicine. (n.d.). Retrieved March 30, 2025, from https://traditionalmedicine.actabotanica.org/nanoparticle-based-drug-delivery-systems-advances-and-challenges-in-nanomedicine/

Neophytou, C. M., Trougakos, I. P., Erin, N., & Papageorgis, P. (2021). Apoptosis Deregulation and the Development of Cancer Multi-Drug Resistance. *Cancers (Basel), 13*(17), 4363. DOI: 10.3390/cancers13174363 PMID: 34503172

Pavitra, E., Kancharla, J., Gupta, V. K., Prasad, K., Sung, J. Y., Kim, J., Tej, M. B., Choi, R., Lee, J. H., Han, Y. K., Raju, G. S. R., Bhaskar, L. V. K. S., & Huh, Y. S. (2023). The role of NF-κB in breast cancer initiation, growth, metastasis, and resistance to chemotherapy. *Biomedicine and Pharmacotherapy, 163*, 114822. DOI: 10.1016/j.biopha.2023.114822 PMID: 37146418

Raheem, M. A., Rahim, M. A., Gul, I., Zhong, X., Xiao, C., Zhang, H., Wei, J., He, Q., Hassan, M., Zhang, C. Y., Yu, D., Pandey, V., Du, K., Wang, R., Han, S., Han, Y., & Qin, P. (2023). Advances in nanoparticles-based approaches in cancer theranostics. *OpenNano, 12*, 100152. DOI: 10.1016/j.onano.2023.100152

Salari, N., Faraji, F., Torghabeh, F. M., Faraji, F., Mansouri, K., Abam, F., Shohaimi, S., Akbari, H., & Mohammadi, M. (2022). Polymer-based drug delivery systems for anticancer drugs: A systematic review. *Cancer Treatment and Research Communications, 32*, 100605. DOI: 10.1016/j.ctarc.2022.100605 PMID: 35816909

Şen, Ö., Armanetti, P., Carmignani, A., Catalano, F., Pugliese, G., Menichetti, L., & Ciofani, G. (2024). Photoacoustic features of nylon-11 nanoparticles for breast cancer imaging, and their modification with trastuzumab, sorafenib, and nutlin-3a for theranostic applications. *Nano Trends, 7*, 100047. DOI: 10.1016/j.nwnano.2024.100047

Tang, X., Loc, W. S., Dong, C., Matters, G. L., Butler, P. J., Kester, M., Meyers, C., Jiang, Y., & Adair, J. H. (2017). The use of nanoparticulates to treat breast cancer. *Nanomedicine (London), 12*(19), 2367–2388. DOI: 10.2217/nnm-2017-0202 PMID: 28868970

Tang, Y., Soroush, F., Tong, Z., Kiani, M. F., & Wang, B. (2017). Targeted multidrug delivery system to overcome chemoresistance in breast cancer. *International Journal of Nanomedicine, 12*, 671–681. DOI: 10.2147/IJN.S124770 PMID: 28176940

Wang, H., Guo, M., Wei, H., & Chen, Y. (2021). Targeting MCL-1 in cancer: Current status and perspectives. *Journal of Hematology & Oncology*, *14*(1), 67. DOI: 10.1186/s13045-021-01079-1 PMID: 33883020

Wang, J., Wang, F., Li, F., Zhang, W., Shen, Y., Zhou, D., & Guo, S. (2016). A multifunctional poly(curcumin) nanomedicine for dual-modal targeted delivery, intracellular responsive release, dual-drug treatment and imaging of multidrug resistant cancer cells. *Journal of Materials Chemistry. B*, *4*(17), 2954–2962. DOI: 10.1039/C5TB02450A PMID: 27152196

Wei, X., Song, M., Li, W., Huang, J., Yang, G., & Wang, Y. (2021a). Multifunctional nanoplatforms co-delivering combinatorial dual-drug for eliminating cancer multidrug resistance. *Theranostics*, *11*(13), 6334–6354. DOI: 10.7150/thno.59342 PMID: 33995661

Wei, X., Song, M., Li, W., Huang, J., Yang, G., & Wang, Y. (2021b). Multifunctional nanoplatforms co-delivering combinatorial dual-drug for eliminating cancer multidrug resistance. *Theranostics*, *11*(13), 6334–6354. DOI: 10.7150/thno.59342 PMID: 33995661

Wind, N. S., & Holen, I. (2011). Multidrug Resistance in Breast Cancer: From In Vitro Models to Clinical Studies. *International Journal of Breast Cancer*, *967419*, 1–12. Advance online publication. DOI: 10.4061/2011/967419 PMID: 22332018

Xiao, B., Ma, L., & Merlin, D. (2016). Nanoparticle-mediated co-delivery of chemotherapeutic agent and siRNA for combination cancer therapy. *Expert Opinion on Drug Delivery*, *14*(1), 65–73. DOI: 10.1080/17425247.2016.1205583 PMID: 27337289

Xue, X., & Liang, X. J. (2012). Overcoming drug efflux-based multidrug resistance in cancer with nanotechnology. *Chinese Journal of Cancer*, *31*(2), 100–109. DOI: 10.5732/cjc.011.10326 PMID: 22237039

Xue, X., & Liang, X. J. (n.d.). *Chinese A nti Cancer A ssociation CACA*. DOI: 10.5732/cjc.011.10326

Yadav, P., Ambudkar, S. V., & Rajendra Prasad, N. (2022). Emerging nanotechnology-based therapeutics to combat multidrug-resistant cancer. *Journal of Nanobiotechnology 2022 20:1, 20*(1), 1–35. DOI: 10.1186/s12951-022-01626-z

Zhang, S., Guo, N., Wan, G., Zhang, T., Li, C., Wang, Y., Wang, Y., & Liu, Y. (2019). PH and redox dual-responsive nanoparticles based on disulfide-containing poly(β-amino ester) for combining chemotherapy and COX-2 inhibitor to overcome drug resistance in breast cancer. *Journal of Nanobiotechnology*, *17*(1), 1–17. DOI: 10.1186/s12951-019-0540-9 PMID: 31623608

Zhao, M. X., & Zhu, B. J. (2016). The Research and Applications of Quantum Dots as Nano-Carriers for Targeted Drug Delivery and Cancer Therapy. *Nanoscale Research Letters*, *11*(1), 1–9. DOI: 10.1186/s11671-016-1394-9 PMID: 27090658

Zhao, Y., Huan, M. L., Liu, M., Cheng, Y., Sun, Y., Cui, H., Liu, D. Z., Mei, Q. B., & Zhou, S. Y. (2016). Doxorubicin and resveratrol co-delivery nanoparticle to overcome doxorubicin resistance. *Scientific Reports*, *6*(1), 35267. DOI: 10.1038/srep35267 PMID: 27731405

Zhao, Y., Liu, T., Ardana, A., Fletcher, N. L., Houston, Z. H., Blakey, I., & Thurecht, K. J. (2022). Investigation of a Dual siRNA/Chemotherapy Delivery System for Breast Cancer Therapy. *ACS Omega*, *7*(20), 17119–17127. DOI: 10.1021/acsomega.2c00620 PMID: 35647423

Zhou, L., Wang, H., & Li, Y. (2018a). Stimuli-Responsive Nanomedicines for Overcoming Cancer Multidrug Resistance. *Theranostics*, *8*(4), 1059–1074. DOI: 10.7150/thno.22679 PMID: 29463999

Zhou, L., Wang, H., & Li, Y. (2018b). Stimuli-Responsive Nanomedicines for Overcoming Cancer Multidrug Resistance. *Theranostics*, *8*(4), 1059–1074. DOI: 10.7150/thno.22679 PMID: 29463999

Chapter 13
Life Cycle Assessment of Biocomposites:
Environmental Impacts and Sustainability Perspectives

Sunandani Chandel
https://orcid.org/0000-0002-7194-4063
Kerala Agricultural University, Thrissur, India

Ashline Shaji
https://orcid.org/0009-0001-2293-5806
Kerala Agricultural University, Thrissur, India

Mahesh Chutturi
https://orcid.org/0009-0009-3201-5825
Kerala Agricultural University, Thrissur, India

Adithya Raj U
https://orcid.org/0009-0003-6686-6149
Kerala Agricultural University, Thrissur, India

ABSTRACT

The growing global emphasis on sustainability and the circular economy has highlighted the potential of biocomposites as environmental friendly alternatives to traditional materials. This chapter explores the application of Life Cycle Assessment (LCA) to evaluate the environmental performance of biocomposites, focusing on various system boundary scenarios and their impact on ecological footprints. By systematically analyzing the environmental consequences of biocomposites at different stages of their life cycle, the chapter offers valuable insights into their sustainability potential. It discusses key challenges and methodological considerations in conducting LCA,

DOI: 10.4018/979-8-3373-1305-4.ch013

while also highlighting the role of LCA in guiding sustainable material design and policy-making. Case studies are presented to demonstrate practical applications and comparative analyses of biocomposites versus conventional materials. The chapter concludes with recommendations for optimizing biocomposite processes and informed material selection to improve their sustainability.

1. INTRODUCTION

The increasing environmental concerns associated with synthetic composites have driven the transition toward sustainable materials. Biocomposites, which incorporate natural fibers and bio-based polymers, have emerged as a viable alternative, offering reduced dependence on fossil-based materials, lower greenhouse gas emissions, and improved biodegradability (Table 1) (Pecas et al., 2018; Shanmugam et al., 2022). These materials have gained significant attention in various industries, including automotive, packaging, and healthcare, where sustainability and performance must be balanced. However, the true environmental impact of biocomposites extends beyond their composition and requires a holistic assessment of their entire life cycle, from raw material extraction to end-of-life disposal.

Life Cycle Assessment (LCA) has become an essential tool in evaluating the environmental performance of biocomposites. Originating in the 1960s and formalized through the ISO 14040 standards in the 1990s, LCA provides a systematic framework to assess environmental impacts such as carbon footprint, water consumption, land use, and energy demands. Early applications of LCA in biocomposites primarily focused on comparing their carbon footprint with petroleum-based composites (Rebitzer et al., 2004). However, with increasing emphasis on sustainability, modern LCA studies now integrate broader indicators, including material circularity, recyclability, and waste reduction strategies (Korol et al., 2016).

The application of LCA in biocomposite research and industry is crucial for sustainable product development. By adopting different system boundaries, such as cradle-to-gate, cradle-to-grave, or cradle-to-cradle, LCA enables industries to quantify the trade-offs between sustainability benefits and potential drawbacks, such as agricultural land use and energy-intensive processing (Ahmad et al., 2022). Furthermore, regulatory frameworks such as the EU Green Deal, Environmental Product Declarations (EPDs), and ISO certifications increasingly mandate LCA-based sustainability assessments for material compliance (Coltelli et al., 2023).

As biocomposites continue to evolve, LCA plays a pivotal role in optimizing production processes, minimizing waste, and enhancing product design to align with circular economy principles (Meng et al., 2018). Despite growing interest in biocomposites, their environmental trade-offs remain underexplored. A systematic

LCA is crucial to quantify the real sustainability advantages over synthetic alternatives. This chapter explores the integration of LCA in biocomposite research and industry, examining its methodologies, applications, and implications for sustainable materials development. By understanding the full life cycle impact of biocomposites, researchers, policymakers, and manufacturers can make informed decisions to advance sustainable material solutions.

Table 1. Comparative energy and environmental performance of different composites

Composite	ER (MJ/kg)	GWP (kg CO_2-eq)	GGE (kg CO_2-eq/kg)	Reference
Carbon Composite				
Polyacrylonitrile (PAN)/Epoxy	1100 (MJ)	~54	N.D.	Ramachandran et al. (2023)
Carbon fiber/Epoxy	N.D.	7.84	N.D.	Watjanatepin et al. (2023)
Glass fiber/Epoxy	N.D.	3.55	N.D.	Watjanatepin et al. (2023)
Glass fiber/PP	70	N.D.	3.76 (kg CO_2 eq.)	Toffe et al. (2019)
Triaxial glass fiber/Epoxy	82.04	N.D.	4.42 (kg CO_2 eq.)	Toffe et al. (2019)
Biocomposites				
Sugarcane bagasse/Bio -epoxy	~178 (MJ)	~30.93	N.D.	Ramachandran and Gnanasagaran (2024)
Sugarcane bagasse/Bio- PE	N.D.	3.01 (kgCO_2/kg)	1.81	Nagy et al. (2020)
Wood fiber/PLA + TPS	65 (MJ)	N.D.	N.D.	Mahalle et al. (2014)
Wood fiber/PLA	78 (MJ)	N.D.	N.D.	Mahalle et al. (2014)
Flax/PLA	15	N.D.	2.02 (kg CO_2 eq.)	Toffe et al. (2019)
Hemp/PLA	N.D.	1.72 (kgCO_2/kg)	N.D.	Seile et al. (2022)
Sprinula bioplastic	3.83	1.99	N.D.	Chalermthai et al. (2024)
Cyanobacterial bioplastic	8.6	N.D.	N.D.	Rueda et al. (2023)
Scenedesmus acutus (UTEX B72) bioplastic	N.D.	0.656	N.D.	Beckstrom et al. (2020)
Aramid nanofiber/PEGDA	N.D.	2.33	N.D.	Tajurahim et al. (2025)

(ER- Energy Requirement; GWP- Global Warming Potential; GGE- Greenhouse Gas Emissions; PE- Polyethylene; PEGDA- polyethylene glycol diacrylate; PLA- Polylactic acid; PP- Polypropylene; TPS- Thermoplastic starch; N.D.- Not determined)

2. ENVIRONMENTAL LCA FOR BIOCOMPOSITES

Despite the environmental benefits of biocomposites, their sustainability is influenced by various factors, including raw material sourcing, energy-intensive processing, durability, and end-of-life cycle disposal. Thus, systematic evaluation of their environmental performance can be assessed through Life Cycle Assessment (LCA). It has become an essential tool in material sustainability analysis. The LCA consists of three important phases (Figure 1):

Figure 1. Different stages of environmental LCA of biocomposites

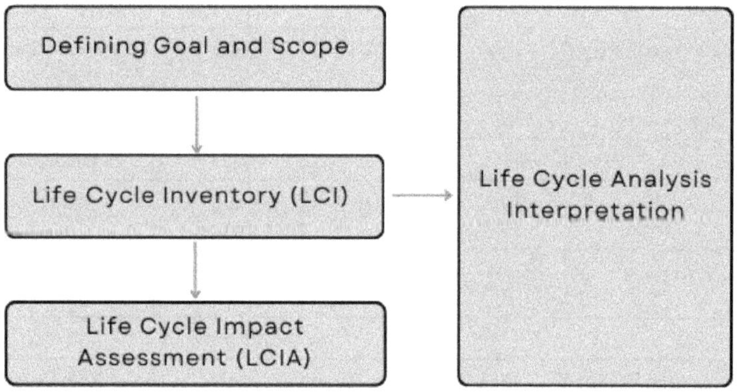

2.1 Life Cycle Assessment

I) **Defining Goal and Scope**

The first phase of LCA involves setting clear objectives and defining the study boundaries. The goal definition and scoping phase of LCA is a crucial step that defines the objectives and methodology for incorporating environmental impacts throughout a product's life cycle into decision-making processes. During this phase, it is essential to determine several key aspects: first, the type of information required to inform and enhance decision-making; second, the level of accuracy needed in the results to ensure they are valuable; and third, how the results should be interpreted and presented to make them both meaningful and actionable (Hauschild et al., 2018). At the beginning of the LCA process following key decisions are made:

System Boundary

The first fundamental concept of LCA is the life cycle perspective, which involves defining system boundaries that encompass all phases of a product's existence from raw material extraction (cradle) to manufacturing, distribution, use, and end-of-life disposal (grave). In the case of biocomposites, the system boundary can vary depending on the scope of the assessment (Figure 2):

- **Cradle to Gate**: This approach includes raw material extraction, processing, and manufacturing but excludes the product's use and end-of-life stages.
- **Cradle to Grave**: This comprehensive approach encompasses the entire life cycle, from raw material extraction, processing, manufacturing, and transportation to the use phase and end-of-life management (e.g., recycling, disposal, or energy recovery).
- **Gate to Gate**: This method focuses on a specific stage within the production process, such as fiber extraction, composite manufacturing, or processing. It is often used to assess improvements within a particular phase of biocomposite production.
- **Well to wheel**: This method is often used for biocomposites used in the transportation industry. It focuses on the entire life cycle, from raw material extraction, processing, manufacturing, and transportation to its use in vehicles and end-of-life management (e.g., recycling, disposal, or energy recovery).

Figure 2. Different stages of LCA for biocomposites based on system boundary

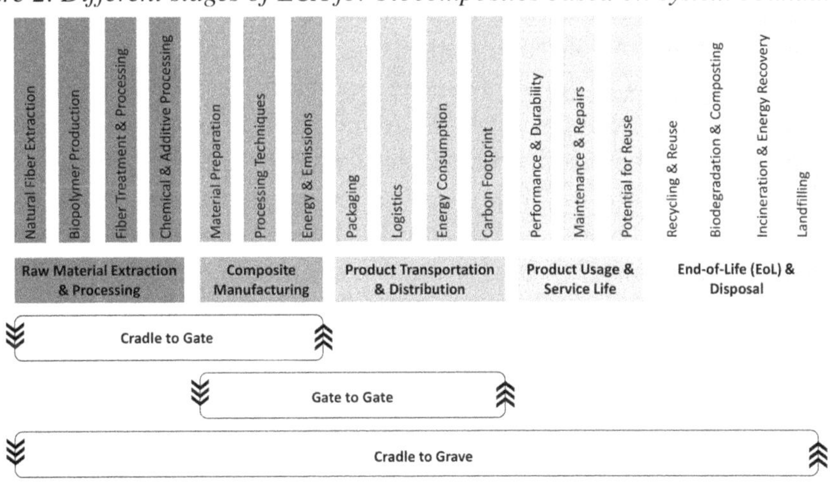

Functional Unit

The functional unit (FU) is critical for enabling accurate and meaningful comparisons across different materials, processes, or product systems. It serves as the basis for assessing environmental impacts by concentrating on the purpose of the product rather than just its volume or dimensions. This is particularly important in the case of biocomposites, where the mechanical properties and durability may differ significantly from those of conventional composites. For instance, comparing 1 kg of a biocomposite to 1 kg of a synthetic composite may be misleading if their mechanical characteristics are not aligned. Instead, defining the FU in terms of functional performance, such as tensile strength per unit weight or longevity, ensures a fair comparison. Additionally, poorly defined FUs can lead to inaccurate conclusions. For example, if a biocomposite has a shorter lifespan than a traditional material, measuring its impact per kilogram rather than over its entire lifespan could exaggerate its sustainability. Common functional units used in biocomposite LCA include per kilogram of material, per cubic meter, per unit of mechanical performance (like stiffness or strength), and product lifespan. Ultimately, a well-defined FU ensures that sustainability assessments are equitable, meaningful, and aligned with the actual performance and application of biocomposites, rather than just highlighting their bio-based features.

II) **Life Cycle Inventory (LCI)**

It includes all the workflows of the inputs and outputs associated with biocomposites throughout its life cycle. The data utilized in the life cycle inventory (LCI) of biocomposites is divided into primary, secondary, and tertiary categories. Primary data comes from direct collection methods involving manufacturers, processing facilities, or laboratory tests, encompassing aspects such as fiber and resin usage, energy consumption, emissions, and waste output. Secondary data is obtained from pre-existing LCI databases (like Ecoinvent, GaBi, SimaPro), industry publications, or scholarly articles. This type of data is especially valuable when direct measurements cannot be obtained. Tertiary data is based on estimations, models, or assumptions, such as anticipated transportation emissions or energy use associated with emerging production technologies (Bouman et al., 2024). It includes valuable information regarding:

i) Raw Material Acquisition

Agricultural Feedstocks

Biocomposites often utilize agricultural feedstocks as primary raw materials. These include natural hemp, flax, jute, kenaf, and cotton fibers. Agricultural residues, such as wheat straw, rice husks, and coconut coir, are also widely used. These renewable materials offer significant environmental advantages over synthetic alternatives due to their biodegradability and lower carbon footprint. The selection of raw materials from agricultural waste plays a crucial role in determining the environmental performance of biocomposites. Factors such as crop yield, land use intensity, and climate adaptability influence the sustainability of fiber production. Additionally, integrating multi-functional cropping systems can enhance resource efficiency by optimizing soil nutrient cycles and minimizing external inputs. LCA studies have been previously conducted to compare the impact of different organic and inorganic fertilization or other farming practices on environmental impacts in different crops, such as wheat and asparagus (Williams et al. 2010; Zafiriou et al. 2012). Similar studies can be practices while selecting the raw material for the biocomposite. Furthermore, the environmental footprints varies among different species of fiber due to different production systems (Table 2).

Table 2. Environmental footprints of different natural fiber production systems (Korol et al. 2020)

Production System	Carbon Footprint kg CO_2eq/kg	Ecological Footprint $m^2 \cdot a$/kg	Water Footprint m^3/kg
Jute	0.58	4.73	1.55
Kenaf	0.55	4.21	0.69
Cotton	2.95	31.32	2.07

Forestry-Based Feedstocks

Forestry-based feedstocks include wood fibers, sawdust, and other lignocellulosic materials derived from sustainably managed forests. These materials are commonly sourced from industrial by-products, reducing waste and maximizing resource efficiency. Certification systems such as the Forest Stewardship Council (FSC) and Programme for the Endorsement of Forest Certification (PEFC) help ensure responsible forest management and sustainable biomass sourcing. Recent advancements in forestry biotechnology, such as genetically modified fast-growing trees and optimized lignin structures, have enhanced feedstock availability while reducing environmental trade-offs. However, concerns remain regarding monoculture plantations, biodiversity loss, and water consumption in large-scale afforestation projects.

The heterogeneity of biomass feedstock sources from different sectors presents several challenges in LCA, particularly in energy consumption, carbon footprint, material properties, and supply chain logistics. High-lignin biomass demands aggressive pretreatment, increasing electricity and heat use, while variability in sugar yields from fermentation leads to inconsistent CO_2 emissions. Feedstock purity also affects the mechanical and thermal performance of biocomposites, and fluctuating biomass quality complicates transportation and storage, raising environmental costs. Strategies to mitigate these issues include standardized biomass pretreatment, blending feedstocks for composition balance, advanced biorefinery techniques to improve sugar yields, and dynamic LCA modeling to incorporate feedstock variability for accurate assessments (Sgarbossa et al., 2020; Shi & Guest, 2020).

Green Polymers

Green polymers, also known as biopolymers or sustainable polymers, are derived from renewable biomass sources such as plant-based starches, lignocellulosic materials, microbial fermentation, and algae. These polymers offer lower carbon footprints compared to conventional fossil-based plastics, contributing to the transition toward a circular bioeconomy. Common green polymers include polylactic acid (PLA), polyhydroxyalkanoates (PHA), bio-based polyethylene (bio-PE), starch algal based polymers. Recent advancements in polymer engineering focus on enhancing biodegradability, mechanical strength, and recyclability to improve performance across diverse applications. However, challenges persist in competing with food production for feedstock, energy-intensive processing, and managing end-of-life waste. Comparative environmental impact and energy requirements of petroleum-based and bio-based plastics as shown in Table 3.

ii) Manufacturing Processes

Energy Consumption

The energy demand during biocomposite manufacturing varies depending on the type of matrix (e.g., thermoplastic or thermosetting) and fiber processing methods.

Table 3. Comparative environmental impact and energy requirements of petroleum-based and bio-based plastics

Material Type	ER (MJ/kg)	CF (kg CO_2eq/kg)	GWP (kg CO_2-eq/kg)	GGE (kg CO_2-eq/kg)	References
Petroleum-Based Plastics					
ABS (Acrylonitrile Butadiene Styrene)	95.78	N.D.	N.D.	4.2	Papong et al. (2014)
HDPE (High-Density Polyethylene)	81.83	N.D.	N.D.	1.81	Papong et al. (2014)
LDPE (Low-Density Polyethylene)	82.9	N.D.	1.94	1.94	Papong et al. (2014); Amponsah et al. (2024)
PE	N.D.	N.D.	2.01	N.D.	Nagy et al. (2020); Amponsah et al. (2024)
PET (Polyethylene Terephthalate)	76.63	N.D.	2.92	3.3	Papong et al. (2014); Amponsah et al. (2024)
PP (Polypropylene)	79.53	N.D.	N.D.	1.67	Papong et al. (2014)
PS (Polystyrene)	90.55	N.D.	3.23	3.44	Papong et al. (2014); Amponsah et al. (2024)
PVC (Polyvinyl Chloride)	77.21	N.D.	1.94	2.11	Papong et al. (2014); Amponsah et al. (2024)
Biodegradable/Bio-based Plastics					
Bio PE	N.D.	N.D.	1.38	N.D.	Nagy et al. (2020)
PHA	N.D.	N.D.	0.2	N.D.	Amponsah et al. (2024)
PHBV	N.D.	N.D.	3.47	N.D.	David et al. (2021)
PLA	N.D.	N.D.	1.87	N.D.	Amponsah et al. (2024)
Saccharina latissimi Biopolymer	N.D.	N.D.	1.25	N.D.	Amponsah et al. (2024)
Starch	N.D.	0.88	N.D.	N.D.	Broeren et al. (2017)
TPS	N.D.	N.D.	2	N.D.	Amponsah et al. (2024)

(ER- Energy Requirement; CF- Carbon Footprint; GWP- Global Warming Potential; GGE- Greenhouse Gas Emissions; ABS- Acrylonitrile Butadiene Styrene; HDPE - High-Density Polyethylene; LDPE- Low-Density Polyethylene; PET- Polyethylene Terephthalate; PP- Polypropylene; PS- Polystyrene; PVC- Polyvinyl Chloride; PE- Polyethylene; Bio-PE- Biobased polyethylene; PHBV- Virgin poly(3-hydroxybutyrate-co-3-hydroxyvalerate); PLA- Polylactic acid; PHA- Polyhydroxyalkanoate; TPS- Thermophilic starch; N.D.- Not determined)

Natural fiber processing typically requires less energy compared to synthetic fibers, but factors such as drying, grinding, and resin impregnation influence overall energy requirements. Recent advancements in green manufacturing techniques, including low-temperature resin curing and enzymatic fiber treatment, have shown promise in reducing energy inputs. Furthermore, life cycle optimization models integrate renewable energy sources such as solar and biomass-based power to minimize fossil fuel reliance in production (Roy et al., 2020).

Emissions and Waste Generation

The environmental footprint of biocomposites includes emissions from fiber processing, resin synthesis, and composite fabrication. While biocomposites generally exhibit lower greenhouse gas emissions than traditional composites, volatile organic compounds (VOCs) and other pollutants can be released during resin curing and fiber treatment. To improve LCA outcomes, alternative bio-based resins derived from lignin, starch, and algae have been explored, offering significant reductions in hazardous emissions. Circular economy approaches, such as closed-loop solvent recovery systems and biopolymer reprocessing, have also enhanced material efficiency and emission control (Rodriguez et al., 2020).

iii) Use Phase

Performance and Durability

The performance and durability of biocomposites depend on factors such as fiber-matrix adhesion, moisture resistance, and mechanical properties. While biocomposites offer advantages such as lightweight construction and impact resistance, challenges include susceptibility to biodegradation and reduced strength under humid conditions. Emerging technologies, such as nanocellulose reinforcements and plasma surface treatments, have improved the mechanical performance and longevity of biocomposites. Digital twin simulations have also been employed to predict failure points and optimize real-world performance (Castillo et al., 2022).

iv) End-of-Life Scenarios

Biodegradation

The biodegradability of biocomposites is largely determined by fiber composition, matrix type, and environmental conditions. Fully biodegradable composites, composed of natural fibers and bio-based resins, can break down in composting conditions, reducing waste accumulation. Recent studies have explored microbial-assisted degradation processes to enhance breakdown efficiency, while material coding via blockchain has been proposed to improve traceability in disposal pathways (Nair et al., 2013).

III) **Life Cycle Impact Assessment (LCIA)**

Life Cycle Impact Assessment (LCIA) evaluates the environmental impacts of products or systems across their life cycle. It begins with the selection of impact categories, identifying key areas like global warming and toxicity. The next step, classification, assigns inventory data (e.g., emissions) to these categories. In characterization, scientific models quantify the impact of emissions, such as CO_2 and methane, on environmental issues. Normalization compares different impacts to determine their relative significance, often by adjusting to global reference values. Grouping organizes impacts based on criteria like geographical scale. The weighting step assigns relative importance to each impact, guiding decision-making. Finally, evaluation and reporting assess the reliability of results and communicate findings transparently, ensuring informed decision-making for environmental sustainability. These steps provide a structured approach to understanding the environmental implications of products and processes (ISO, 2006). Different impact categories are considered for LCA of biocomposites (Figure 3).

Figure 3. Different impact categories used in LCA of biocomposites

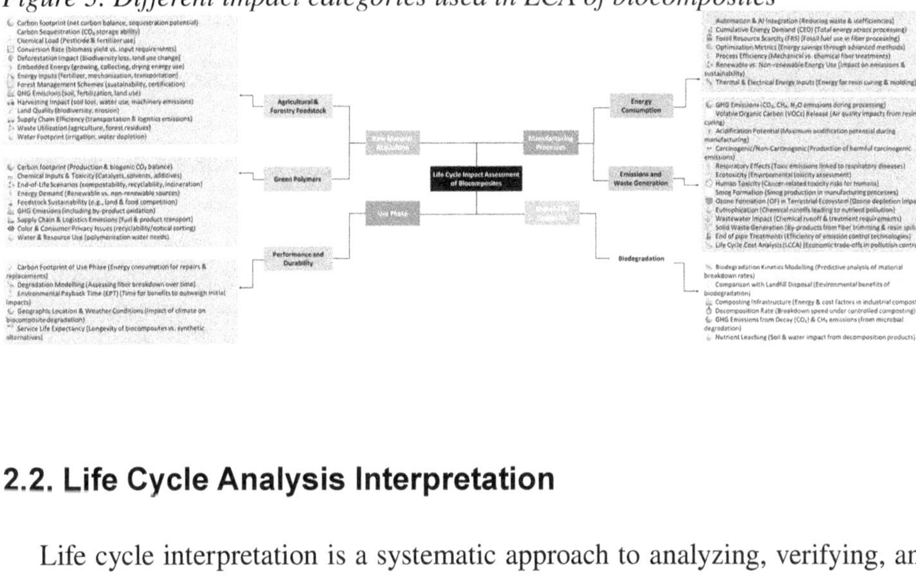

2.2. Life Cycle Analysis Interpretation

Life cycle interpretation is a systematic approach to analyzing, verifying, and evaluating data from the Life Cycle Inventory (LCI) and Life Cycle Impact Assessment (LCIA) to effectively communicate findings. As the final phase of the LCA process, it aims to analyze results, draw conclusions, acknowledge limitations, and provide recommendations transparently. According to ISO, its objectives include presenting LCA results clearly, comprehensively, and consistently while aligning with the study's goal and scope. When comparing alternatives, interpreting LCA results is complex, as assumptions, engineering estimates, and stakeholder values influence decisions. Each of these factors must be transparently documented to support conclusions. Due to uncertainties, it may not always be possible to determine a definitive best alternative, but the process enhances understanding of environmental and health impacts at local, regional, and global scales, helping decision-makers weigh the pros and cons of each option. While LCA provides valuable insights, it does not consider factors like technical performance, cost, or social and political acceptance. Therefore, it should be used alongside these parameters to make well-rounded, informed decisions. The key steps for interpreting the results of a LCA are based on the guidelines outlined by the International Standard Organization (ISO, 2006).

Identification of Significant Issues

The first step in life cycle interpretation involves reviewing data from the initial LCA phases to identify significant issues—key elements influencing the LCI and LCIA results. Given the extensive data collected, only elements with substantial impact are assessed. A comprehensive review of study objectives, methodology, impact weights, results, and external inputs ensures alignment with the LCA's goal and scope. Once confirmed, the significance of the results can be determined.

Evaluation of Results

The evaluation of results is composed of completeness, sensitivity, and consistency checks.

- ***Completeness Check*:** It verifies whether the study is comprehensive and includes all necessary data. The completeness check ensures all relevant data are available and align with system boundaries. A checklist should cover key areas such as life cycle stages, processes, and emissions to verify data representativeness (e.g., covering 90% of raw materials and releases). If gaps exist, fair comparison is compromised, requiring additional data collection. When missing data cannot be filled, differences must be reported, with their impact estimated quantitatively (e.g., uncertainty percentage) or qualitatively (e.g., explaining missing factors affecting results).
- ***Sensitivity Check:*** It Assesses how variations in significant data elements affect the results. It aims to assess the reliability of LCA results by evaluating whether uncertainties in significant issues, identified in the previous step affect decision-making. It can be conducted using three common techniques:

  a) **Contribution Analysis**: It Identifies data with the greatest influence on impact indicators.

b) **Uncertainty Analysis**: It examines the variability in LCIA data to assess the significance of impact indicators.

c) **Sensitivity Analysis**: It Measures how changes in LCI results and models affect impact indicators. If sensitivity, uncertainty, or contribution analyses were conducted during earlier LCA phases, those results can be used here. The sensitivity check should verify that data quality and accuracy goals, defined during the goal and scope phase, are met. If deficiencies are found, further efforts are needed to improve data or impact models. If better data is unavailable, the deficiencies should be reported, with their impact estimated either quantitatively or qualitatively.

- ***Consistency Check:*** It evaluates the uniformity of system boundaries, data collection, assumptions, and impact category allocations across alternatives. The consistency check ensures that the assumptions, methods, and data align with the LCA's goals and scope for each product/process. A formal checklist should document the evaluation, with categories defined by the goal and scope. Inconsistencies, if any, must be documented and assessed. It confirms that the results are complete, comparable, and acceptable, and conclusions can be drawn. If not, repeat the steps until the results meet the study's objectives.
- ***Conclusion and Reporting*:** Upon reviewing the LCA findings for biocomposites, we can conclude their environmental performance. If the data is thorough and precise, it will be possible to identify the most sustainable biocomposite system. However, should there be any data gaps or inconsistencies, the analysis needs to be revisited to ensure it aligns with the study's goals. Important suggestions for enhancing sustainability include refining production processes to minimize energy use, such as implementing energy-efficient technologies and lower-temperature curing methods. Utilizing bio-based resins with reduced environmental impacts, sourced from renewable materials, can also enhance the sustainability of biocomposites. Furthermore, improving end-of-life management through more effective recycling or composting options will contribute to waste reduction and lessen environmental impacts. Finally, emphasizing the use of renewable energy in production processes will lead to a significant decrease in carbon emissions. The final report should meticulously outline the methodology, data sources, and assumptions to guarantee the transparency and reliability of the findings while providing practical recommendations for advancing biocomposite sustainability.

2.3. Limitations of Environmental LCA for Biocomposites

The adoption of standardized methodological frameworks, such as ISO 14040, is fundamental for conducting LCAs consistently and comparably across different studies and applications (Ead et al., 2021). These frameworks provide structured guidelines for assessing environmental impacts, ensuring methodological robustness, and facilitating comparative analysis in biocomposite research. Standardization of LCA methodology is particularly critical in the context of biocomposites, given the diverse range of raw materials, processing techniques, and end-of-life scenarios involved. Integrating LCA with life cycle cost (LCC) assessments enhances the holistic evaluation of biocomposites by providing insights into both environmental and economic aspects (Gkoloni et al., 2022). This approach aids in decision-making processes related to sustainable material development and production. Additionally, assumptions regarding material composition and structural attributes significantly influence LCA outcomes. For instance, the selection of fibers; natural or synthetic, can result in distinct environmental trade-offs due to variations in energy use, processing requirements, and end-of-life disposal strategies.

Another key challenge in LCA studies of biocomposites is input variability. Variations in energy consumption, emissions, and resource utilization during production introduce uncertainties in LCA results. Sensitivity analysis is often employed to assess the extent to which these variations influence overall environmental impact assessments (Andersen et al., 2023). Moreover, advanced modelling techniques, such as micromechanics and finite element analysis, are increasingly being used to predict the behaviour of biocomposites. These models must account for the inherent complexities of biocomposite microstructures, which can introduce additional uncertainties to LCA calculations (Seile et al., 2022; Gkoloni et al., 2022). Current modelling tools may not adequately predict the behaviour of biocomposite materials, necessitating the development of advanced models that incorporate nonlinear responses and material interactions (Elmasry et al., 2024).

Despite ongoing standardization efforts, challenges persist in fully capturing the environmental impacts of biocomposites due to the intrinsic variability of natural materials and the multifaceted nature of their life cycles. Enhancing the reliability of LCA outcomes requires continuous improvements in modelling techniques, data collection methodologies, and sensitivity analyses. Addressing these uncertainties is crucial for ensuring that biocomposites are accurately evaluated and effectively positioned as sustainable alternatives to conventional composite materials.

A) **Methodological Challenges** Standardized methodologies are essential for reliable Life Cycle Assessment (LCA) studies, especially for biocomposites, where variability in raw materials, processing, and end-of-life (EoL) scenarios complicates assessments. Key challenges include:

Data Availability and Quality

The reliability of LCA depends on high-quality data, yet biocomposites pose challenges due to their natural variability.

- **Feedstock Variability**: Agricultural and forestry residues (e.g., hemp, wheat straw) vary in properties based on geography, climate, and farming practices, complicating standardized datasets (Syduzzaman et al., 2020; Akras et al., 2024).
- **EoL Data Gaps**: Limited studies assess biocomposite biodegradability, recyclability, or reuse, leading to incomplete sustainability evaluations (Volk et al., 2024; Gomez-Campos et al., 2020).

Functional Unit Selection

- **Diverse Applications**: Biocomposites serve multiple industries (automotive, packaging, construction), each with different performance criteria (Vinod et al., 2020; Andrew & Dhakal, 2021).
- **Material Composition Variability**: Different fiber-polymer compositions and treatments affect environmental impacts.
- **Durability Considerations:** Environmental exposure alters performance over time, requiring a holistic LCA approach (Fitzgerald et al., 2021).

Allocation of Environmental Burdens

- **Multifunctional Agricultural Systems:** Feedstocks like rice husks have multiple uses (animal feed, soil amendment), requiring careful allocation (Cherubini et al., 2011).
- **Shared Environmental Burdens**: By-products from cultivation and processing influence sustainability assessments.
- **Co-Product Systems:** Manufacturing often generates multiple outputs, necessitating standardized allocation methods.

Addressing these challenges through improved data collection and standardized methodologies will enhance the accuracy and comparability of biocomposite LCA studies.

B) **Geographical Variation in LCA**

Agricultural Practices and Resource Requirements

Geographical differences in agricultural practices, such as climate, soil composition, local resources, farming techniques, and land management strategies, can significantly influence the outcomes of life cycle assessments (LCA) by altering factors like resource consumption, emissions, and environmental impact. To obtain a more accurate evaluation of the environmental effects across different regions, it is crucial to consider these regional variations. For example, Yang et al. (2017) found that differences in agricultural practices and crop types lead to substantial variations in emissions due to differing requirements for nutrients, herbicides, fuel, and electricity in the United States. Similarly, Heidari et al. (2019) highlighted the importance of conducting region-specific LCAs to assess the environmental consequences of bio-based materials like hempcrete effectively. By incorporating site-specific factors, regional LCAs provide more relevant data for making informed decisions, ensuring that the actual ecological impact of materials is accurately evaluated in the context of local production practices and environmental conditions.

Energy Sources and Carbon Footprint

Geographical variations in energy sources and the efficiency of local power grids play a crucial role in the LCA of biocomposites. Regions that rely on cleaner, renewable energy sources contribute to a lower carbon footprint in the production and transportation of biocomposites, whereas areas dependent on fossil fuels tend to exhibit higher emissions. Consequently, incorporating geographical differences in electricity generation into LCAs leads to more accurate and realistic assessments of both environmental and economic outcomes. By focusing on more localized scales, such as site-specific data or hourly emissions, LCAs can more effectively evaluate the localized environmental impacts, including land use and eutrophication, and support the development of more targeted sustainability initiatives. Furthermore, the majority of existing research has been concentrated in Europe, Asia, and North America, with countries such as the United States, Italy, Germany, and China being the most frequently studied. This geographic focus underscores the need for greater research attention in regions like Africa and South America, which are often underrepresented in LCA studies. As such, there is considerable potential for further exploration in these underrepresented regions, fuel types, and impact categories. Additionally, the increasing application of optimization techniques and Geographic Information System (GIS) tools offers opportunities to refine LCAs, enabling them to better capture the complexities of localized environmental and economic contexts (Jordaan et al., 2021).

Transportation Routes and Logistics

Transportation pathways and overall transport distances can vary significantly, ranging from a few kilometers in certain areas to several kilometers in others, thereby having a substantial impact on life cycle assessments (LCA). Incorporating transportation factors into LCA is essential for accurately evaluating the environmental consequences of biocomposites, underscoring the importance of considering transportation methods, distances, and regional infrastructure. Key insights emphasize the necessity of including detailed information in the life cycle inventory. The selection of transportation mode plays a critical role in influencing emissions. Although air transport offers speed, it is associated with a larger carbon footprint when compared to road or rail transport. For instance, transporting raw materials for biocomposites by road may result in significantly higher emissions in countries where long-haul freight relies heavily on diesel trucks. In contrast, rail or maritime transport generally leads to lower emissions per ton-kilometer, though this is contingent upon regional infrastructure and energy sources, including both renewable and non-renewable options. For example, Norway's extensive hydropower system substantially reduces the environmental impact of transportation when compared to countries like China or India, where transportation relies more on fossil fuels, resulting in higher emissions. The complexity of the supply chain, often involving multiple countries or regions, exacerbates environmental effects due to the need for multiple transportation stages and pathways. For example, biocomposites produced in Europe, sourced from fibers in Africa and resins in Asia, are likely to exhibit a much larger carbon footprint than those manufactured entirely within the same region. However, in regions such as Italy, Ferronato et al. (2021) successfully employed ArcGIS to determine the optimal transportation route for raw material collection. Similarly, various studies have developed specific algorithmic models to optimize transportation logistics, such as linear programming in Turkey (Rızvanoglu et al., 2020) and the green vehicle routing problem (PCGVRP) model in China (Wu et al., 2020).

C) **Temporal Variation in LCA of Biocomposites**

Technological Advances and Energy Transitions

Advancements in technology and the ongoing shift toward renewable energy sources are key drivers in reducing the environmental footprint of biocomposite production. Dynamic LCA studies that incorporate time-sensitive data demonstrate how shifts in technology and energy sources can significantly affect LCA outcomes. Over time, the transition from fossil fuels to renewable energy, illustrated by Germany's energy transformation, has led to substantial reductions in carbon emissions associated with biocomposite production. The time-dependent nature of renewable energy sources, particularly those that are intermittent, plays a crucial role, as their variability can considerably influence both emissions and economic outcomes. By integrating temporal resolution into LCA frameworks, alongside Geographic Information Systems (GIS) and economic evaluations, more accurate and context-specific assessments can be achieved. These refined evaluations are instrumental in identifying effective mitigation strategies and fostering more informed policy-making (Jordaan et al., 2021). Furthermore, advancements in manufacturing technology, innovations in materials, and improvements in biocomposite processing techniques contribute to substantial reductions in energy consumption, enhanced performance, and minimized environmental impacts. As bio-resins and bio-based polymers become increasingly efficient over time, the environmental burdens associated with biocomposite production are reduced. The adoption of more efficient machinery and automated processes further lowers carbon emissions per unit of biocomposite produced. Consequently, an LCA conducted today may yield different conclusions compared to one performed in previous years, reflecting the cumulative effect of technological advancements (Korol et al., 2016).

Climate and Seasonal Changes

Changes in climate and seasonal trends significantly influence the life cycle assessment (LCA) of biocomposites, especially during the stages of raw material production, manufacturing, and end-of-life management. Climate change can alter agricultural practices by affecting crop yields, quality, and the resources needed for cultivation. Fluctuations in temperatures and precipitation can lead to reduced crop yields and lower fiber quality, resulting in greater resource consumption, such as an increased use of water and fertilizers, along with higher land requirements. Extreme weather conditions can also heighten the energy demands of manufacturing processes. In areas dependent on fossil fuels, additional energy is necessary for heating or cooling during production, which contributes to elevated emissions. Seasonal changes can impact the physical characteristics of biocomposites, including fiber strength and moisture levels, which may hinder processing efficiency and raise waste levels. Moreover, the performance of biocomposites under varying climatic conditions, such as degradation in high humidity or drastic temperature shifts, can shorten their lifespan, requiring more regular maintenance or earlier replacements, thereby amplifying their environmental effects over time.

Supply Chain and Material Availability

Variations in the availability of materials and the dynamics of supply chains can greatly affect the environmental impact of biocomposite manufacturing over time. As the demand for biomass feedstocks such as hemp, flax, or bamboo rises, the ecological effects of acquiring these materials change. Over time, implementing more sustainable practices, like minimizing land use or conserving water, can reduce the environmental effects related to sourcing raw materials. Conversely, if practices that are not sustainable, such as monoculture farming or deforestation, are utilized, the outcomes of life cycle assessments may deteriorate. These transitions are particularly crucial in the long run, as they represent global shifts in the availability of raw materials and supply chain dynamics.

Regulatory and Policy Changes

Regulatory and policy modifications are vital factors influencing the outcomes of Life Cycle Assessments (LCA), as governments and international bodies consistently implement new regulations, standards, and incentives aimed at fostering sustainable practices. Policies concerning carbon pricing, waste management, and renewable energy goals can have a direct impact on the LCA of biocomposites, particularly during their production and disposal phases. More stringent emissions controls or incentives for sustainable methods can significantly lessen the environmental footprint of biocomposites. Worldwide, LCA is an important aspect in policy formulation, with significant instances seen in the USA, China, Thailand, various European nations, and Latin American countries such as Mexico, Chile, Colombia, and Brazil (Sala et al. 2021). Additionally, forthcoming regulatory adjustments pertaining to recycling and end-of-life management for biocomposites may change the methods for disposing of or reusing these materials, thereby potentially minimizing waste and improving their circularity. An LCA conducted at present might not fully account for the impacts of carbon taxes or anticipated green energy incentives, which could decrease the environmental impact of biocomposites in future evaluations.

Therefore, incorporating geographical and temporal variations into LCA is vital for precise evaluations of environmental impacts. Areas abundant in renewable energy sources generally display smaller carbon footprints, while regions reliant on fossil fuels tend to produce higher emissions. Likewise, temporal elements like advancements in technology, fluctuations in climate, and policy changes can greatly affect environmental outcomes. By tackling these variations with dynamic and region-specific LCA approaches, decision-making can be refined towards more sustainable practices in product design, manufacturing, and consumption.

2.4. Software Tools for LCA of Biocomposites

A variety of LCA software tools are available, each with distinct features, databases, and areas of application. The are specific specialized software's designed specifically for LCA of biocomposites (Table 4).

Table 4. Different tools and software used for LCA of biocomposites

Software	Key Features	Databases (Regional Relevance)	Applications
ACMA LCA+EPD Generator	Composite manufacturers can efficiently create reliable, cost-effective Environmental Product Declarations (EPDs) and climate impacts through LCA	U.S. and global composite materials databases	Assessing the environmental performance of fiber-reinforced composites EPD certification for sustainability reporting
Brightway2	Python-based for high customization, large-scale uncertainty analysis, academic, and research-focused	Ecoinvent, FORWAST, USLCI (Global)	Advanced biocomposite scenario modelling Regional comparisons with Monte Carlo simulations
C3R'IMPACT	LCA tool for the plastics and composites industry, facilitates eco-design and product development for manufacturers and designers	Internal datasets and Ecoinvent (France, EU)	Optimizes the environmental performance of plastic and biocomposite products and identifies key impact categories
EcoChain	Cloud-based, real-time footprint tracking, designed for businesses and supply chains with easy-to-use interface	Ecoinvent, EF 3.0 (EU-focused)	Quick assessment of biocomposites in supply chains Corporate sustainability
GaBi	Large industrial database, hybrid modelling (process and input-output), and circular economy integration	GaBi Professional, Ecoinvent (Europe, North America)	Regional sensitivity analysis Waste management and end-of-life analysis
GREET (Argonne National Lab)	Focuses on energy, transportation, LCA, such as Well-to-wheel and cradle-to-grave analysis	U.S. and global transport databases	Assessing transport emissions of bio-based composites Life cycle energy use analysis

continued on following page

Table 4. Continued

Software	Key Features	Databases (Regional Relevance)	Applications
One Click LCA	An AI-powered, cloud-based platform that integrates with Building Information Modelling (BIM) and sustainability criteria while ensuring compliance with industry certifications.	Ecoinvent, GaBi, National EPD databases (Global)	LCA for biocomposites in construction Automated data analysis and sustainability compliance
OpenLCA	Open-source, highly customizable, supports multiple databases and ideal for academic research	Ecoinvent, Agribalyse, Social Hotspot Database (Global, EU)	LCA of small-scale biocomposite production Developing new material-specific LCI datasets
SimaPro	Advanced LCA modelling, multi-impact assessment (carbon, water, land use, etc.) and supports consequential LCA	Ecoinvent, Agri-footprint, USLCI (Europe, US, Global)	Comparing fossil-based vs. bio-based composites Land-use impact analysis
Sustainable Minds	Suitable for product designers, it focuses on carbon footprint and eco-labelling.	Internal databases and public datasets (North America, EU)	Quick sustainability assessments of biocomposites Product development and marketing
Umberto LCA+	Integration of material flow analysis (MFA), resource efficiency, and circular economy impacts	Ecoinvent, GaBi (Global, EU)	Biocomposite production flow analysis Optimization of industrial production

For comprehensive life cycle modelling and environmental impact assessment, SimaPro, GaBi, and Brightway2 offer advanced analytical tools. OpenLCA and Brightway2 are ideal for academic research due to their open-source flexibility. In industry, C3R'IMPACT and ACMA's LCA+EPD Generator support biocomposites manufacturers in optimizing sustainability and creating Environmental Product Declarations (EPDs). For real-time corporate assessments, EcoChain and Sustainable Minds provide user-friendly, cloud-based solutions. GREET specializes in energy and transportation-related LCA, while One Click LCA is designed for construction materials, integrating seamlessly with Building Information Modelling (BIM) tools.

3. SOCIAL LIFE CYCLE ASSESSMENT (S-LCA) OF BIOCOMPOSITES

It evaluates the social and socio-economic impacts associated with biocomposites throughout their life cycle, from raw material extraction to disposal. Unlike traditional Life Cycle Assessment (LCA), which focuses on environmental impact,

S-LCA considers human and societal factors, such as labour rights, health and safety, and community well-being (Zarauz et al., 2024). This assessment helps identify potential social risks and benefits in the biocomposite sector.

3.1. Key Aspects of S-LCA for Biocomposites

1. **Stakeholders Considered** (Aybar et al., 2025)
    - *Workers*: Fair wages, occupational health & safety, working conditions.
    - *Local Communities*: Land use implications, cultural impacts, job creation.
    - *Consumers*: Product safety, affordability, ethical considerations.
    - *Governments & Institutions*: Regulatory policies, labour laws, fair trade agreements.
2. **Life Cycle Stages Assessed**
    - *Raw Material Extraction*: Farming of natural fibers, resin production, forestry for lignin-based composites.
    - *Manufacturing & Processing*: Ethical supply chains, factory labour conditions, worker rights.
    - *Distribution & Use*: Fair trade practices, consumer health, and safety.
    - *End-of-Life*: Biodegradability, recyclability, impacts on waste management systems.
3. **Key Indicators** (Bouillass et al., 2021)
    - *Working Conditions*: Fair wages, elimination of child labour, safe workplaces.
    - *Community Well-being*: Contributions to local economies, land tenure security.
    - *Human Health & Safety*: Exposure to hazardous chemicals, ergonomic risks.
    - *Governance & Ethics*: Compliance with labour laws, supply chain transparency.
    - *Consumer Rights & Product Responsibility*: Ethical marketing, access to sustainable alternatives.

3.2. Methodologies Used (Huang et al., 2025)

- *UNEP/SETAC Guidelines for S-LCA*: A widely accepted framework for assessing social impacts at each life cycle stage.
- *Social Hotspot Database (SHDB)*: A tool for identifying high-risk supply chain regions based on labor conditions and governance factors.

- *Multi-Criteria Decision Analysis (MCDA)*: Used to assign weightings to different social factors, facilitating decision-making in complex scenarios.
- *Social Impact Assessment (SIA)*: Provides qualitative and quantitative evaluations of social consequences.

3.3. Challenges in S-LCA of Biocomposites (Lehmann et al., 2013)

- *Data Availability*: Social data are harder to quantify than environmental data, requiring qualitative assessments.
- *Subjectivity*: Different regions prioritize different social factors, complicating standardization.
- *Complex Supply Chains*: Biocomposites involve multiple industries (agriculture, forestry, chemicals), making traceability difficult.

Thus, there is a growing need to develop and standardize S-LCA databases to improve data accessibility. Blockchain technology is gaining immense attention for enhancing supply chain transparency and integrating participatory approaches involving affected communities.

4. ECONOMIC LIFE CYCLE ASSESSMENT (E-LCA) OF BIOCOMPOSITES

An Economic Life Cycle Assessment (E-LCA) evaluates the financial costs and benefits associated with biocomposites from raw material extraction to disposal. This assessment helps determine the feasibility and competitiveness of biocomposites compared to conventional materials, such as plastics, metals, and synthetic composites (La Rosa et al., 2024).

4.1. Key Aspects of E-LCA for Biocomposites

1. **Life Cycle Stages & Cost Components**
    - *Raw Material Sourcing* (Safi Jahanshahi et al., 2024)
        - o Costs of natural fiber or bio-based resin production (e.g., lignin, cellulose, PLA, bio-epoxies).
        - o Agricultural or forestry costs (land use, fertilizers, labour).
        - o Price fluctuations of bio-based raw materials.
    - *Processing & Manufacturing* (Nutrizio et al., 2024)

    - Processing costs: Fiber extraction, chemical modifications, and resin synthesis.
    - Energy consumption comparison between biocomposite and synthetic material production.
    - Equipment and labour costs (e.g., compression molding, extrusion).
- *Distribution & Market Entry* (Ali et al., 2022)
    - Transportation and logistics expenses.
    - Trade barriers and tariffs on bio-based products.
    - Consumer demand and willingness to pay for sustainable alternatives.
- *Use Phase* (Stillitano, 2022)
    - Performance benefits (e.g., lightweight materials reducing fuel consumption in automotive applications).
    - Durability and maintenance costs versus traditional materials.
- *End-of-Life* (Stillitano, 2022)
    - Recycling or biodegradation costs compared to landfill disposal.
    - Potential revenue from recovered bio-based materials (circular economy models).

2. **Economic Indicators in E-LCA** (Safi Jahanshahi et al., 2024)
    - Life Cycle Costing (LCC): Total cost of ownership over the product life cycle.
    - Return on Investment (ROI): Profitability of biocomposite adoption.
    - Net Present Value (NPV): Discounted value of future earnings from biocomposites.
    - Payback Period: Time required to recover initial investment.
    - Cost-Benefit Analysis (CBA): Comparison of economic benefits against production costs.

4.2. Challenges in E-LCA of Biocomposites (Pacheco-Torgal, 2025)

- Data Uncertainty: Variability in bio-based feedstock prices due to climate and market conditions.
- Regional Differences: Cost disparities based on local policies, subsidies, and labor expenses.
- External Costs: Incorporating environmental and social benefits into economic calculations remains complex.
- Potential Solutions:
    - Development of economic models that integrate external benefits (e.g., carbon sequestration, job creation).

- Improved life cycle databases specific to biocomposite industries.
- Policy incentives (e.g., tax credits, subsidies) to enhance market adoption.

The E-LCA evaluates financial feasibility. Addressing the challenges in both assessments through improved data availability, methodological standardization, and policy support can facilitate the widespread adoption of biocomposites as sustainable alternatives to conventional materials.

5. INTEGRATED ENVIRONMENTAL, SOCIAL, AND ECONOMIC LCA FOR BIOCOMPOSITES

Furthermore, there is a growing need for hybrid LCA that integrates the environmental, social, and economic aspects of biocomposites to drive the growing impact towards a sustainable economy. Calado et al. (2018) combined environmental life cycle assessment (LCA) with life cycle cost analysis to enhance the configuration of carbon fiber-reinforced composites in aircraft structures. Their findings indicated a significant relationship between CO_2 emissions and life cycle costs, both of which are primarily driven by fuel consumption, especially kerosene use. Although life cycle costs and CO_2 emissions display a similar pattern, the overall environmental impact score (a single score) incorporates emissions from air, water, and soil, resulting in minor discrepancies. Chen et al. (2020) demonstrated a hybrid LCA approach model to evaluate the economic, social, and environmental effects of integrating potato pulp with PLA and PHA to develop biocomposites. The results demonstrated that utilizing potato pulp leads to enhanced socio-economic advantages, especially in PLA-based systems, with a possible gross value added of €4.24 and 0.19 hours of employment for each kilogram of biocomposite produced. Nonetheless, this process also results in increased greenhouse gas (GHG) emissions across both supply chains, chiefly due to the energy-intensive drying process of potato pulp. Implementing mitigation measures, such as optimizing thermal energy usage or employing low-carbon solutions, can effectively lower environmental impacts. Biocomposites made from PLA present a greater opportunity for enhancing sustainability, considering their prominent market presence in bioplastics. Furthermore, the addition of potato pulp improves biodegradability and aids in reducing agricultural waste, thereby reinforcing its significance in circular bioeconomy initiatives. Future studies should look into other agricultural residues for PHA systems and cutting-edge PHA production methods to further lessen GHG emissions. With ongoing research, financial backing, and supportive policies, the valorization of potato pulp in biocomposites has the potential to play a role in advancing a more sustainable bioplastic industry.

6. LCA BASED CASE STUDIES OF BIOCOMPOSITES

LCA is a systematic method used to evaluate the environmental impacts of a product or process throughout its entire life cycle, from raw material extraction to disposal. LCA provides critical insights into sustainability and environmental performance in biomedical and engineering fields. Below are detailed case studies highlighting the application of LCA in different industries (Figure 4).

Figure 4. Application of LCA for biocomposites in different industries

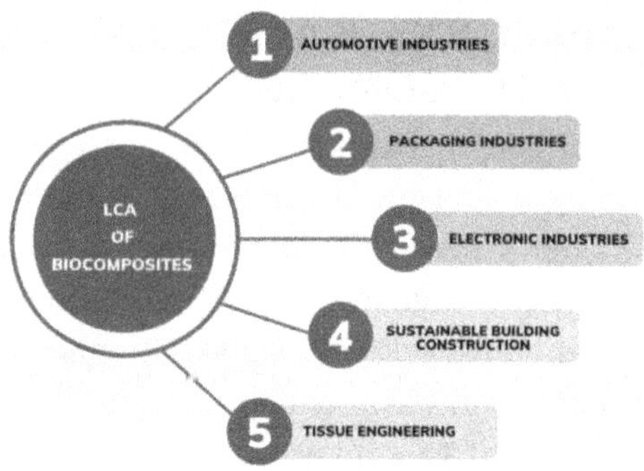

6.1. Biocomposites for Automotive Industries

Tadele et al. (2019) conducted a LCA to evaluate the environmental impact of a biocomposite synthesized from biochar derived from *Miscanthus* fiber, compared to a traditional composite incorporating talc into a polypropylene matrix at a ratio of 30%:70%. The study followed the standard protocol established by the International Organization for Standardization (ISO, 2006) and used a functional unit of 982 cm^3 of composite material. The researchers assessed environmental impacts across all life cycle stages, including raw material extraction, transportation, manufacturing, usage, and end-of-life disposal. The LCA results revealed that during the manufacturing phase, ozone depletion potential (ODP) was the major environmental impact, contributing up to 105.6% in biocomposites and 105.5% in talc-based composites. The substitution of talc with biochar, produced through slow pyrolysis of *Miscanthus* grass, aligns with the automotive industry's goal of reducing vehicle component weight to improve fuel efficiency while increasing the use of renewable materials for environmental benefits. However, during the use phase, both traditional (85.5%) and biocomposite materials (85.2%) were the highest contributors to global warming potential (GWP). At the end of life, biocomposites exhibited a higher GWP contribution than talc-based composites due to the greater degradation capacity of biochar and polypropylene. The study concluded that conducting an LCA across all life cycle stages is crucial for assessing the sustainable production and application of biocomposites in automotive industries. Similarly, Roy et al. (2020) conducted a LCA to evaluate the environmental impact of a biocomposite synthesized from biocarbon and *Miscanthus* fiber, incorporated into a polypropylene matrix, for advanced applications in the automotive industry. The study used a functional unit of 441 cm^3 of composite material. The researchers assessed environmental impacts across all life cycle stages, including raw material extraction, transportation, manufacturing, usage, and end-of-life disposal. LCA results indicated that the use phase was the primary contributor to global warming potential (GWP), followed by manufacturing, raw materials, transportation, and end-of-life processes. The GWP of the biocomposite component was 11.3 kg CO_2 eq., compared to 12.8 kg CO_2 eq. for the traditional composite incorporated with talc and colorant. As biocarbon and *Miscanthus* fiber are lighter than talc and conventional colorants, the biocomposites were lighter in weight. Furthermore, the findings suggest that adopting the biocomposites in automotive applications could not only reduce environmental impacts but also mitigate fossil fuel depletion. The reduction in environmental impact is primarily attributed to fuel savings by 11% during the use phase (27.13 MJ to 24.04 MJ).

Castillo et al. (2022) optimized the LCA study to compare the environmental impact analysis of neat polypropylene (PP) composites as well as fillers such as biogenic chicken feathers (PP-CFs) and glass fibers (PP-GF). The study followed the Cradle-to-Grave approach across all the life stages *viz.* extraction and processing of raw materials; manufacturing of the different materials considered, use, and end of life (EoL), and used a functional unit of 20 Kg of composite material for internal panels of the car having a lifetime of 10 years. The findings indicated that in the context of automotive applications, all materials examined (PP-GF, PP-CFs, and PP) significantly impacted the environmental impact categories evaluated during their use phase. This demonstrates that the newly developed material utilizing CFs (PP-CFs) is suitable for stationary applications but not for automotive or mobile uses. Furthermore, the end-of-life scenario analyzed, which involved incineration with energy recovery, has been shown to yield additional environmental benefits.

6.2. Biocomposites for Packaging Industries

Saraiva et al. (2016), reported an improved composite for mango packaging when integrated with 30% wood fiber in comparison to the traditional HDPE composite packing. The research adhered to the standard protocols set by the International Organization for Standardization (ISO 14040, 2006) with a functional unit of 10 mangoes per packaging. The findings from the LCA study showed that composite packaging boards containing 30% wood fiber exhibited a reduced environmental impact across different categories, including global warming potential (GWP), particulate matter (PM), acidification (A), photochemical ozone formation (POF), and eutrophication in both marine (Emw) and freshwater (Efw) environments, as well as human toxicity (HT) in both carcinogenic and non-carcinogenic forms, along with ecotoxicity (ET). Similarly, Rodriguez et al. (2020) studied the comparative LCA to evaluate the environmental impacts of biocomposites used as a coffee jar lid made from banana fiber reinforced into polylactic acid. These biocomposites were compared with conventional lids synthesized using high density polyethylene (HDPE). The research adhered to the standard protocols set by the International Organization for Standardization (ISO 14040, 2006) and ReCiPe with a functional unit of the circular lid having a diameter of 53 mm. The LCA findings revealed that the integration of 40% of banana fiber with PLA had a lower environmental impact compared with the HDPE. They concluded that the inclusion of natural fiber in green polymer matric can significantly reduce its harmful impact on the environment in comparison to plastic composite used for packaging.

Majewski and Sobolewska (2018) evaluated a comparative LCA study to optimize the best packaging material for apples. They compared three packing materials polypropylene (PP), recycled HDPE, and cardboard using standard ISO protocols with a functional unit of 12 apples per packaging. The results from the LCA study revealed that more than 50% of the environmental impact among all three packing materials contributes to the production phase. The highest environmental impact in terms of impact point (Pt) was observed for the polypropylene (2.33 Pt) based packaging, followed by recycled HDPE (0.9 Pt) and cardboard box (0.06 Pt). However, using the usage phase maximum impact on the environment was observed due to the usage of fossil fuels in the manufacturing and transportation sector. Thus, they concluded that depending upon the requirement of strength and durability of the packaging optimum choice can be made for the least environmental impact.

6.3. Biocomposites for Electronic Industries

Deng et al. (2016) conducted a comparative LCA to evaluate the environmental impacts of biocomposites made from flax fibers reinforced with epoxidized linseed oil, incorporating melamine polyphosphate (MPP) as a flame retardant. This biocomposite was compared to a conventional fiberglass-reinforced composite created with brominated epoxy resin, specifically tetrabromobisphenol-A (TBBPA). The goal of the study was to analyze the sustainability of these materials by assessing their environmental performance across various life cycle stages. The assessment utilized a cradle-to-grave approach, employing the ReCiPe method with a functional unit of 1 m^2 and a thickness of 1.6 mm for producing standard printed circuit boards (PCBs) in the electronics industry. The LCA findings indicated that the bio-based PCB had a lower impact on climate change, ozone depletion, human toxicity, photochemical toxicity, particulate matter, ionizing radiation, terrestrial acidification, terrestrial ecotoxicity, marine ecotoxicity, nature land use, and the depletion of metals, fossil fuels, and water resources. Conversely, the traditional plastic-based PCB demonstrated a reduced impact concerning eutrophication, freshwater ecotoxicity, and land use. The elevated contribution of the biobased PCB to eutrophication was primarily linked to the significant use of fertilizers and pesticides during flax cultivation, issues commonly associated with agro-products that utilize such chemicals. While the end-of-life impacts were negligible for both materials, the bio-based substrate exhibited higher embodied energy, which might offer advantages in incineration scenarios. They also noted that the impact of the biobased PCB was lower when assessed through mass allocations compared to economic allocations. The study concluded that the design of the bio-based PCB achieved a 42% reduction in the aggregated eco-points score (according to the ReCiPe methodology) compared to the conventional TBBPA-based design. Given its alignment with numerous international standards, the bio-based PCB presents a promising, sustainable alternative for further exploration and practical application in electronic industries.

6.4. Biocomposites for Sustainable Building Construction

Several previous studies have reported the use of wood-plastic composites for non-structural purposes in building construction. However, due to sustainability issues, these wood plastic composites can be replaced with biocomposites. Thus, LCA can provide the key areas for overall improving the sustainability of biocomposites for its commercial application in buildings. Khoshnava et al. (2018) performed a comparative LCA to investigate the environmental effects of hybrid biocomposites that consist of kenaf and oil palm empty fruit branch fiber mats reinforced with polyhydroxybutyrate (PHB) to form an eleven layered composite. This biocomposite was evaluated against a traditional fiberglass-reinforced composite made with polypropylene (PP) and polyethylene (PE). The study aimed to examine the sustainability of these materials by analyzing their environmental impact throughout different stages of the life cycle. The analysis applied cradle to gate approach along with ReCiPe as the common method for appraising and comparing impact assessment with a functional unit of 1.14 kg having a sample size $0.3 \times 0.2\ m^2$. The findings from the weighted indicator across various damage categories indicated that biocomposites inflict the least harm to the ecosystem (0.21), followed by resources (0.25) and human health (0.26), when compared to fiberglass-reinforced composite materials made with polypropylene (PP) and polyethylene (PE). Their findings indicated that substituting biocomposite for a completely petroleum-based composite led to a 30%

reduction in the single score outcome. This information offers significant insights for policymakers and manufacturers moving forward.

6.5. Biocomposites for Tissue Engineering

LCA is a vital tool for evaluating the environmental impact of biocomposites in tissue engineering, by analyzing the entire lifecycle from raw material extraction to disposal. LCA helps to identify key areas for improving sustainability. In tissue engineering, scaffolds are critical in supporting cell growth and tissue regeneration. These scaffolds can be derived from natural or synthetic materials and may be biodegradable or non-biodegradable. However, biocompatibility is essential to prevent adverse cellular responses. Common scaffold materials include polylactic acid (PLA), polyglycolic acid (PGA), and polycaprolactone (PCL), each exhibiting distinct degradation rates suited to specific tissue engineering applications (Barbier et al., 2017). Tajurahim et al. (2025) performed a LCA of biocomposites (PEGDA/ANFs) that were created from polyethylene glycol diacrylate (PEGDA) combined with aramid nanofibers (ANFs) using advanced digital light processing (DLP) to fabricate scaffolds for tissue engineering applications. The research adhered to the standard protocols set by the International Organization for Standardization (ISO 14040, 2006; 14044, 2006) i.e. cradle to gate and employed a functional unit of 0.188 kg of 3D aerogel scaffold. The LCA findings revealed a notable global warming potential (GWP) of 2.33 kg CO_2-equivalent, mainly related to the processes of preparation, printing, and additive manufacturing of scaffolds. In addition, the acidification potential (AP) was recorded at 2.74×10^3 kg SO_2-equivalent, primarily resulting from emissions of sulfur dioxide and nitrogen oxides during the acquisition, processing, and fabrication of raw materials and scaffolds. Moreover, the eutrophication potential was calculated at 6.23×10^{-4} kg phosphate-equivalent, stemming from the discharge of phosphate ions (PO_4), biological oxygen demand (BOD), and chemical oxygen demand (COD). The analysis also found a human toxicity potential (HTP) of 0.079 kg dichlorobenzene (DCB)-equivalent, predominantly linked to nitrogen oxides (NO_x) and non-methane volatile organic compounds (NMVOCs).

7. INDUSTRIAL APPLICATIONS OF BIOCOMPOSITES

Automotive Industry

Bcomp Ltd., a company based in Switzerland, has created natural fiber composites utilizing flax to produce strong, lightweight, and environmentally friendly automotive components. These materials, named ampliTex™ and powerRibs™, are formed into car interior panels, substituting as much as 70% of plastic and reducing component weight by up to 50%. This advancement also significantly lowers environmental impact. When compared to conventional carbon fiber, Bcomp's biocomposites can cut CO_2 emissions by up to 85% from material sourcing through manufacturing (cradle-to-gate). The reduced weight contributes to better fuel efficiency in conventional vehicles and prolongs battery duration in electric cars. Numerous leading automotive brands have embraced these sustainable materials, including the Porsche Cayman 718 GT4 CS MR, Tesla's Model S P100DL racecar (produced by Electric GT), Volvo's XC60 hybrid SUV, and the Polestar Precept. In addition to their lighter weight and reduced carbon footprint, these biocomposites provide practical end-of-life options. Instead of generating waste, they can be repurposed into new materials or utilized for energy recovery from renewable sources. By replacing plastics and carbon fiber, Bcomp's products are contributing to a more sustainable future within the automotive sector (Bcomp, n.d.). Ford has been at the forefront of utilizing sustainable materials in vehicle production since 2000, employing various plant-based fibers and agricultural by-products to minimize plastic usage and foster a circular economy. Currently, eight sustainable materials are featured in Ford vehicles, such as soy foam, castor oil, wheat straw, kenaf fiber, cellulose, wood, coconut fiber, agave, and rice hulls. To build on these initiatives, Ford has formed partnerships and research projects aimed at enhancing the sustainability of its vehicle components. Recently, they are making progress in using waste from olive trees—including branches, twigs, and leaves by combining them with biocomposites to create automobile parts. This effort was inspired by experiments carried out under the COMPOlive project (Ford, n.d.). Several companies are increasingly adopting greener composite materials. GM has recently submitted multiple patent applications for the incorporation of natural fiber composites in vehicle interior elements. Daimler utilizes bast fibers (derived from the phloem, or "inner bark," of plants) combined with Acrodur (a water-based acrylic) resin, sourced from BASF, for the roof structures of their Mercedes-Benz E Class model. Ford is partnering with Heinz (famous for ketchup) to create composites made from tomato peels suitable for various components in upcoming vehicles. Lastly, Toyota supports the development of composites from kenaf (a type of hibiscus) fibers for future automobiles in collaboration with Covestro (Walker, 2024).

Building Construction

Miniwiz, a Taiwan-based company, upcycles waste like PET bottles into construction materials. Its EcoARK Pavilion, built with 1.5 million PET bottles, reduced carbon emissions by 90% in a life cycle assessment (LCA) compared to conventional materials while maintaining durability and insulation. In a similar way, Barzakh presents the UAE's first enduring architecture constructed from waste materials, employing discarded wood and bio-based adhesive, as well as brine—a byproduct of the desalination process—potentially serving as a binder for the coral modules at the Public Art Abu Dhabi Biennial, highlighting the structure with the lowest carbon footprint (Designboom, 2025). Lingrove's Ekoa®, a flax-based biocomposite, replaces plastics and engineered wood. Its carbon-negative LCA highlights reduced deforestation and embodied carbon while ensuring high durability (Lingrove, 2024).

Electronics

Casio is one of the companies effectively employing biocomposites in their commercial products by integrating bio-based resins sourced from castor seeds and corn, reinforced with glass fiber. These eco-friendly materials are utilized in the case, band, and case back of watches such as the PRO TREK series, lowering environmental impact while promoting the principles of a circular economy. This strategy illustrates the real-world use of biocomposites in the consumer electronics sector, striking a balance between durability, performance, and sustainability. The G-Shock G-5600BG showcases an innovative sustainability approach by reusing surplus resin scraps generated from producing other bezels and bands. This design reduces material waste while maintaining the watch's durability and iconic toughness (Casio, n.d.)

Packaging Industry

Ecovative Design, based in New York, develops mycelium-based biocomposites for insulation and biodegradable structures. An LCA of its Mushroom Packaging found that drying processes caused over 50% of emissions, prompting the company to develop an energy-efficient drying method that cut energy use by two-thirds for packing different items such as soaps, perfumes, etc. (Ecovative, n.d.).

8. CHALLENGES ASSOCIATED WITH BIOCOMPOSITES

Biocomposites, which consist of natural fibers and biopolymers, offer an eco-friendly alternative to synthetic, petroleum-derived materials. Nonetheless, their broader acceptance faces numerous challenges that influence their efficacy, market viability, and application scope.

8.1. Material and Structural Challenges

Material Variability

Natural fibers like flax, hemp, jute, and kenaf show considerable differences in their characteristics due to variations in plant species, growing conditions, and extraction techniques. This inconsistency affects the mechanical properties of biocomposites and complicates efforts to maintain quality control.

Moisture Absorption and Durability

The hydrophilic properties of natural fibers lead to significant moisture uptake, which can cause swelling, diminished mechanical characteristics, and potential degradation over time. Research indicates that water absorption may lead to interface failure and matrix embrittlement in biocomposites, limiting their effectiveness in humid conditions.

Compatibility Issues

Establishing strong interfacial bonding between hydrophilic natural fibers and hydrophobic polymer matrices presents challenges. Inadequate adhesion can result in weakened mechanical performance. Chemical treatments like alkalization and silane coupling are used to improve fiber-matrix compatibility.

Biodegradability vs. Longevity

While the environmental benefits of biocomposite biodegradability are clear, concerns arise regarding their long-term stability in applications that demand durability. Finding a balance between biodegradability and longevity remains a significant challenge. Natural fiber composites typically show inferior mechanical properties when compared to synthetic fiber-reinforced composites. The tensile strength and impact resistance of biocomposites are generally less favourable, requiring modifications or hybrid approaches to satisfy specific application needs.

8.2. Manufacturing and Processing Challenges

Processing Constraints

Natural fibers are prone to damage from high temperatures, limiting the processing methods like injection molding or extrusion, that can be utilized. Furthermore, achieving uniform fiber dispersion and orientation during manufacturing is complicated, impacting the final product's consistency.

Cost and Market Competition

Though they are sustainable, biocomposites frequently face higher production costs than traditional composites. The processing and treatment of natural fibers add to overall expenses, making competition with established, cost-effective synthetic composites difficult.

8.3. Environmental and Sustainability Challenges

Recycling and End-of-Life Management

Recycling biocomposites becomes complex when paired with non-biodegradable polymers. To fully harness their environmental advantages, developing effective recycling strategies and infrastructure is crucial.

Standardization and Regulations

The absence of universally accepted standards for biocomposites hampers their industrial adoption. Regulatory differences regarding sustainability claims and biodegradability further hinder commercialization efforts.

8.4. Consumer Perception Challenges

Aesthetic and Functional Perceptions

Consumers often view biobased composites as less attractive and valuable due to their visual and tactile characteristics. Attributes such as beauty, naturality, and value are influenced by these sensory evaluations, which can lead to perceptual incongruities between designers and consumers.

Awareness and Information

There is a general lack of awareness and understanding among consumers about biobased products, which complicates their market access. This lack of information can lead to confusion and skepticism about the environmental benefits of biobased composites (Fletcher, 2022).

Consumer Preferences and Resistance to Change

Users and industries are often reluctant to shift to new materials, particularly when current solutions are effective and widely accepted. To address this resistance, targeted marketing strategies, practical demonstrations of performance, and policy incentives that support the transition to biocomposites are essential.

8.5. Market Challenges

Limited Market Availability and Infrastructure

The restricted availability of production facilities and supply chains for biocomposites inhibits their adoption. In contrast to conventional composites, which have well-established distribution networks, biocomposites need enhanced manufacturing scalability and integration into mainstream markets. Investments from the public and private sectors in biocomposite production infrastructure can assist in overcoming this barrier.

Consumer Preferences and Resistance to Change

Users and industries are often reluctant to shift to new materials, particularly when current solutions are effective and widely accepted. To address this resistance, targeted marketing strategies, practical demonstrations of performance, and policy incentives that support the transition to biocomposites are essential.

Economic and Supply Challenges

High costs and limited availability of biobased composites are major barriers. Consumers are often price-sensitive, and the premium prices of biobased products can deter purchase intentions (Dawson, 2023).

Industry and Consumer Dynamics

Industry stakeholders' express concerns about the potential conflict between food security and the cultivation of feedstock crops for biobased materials. Additionally, there is a preference for drop-in bioplastics over biodegradable options, indicating a need for better alignment between consumer preferences and industry offerings (Molina-Besch & Keszleri, 2022).

9. OPPORTUNITIES FOR INNOVATION

9.1. Process Optimization

Optimizing biocomposite manufacturing processes can significantly enhance both their economic and environmental performance. This involves refining manufacturing techniques to reduce energy consumption and waste generation while improving efficiency (Mujtaba et al., 2023).

Energy-Efficient Processing Techniques

Traditional manufacturing methods for biocomposites can be energy-intensive, requiring high temperatures and long processing times. However, emerging technologies are helping reduce these energy demands. Examples include:

- *Microwave-Assisted Processing*: This technique uses microwave energy to accelerate the curing process of resins, reducing energy consumption and processing time. It is particularly useful for composite materials with complex structures or those requiring precise curing (Nodehi et al., 2022).
- *Enzymatic Fiber Modification*: Enzymatic treatments offer a greener alternative to traditional chemical treatments for natural fibers. These treatments improve fiber adhesion to polymer matrices without the need for harsh chemicals or high temperatures, thereby reducing both environmental impact and energy consumption (Filgueira et al., 2017).
- *Supercritical Fluid Processing*: This involves using supercritical fluids (e.g., carbon dioxide) to extract or modify materials at lower temperatures. Compared to conventional solvents or heat-based methods, this process consumes less energy and produces fewer harmful by-products (Knez et al., 2014). Such innovations hold significant potential for improving biocomposite processing and addressing existing research gaps.

Optimizing Fiber Treatment

Natural fibers such as hemp, flax, and jute require treatment to improve compatibility with synthetic or bio-based polymers (Alamry et al., 2024). Traditional treatments often involve harsh chemicals or mechanical processes, but newer sustainable methods aim to reduce environmental impact while improving fiber properties. Notable innovations include:

- *Coatings*: Coating hemp fibers with bio-based waxes from pine bark has been explored. However, the mechanical improvements were not as pronounced as expected, indicating the need for optimized processing conditions (Abbel et al., 2024). Further research into bio-based coatings and nanocomposite reinforcements could enhance fiber durability while maintaining biodegradability.
- *Coupling Agents*: The use of maleic anhydride (MAH) coupling agents has significantly improved mechanical properties, with increases in tensile strength (35%) and impact strength (20%) observed in treated jute and kenaf fibers (Alamry et al., 2024). Bio-based pyrrole compounds containing sulfur atoms have also been used to functionalize carbon black, improving curing efficiency and mechanical properties in elastomer composites, thereby reducing hysteresis and enhancing dynamic rigidity (Dong et al., 2022).
- *Surface Treatments*: Surface treatments play a crucial role in enhancing the performance of natural fiber-reinforced biocomposites. Tannin-based treatments, such as quebracho tannins with NaOH, improve fiber-matrix adhesion and mechanical properties in flax fiber epoxy composites (Tilouche-Guerdelli et al., 2024). Similarly, sustainable chemicals like sodium bicarbonate and borax enhance the crystallinity, strength, and thermal stability of pineapple leaf fiber composites (Thirumalaisamy et al., 2023). Alkaline and silane treatments enhance interfacial bonding in polyhydroxyalkanoate-based biocomposites, reducing water uptake in Aloe Vera fibers (Komal & Singh, 2022). Additionally, cellulose modified with diisocyanates (MDI, TDI) improves hydrophobicity and mechanical strength (Hejna et al., 2023). Biological and physical treatments offer eco-friendly alternatives. These strategies collectively enhance durability, strength, and sustainability in biocomposites.

Waste Utilization in Biocomposite Manufacturing

The use of agricultural and industrial waste residues as sustainable feedstock for biocomposites reduces reliance on virgin materials and contributes to a circular economy (Phiri et al., 2023).

Development of Bio-Based Resins

A major challenge for biocomposites is their reliance on petroleum-derived resins. Transitioning to bio-based resins improves the environmental footprint of biocomposites while enhancing sustainability by reducing dependence on fossil fuels. Notable advancements include:

- *Lignin-Based Resins*: Lignin, a complex polymer found in plant cell walls and a by-product of the pulp and paper industry, is being explored as a bio-based alternative to petroleum-derived resins. Its renewable nature and potential to provide strong mechanical properties make it suitable for applications in automotive parts and construction materials (Lu & Gu, 2023).
- *Starch and Protein-Based Resins*: Derived from natural sources such as corn starch and soy protein, these resins offer biodegradable and renewable alternatives to synthetic resins. Starch-based resins are particularly useful in packaging and disposable products, while protein-based resins, made from soy or wheat gluten, provide mechanical properties comparable to synthetic resins (Mekonnen et al., 2015).
- *Fungal Mycelium*: Mycelium, the root structure of fungi, is gaining attention as a biodegradable, renewable matrix material for biocomposites. It can grow in molds to form lightweight and strong composite structures suitable for applications in packaging, construction, and furniture (Elsacker et al., 2020).

9.2. Advanced Recycling and Upcycling Technologies

As biocomposites gain popularity, addressing their end-of-life (EOL) options is crucial for ensuring long-term sustainability. Advanced recycling and upcycling technologies extend their lifecycle and minimize environmental impact. Several types of advanced recycling techniques are being employed for overall enhancing the circular economy of the biocomposites (Table 5).

Table 5. Advanced recycling methods for biocomposites

Recycling Method	Description	Inference
Mechanical Recycling	Shredding, grinding, and reprocessing biocomposites into reusable materials.	Cost-effective, retains fiber integrity, and enables closed-loop recycling.
Pyrolysis	Thermal decomposition in an oxygen-free environment to produce bio-oil, syngas, and biochar.	Generates renewable energy, reduces landfill waste, and recovers valuable by-products.
Hydrothermal Carbonization	Uses superheated water to convert waste into hydrochar.	Enhances carbon sequestration and produces valuable fuel alternatives.
Gasification	Converts composite waste into synthetic gas (syngas) for energy production.	High energy recovery potential and reduces dependency on fossil fuels.
Solvolysis	Chemical dissolution of polymer matrices to recover fibers.	Allows selective fiber recovery and enables high-value recycling of hybrid composites.
Enzymatic Depolymerization	Uses enzymes to break down biodegradable polymers and fibers.	Eco-friendly, selective decomposition, and supports circular economy.
Depolymerization & Monomer Recovery	Breaks down composite matrices into base monomers for repolymerization.	Enables high-purity recycling and extends material lifespan.
Microbial Biodegradation	Uses bacteria and fungi to decompose biocomposites naturally.	Low-energy process, sustainable, and ideal for fully biodegradable materials.
Vermicomposting	Employs earthworms to degrade biodegradable biocomposites into organic compost.	Promotes soil health, waste-to-nutrient conversion, and supports agricultural applications.
Selective Fiber Recovery	Ultrasonic and chemical separation of fibers in hybrid composites.	Preserves fiber properties for reuse in advanced applications.
Smart Self-Healing Materials	Development of reversible-bond composites that can be repaired or reprocessed multiple times.	Enhances material durability and minimizes waste generation.
Additive Manufacturing (3D Printing)	Uses recycled biocomposite materials for 3D printing applications.	Supports customized production and reduces material wastage.

In recent years, several closed-loop recycling systems have been implemented to recover and reuse materials while maintaining their quality. For example, biocomposites made from epoxidized waste flour and recycled carbon fibers can be efficiently recycled using non-toxic solvents, which preserve fiber integrity and facilitate matrix reuse (Ferjan et al., 2023). Advanced recycling technologies, such as solvolysis and pyrolysis, also present viable end-of-life solutions for biocomposites in industries like aviation (Vu et al., 2022).

Recycling of Hybrid Biocomposites

The management of hybrid biocomposites composed of natural fibers combined with synthetic polymers poses notable difficulties at the end of their life cycle due to their intricate structure. The incompatibility of these materials complicates their separation and recycling, as distinct processing methods are often required for various components. Although natural fibers are biodegradable, the durability of synthetic matrices diminishes the overall ecological advantages. Moreover, the lack of standardized recycling methods for such heterogeneous materials obstructs effective waste management. Conventional recycling techniques, including mechanical and thermal processes, may damage natural fibers, restricting their opportunity for reuse. Additionally, the inclusion of additives and crosslinking agents raises further barriers to recyclability and may emit harmful substances during the recycling process. Tackling these issues necessitates improvements in mixed-material recovery approaches and the creation of more sustainable alternatives.

To enhance the recyclability of hybrid biocomposites, researchers are investigating bio-based resins to improve biodegradability. Techniques like selective solvent dissolution allow for the extraction of polymer components while maintaining the integrity of natural fibers. For example, Zhao et al. (2023) established a method for recycling carbon-fiber-reinforced bismaleimide resin composites using monoethanolamine solvent, resulting in considerable recovery of fibers. Likewise, enzymatic and microbial degradation methods are being explored more eco-friendly waste disposal option by selectively breaking down biocomposite matrices. Thermochemical recycling processes, such as pyrolysis, can reclaim valuable materials from hybrid composites, although they often require a significant amount of energy. Ferjan et al. (2023) emphasized the potential of these methods despite their high energy consumption. At the same time, manufacturers are adopting closed-loop systems to simplify disassembly and material separation, thus improving recycling efficiency. Kamble and Behera (2021) created sustainable hybrid composites reinforced with textile waste for use in construction, thereby advocating for the repurposing of waste into new products. Innovations in end-of-life management are pivotal for enhancing the sustainability of hybrid biocomposites. Future developments in material science, recycling infrastructure, and policy initiatives will further solidify their position in a circular economy. Xu et al. (2019) showcased advances in this domain by crafting self-healing and recyclable epoxidized natural rubber/carboxymethyl chitosan biobased composites featuring hydrogen bonding supramolecular hybrid networks, which displayed improved mechanical properties and recyclability. The ongoing progression of sustainable approaches for hybrid biocomposite recycling will be vital in mitigating environmental impacts and fostering circularity. Continuous research and policy advocacy will be essential to ensure that these materials effectively contribute to a more sustainable future.

Factors Affecting the Recycling of Biocomposites

Recycling of composites, including biocomposites, is affected by a variety of interrelated elements, such as policy, financial, technical, material, chemical, and market factors. Legislative frameworks are essential for promoting biocomposite recycling by enacting practical laws and updating product and technology certification criteria to improve recyclability (Figure 5). Financial motivation is another key driver in this area, as lowering recycling process costs and boosting investment opportunities can lead industries to embrace sustainable waste management practices. Advancements in technology are vital for enhancing the efficiency of biocomposite recycling. An effective collection and distribution system, along with the incorporation of recycling and reuse concepts in product design, can greatly improve the sustainability of biocomposites. Additionally, the accessibility of scrap materials and accurate documentation of material management processes are essential in ensuring a reliable supply of recyclable inputs and streamlining the recycling procedure. Chemical aspects are also crucial for biocomposite recycling. Reducing the complexity of product compositions by decreasing the variety of materials used can make recycling easier, while incorporating certain chemical additives can improve the efficiency of material separation and recovery. From a market standpoint, it is important that recycled biocomposites remain cost-competitive with virgin materials and retain their quality to encourage broad industry acceptance. A comprehensive approach addressing these factors through policy encouragement, financial incentives, technological advancements, and market-driven strategies can support the transition to a circular economy for biocomposites, minimizing environmental impacts while fostering sustainable material utilization.

Innovation in biocomposites through energy-efficient processing, waste utilization, bio-based resins, and advanced recycling improves environmental performance. LCA plays a crucial role in quantifying sustainability benefits, highlighting reductions in carbon emissions, energy use, and waste generation. Future research should focus on:

- Expanding LCA datasets for different biocomposite applications.
- Improving closed-loop recycling technologies.
- Developing standardized LCA methodologies for biocomposites.
- Enhancing market acceptance through policy and consumer education.

By integrating LCA insights into biocomposite development, industries can accelerate the transition toward sustainable materials and circular economy models.

Figure 5. Factors affecting composite recycling (Adapted from "Circular Economy in Biocomposite Development: State-of-the-Art, Challenges and Emerging Trends," by Shanmugam et al., 2021, Composites Part C: Open Access, 5, 100138. © 2021 by Elsevier)

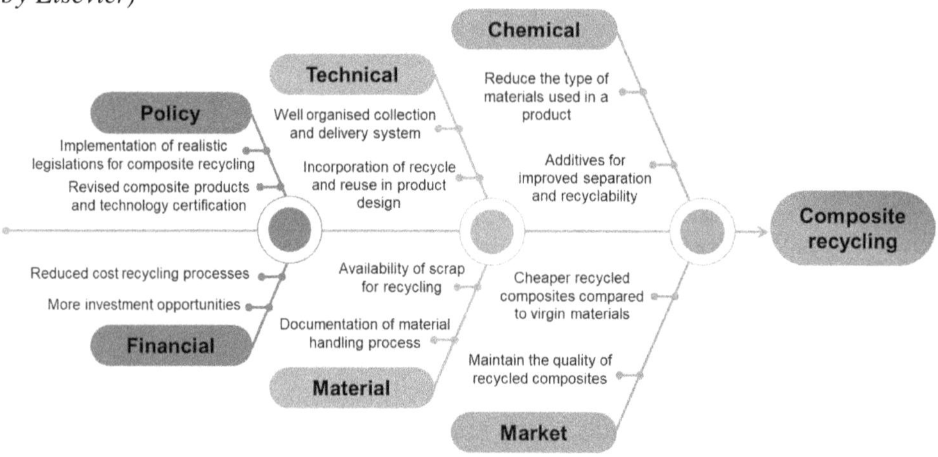

10. POLICY IMPLICATIONS

Promotion of Sustainable Materials and Regulatory Frameworks

To ensure long-term sustainability, policies should encourage the use of renewable resources, streamline regulatory procedures, and establish clear oversight mechanisms to facilitate the market entry of biocomposite products. Encouraging the use of biomass and industrial waste as raw materials can significantly reduce dependence on non-renewable resources (Rylko-Polak et al., 2022). Additionally, supporting the development of biodegradable polymers derived from natural fibers can offer sustainable alternatives to conventional materials in construction and other industries (Yazdi et al., 2014). Simplifying approval processes to minimize delays and costs associated with commercialization is essential, as is establishing a single coordinating agency responsible for overseeing biocomposite regulations to ensure clarity and efficiency (Coons, 2023). Currently following certification standards are being exclusively used for ensuring the overall sustainability of biocomposites (Table 6).

Table 6. Certifications for LCA studies in different countries and globally

Region/ Country	Certification Program	Year of Release	Description
Germany	Blue Angel	1978	Oldest eco-label, requiring comprehensive LCA analysis for certification.
Canada	Environmental Choice Program (EcoLogo)	1988	Recognizes products with verified LCA sustainability data.
Nordic Countries	Nordic Swan Ecolabel	1989	Requires LCA-based evaluation for product sustainability and environmental impact.
Japan	Eco Mark	1989	Certifies products with low environmental impact, based on LCA results.
France	NF Environnement	1991	French eco-label requiring LCA to validate environmental claims.
European Union	EU Ecolabel	1992	Recognizes products with lower environmental impact, requiring LCA assessments.
China	China Environmental Labelling	1993	Requires LCA data for assessing environmental impact and energy efficiency.
Australia	GECA (Good Environmental Choice)	2000	Requires full LCA-based assessment for sustainable product certification.
United States	USDA BioPreferred	2002	Certifies biobased products, integrating LCA metrics for sustainability.
Global	ISO 14040/14044	2006	International standard for LCA principles and framework.
European Union	European Blue Deal	2019	A sustainability initiative promoting circular economy and LCA-based environmental performance.

To strengthen LCA-based certifications for biocomposites, a unified international framework should be established, integrating standardized LCA metrics in collaboration with regulatory bodies. Mandatory third-party LCA reporting must be enforced to ensure transparency and comparability, supported by digital labelling for consumer awareness. Existing eco-labeling programs such as EU Ecolabel and USDA BioPreferred should incorporate stricter LCA-based impact assessments, prioritizing sustainability indicators like carbon footprint and recyclability. Industry compliance should be incentivized through tax benefits, government procurement preferences, and R&D funding. Consumer engagement can be enhanced through education campaigns and interactive certification databases to promote informed decision-making. Cross-border recognition of LCA certifications and international collaboration will facilitate market expansion and policy harmonization. Periodic updates to certification standards should integrate advancements in sustainability assessment methodologies, ensuring continuous improvement and alignment with global sustainability goals.

Life Cycle Assessment (LCA) is essential for obtaining eco-certifications such as LEED (Leadership in Energy and Environmental Design), Environmental Product Declarations (EPDs), and ISO 14040, as it provides a scientific basis for measuring and reducing environmental impacts. In LEED certification, LCA is used to earn credits in categories like Materials and Resources (MR) and Energy and Atmosphere (EA) by assessing the environmental footprint of construction materials and optimizing whole-building energy performance. Products with third-party verified EPDs, which rely on LCA data, contribute to LEED credits by providing transparent impact assessments, helping architects and developers select low-carbon alternatives like engineered wood, recycled concrete, or energy-efficient insulation. Similarly, EPDs, following ISO 14025 standards, allow manufacturers to communicate a product's environmental footprint based on LCA results, facilitating informed material choices and regulatory compliance. Industries such as construction, automotive, and electronics use EPDs to improve supply chain transparency, carbon footprint reduction, and regulatory compliance with the EU Green Deal and sustainable procurement policies. Additionally, ISO 14040 and ISO 14044 set the global framework for conducting LCA, ensuring consistency in impact assessment methodologies across industries. These standards are widely applied in environmental management systems, helping companies evaluate the sustainability of their products and processes while aligning with international regulations like the EU Ecodesign Directive. Ultimately, LCA-driven certifications promote sustainability by guiding material selection, optimizing resource efficiency, and ensuring that businesses meet environmental performance benchmarks, making them more competitive in an increasingly eco-conscious market.

Inclusion of Closed-Loop Systems

Biocomposites should be designed with sustainability as a priority, ensuring they can be easily disassembled and recycled to facilitate the recovery of fibers and resins for reuse in new products. In a closed-loop system, these materials can be recycled or upcycled at the end of their useful life, which reduces the consumption of new raw materials and improves resource efficiency (John & Thomas, 2023). By incorporating end-of-life recovery considerations into the design phase, manufacturers can optimize material reclamation, making it easier to reclaim and reuse raw materials for new biocomposite production. This approach minimizes reliance on virgin resources and helps mitigate resource depletion. The widespread adoption of biocomposites across various industries necessitates a robust policy framework to enhance sustainability and reduce environmental impact. Effective policies should focus on promoting the use of renewable resources, improving waste management practices, and fostering innovation in biocomposite technologies. The following key recommendations outline essential policy measures to drive the sustainable development of biocomposites.

Investment in Research and Development

A strong emphasis on research and innovation is crucial for enhancing biocomposite performance and expanding their applications. Expanding financial support for research in biocomposite technologies, with a focus on improving material properties and broadening industrial applications, is a key priority. Public-private partnerships can further foster collaborations between government entities, academia, and industry, driving innovation and accelerating market readiness. Despite these proactive measures, challenges such as high initial investments and lengthy commercialization timelines persist. Addressing these issues is critical for maximizing the benefits of biocomposite technologies (Patel et al., 2021; Nagaraju, 2022)

Targeted Policy Actions

The following targeted policy actions can further facilitate this transition:

- **Incentives for Sustainable Materials Development**: Governments can play a pivotal role in accelerating the adoption of bio-based materials through financial and structural incentives. Implementing grants, tax credits, and subsidies can offset the higher initial costs associated with bio-based materials, making them more competitive with conventional alternatives (Cai et al., 2024; Cosentino et al., 2024). Additionally, supporting research to enhance key properties such as thermal conductivity and mechanical strength can increase the commercial viability of biocomposites.
- **Guidelines for Industry and Policymakers**: Establishing standardised benchmarks and certification mechanisms can enhance industry-wide sustainability practices. Developing clear guidelines to define sustainable practices, including responsible sourcing of raw materials and ethical labour standards, is essential. Governments can collaborate with certification bodies to introduce sustainability labels, enabling consumers to identify environmentally friendly biocomposite products (Ersus et al., 2020). These certifications serve as strong incentives for manufacturers to adopt sustainable practices.
- **Legislation on End-of-Life Management**: The responsible disposal and recycling of biocomposite products at the end of their life cycle is a critical concern. Governments should introduce legislation mandating environmentally responsible waste management. Policies such as Extended Producer Responsibility (EPR) can require manufacturers to take responsibility for the

disposal and recycling of their products, promoting the design of biocomposites with end-of-life considerations in mind. This approach reduces landfill waste and encourages the adoption of biodegradable or recyclable materials. Legislative models such as the European and German Packaging Directives provide a structured approach for material recovery in biodegradable packaging, which can be extended to biocomposites (Manthey, 2013). Such regulations can integrate biocomposites into existing waste management systems, ensuring a circular economy approach.

10. FUTURE RESEARCH IMPLICATIONS

While progress has been made, further research is needed to enhance the environmental performance and sustainability of biocomposites. Focusing on key areas can improve the LCA outcomes and expand the application of biocomposites across different industries.

Biodegradability Enhancements

Biocomposites are generally considered more environmentally friendly than traditional composites because they are derived from renewable resources and can be biodegradable. However, some biocomposites may not degrade as efficiently as desired. Research into enhancing biodegradability through the development of additives or processing techniques can address this challenge.

- *Additives for Enhanced Degradation*: Biodegradable additives, such as natural enzymes or biopolymers, could be incorporated into biocomposites to accelerate their breakdown when exposed to environmental factors like moisture, heat, or microbial activity. This would improve the overall environmental impact by reducing waste and preventing long-term pollution (Goni-Ciaurriz et al., 2022)
- *Processing Techniques for Improved Degradability*: Adjusting the processing conditions (e.g., temperature, moisture content, and pressure) or modifying the composite structure can improve the ease with which biocomposites degrade. Research is needed to determine the most effective techniques that balance performance and biodegradability (Samarajeewa, 2022).

Advanced Biomaterials

Emerging biomaterials in biocomposites are revolutionizing sustainable material development by enhancing mechanical properties, biodegradability, and functionality. Nano lignin-based composites, incorporating lignin nanoparticles (LNPs), improve mechanical strength, thermal stability, and water resistance, making them ideal for epoxy polymers, bioadhesives, and coatings. Similarly, nanocellulose-based composites offer a high strength-to-weight ratio and excellent barrier properties, reinforcing thermoplastic polyurethane and biodegradable films for applications in packaging and sustainable materials. Algal-based nanocomposites utilize algal biomass and biochar to enhance mechanical performance in biodegradable plastics and cementitious materials, contributing to eco-friendly alternatives in construction and packaging. Additionally, mycelium-based composites leverage fungal mycelium and agricultural waste to create strong, lightweight, and fully biodegradable materials suited for packaging and insulation. MXene-based biocomposites, incorporating two-dimensional nanomaterials, provide high electrical conductivity and thermal stability, offering potential applications in energy storage and electronics. Polyhydroxyalkanoate (PHA) composites, derived from microbial sources, are reinforced with nanofillers such as graphene to enhance thermal stability and mechanical properties for use in biomedical devices and packaging. Furthermore, advancements in additive manufacturing, such as 3D printing with biocomposites, enable the fabrication of complex structures with self-healing and adaptive properties, broadening their applications in sustainable architecture and product design. Collectively, these innovations are driving the next generation of biocomposites, improving performance while reducing environmental impact across various industries.

Integration of AI in LCA Modelling

Life cycle assessments for biocomposites can be complex due to the large number of variables involved, from raw material sourcing to end-of-life disposal. Integrating artificial intelligence (AI) and machine learning (ML) into LCA models can help analyze large datasets and identify patterns or correlations in environmental performance using different techniques (Figure 6). In the definition of goals and scope, AI simplifies literature reviews and refines system boundaries. For Life Cycle Inventory (LCI), AI facilitates automated data gathering, addresses gaps, and allows for real-time monitoring through integration with IoT. Predictive Modelling for Impact Assessment involves the integration of AI and machine learning into LCA models to handle complex datasets and identify patterns in environmental performance. This can facilitate the development of predictive models that forecast the environmental impact of new biocomposite formulations or manufacturing processes. AI-enhanced models improve Life Cycle Impact Assessment (LCIA) by forecasting environmental effects, optimizing material choices, and enhancing uncertainty evaluations. In the realms of interpretation and optimization, AI pinpoints critical areas, suggests eco-design approaches, and aids in making sustainable decisions. The advantages of comparative LCA are amplified by AI's capability to model scenarios, evaluate trends, and predict the performance of biocomposites. AI also plays a role in end-of-life assessments by streamlining waste management and promoting circular economy initiatives. When integrated into LCA software such as SimaPro and OpenLCA, AI boosts data processing and transparency, rendering LCA more effective and trustworthy for the sustainable development of biocomposites (Samarajeewa, 2022). One Click LCA is a widely used AI-powered, cloud-based platform that integrates with Building Information Modelling (BIM) and sustainability criteria while ensuring compliance with industry certifications.

Figure 6. Different AI and ML techniques used for LCA of biocomposites

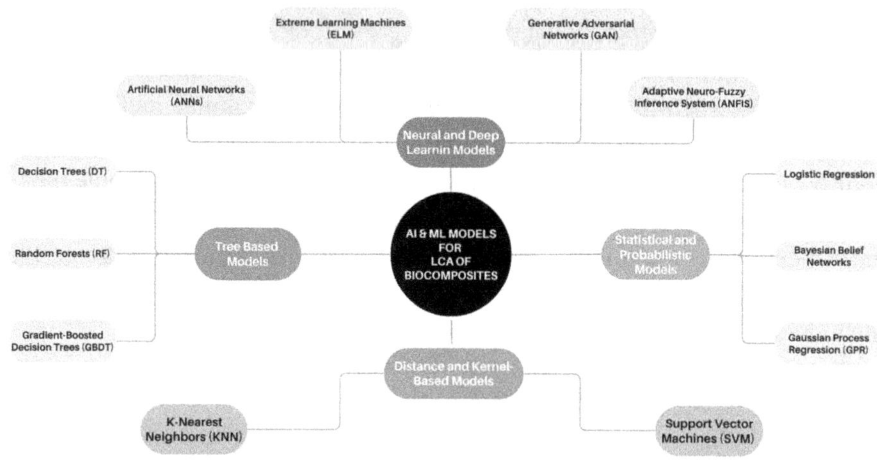

Enhancing Collaborative Efforts Between Academia and Industry

Collaboration between academic researchers and industry stakeholders is essential for translating theoretical advancements into practical, market-ready solutions. By fostering closer ties between researchers, product designers, and manufacturers, the development and commercialization of sustainable biocomposites can be accelerated.

- **Knowledge Transfer and Innovation Ecosystems**: Establishing innovation ecosystems that encourage the exchange of knowledge between academia, industry, and government can stimulate the development of new technologies, business models, and policy frameworks. This collaborative approach can lead to a more rapid adoption of sustainable biocomposites across various sectors (Muller, 2023).
- **Effective Knowledge Transfer**: Successful academia-industry collaborations depend on efficient knowledge transfer mechanisms. Current methods often face challenges such as differing goals and timelines, which can hinder the integration of academic research into industry practices (Rossoni et al., 2023).
- **Barriers and Facilitators**: Common barriers to collaboration include cultural differences, lack of joint platforms, and misaligned objectives between academia and industry (Fortunato et al., 2023). Facilitators include fostering relational social capital, providing tax incentives, and initiating smaller projects to gradually build complexity (Ursic et al., 2022).

Transparent Communication of LCA Results

To maximize the impact of Life Cycle Assessment (LCA) in promoting sustainability, it is essential to ensure clear, accessible, and transparent communication of LCA results to both consumers and policymakers. Standardized reporting formats, easily understandable environmental labels, and digital tools such as QR codes linking to detailed LCA reports can help bridge the gap between scientific assessments and public awareness. Transparency in LCA findings enables informed decision-making, fosters consumer trust, and encourages the adoption of sustainable products and policies.

11. CONCLUSION

The findings of this chapter emphasize the crucial role of including LCA studies to evaluate the sustainability of biocomposites. By systematically analyzing environmental impacts arising from the extraction of raw materials to the ultimate disposal, LCA provides a comprehensive framework useful in decision making process. While biocomposites offer advantages such as a reduced carbon footprint and reliance on renewable resources, challenges remain concerning data availability, method standardization, and end-of-life management. Future advancements should focus on enhancing biodegradability, utilizing artificial intelligence for improved LCA modeling, and fostering stronger collaboration between academia and industry. Additionally, refining production techniques, increasing energy efficiency, and developing innovative recycling methods can further enhance the sustainability of biocomposites. Addressing these issues will not only improve environmental impact but also support the wider adoption of biocomposites among different industries. Ultimately, a holistic approach that integrates technological innovations with sustainable policy frameworks plays a crucial role in enhancing the long-term sustainability of biocomposite materials. Future research should focus on harmonizing LCA databases for biocomposites and integrating circular economy principles to enhance sustainability assessments.

REFERENCES

Abbel, R., Risani, R., Nourtier, M., Donaldson, L., Brunschwig, C., Mayer-Laigle, C., Bridson, J. H., Thumm, A., Dickson, A., Murray, R., Harris, J., Beaugrand, J., & Hill, S. (2024). Coating of Hemp Fibres with Hydrophobic Compounds Extracted from Pine Bark. *Fibers (Basel, Switzerland)*, *12*(11), 96. DOI: 10.3390/fib12110096

Ahmad, H., Chhipi-Shrestha, G., Hewage, K., & Sadiq, R. (2022). A comprehensive review on construction applications and life cycle sustainability of natural fiber biocomposites. *Sustainability (Basel)*, *14*(23), 15905. DOI: 10.3390/su142315905

Akras, L., Silvenius, F., Baniasadi, H., Vahvaselkä, M., Ilvesniemi, H., & Seppälä, J. (2024). A cradle-to-gate life cycle assessment of polyamide-starch biocomposites: Carbon footprint as an indicator of sustainability. *Clean Technologies and Environmental Policy*, *26*(10), 3297–3312. DOI: 10.1007/s10098-024-02884-1

Alamry, A., & Islam, M. S., Hamdan, S., & Abdullah, M. (2024). Enhancing the performance of hybrid biocomposites reinforced with natural fibers by using coupling agents. *Materials Research Express*. Advance online publication. DOI: 10.1088/2053-1591/ad92f4

Ali, S. S., Elsamahy, T., Abdelkarim, E. A., Al-Tohamy, R., Kornaros, M., Ruiz, H. A., Zhao, T., Li, F., & Sun, J. (2022). Biowastes for biodegradable bioplastics production and end-of-life scenarios in circular bioeconomy and biorefinery concept. *Bioresource Technology*, *363*, 127869. DOI: 10.1016/j.biortech.2022.127869 PMID: 36064080

Amponsah, L., Chuck, C., & Parsons, S. (2024). Life cycle assessment of a marine biorefinery producing protein, bioactives and polymeric packaging material. *The International Journal of Life Cycle Assessment*, *29*(2), 174–191. DOI: 10.1007/s11367-023-02239-w

Andrew, J. J., & Dhakal, H. (2021). Sustainable biobased composites for advanced applications: Recent trends and future opportunities – A critical review. *Composites Part C Open Access*, *7*, 100220. DOI: 10.1016/j.jcomc.2021.100220

Aybar, D. M. R., Biswas, W., & John, M. (2025). Development of a Life Cycle Sustainability Assessment Framework for Hemp-Based Building Materials in Australia. *Advances in Environmental and Engineering Research*, *6*(1), 1–34. DOI: 10.21926/aeer.2501014

Bcomp. (n.d.). Bcomp. https://www.bcomp.com/sustainability/

Beckstrom, B. D., Wilson, M. H., Crocker, M., & Quinn, J. C. (2020). Bioplastic feedstock production from microalgae with fuel co-products: A techno-economic and life cycle impact assessment. *Algal Research*, *46*, 101769. DOI: 10.1016/j.algal.2019.101769

Bouillass, G., Blanc, I., & Perez-Lopez, P. (2021). Step-by-step social life cycle assessment framework: A participatory approach for the identification and prioritization of impact subcategories applied to mobility scenarios. *The International Journal of Life Cycle Assessment*, *26*(12), 2408–2435. DOI: 10.1007/s11367-021-01988-w

Bouman, L., Spuhler, D., Bünzli, M.-A., Melad, A., Diop, L., Coelho, O., & Meierhofer, R. (2024). The water flow diagram. *Frontiers in Water*, *6*. Advance online publication. DOI: 10.3389/fwater.2024.000001

Broeren, M. L., Kuling, L., Worrell, E., & Shen, L. (2017). Environmental impact assessment of six starch plastics focusing on wastewater-derived starch and additives. *Resources, Conservation and Recycling*, *127*, 246–255. DOI: 10.1016/j.resconrec.2017.09.001

Cai, S., Zhang, X., Zhang, C., Pan, Z., Zhang, C., & Zhao, Y. (2024). Development of bio-based flexible phase change materials utilizing lauric acid for battery thermal management systems. *Journal of Energy Storage*, *86*, 111382. Advance online publication. DOI: 10.1016/j.est.2024.111382

Calado, E. A., Leite, M., & Silva, A. (2018). Selecting composite materials considering cost and environmental impact in the early phases of aircraft structure design. *Journal of Cleaner Production*, *186*, 113–122. DOI: 10.1016/j.jclepro.2018.02.048

Casio. (n.d.). CASIO Official Website. https://www.casio.com/intl/watches/sustainability/material/

Castillo, M. D. A., Garrido-Soriano, N., Casadesus, M., Maçanàs, J., Molins-Duran, G., & Carrillo-Navarrete, F. (2022). Environmental impact of chicken feather-based polypropylene composites developed for automotive and stationary applications and comparison with glass-fibre analogues. *Waste and Biomass Valorization*, *13*(11), 4585–4598. DOI: 10.1007/s12649-022-01810-0

Chalermthai, B., Nootong, K., Olsen, B. D., Assabumrungrat, S., & Charoensuppanimit, P. (2024). Cradle-to-gate life cycle assessment of *Spirulina* bioplastic produced via plasticization with glycerol. *Environmental Research*, *251*, 118622. DOI: 10.1016/j.envres.2024.118622 PMID: 38442816

Chen, W., Oldfield, T. L., Cinelli, P., Righetti, M. C., & Holden, N. M. (2020). Hybrid life cycle assessment of potato pulp valorisation in biocomposite production. *Journal of Cleaner Production*, *269*, 122366. DOI: 10.1016/j.jclepro.2020.122366

Cherubini, F., Strømman, A. H., & Ulgiati, S. (2011). Influence of allocation methods on the environmental performance of biorefinery products—A case study. *Resources, Conservation and Recycling*, *55*(11), 1070–1077. DOI: 10.1016/j.resconrec.2011.06.001

Coltelli, M. B., Morganti, P., & Lazzeri, A. (2023). Sustainability assessment, environmental impact, and recycling strategies of biodegradable polymer nanocomposites. In *Biodegradable and Biocompatible Polymer Nanocomposites* (pp. 699–737). Elsevier., DOI: 10.1016/B978-0-323-91696-7.00016-7

Coons, R. (2023). Developing Supportive Bioeconomy Policies. [editorial]. *Industrial Biotechnology (New Rochelle, N.Y.)*, *19*(2), 35–36. DOI: 10.1089/ind.2023.29310.editorial

Cosentino, L., Fernandes, J. E. P., & Mateus, R. (2024). Fast-Growing Bio-Based Construction Materials as an Approach to Accelerate United Nations Sustainable Development Goals. *Applied Sciences (Basel, Switzerland)*, *14*(11), 4850. DOI: 10.3390/app14114850

David, G., Croxatto Vega, G., Sohn, J., Nilsson, A. E., Hélias, A., Gontard, N., & Angellier-Coussy, H. (2021). Using life cycle assessment to quantify the environmental benefit of upcycling vine shoots as fillers in biocomposite packaging materials. *The International Journal of Life Cycle Assessment*, *26*(4), 738–752. DOI: 10.1007/s11367-020-01824-7

Dawson, S. (2023). Social Perspectives towards Biobased Products and Textiles. *Sustainability (Basel)*, *15*(3), 2284. DOI: 10.3390/su15032284

Deng, Y., Paraskevas, D., Tian, Y., Van Acker, K., Dewulf, W., & Duflou, J. R. (2016). Life cycle assessment of flax-fiber reinforced epoxidized linseed oil composite with a flame retardant for electronic applications. *Journal of Cleaner Production*, *133*, 427–438. DOI: 10.1016/j.jclepro.2016.05.172

Designboom. (2025, January 21). *wael al awar on reclaiming brine for a new sustainable vernacular at public art abu dhabi*. Designboom | Architecture & Design Magazine. https://www.designboom.com/architecture/wael-al-awar-reclaiming-brine-sustainable-vernacular-public-art-abu-dhabi-interview-12-20-2024/

Dong, J., Su, Y., Jiang, T., Li, D., & Ma, X. (2022). Insight into the complex coupling agents on thermal, mechanical, and barrier properties of lignin-poly(3-hydroxybutyrate-co-3-hydroxyhexanoate) biocomposites. *Polymer Composites*, *43*(4), 2431–2439. DOI: 10.1002/pc.26552

Ead, A. S., Appel, R., Alex, N., Ayranci, C., & Carey, J. P. (2021). Life cycle analysis for green composites: A review of literature including considerations for local and global agricultural use. *Journal of Engineered Fibers and Fabrics*, *16*, 15589250211026940. Advance online publication. DOI: 10.1177/15589250211026940

Ecovative. (n.d.). Mushroom Packaging. https://mushroompackaging.com/pages/about?srsltid=AfmBOooFArkwaZD4DbNVkJaR5ddVJ9RxyfddsMwS_yYod51GeohvJf7S

Elmasry, A., Azoti, W., Ghoniem, E., & Elmarakbi, A. (2024). Modelling of hybrid biocomposites for automotive structural applications. *Composites Science and Technology*, *251*, 110562. Advance online publication. DOI: 10.1016/j.compscitech.2024.110562

Elsacker, E., Vandelook, S., Van Wylick, A., Ruytinx, J., De Laet, L., & Peeters, E. (2020). A comprehensive framework for the production of mycelium-based lignocellulosic composites. *The Science of the Total Environment*, *725*, 138431. DOI: 10.1016/j.scitotenv.2020.138431 PMID: 32298897

Ersus, S., Yalçin Melikoglu, A., & Cesur, S. (2020). Production of Biocomposite Packaging Materials from Fruit Juice Processing Wastes. *Journal of the Institute of Science and Technology*, *10*(1), 250–259. DOI: 10.21597/jist.528965

Ferjan, Š., Jovičić, M., Lardiés Miazza, N., Ligthart, T., Harvey, C., Fita, S., Mehta, R., & Samani, P. (2023). Sustainability Assessment of the End-of-Life Technologies for Biocomposite Waste in the Aviation Industry. *Polymers*, *15*(12), 2689. DOI: 10.3390/polym15122689 PMID: 37376334

Ferjan, S., Lardiss Miazza, N., Ligthart, T. N., Fita, S., & Samani, P. (2023). Sustainability Assessment of the End-of-Life Technologies for Biocomposite Waste in the Aviation Industry. *Polymers*, *15*(12), 2689. DOI: 10.3390/polym15122689 PMID: 37376334

Ferronato, N., Alarcón, G. P. P., Lizarazu, E. G. G., & Torretta, V. (2021). Assessment of municipal solid waste collection in Bolivia: Perspectives for avoiding uncontrolled disposal and boosting waste recycling options. *Resources, Conservation and Recycling*, *167*, 105234. DOI: 10.1016/j.resconrec.2020.105234

Filgueira, D., Holmen, S., Melbø, J. K., Moldes, D., Echtermeyer, A. T., & Chinga-Carrasco, G. (2017). Enzymatic-Assisted Modification of Thermomechanical Pulp Fibers To Improve the Interfacial Adhesion with Poly(lactic acid) for 3D Printing. *ACS Sustainable Chemistry & Engineering*, *5*(10), 9338–9346. DOI: 10.1021/acssuschemeng.7b02351

Fitzgerald, A., Proud, W., Kandemir, A., Murphy, R. J., Jesson, D. A., Trask, R. S., Hamerton, I., & Longana, M. L. (2021). A life cycle engineering perspective on biocomposites as a solution for a sustainable recovery. *Sustainability (Basel)*, *13*(3), 1160. DOI: 10.3390/su13031160

Fletcher, C. (2022). Is the consumer experience creating barriers for the effective uptake and disposal of bioplastics? *Clean Technologies and Recycling*, *2*(4), 308–320. DOI: 10.3934/ctr.2022016

Ford (n.d.).*Finding Sustainability in Surprising Places.* https://corporate.ford.com/

Fortunato, E., Jimenez Saez, F., & Hontoria, E. (2023). Can Industry Counteract the Ecological Crisis? An Approach for the Development of a New Circular Bio-economic Model Based on Biocomposite Materials. *Sustainability (Basel)*, *15*(4), 3382. DOI: 10.3390/su15043382

Gkoloni, N., Golonis, C., & Kostopoulos, V. (2022). Integration of LCA and LCC for decision making in biocomposite production. *IOP Conference Series, 1123*(1), 012071. DOI: 10.1088/1755-1315/1123/1/012071

Gomez-Campos, A., Vialle, C., Rouilly, A., Sablayrolles, C., & Hamelin, L. (2020). Flax fiber for technical textile: A life cycle inventory. *Journal of Cleaner Production*, *281*, 125177. DOI: 10.1016/j.jclepro.2020.125177

Goni-Ciaurriz, L., Durán, A., Penas, F. J., & Velaz, I. (2022). Enhanced biodegradation of polylactic acid and cellulose acetate nanocomposites in wastewater: Effect of TiO2 and β-cyclodextrin. *Research Square(Research Square).* DOI: 10.21203/rs.3.rs-2064652/v1

Heidari, M. D., Lawrence, M., Blanchet, P., & Amor, B. (2019). Regionalised life cycle assessment of bio-based materials in construction; the case of hemp shiv treated with sol-gel coatings. *Materials (Basel)*, *12*(18), 2987. DOI: 10.3390/ma12182987 PMID: 31540180

Hejna, A., Barczewski, M., Kosmela, P., Mysiukiewicz, O., Tercjak, A., Piasecki, A., Saeb, M. R., & Szostak, M. (2023). Sustainable Chemically Modified Mater-Bi/Poly(ε-caprolactone)/Cellulose Biocomposites: Looking at the Bulk through the Surface. *Research Square(Research Square).* DOI: 10.21203/rs.3.rs-3064683/v1

Huang, Q., Sun, Y., Guo, Q., Li, Q., Zhang, Y., Li, X., & Wang, L. (2025). Social life cycle assessment and its methodological challenges: A bibliometric and content analysis. *Journal of Industrial Ecology*, *29*(1), 264–278. DOI: 10.1111/jiec.13605

International Organization for Standardization. (2006). Environmental management – Life cycle assessment – Requirements and guidelines (ISO 14044:2006). International Organization for Standardization. https://www.iso.org/standard/38498.html

International Organization for Standardization. (14040). ISO 14040:2006/Amd 1:2020: Environmental management – Life cycle assessment – Principles and framework – Amendment 1. https://www.iso.org/standard/76121.html

International Organization for Standardization. (14044). ISO 14044:2006/Amd 2:2020: Environmental management – Life cycle assessment – Requirements and guidelines – Amendment 2. https://www.iso.org/standard/76122.html

John, M. J., & Thomas, S. (2023). Bio-Based Materials: Contribution to advancing Circular economy. In *MDPI eBooks*. DOI: 10.3390/books978-3-0365-6048-9

Jordaan, S. M., Combs, C., & Guenther, E. (2021). Life cycle assessment of electricity generation: A systematic review of spatiotemporal methods. *Advances in Applied Energy*, *3*, 100058. DOI: 10.1016/j.adapen.2021.100058

Kamble, Z., & Behera, B. K. (2021). Sustainable hybrid composites reinforced with textile waste for construction and building applications. *Construction & Building Materials*, *284*, 122800. DOI: 10.1016/j.conbuildmat.2021.122800

Khoshnava, S. M., Rostami, R., Ismail, M., Rahmat, A. R., & Ogunbode, B. E. (2017). Woven hybrid Biocomposite: Mechanical properties of woven kenaf bast fibre/oil palm empty fruit bunches hybrid reinforced poly hydroxybutyrate biocomposite as non-structural building materials. *Construction & Building Materials*, *154*, 155–166. DOI: 10.1016/j.conbuildmat.2017.07.189

Knez, Z., Markocic, E., Leitgeb, M., Primozic, M., Hrncic, M. K., & Skerget, M. (2014b). Industrial applications of supercritical fluids: A review. *Energy*, *77*, 235–243. DOI: 10.1016/j.energy.2014.07.044

Komal, U. K., & Singh, I. (2022). Sustainable Treatments of Pineapple Leaf Fibers for Polylactic Acid Based Biocomposites. *Journal of Natural Fibers*, *19*(16), 13438–13456. DOI: 10.1080/15440478.2022.2095550

Korol, J., Burchart-Korol, D., & Pichlak, M. (2016). Expansion of environmental impact assessment for eco-efficiency evaluation of biocomposites for industrial application. *Journal of Cleaner Production*, *113*, 144–152. DOI: 10.1016/j.jclepro.2015.11.101

Korol, J., Hejna, A., Burchart-Korol, D., & Wachowicz, J. (2020). Comparative analysis of carbon, ecological, and water footprints of polypropylene-based composites filled with cotton, jute and kenaf fibers. *Materials (Basel)*, *13*(16), 3541. DOI: 10.3390/ma13163541 PMID: 32796660

La Rosa, A. D., Valente, C., & Aradoaei, M. (2024, October). Environmental, Economic, and Social Life Cycle Assessment in the Polymer Composites Sector. In *2024 IEEE International Conference And Exposition On Electric And Power Engineering (EPEi)* (pp. 29-36). IEEE. DOI: 10.1109/EPEi63510.2024.10758166

Lehmann, A., Zschieschang, E., Traverso, M., Finkbeiner, M., & Schebek, L. (2013). Social aspects for sustainability assessment of technologies—Challenges for social life cycle assessment (SLCA). *The International Journal of Life Cycle Assessment*, *18*(8), 1581–1592. DOI: 10.1007/s11367-013-0594-0

Lingrove. (2024, February 6). From flax to furniture: new, plant-based decor - Lingrove. *Lingrove*. https://lingrove.com/from-flax-to-furniture-new-plant-based-decor/

Lu, X., & Gu, X. (2023). A review on lignin-based epoxy resins: Lignin effects on their synthesis and properties. *International Journal of Biological Macromolecules*, *229*, 778–790. DOI: 10.1016/j.ijbiomac.2022.12.322 PMID: 36603715

Mahalle, L., Alemdar, A., Mihai, M., & Legros, N. (2014). A cradle-to-gate life cycle assessment of wood fibre-reinforced polylactic acid (PLA) and polylactic acid/thermoplastic starch (PLA/TPS) biocomposites. *The International Journal of Life Cycle Assessment*, *19*(6), 1305–1315. DOI: 10.1007/s11367-014-0731-4

Majewski, J., & Sobolewska, A. (2018). Comparative life cycle assessment of apple packaging. In Proceedings of the 2018 International Scientific Conference "Economic Sciences for Agribusiness and Rural Economy" (No. 2) (pp. 340–346). Warsaw, 7–8 June 2018.

Manthey, N. W. (2013). *Development of hemp oil based bioresins for biocomposites*. https://eprints.usq.edu.au/23672/

Mekonnen, T., Misra, M., & Mohanty, A. (2015). Processing, performance, and applications of plant and animal protein-based blends and their biocomposites. In *Elsevier eBooks* (pp. 201–235). DOI: 10.1016/B978-1-78242-373-7.00017-2

Meng, F., Olivetti, E. A., Zhao, Y., Chang, J. C., Pickering, S. J., & McKechnie, J. (2018). Comparing life cycle energy and global warming potential of carbon fiber composite recycling technologies and waste management options. *ACS Sustainable Chemistry & Engineering*, *6*(8), 9854–9865. DOI: 10.1021/acssuschemeng.8b01026

Molina-Besch, K., & Keszleri, H. (2022). Exploring the industrial perspective on biobased plastics in food packaging applications – Insights from Sweden. Sustainable Production and Consumption, *MDPI,* 35, 72–84. DOI: 10.1016/j.spc.2022.10.018

Mujtaba, M., Fraceto, L. F., Fazeli, M., Mukherjee, S., Savassa, S. M., De Medeiros, G. A., Pereira, A. D. E. S., Mancini, S. D., Lipponen, J., & Vilaplana, F. (2023). Lignocellulosic biomass from agricultural waste to the circular economy: A review with focus on biofuels, biocomposites and bioplastics. *Journal of Cleaner Production*, *402*, 136815. DOI: 10.1016/j.jclepro.2023.136815

Muller, M. (2023). Transferring Knowledge from Academia to the Companies: A New Method. *Research for Development*, •••, 65–80. DOI: 10.1007/978-3-031-25207-5_4

Nagaraju, D. H. (2022). *Biopolymer-Based Composites.*, DOI: 10.1007/978-981-16-6603-2_18-1

Nagy, D. I., Rowe, I. V., Kahhat, R., Quispe, I., Carrasco, G. C., Clauser, N. M., & Area, M. C. (2020). Life cycle assessment of bagasse fiber reinforced biocomposites. *The Science of the Total Environment*, *720*, 137586. DOI: 10.1016/j.scitotenv.2020.137586 PMID: 32325583

Nair, A. B., Sivasubramanian, P., Balakrishnan, P., Ajith Kumar, K. A. N., & Sreekala, M. S. (2013). Environmental effects, biodegradation, and life cycle analysis of fully biodegradable "green" composites. *Polymer Composites*, •••, 515–568.

Nodehi, M., Ozbakkaloglu, T., Gholampour, A., Mohammed, T., & Shi, X. (2022). The effect of curing regimes on physico-mechanical, microstructural and durability properties of alkali-activated materials: A review. *Construction & Building Materials*, *321*, 126335. DOI: 10.1016/j.conbuildmat.2022.126335

Nutrizio, M., Dukić, J., Sabljak, I., Samardžija, A., Fučkar, V. B., Djekić, I., & Jambrak, A. R. (2024). Upcycling of food by-products and waste: Nonthermal green extractions and life cycle assessment approach. *Sustainability (Basel)*, *16*(21), 9143. DOI: 10.3390/su16219143

Pacheco-Torgal, F. (2025). An introductory overview of bio-based construction materials. *Advances in Bio-Based Materials for Construction and Energy Efficiency*, 1-14.

Papong, S., Malakul, P., Trungkavashirakun, R., Wenunun, P., Chom-in, T., Nithitanakul, M., & Sarobol, E. (2014). Comparative assessment of the environmental profile of PLA and PET drinking water bottles from a life cycle perspective. *Journal of Cleaner Production*, *65*, 539–550. DOI: 10.1016/j.jclepro.2013.09.030

Patel, P., Gohil, P. P., & Parmar, V. (2021). *Bio Composite Material: Review and its Applications in Various Fields*. Elsevier., DOI: 10.1016/B978-0-12-819724-0.00011-2

Pecas, P., Carvalho, H., Salman, H., & Leite, M. (2018). Natural fiber composites and their applications: A review. *Journal of Composites Science*, *2*(4), 66. DOI: 10.3390/jcs2040066

Phiri, R., Rangappa, S. M., Siengchin, S., Oladijo, O. P., & Dhakal, H. N. (2023). Development of sustainable biopolymer-based composites for lightweight applications from agricultural waste biomass: A review. *Advanced Industrial and Engineering Polymer Research*, *6*(4), 436–450. DOI: 10.1016/j.aiepr.2023.04.004

Ramachandran, K., & Gnanasagaran, C. L. (2024). Life cycle assessment of sugarcane bagasse based natural composites prepared via vacuum bagging technique. *Bioresource Technology Reports*, *26*, 101811. DOI: 10.1016/j.biteb.2024.101811

Ramachandran, K., Gnanasagaran, C. L., & Vekariya, A. (2023). Life cycle assessment of carbon fiber and bio-fiber composites prepared via vacuum bagging technique. *Journal of Manufacturing Processes*, *89*, 124–131. DOI: 10.1016/j.jmapro.2023.01.068

Rebitzer, G., Ekvall, T., Frischknecht, R., Hunkeler, D., Norris, G., Rydberg, T., Schmidt, W. P., Suh, S., Weidema, B. P., & Pennington, D. W. (2004). Life cycle assessment: Part 1: Framework, goal and scope definition, inventory analysis, and applications. *Environment International*, *30*(5), 701–720. DOI: 10.1016/j.envint.2003.11.005 PMID: 15051246

Rızvanoglu, O., Kaya, S., Ulukavak, M., & Yeşilnacar, M. İ. (2020). Optimization of municipal solid waste collection and transportation routes, through linear programming and geographic information system: A case study from Şanlıurfa, Turkey. *Environmental Monitoring and Assessment*, *192*(1), 1–12. DOI: 10.1007/s10661-019-7975-1 PMID: 31802257

Rodriguez, L. J., Fabbri, S., Orrego, C. E., & Owsianiak, M. (2020). Comparative life cycle assessment of coffee jar lids made from biocomposites containing poly(lactic acid) and banana fiber. *Journal of Environmental Management*, *266*, 110493. DOI: 10.1016/j.jenvman.2020.110493 PMID: 32310114

Rossoni, A. L., De Vasconcellos, E. P. G., & De Castilho Rossoni, R. L. (2023). Barriers and facilitators of university-industry collaboration for research, development and innovation: A systematic review. *Management Review Quarterly*, *74*(3), 1841–1877. DOI: 10.1007/s11301-023-00349-1

Roy, P., Defersha, F., Rodriguez-Uribe, A., Misra, M., & Mohanty, A. K. (2020). Evaluation of the life cycle of an automotive component produced from biocomposite. *Journal of Cleaner Production*, *273*, 123051. DOI: 10.1016/j.jclepro.2020.123051

Rueda, E., Senatore, V., Zarra, T., Naddeo, V., García, J., & Garfí, M. (2023). Life cycle assessment and economic analysis of bioplastics production from cyanobacteria. *Sustainable Materials and Technologies*, *35*, e00579. DOI: 10.1016/j.susmat.2023.e00579

Rylko-Polak, I., Komala, W., & Bialowiec, A. (2022). The Reuse of Biomass and Industrial Waste in Biocomposite Construction Materials for Decreasing Natural Resource Use and Mitigating the Environmental Impact of the Construction Industry: A Review. *Materials (Basel)*, *15*(12), 4078. DOI: 10.3390/ma15124078 PMID: 35744137

Safi Jahanshahi, S., Sharafati, A., Vahidi, H., & Hosseini, S. A. (2024). Life Cycle Analysis of Polypropylene Product in Industry Petrochemicals in Iran. *Pollution*, *10*(4), 1019–1031. DOI: 10.22059/poll.2024.375323.2344

Sala, S., Amadei, A. M., Beylot, A., & Ardente, F. (2021). The evolution of life cycle assessment in European policies over three decades. *The International Journal of Life Cycle Assessment*, *26*(12), 2295–2314. DOI: 10.1007/s11367-021-01893-2

Samarajeewa, N. U. (2022). The researcher and the future. *Vidyodaya Journal of Science*, *25*(02). Advance online publication. DOI: 10.31357/vjs.v25i02.6171

Saraiva, A. B., Pacheco, E. B., Gomes, G. M., Visconte, L. L., Bernardo, C. A., Simões, C. L., & Soares, A. G. (2016). Comparative life cycle assessment of mango packaging made from a polyethylene/natural fiber-composite and from cardboard material. *Journal of Cleaner Production*, *139*, 1168–1180. DOI: 10.1016/j.jclepro.2016.08.135

Seile, A., Spurina, E., & Sinka, M. (2022). Reducing global warming potential impact of bio-based composites based of LCA. *Fibers (Basel, Switzerland)*, *10*(9), 79. DOI: 10.3390/fib10090079

Sgarbossa, A., Boschiero, M., Pierobon, F., Cavalli, R., & Zanetti, M. (2020). Comparative life cycle assessment of bioenergy production from different wood pellet supply chains. *Forests*, *11*(11), 1127. DOI: 10.3390/f11111127

Shanmugam, V., Mensah, R. A., Forsth, M., Sas, G., Restas, A., Addy, C., Xu, Q., Jiang, L., Neisiany, R. E., Singha, S., George, G., Jose, L., Berto, F., Hedenqvist, M. S., Das, O., & Ramakrishna, S. (2021). Circular economy in biocomposite development: State-of-the-art, challenges and emerging trends. *Composites Part C: Open Access, 5*, 100138. DOI: 10.1016/j.jcomc.2021.100138

Shi, R., & Guest, J. S. (2020b). BioSTEAM-LCA: An integrated modeling framework for agile life cycle assessment of biorefineries under uncertainty. *ACS Sustainable Chemistry & Engineering*, *8*(51), 18903–18914. DOI: 10.1021/acssuschemeng.0c05998

Stillitano, T., Spada, E., Iofrida, N., Falcone, G., & De Luca, A. I. (2021). Sustainable agri-food processes and circular economy pathways in a life cycle perspective: State of the art of applicative research. *Sustainability (Basel), 13*(5), 2472. DOI: 10.3390/su13052472

Syduzzaman, M., Al Faruque, M. A., Bilisik, K., & Naebe, M. (2020). Plant-Based Natural Fibre Reinforced Composites: A Review on Fabrication, Properties and Applications. *Coatings*, *10*(10), 973. DOI: 10.3390/coatings10100973

Tadele, D., Roy, P., Defersha, F., Misra, M., & Mohanty, A. K. (2020). A comparative life-cycle assessment of talc- and biochar-reinforced composites for lightweight automotive parts. *Clean Technologies and Environmental Policy*, *22*(3), 639–649. DOI: 10.1007/s10098-019-01807-9

Tajurahim, N. A. N., Mahmood, S., Ngadiman, N. H. A., & Sing, S. L. (2025). Biomaterials for tissue engineering scaffolds: Balancing efficiency and eco-friendliness through life cycle assessment. [M.]. *Cleaner Environmental Systems*, *16*, 100253. DOI: 10.1016/j.cesys.2024.100253

Thirumalaisamy, R., Kumar, S. S., Chelladurai, S. J. S., Gnanasekaran, S., Sivananthan, S., Geetha, N. K., Ramesh, A., & Assefa, G. (2023). Study on Water Absorption Characteristics, Various Chemical Treatments, and Applications of Biological Fiber-Reinforced Polymer Matrix Composites. *Journal of Nanomaterials, 2023*, 1–7. DOI: 10.1155/2023/9903119

Tilouche-Guerdelli, K., Lacoste, C., Perrin, D., Liotier, P.-J., Ouagne, P., Tirillò, J., Sarasini, F., & Bergeret, A. (2024). Tannins as Biobased Molecules for Surface Treatments of Flax Wrapped Rovings for Epoxy/Flax Fabrics Biocomposites: Influence on Mechanical Properties through a Multi-Scale Approach. *Journal of Composites Science*, *8*(2), 75. Advance online publication. DOI: 10.3390/jcs8020075

Toffe, G. T., Oluwarotimi Ismail, S., Montalvão, D., Knight, J., & Ren, G. (2019). A scale-up of energy-cycle analysis on processing non-woven flax/PLA tape and triaxial glass fibre fabric for composites. *Journal of Manufacturing and Materials Processing*, *3*(4), 92. DOI: 10.3390/jmmp3040092

Ursic, L., Baldacchino, G., Bacic, Z., Sainz, A. B., Buljan, I., Hampel, M., Kruzic, I., Majic, M., Marusic, A., Thetiot, F., Tokalic, R., & Markic, L. V. (2022). Factors Influencing Interdisciplinary Research and Industry-Academia Collaborations at Six European Universities: A Qualitative Study. *Sustainability (Basel)*, *14*(15), 9306. DOI: 10.3390/su14159306

Vinod, A., Sanjay, M. R., Suchart, S., & Jyotishkumar, P. (2020). Renewable and sustainable biobased materials: An assessment on biofibers, biofilms, biopolymers and biocomposites. *Journal of Cleaner Production*, *258*, 120978. DOI: 10.1016/j.jclepro.2020.120978

Volk, R., Schroter, M., Saeidi, N., Steffl, S., Javadian, A., Hebel, D. E., & Schultmann, F. (2024). Life cycle assessment of mycelium-based composite materials. *Resources, Conservation and Recycling*, *205*, 107579. DOI: 10.1016/j.resconrec.2024.107579

Vu, D. H., Mahboubi, A., Ferreira, J. A., Taherzadeh, M. J., & Akesson, D. (2022). Polyhydroxybutyrate-Natural Fiber Reinforcement Biocomposite Production and Their Biological Recyclability through Anaerobic Digestion. *Energies*, *15*(23), 8934. DOI: 10.3390/en15238934

Walker, R. (2024, July 9). *Composites in Automotive Applications: Accelerating towards a greener future?*https://www.mewburn.com/. https://www.mewburn.com/news-insights/composites-in-automotive-applications-accelerating-towards-a-greener-future

Watjanatepin, P., Lepelaar, M., Verbruggen, J., Ouagne, P., De Luca, R., Li, Q., Scarpa, F., Placet, V., & Van Acker, K. (2023). Environmental assessment of woven hemp fibre reinforced epoxy composites and potential applications in aerospace and electric scooter industries. *Results in Materials*, *20*, 100474. DOI: 10.1016/j.rinma.2023.100474

Williams, A. G., Audsley, E., & Sandars, D. L. (2010). Environmental burdens of producing bread wheat, oilseed rape and potatoes in England and Wales using simulation and system modelling. *The International Journal of Life Cycle Assessment*, *15*(8), 855–868. DOI: 10.1007/s11367-010-0212-3

Wu, H., Tao, F., & Yang, B. (2020). Optimization of vehicle routing for waste collection and transportation. *International Journal of Environmental Research and Public Health*, *17*(14), 4963. DOI: 10.3390/ijerph17144963 PMID: 32660117

Xu, C., Nie, J., Wu, W., Zheng, Z., & Chen, Y. (2019). Self-healable, recyclable, and strengthened epoxidized natural rubber/carboxymethyl chitosan biobased composites with hydrogen bonding supramolecular hybrid networks. *ACS Sustainable Chemistry & Engineering*, *7*(18), 15778–15789. DOI: 10.1021/acssuschemeng.9b04324

Yang, Y., Tao, M., & Suh, S. (2018). Geographic variability of agriculture requires sector-specific uncertainty characterization. *The International Journal of Life Cycle Assessment*, *23*(8), 1581–1589. https://link.springer.com/article/10.1007/s11367-017-1388-6. DOI: 10.1007/s11367-017-1388-6

Yazdi, M. F. A., Zakaria, R., Mustaffar, M., Majid, M. Z. A., Zin, R. M., Ismail, M., & Yahya, K. (2014). Biocomposite materials potential in enhancing sustainable construction. *Desalination and Water Treatment*, *52*, 3631–3636. DOI: 10.1080/19443994.2013.854105

Z., Rosenbaum, R. K., & Olsen, S. I. (2018). Life cycle assessment: Theory and practice. Springer.

Zafiriou, P., Mamolos, A. P., Menexes, G. C., Siomos, A. S., Tsatsarelis, C. A., & Kalburtji, K. L. (2012). Analysis of energy flow and greenhouse gas emissions in organic, integrated and conventional cultivation of white asparagus by PCA and HCA: Cases in Greece. *Journal of Cleaner Production*, *29*, 20–27. DOI: 10.1016/j.jclepro.2012.01.040

Zarauz, I., Sanz-Hernández, A., & Rivera-Lirio, J. M. (2024). Social sustainability in a good bioeconomy paradigm: A systematic review of social life cycle assessment (S-LCA). *Journal of Cleaner Production*, *144570*. Advance online publication. DOI: 10.1016/j.jclepro.2024.144570

Zhao, Q., Jiang, J., Zhang, L., Wang, S., Chen, J., Yao, X., & Li, Y. (2023). Simple and mild method for the recycling of carbon-fiber-reinforced bismaleimide resin composite waste. *ACS Sustainable Chemistry & Engineering*, *11*(7), 2830–2839. DOI: 10.1021/acssuschemeng.2c06090

Chapter 14
Advancing Cancer Therapy with Nanomaterials Targeting Metalloptosis Mechanisms

Girish Sharma
https://orcid.org/0000-0003-2127-5700
Amity University, Noida, India

Anusha Mittal
https://orcid.org/0009-0004-7874-3653
Amity University, Noida, India

Tejasvi Batra
https://orcid.org/0009-0006-7103-5253
Amity University, Noida, India

Jasmine Kaur
https://orcid.org/0009-0006-5962-6085
Amity University, Noida, India

Banashree Bandhopadhyay
https://orcid.org/0000-0002-6679-7791
Amity University, Noida, India

ABSTRACT

Despite the widespread use of traditional cancer therapies such as surgery, chemo-

DOI: 10.4018/979-8-3373-1305-4.ch014

therapy, and radiation, these approaches often suffer from significant drawbacks. Nanomaterials (NMs) are a promising alternative due to their distinct nanoscale properties which enable more precise drug delivery and reduced off-target effects. Recently, cuproptosis and ferroptosis have emerged as novel forms of programmed cell death regulated by metal ions, offering novel pathways for cancer therapy. Cuproptosis, caused by copper ion accumulation, leads to mitochondrial dysfunction, while ferroptosis, driven by iron-mediated lipid peroxidation, disrupts cellular integrity through oxidative stress. Here, we propose to explore how NMs can be harnessed to induce metalloptosis, for advanced cancer treatment strategies. Variations in NM size, morphology, and the synergistic effects of composite NMs complicate the identification of individual mechanisms. Use of NMs in cancer therapy, requires focusing on the precise design and regulation of metalloptosis pathways.

INTRODUCTION

Cancer has long been established as a global health burden and its complex pathology and disease progression makes it extremely complicated to manage and cure. Conventional cancer therapies, including surgery, chemotherapy, and radiation, face significant limitations despite their widespread use. These treatment modalities often induce systemic toxicity due to their lack of selectivity, multi-drug resistance and immune suppression, usually with results ranging from recurrence to mortality. This predicament has urged scientists and clinicians around the world to continuously develop and come up with more precise and optimal treatment alternatives for cancer. One such revolution has been the integration of nanotechnology with biologically active components to target malignancy at the sub-cellular scale. As materials shrink to the nanoscale, they exhibit unique optical, magnetic, and electrical properties that distinguish them from traditional macromolecules. Nanomaterials typically share several defining characteristics, including a high surface-to-volume ratio, enhanced electrical conductivity, superparamagnetic behaviour, shifted optical absorption spectra, and distinctive fluorescence properties (Cheng et al., 2021).

In the medical field, nanomaterials have found extensive applications, particularly in drug delivery and controlled release systems. Their ability to increase permeability allows them to traverse biological barriers more effectively, enhancing drug targeting to specific sites. Additionally, nanomaterials offer improved biocompatibility, making them highly suitable for biomedical applications. Another key advantage of nanoparticle-based drug delivery systems is their ability to shield encapsulated drugs from metabolic degradation while minimizing toxicity to surrounding tissues (Rawat et al., 2023). Additionally, the nanoscale of these materials provides a substantial surface area, allowing for the attachment and delivery of a larger number of drug molecules. For instance, a single polymeric nanoparticle with an average diameter of 70 nm can accommodate approximately 2,000 drug molecules, compared to polymer–drug conjugates, which can typically bind only 9 drug molecules per unit (Lungu et al., 2019). This increased drug-loading capacity represents a significant advantage for cancer therapies. These attributes collectively position nanomaterials as transformative tools in advancing medical science and therapeutics.

Since the dawn of their potential in cancer therapy, several strategies and combinations have emerged in the past two decades. The main objective of this chapter is to explore the utilization of nanomaterials for eradicating cancer cells via "metalloptosis" – a newly emerged target in cancer therapy (Wang et al., 2024). The term, proposed by Wang et al., refers to that subset of programmed cell death pathways that is initiated by metal ions. Programmed cell death (PCD) is a crucial biological process that regulates cellular homeostasis, development, and response to stress. Among the various forms of PCD, cuproptosis, ferroptosis, and calcium overload have gained attention due to their peculiar involvement of metal ions in orchestrating cell death pathways. Cuproptosis is a recently discovered form of cell death driven by the accumulation of copper ions, which leads to mitochondrial dysfunction, oxidative stress, and proteotoxicity. This copper-induced cell death is characterized by the dysregulation of the TCA cycle and disruption of mitochondrial integrity (Xie et al., 2023). On the other hand, ferroptosis is a cell death mechanism dependent on iron and lipid peroxidation, where excess iron catalyses the formation of reactive oxygen species (ROS), leading to lipid membrane damage and eventual cellular demise (Lei et al., 2022). These novel targets are now being incorporated with nanomaterials-based solutions to discover better, more selective and more potent avenues for cancer treatment, ranging from stimuli-responsive nanocarriers to magnetically manipulable nanoparticles that also allow for real-time diagnosis and monitoring of treatment efficacy, i.e., an aspect of theranostics (Huang et al., 2024; Ko et al., 2024; Liu et al., 2023).

With that in consideration, all innovations bring their own set of challenges. Innovating the regulation of metalloptosis signalling pathways from a mechanistic perspective is a highly challenging task. Therefore, conducting in-depth studies on the interactions between different nanomaterial (NM) components and cancer cells is essential for a comprehensive understanding of metalloptosis. For example, the size and morphology of NMs can significantly influence their phagocytic efficiency, which in turn affects how they interact with cancer cells. Moreover, when investigating the anticancer mechanisms of NM-induced metalloptosis, it is important to consider the degradation and release properties of the metals within the NMs. Understanding the specific concentrations of metals, incubation times, and their effects on cellular morphology, metabolism, intracellular and extracellular ion balance, and cell death markers is crucial. Consequently, an interdisciplinary approach is essential for advancing the use of nanomaterials in cancer therapy. Current research and development have increasingly focused on these nano systems, and innovations in materials science, combined with biological materials, could lead to more practical applications of nanomaterial platforms for the induction of programmed cell death (metalloptosis).

CUPROPTOSIS

Cuproptosis is a recently discovered mode of cell death triggered by the excessive buildup of copper (Cu) within cells. This process is driven by Cu-induced aggregation of dihydrolipoamide S-acetyltransferase, a key enzyme linked to the mitochondrial tricarboxylic acid cycle, alongside the degradation of iron–sulphur cluster proteins (Zhang et. al., 2024). These disruptions lead to proteotoxic stress, ultimately initiating cell death. In recent years, cuproptosis has attracted considerable attention in cancer research, as it presents a promising avenue for therapeutic intervention against tumours (Cong et. al., 2025; Zhang et. al., 2024).

Introduction

The concept of cuproptosis was first introduced by Tsvetkov and colleagues in 2022 (Zhang et. al., 2024). Their pioneering research provided foundational insights into copper-induced cell death, revealing its potential as a novel therapeutic strategy in cancer treatment. Previous studies had already established key observations regarding copper's role in cellular toxicity. For instance, disulfiram (DSF) was identified as an anticancer agent (Wang et. al., 2022; Beaudoin et. al., 2024), while earlier reports confirmed that copper exposure alone could trigger cell death (Triboulet et. al., 2013). Further studies demonstrated that copper accelerates cancer cell death and that copper-based anticancer compounds effectively induce tumour cell apoptosis (Abdolmaleki et al., 2024; Zhao et al., 2022). Additionally, elesclomol (ES), a known Cu ionophore, was shown to selectively transport copper into mitochondria, enhancing its cytotoxic effects against cancer cells (Nagai et al., 2012; Huang et al., 2024). Research also found that copper enhances the anti-tumour efficacy of disulfiram (Beaudoin et. al., 2024). Notably, ferredoxin 1 (FDX1) and lipoyl synthase (LIAS) were identified as crucial regulators of copper toxicity, further contributing to the mechanistic understanding of copper-induced cell death (Tang et al., 2023; Tsvetkov et al., 2023).

Cuproptosis differs significantly from other programmed cell death mechanisms, including necroptosis, apoptosis, pyroptosis, and ferroptosis (Zhao et al., 2025). As an essential trace metal, copper is vital for numerous biological functions. It acts as a redox-active cofactor for various enzymes and plays a crucial role in processes such as oxidative phosphorylation (OXPHOS), iron homeostasis, connective tissue cross-linking, detoxification of reactive oxygen species (ROS), and cellular signalling. However, copper can also be cytotoxic when its intracellular levels become excessive (Zhao et al., 2022). Copper overload stimulates ROS production through Cu-mediated Fenton reactions, leading to oxidative stress and the disruption of iron–sulphur cluster proteins (Macomber et al., 2009). Chronic exposure to elevated copper levels has been linked to various diseases, including cancer, due to its role in tumour growth and metastasis (Turski et al., 2015). Despite extensive research, the precise molecular mechanisms underlying copper-induced cytotoxicity remain incompletely understood, and the known cellular targets of copper toxicity do not fully explain the cellular response to its accumulation (Kumari et al., 2023).

Cuproptosis as a Target in Cancer Therapy

Intracellular Cu^{2+} can be transported to the mitochondria by copper ionophores such as CRT1, where it is reduced by FDX1 to Cu^{+}. This reduction triggers the direct binding of Cu^{+} to lipoylated dihydrolipoamide S-acetyltransferase (DLAT), leading to protein aggregation and the destabilization of iron–sulphur cluster proteins (Zhao et al., 2024). These molecular events induce proteotoxic stress, ultimately resulting in cuproptotic cell death (Zhao et al., 2023). Notably, neither genetic nor pharmacological inhibition of apoptosis, ferroptosis, or necroptosis was able to prevent ES-Cu-induced cell death across multiple cancer cell lines (Zhao et al., 2022). Furthermore, common antioxidants such as N-acetylcysteine, α-tocopherol, ebselen, and JP4-039 failed to mitigate ES-Cu-mediated cytotoxicity, suggesting that ROS (including mitochondrial ROS) are not essential for cuproptosis (Tsvetkov et al., 2022). However, the hydrophilic antioxidant glutathione (GSH) successfully inhibited ES-Cu toxicity by chelating intracellular copper, reinforcing the notion that cuproptosis is mechanistically distinct from other known forms of cell death (Zhao et al., 2023).

Further studies by Tsvetkov et al. established a strong connection between mitochondrial metabolism and copper toxicity. They observed that lung cancer cells dependent on galactose-driven mitochondrial respiration exhibited nearly 1,000-fold greater sensitivity to ES-Cu-induced cell death compared to those relying on glucose-fuelled glycolysis (Zhao et al., 2022). Consistent with this observation, inhibitors of mitochondrial respiration—including rotenone and antimycin A (targeting respiratory chain complexes I and III, respectively)—as well as UK5099 (an inhibitor of mitochondrial pyruvate uptake), effectively blocked cuproptosis. In contrast, ES-Cu treatment did not impact basal or ATP-linked respiration in cells (Zhao et al., 2024). Moreover, hypoxic conditions (1% O_2), which force cells to rely on glycolysis instead of OXPHOS, significantly reduced their sensitivity to cuproptosis (Zhao et al., 2022; Huang et al., 2024). These findings distinguish cuproptosis from ferroptosis, which relies on glucose uptake and pyruvate oxidation (Cong et al., 2025). Thus, while both pathways involve metal-induced cell death, cuproptosis and ferroptosis are driven by distinct alterations in energy metabolism and mitochondrial function (Zhao et al., 2024). Collectively, these discoveries define cuproptosis as a novel, oxidative stress-independent, mitochondria-mediated form of cell death (Figure 1).

Figure 1. Metabolic pathways of Ferroptosis and their interplay with other cell death mechanisms.

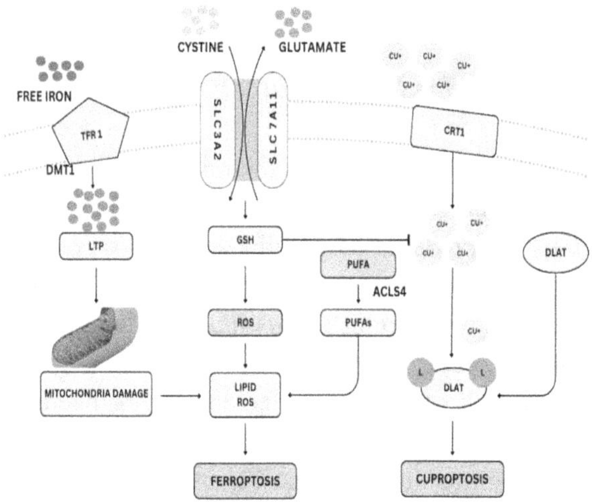

Abbreviations: PUFA polyunsaturated fatty acids, GSH glutathione, ROS reactive oxygen species, ACSL4 acyl-CoA synthetase long-chain family member 4, DLAT recombinant dihydrolipoyl transacetylase, TFR1 transferrin receptor 1.

Recent Innovations in Nanomaterial Engineering Harnessing Cuproptosis

Recent propositions have been made in introducing nanoplatforms integrating ferroptosis, cuproptosis, and chemodynamic therapy (CDT) for targeted tumour imaging and treatment (Table 1). Despite the therapeutic promise of these mechanisms, their clinical efficacy has been hindered by the inefficient delivery of catalytic ions and the tumour microenvironment's (TME) unfavourable conditions, including excess glutathione (GSH), limited acidity, and insufficient hydrogen peroxide (H_2O_2). To address these limitations, p-carboxybenzenesulfonamide (BS), a carbonic anhydrase IX (CA IX) inhibitor, was conjugated to generation-5 poly(amidoamine) dendrimers for the controlled delivery of copper peroxide (CuO_2) nanoparticles, which were further stabilized by iron-tannic acid (TF) networks. The resulting CuO_2@G5-BS/TF nanocomplexes (~39.4 nm) exhibited selective accumulation in tumours via CA IX-mediated targeting, enabling precise magnetic resonance (MR) imaging and enhanced therapeutic efficacy. Mechanistically, CA IX inhibition decreased intracellular pH, accelerating Fe^{3+}/Cu^{2+} release, promoting endogenous H_2O_2 production, and boosting Fenton reactivity while simultaneously suppressing tumour metastasis by neutralizing extracellular acidity. In vivo studies confirmed that CuO_2@G5-BS/TF nanocomplexes significantly improved tumour MR imaging, effectively suppressed both primary tumour growth and metastasis in a 4T1 breast cancer model and exhibited minimal systemic toxicity. These findings highlight the potential of this multifunctional nanoplatform as a promising approach for targeted MR imaging and synergistic ferroptosis/cuproptosis/CDT in triple-negative breast cancer therapy (Huang et al., 2024).

Another study exhibited an innovative near-infrared-II (NIR-II) excitation multifunctional nanomedicine designed to overcome key challenges in cuproptosis-based phototheranostics for triple-negative breast cancer (TNBC), including poor copper retention, inadequate tumour-targeting, and limited light penetration depth. The nanoplatform is constructed through the self-assembly of AS1411 aptamers using metallic copper ions as coordination nodes, followed by encapsulation with ultrasmall NIR-II polymer dots (Pdots) exhibiting superior optical properties. This results in a carrier-free hybrid nanosystem with enhanced targeting and imaging capabilities. Upon selective accumulation in TNBC cells via aptamer-mediated recognition of cell surface nucleolin, the Pdots facilitate NIR-IIa fluorescence and NIR-II photoacoustic imaging, enabling precise tumour visualization and guiding NIR-II photothermal therapy (PTT) under 1064 nm excitation. Simultaneously, intracellular glutathione (GSH) and ferredoxin 1 (FDX1) reduce Cu(II) to cytotoxic Cu(I), triggering chemodynamic therapy (CDT) and inducing cuproptosis. Moreover, NIR-II PTT and GSH depletion further potentiate CDT and cuproptosis by enhancing cancer cell susceptibility to treatment (Dai et al., 2023).

Research by Yang et al. elucidated a high-performance plasmonic-thermoelectric catalytic therapy leveraging urchin-like $Cu_{2-X}Se$ hollow nanospheres (HNSs) to overcome the limitations of conventional thermoelectric therapy, particularly the restricted temperature gradient in biological systems. The designed $Cu_{2-X}Se$ HNSs, enriched with copper vacancies (VCu), exhibit exceptional plasmonic photothermal conversion efficiency (67.0%), enabling rapid localized heating under 1064 nm laser irradiation. This temperature gradient subsequently activates thermoelectric catalysis, leading to the generation of reactive oxygen species (ROS) for targeted cancer cell destruction. In vivo studies using tumour-bearing BALB/c mice validate the high therapeutic efficacy of this nanoplatform. This work pioneers the integration of plasmonic-thermoelectric catalysis within a single nanostructure, utilizing dual mitochondrial dysfunction mechanisms—membrane potential reduction and thioctylated protein aggregation—for enhanced cancer therapy. These findings open new pathways for energy-converting nanomedicines in oncological applications (Yang et al., 2024).

The application of targeting cuproptotic pathways in developing a immunotherapeutic strategy was also explored, by leveraging cuproptosis-lactate regulation to overcome immune cell proliferation limitations and the immunosuppressive tumour microenvironment (Wang et al. 2024). A multifunctional nanoplatform, BAu-CuNCs, was developed by integrating copper-human serum albumin (Cu-HSA) nanocomplexes into gold nanocages (AuNCs) coated with a bacterial membrane for targeted tumour therapy (Liu et al. 2024). Upon tumour cell internalization, BAu-CuNCs underwent controlled disassembly, initiating a cascade of therapeutic effects. Near-infrared (NIR) laser irradiation enhanced Cu-HSA release, which reacted with intracellular glutathione (GSH) via a disulfide exchange reaction, liberating Cu^{2+} ions to induce cuproptosis. This process triggered immunogenic cell death (ICD), marked by the release of damage-associated molecular patterns (DAMPs), subsequently activating robust anti-tumour immunity through increased cytotoxic CD^{8+} T cells and helper CD^{4+} T cells. Simultaneously, NIR irradiation amplified ROS production via AuNCs, disrupting glycolysis and reducing lactate and ATP levels. The combined effects of lactate depletion, ATP reduction, and GSH exhaustion sensitized tumour cells to cuproptosis. Notably, the decreased lactate concentration led to significant suppression of immunosuppressive regulatory T cells (Tregs), further enhancing anti-tumour immunity. In vivo studies demonstrated that BAu-CuNCs + NIR therapy effectively inhibited tumour growth, remodelled the immunosuppressive tumour microenvironment, and suppressed breast cancer metastasis to the lungs (Zafar et al., 2024).

Another interesting study showcased a tumour microenvironment (TME)-responsive core-shell tecto dendrimer (CSTD) nanoplatform for targeted magnetic resonance (MR) imaging and enhanced cuproptosis-promoted chemo-chemodynamic therapy. The CSTD was engineered by conjugating phenylboronic acid- and mannose-modified poly(amidoamine) dendrimers via phenylboronic ester bonds, making it responsive to both acidic pH and reactive oxygen species (ROS). This nanoplatform efficiently encapsulated copper ions (CuII) and the chemotherapeutic agent disulfiram (DSF) to achieve tumour-specific drug delivery. Following systemic circulation, CSTD-Cu(II)@DSF selectively accumulated in MCF-7 breast cancer cells, where it underwent TME-triggered drug release. The elevated intracellular CuII levels promoted lipoylated protein oligomerization and proteotoxic stress, inducing cuproptosis. Concurrently, CuII catalysed lipid peroxidation, amplifying chemodynamic therapy. Additionally, mitochondrial dysfunction and G2/M cell cycle arrest enhanced DSF-mediated apoptosis, resulting in potent tumour inhibition through the combined effects of chemotherapy, cuproptosis, and chemodynamic therapy. Beyond its therapeutic efficacy, CSTD-Cu(II)@DSF exhibited CuII-associated r1 relaxivity, enabling real-time T1-weighted MR imaging for precise tumour diagnosis (Ni et al., 2023).

FERROPTOSIS

In 2012, Brent R. Stockwell characterized ferroptosis as a form of iron-dependent cell death driven by the accumulation of lipid reactive oxygen species (ROS) (Dixon et al., 2012).

Ferroptosis as a Target for Cancer Therapy

Growing evidence suggests that ferroptosis functions as a tumour suppressor, playing a pivotal role in regulating the cell cycle, proliferation, and progression of cancer. Beyond its impact on hematologic malignancies, ferroptosis has been identified as a suppressor in several solid tumours, including lung, breast, pancreatic, colorectal, liver, oesophageal squamous cell carcinoma, gastric, and melanoma (Cui et al. 2024; Hua et al. 2024).

Both the extrinsic and intrinsic pathways play a crucial role in ferroptosis regulation (Figure 1). The extrinsic pathway is activated by inhibiting the cystine-glutamate antiporter (system Xc^-) (Stockwell et al. 2020). Reduced system Xc^- activity hinders extracellular cystine uptake, thereby disrupting glutathione (GSH) synthesis and compromising cellular antioxidant capacity (Zhang et. al.,2023). This depletion of GSH leads to lipid reactive oxygen species (ROS) accumulation, ultimately triggering ferroptosis (Li et al. 2020). Additionally, the activation of iron transporters, such as serum transferrin and lactotransferrin, can induce ferroptosis by increasing intracellular iron levels, enhancing iron accumulation, and promoting oxidative stress (Zhou et al. 2024). In contrast, the intrinsic pathway is primarily driven by the inhibition of intracellular antioxidant enzymes (Zhang et al. 2023). For instance, glutathione peroxidase 4 (GPX4) plays a crucial role in reducing cytotoxic lipid peroxides (L-OOH) into non-toxic lipid alcohols (L-OH) (Li et al. 2020). Inhibition of GPX4 results in the accumulation of lipid peroxides in the cell membrane, leading to ferroptotic cell death. Additionally, long-chain fatty acid coenzyme A ligase 4 (ACSL4) facilitates the incorporation of polyunsaturated fatty acids (PUFAs) into phospholipids, forming polyunsaturated fatty acid phospholipids (PUFA-PLs) (Zhou et al. 2024). These PUFA-PLs are highly susceptible to oxidation mediated by lipoxygenases (ALOXs), which destabilizes the lipid bilayer, disrupts membrane integrity, and ultimately induces ferroptosis.

Both the extrinsic and intrinsic pathways can be selectively activated by small molecules, such as RAS-selective lethal 3 (RSL3) and erastin. However, the development and clinical application of ferroptosis-inducing compounds remain challenging. Some small molecules, such as ferristatin-1, exhibit poor solubility, stability, pharmacokinetics, and bioavailability, making them unsuitable for in vivo applications and limiting their therapeutic potential (Wan et al. 2008)

Beyond its role in limiting tumour growth, ferroptosis also restricts cancer cell migration and invasion. For instance, Krüppel-like factor 2 (KLF2) has been shown to regulate ferroptosis through glutathione peroxidase 4 (GPX4), thereby suppressing cancer cell migration and invasion in clear cell renal cell carcinoma. Conversely, SLC7A11 has been found to promote renal cancer cell migration and invasion by enhancing GPX4 export (Zhou et al. 2021). In colorectal cancer, acyl-coenzyme A dehydrogenase, short/branched chain (ACADSB), negatively regulates GPX4. Overexpression of ACADSB reduces SW620 and LoVo cell migration and invasion by increasing intracellular Fe^{2+} levels and downregulating GPX4 and glutathione reductase expression. Additionally, in hepatocellular carcinoma (HCC), miR-211-5p directly targets ACSL4, suppressing cell proliferation, migration, and invasion through its inhibitory effect on ACSL4 expression (Qin et al. 2020).

Further supporting ferroptosis' role in limiting tumour progression, a study by the Feng group revealed that ferroptosis is inversely correlated with metastasis. They observed a higher prevalence of lymph node metastases in SLC7A11-positive oesophageal squamous cell carcinoma patients, suggesting a link between SLC7A11 expression and tumour progression (Feng et al. 2021). In human HCC, SLC7A11 overexpression correlates with poor differentiation, advanced tumour-nodule-metastasis (TNM) stage, and worse prognosis (Zhang et al. 2024). Additionally, Liu et al. demonstrated that ferroptosis resistance increases metastatic potential, identifying 27-hydroxycholesterol (27HC) as a key metabolite promoting lipid biosynthesis in cancer cells (Liu et al. 2024). Notably, inhibiting GPX4 reverses the tumorigenic and metastatic effects of 27HC-resistant cells. Similarly, neratinib, an irreversible pan-tyrosine kinase inhibitor, has been shown to induce ferroptosis and suppress brain metastases in a HER2-positive breast cancer model (Nagpal et al. 2019). These findings further underscore the critical role of ferroptosis in inhibiting tumour metastasis.

Emerging clinical data suggest that ferroptosis is strongly associated with cancer prognosis and overall survival. One of the most direct indicators is the overexpression of SLC7A11 in renal cell carcinoma (RCC), where it serves as an independent prognostic marker linked to poor clinical outcomes. Similarly, ATP-binding cassette subfamily C member 5 (ABCC5) has been found to be upregulated in HCC, negatively regulating ferroptosis by increasing intracellular GSH levels and stabilizing SLC7A11 (Tang et al. 2024). Notably, HCC cells resistant to sorafenib exhibit elevated ABCC5 expression, which is associated with poorer prognosis. Moreover, ACSL4 and GPX4, key regulators of ferroptosis, exert opposing effects on cancer progression. Unlike GPX4, which is downregulated in breast cancer cells, ACSL4 is highly expressed in breast cancer tissues. Interestingly, the expression levels of ACSL4 and GPX4—individually or in combination—serve as independent prognostic markers for disease-free survival. High ACSL4 expression correlates with improved overall survival, whereas elevated GPX4 levels are associated with better distant metastasis-free survival (Zhang et al. 2023). Collectively, these findings highlight ferroptosis as a tumour suppressor through multiple molecular and cellular mechanisms, offering promising therapeutic implications for cancer treatment.

Table 1. Summary of some nanomaterial advances in cancer therapy

S. No.	Type	Composition of Nano Material	Therapy	Tumour Type	Model	References
1	Pt/pFeS_2@GOX@ 4T1 nanovesicles	Pt-doped porous FeS2 nanoparticles (Pt/pFeS2 NPs),with glucose oxidase (GOX)-loaded and 4T1 cell membrane-coated	Photothermal-enhanced photodynamic/ferroptosis antitumor combination therapy	Breast	*in vivo*	Feng et al. (2023)
2	Fe3O4-αPD-L1	Anti-PD-L1 antibody-conjugated iron oxide nanoprobe	RT-Sensitization	Breast	*in vivo*	Zhu et al. (2024)
3	CuO_2@G5-BS/TF nanocomplex	p-carboxybenzenesulfonamide (BS), a carbonic anhydrase IX (CA IX) inhibitor, modified on the surface of generation-5 poly(amidoamine) dendrimer to load copper peroxide nanoparticles, which were complexed with iron (Fe)-tannic acid (TF) networks	Enhanced ferroptosis/cuproptosis/ CDT	TNBC	*in vivo*	Huang et al. (2024)
4	PAA/mCaP/mCuP NS	Poly(acrylic acid)/ mesoporous calcium phosphate/mesoporous copper phosphate nanosphere	Multimodal therapy	Breast	*in vitro/ in vivo*	Sun et al. (2024)
5	ACP NP	Self-assembly of targeting aptamers (AS1411) utilizing metallic copper ions as coordination nodes, followed by coating with ultrasmall NIR-II polymer dots (Pdots)	NIR-IIa fluorescence/ NIR-II photoacoustic imaging-guided NIR-II photothermal therapy (PTT)	TNBC	*in vivo*	Dai et al. (2023)
6	AuPt@Cu-PDA Nanocomposite	AuPt-loaded Cu-doped polydopamine nanocomposite	Photothermal and photoacoustic imaging (PTI/PAI)-guided cuproptosis-enhanced NCT/PTT	Breast	*in vitro/ in vivo*	Wang et al. (2023)

continued on following page

Table 1. Continued

S. No.	Type	Composition of Nano Material	Therapy	Tumour Type	Model	References
7	CNSI-Fe	Carbon nanoparticles-Fe(II) complex	Apoptosis and Ferroptosis	Colon	*in vitro/ in vivo*	Xie et al. (2023)
8	R-PtMn-1	pH-ultrasensitive PtMn nanoparticles	Enhanced ferroptosis-based cancer theranostics.	Breast, Colorectal	*in vitro/ in vivo*	Guan et al. (2023)
9	PEG@Cu2O-ES nanocomposite	Elesclomol (ES) loaded cuprous oxide (Cu2O) nanocomposite	Immunotherapy Sensitization	Breast	*in vivo*	Li et al. (2024)
10	ZnPc-TK-DOX CCNA	Incorporating a photosensitizer Zinc Phthalocyanine (ZnPc)-chemotherapeutic (DOX) prodrug with a thioketal (TK) spacer and an IDO inhibitor (1-methyl tryptophan, 1-MT) as building blocks for Cu2+-coordination self-assembly	Combinational apoptosis-cuproptosis and immunotherapy	Prostate	*in vitro/ in vivo*	Liang et al. (2023)
11	BAu-CuNCs	Copper-human serum albumin nanocomplex loaded gold nanocages with bacterial membrane coating	Immunogenic cell death (ICD)	Breast	*in vivo*	Zafar et al. (2024)
12	Cu-IR783 NPs	Cu2+-induced IR783 assembly	SDT Visualiziation/CDT			Hu et al. (2024)
13	Cu2−xSe HNS	Urchin-like Cu2−xSe hollow nanospheres (HNSs) featuring rich copper vacancies (VCu)	Thermoelectric catalytic cancer therapy	Colon	*in vitro/ in vivo*	Yang et al. (2024)
14	CSTD-Cu(II)@DSF	Tumour microenvironment (TME)-responsive core-shell tecto dendrimer (CSTD) assembled by phenylboronic acid- and mannose-modified poly(amidoamine) dendrimers via the phenylboronic ester bonds, efficiently loaded with copper ions and chemotherapeutic drug disulfiram (DSF)	Tumour-targeted magnetic resonance (MR) imaging/Cuproptosis-promoted chemo-chemodynamic therapy	Breast	*in vitro/ in vivo*	Ni et al. (2023)
15	CuET@PHF	Copper ionophores CuET nanocrystals stabilized with polydopamine and hydroxyethyl starch	Mild PTT with Cuproptosis and ICD	TNBC	*in vitro*	Xiao et al. (2024)
16	HMCPN17	Hollow mesoporous calcium peroxide nanoparticles	Calcicoptosis	Breast	*in vitro/ in vivo*	Zhou et al. (2024)
17	Ca/DHA@Afn	Biomineralized apoferritin-based nanovector, encapsulating the ferroptosis inducer dihydroartemisinin (DHA)	Dual-mode calcicoptosis and ferroptosis therapy	Breast	*in vitro*	Zhao et al. (2024)

Recent Innovations in Nanomaterial Engineering Harnessing Ferroptosis

To enhance the cargo-loading capacity of nanoparticles and integrate ferroptosis with apoptosis, the synthesis of platinum-doped porous FeS_2 nanoparticles (Pt/pFeS_2 NPs) was reported by Feng and colleagues (Feng et al., 2023) (Table 1). The porous architecture of Pt/pFeS_2 NPs provides abundant active sites for the Fenton reaction and photodynamic processes, significantly increasing reactive oxygen species (ROS) generation. The incorporation of GOX further amplifies endogenous hydrogen peroxide (H_2O_2) production while lowering the tumour microenvironment pH, thereby enhancing Fenton reaction-driven ferroptosis. Moreover, the incorporation of the 4T1 cell membrane increases its cellular uptake with in vivo studies confirming their accumulation at tumour sites, enabling precise photoacoustic imaging.

Another study conducted by Guan et al. presents a novel approach to enhancing ferroptosis-based cancer theranostics through the development of pH-ultrasensitive platinum-manganese (PtMn) nanoparticles. Traditional manganese-based nanomaterials (Mn-nanomaterials) have been hindered by their low sensitivity and inefficiency under the mildly acidic conditions of the tumour microenvironment (pH 6.4–6.8), resulting in suboptimal therapeutic efficacy and limited MRI performance. To overcome these limitations, PtMn nanoparticles with controlled core sizes (ranging from 5.3 to 2.7 nm) were synthesized and modified with an acidity-responsive polymer, enabling precise pH-sensitive activation. Among the variants, R-PtMn-1 (3 nm core) demonstrated superior "turn-on" oxidase-like activity, achieving a 6.7-fold enhancement in catalytic performance at pH 6. Additionally, R-PtMn-1 exhibited exceptional dual-mode contrast enhancement in high-field MRI, with a notable increase in T1- and T2-weighted imaging contrast at pH 6.4 (3.0- and 3.2-fold, respectively). This heightened pH sensitivity enabled selective activation within the tumour microenvironment, minimizing off-target effects in normal tissues (Guan et al., 2023).

There have also been attempts to demonstrate the potential of ferroptosis in radiotherapy sensitization. A study conducted by Zhu and coworkers (Zhu et al., 2024) hypothesized and validated a novel strategy to overcome tumour radiotherapy (RT) resistance by targeting myeloid-derived suppressor cells (MDSCs), which contribute to post-RT immunosuppression through their massive accumulation in tumours. To address this challenge, an anti-PD-L1 antibody-conjugated iron oxide nanoprobe (Fe_3O_4-αPD-L1) was developed to selectively target MDSCs and induce ferroptosis, thereby restoring immune function and enhancing RT efficacy. The overexpression of PD-L1 in MDSCs following RT enabled precise, non-invasive tracking via magnetic resonance imaging (MRI) and positron emission tomography (PET) using ^{89}Zr-labelled Fe_3O_4-αPD-L1 nanoprobes. Once internalized by tumour-infiltrating MDSCs, these nanoprobes predominantly localized within lysosomes, where they catalysed the Fenton reaction, generating excessive reactive oxygen species (ROS). This oxidative stress induced ferroptosis in MDSCs, as evidenced by lipid peroxidation and mitochondrial dysfunction, effectively disrupting the immunosuppressive tumour microenvironment. By integrating imaging and therapeutic functions, this approach enables real-time monitoring and precise modulation of MDSC immunosuppressive effects, offering a promising strategy to mitigate RT resistance and improve clinical outcomes. These findings underscore the potential of ferroptosis induction in MDSCs as a targeted immunomodulatory therapy for enhancing radiotherapy efficacy (Zhu et al., 2024).

CALCICOPTOSIS

Introduction

Calcium serves both structural and physiological functions in the body. Structurally, it is an essential component of bones and teeth, contributing to their strength and durability. On a functional level, calcium is crucial for various biological processes, including muscle contraction in skeletal, cardiac, and smooth muscle tissues (Berchtold et al., 2000). An imbalance in calcium levels, whether deficiency (hypocalcaemia) or excess (hypercalcemia), can lead to a range of health complications, such as bone demineralization, cardiac arrhythmias, hypertension, convulsions, muscle weakness, kidney stones, and inflammation. Furthermore, dysregulated calcium homeostasis has been associated with several disorders, including osteoporosis, tetany, metabolic dysfunctions, cardiovascular diseases, and cancer (Razzaque et al., 2025).

Calcium signalling is a key regulator of cancer progression, influencing cellular processes essential for tumour development and metastasis. Disruptions in calcium homeostasis within cancer cells contribute to uncontrolled proliferation, enhanced survival, and increased migratory capacity—hallmarks of malignant transformation. Specifically, modifications in calcium transport mechanisms, particularly within store-operated calcium entry (SOCE) pathways, lead to elevated calcium influx, promoting cancer cell invasion (Shapovalov et al., 2021). Research indicates that calcium channels such as transient receptor potential melastatin 7 (TRPM7) and transient receptor potential cation channel subfamily V member 4 (TRPV4) play a significant role in endothelial cell migration, thereby supporting angiogenesis—a critical process in tumour expansion. Additionally, alterations in calcium signalling pathways influence the epithelial-to-mesenchymal transition (EMT), a key mechanism enabling cancer cells to spread and establish secondary tumours (Kaouri et al. 2020). A deeper understanding of these calcium-dependent mechanisms offers promising therapeutic prospects. Selectively targeting calcium-related pathways could hinder tumour growth and metastasis while preserving normal cellular functions, presenting a potential strategy for more effective cancer treatment.

Calcicoptosis as a Target for Cancer Therapy

Excessive intracellular calcium levels have been linked to disturbances in metabolic and proliferative processes. Recently, Zhang et al. introduced the concept of "calcicoptosis" as a novel form of cell death. Their research involved the development of calcium peroxide nanoparticles (SH-CaO2 NPs) coated with sodium hyaluronate (Zhang et al. 2023). These nanoparticles remained stable in physiological fluids but, when exposed to the acidic tumour microenvironment, triggered the release of calcium ions and hydrogen peroxide, contributing to cell death. Chemotherapy and radiation therapy generate significant amounts of free radicals within cancer cells, potentially leading to calcium ion accumulation and tissue calcification (Zhang et al. 2024). The interplay between excess calcium and reactive oxygen species (ROS) amplifies their anticancer effects, ultimately driving cancer cell death. Although the precise mechanisms underlying this process remain unclear, calcium signalling is known to regulate critical cellular functions such as metabolism, proliferation, and cell death.

Calcium ion overload has been implicated in various forms of programmed cell death, including apoptosis, necrosis, necroptosis, pyroptosis, and autophagy (Zhang et al. 2024). Notably, certain cancer types, such as acute lymphoblastic leukaemia (ALL) and acute myeloid leukaemia (AML), exhibit a heightened dependence on mitochondrial calcium homeostasis (Smith et al. 2024). This reliance is particularly evident in aggressive subtypes like T-cell ALL, where mitochondrial function is essential for sustaining metabolic processes, energy production, biosynthesis, and survival under stress. Unlike normal cells that tightly regulate calcium homeostasis, cancer cells frequently exploit dysregulated calcium signalling to adapt their metabolic processes and evade apoptosis.

Mitochondrial calcium dysregulation not only enhances cancer cell survival but also contributes to metabolic plasticity, exemplified by the Warburg effect—where cancer cells preferentially use glycolysis over oxidative phosphorylation even in oxygen-rich conditions (Zabala et al. 2020). In venetoclax-resistant leukaemia stem cells (LSCs), increased mitochondrial calcium uptake supports oxidative phosphorylation, enabling their survival despite chemotherapy. Targeting mitochondrial calcium uptake in these resistant LSCs has shown therapeutic potential by effectively eliminating them. Similarly, mitochondria play a crucial role in T-cell ALL by regulating ROS generation, calcium signalling, and cell death pathways. Therapeutic strategies that exploit mitochondrial vulnerabilities—such as promoting mitochondrial calcium overload or disrupting voltage-dependent anion channel 1 (VDAC1)—have been proposed as effective approaches (Shoshan et al. 2019). By selectively disrupting mitochondrial calcium homeostasis, these targeted interventions could induce cancer cell death while sparing healthy tissue. Consequently, therapies aimed at modulating mitochondrial calcium signalling present a promising avenue for overcoming resistance mechanisms and enhancing the efficacy of conventional cancer treatments.

Recent Innovations in Nanomaterial Engineering Harnessing Calcicoptosis

A study introduced hollow mesoporous calcium peroxide nanoparticles (HMCPN) as a drug-free nanoplatform for inducing calcicoptosis, a cell death mechanism triggered by intracellular calcium overload (Table 1). Developed through a hydrolysis-precipitation method, the optimized HMCPN17 nanoparticles possess a high surface area (81.3 m^2/g) and an average pore size of 6.4 nm, allowing for efficient drug loading. HMCPN17 exhibits pH-responsive decomposition, releasing calcium ions (Ca^{2+}) and hydrogen peroxide (H_2O_2) more rapidly in the tumour microenvironment (pH 6.8) compared to physiological conditions (pH 7.4). This acid-triggered (Ca^{2+}) surge effectively promotes calcicoptosis without requiring additional therapeutic agents. Moreover, HMCPN17 demonstrates a high capacity for loading chemotherapeutics such as doxorubicin (DOX) and sorafenib (SFN), highlighting its versatility as a multifunctional drug delivery system. Both in vitro and in vivo experiments confirm the potent tumour inhibition capability of HMCPN17, attributed to its efficient tumour accumulation and localized Ca\(^{2+}\) and H\(_2\)O\(_2\) generation. This work underscores the potential of HMCPN17 as a promising nanoplatform for drug-free calcicoptosis therapy and as a foundation for constructing multifunctional nanocomposites with enhanced therapeutic efficacy (Zhou et al., 2024).

While ferroptosis therapy has emerged as a promising treatment strategy by promoting intracellular reactive oxygen species (ROS) accumulation and lipid peroxidation (LPO), its clinical efficacy is hindered by inadequate ROS levels and poor drug accumulation at tumour sites. To address these limitations, Zhao and colleagues (Zhao et al., 2024) propose a biomineralized apoferritin-based nanovector (Ca/DHA@AFn) designed to achieve synergistic ferroptosis and calcicoptosis for enhanced breast cancer therapy. The nanoplatform encapsulates dihydroartemisinin (DHA), a ferroptosis inducer, within an apoferritin (AFn) carrier mineralized with calcium ions (Ca^{2+}), forming uniformly distributed nanoparticles (~20 nm) with a drug loading efficiency of 2.32%. Cell viability assays demonstrated that Ca/DHA@AFn exhibited significantly greater cytotoxicity against 4T1 breast cancer cells compared to control formulations (DHA, Ca@AFn, and DHA@AFn), confirming its enhanced therapeutic potency. In vivo studies further validated its superior antitumor efficacy, as the combined ferroptosis and calcicoptosis mechanisms effectively inhibited tumour growth, prolonged survival, and exhibited high biocompatibility.

Nanoconjugates have emerged as advanced theranostic platforms, integrating precise diagnostics with targeted therapeutic potential to enhance cancer treatment strategies. The following study presents the design and synthesis of a novel nanoconjugate, NIONP-CaCD, formed by conjugating naphthalimide-based organic nanoparticles (NIONPs) with calcium-doped carbon dots (CaCDs). This nanoplatform demonstrated potential in bioimaging and pro-drug–free combination cancer therapy (Ghosh et al., 2024). Hydroxychloroquine (HCQ) was efficiently encapsulated within the NIONP-CaCD conjugate, exhibiting significantly higher loading capacity compared to individual carriers (NIONPs or CaCDs). Upon exposure to the lysosomal pH range (4.5–5.0), the boronate–diol bond was cleaved, triggering the disintegration of the nanoconjugate and the controlled release of HCQ and CaCDs. The resulting NIONP-CaCD-HCQ nanoformulation enhanced therapeutic efficacy, achieving approximately a threefold increase in cancer cell death compared to standalone cargo-loaded therapies. Notably, it exhibited a twofold higher cytotoxicity against cancer cells (A549 and HepG2) compared to normal cells (NIH3T3). This superior anticancer activity is attributed to a synergistic mechanism involving calcium overload-induced apoptosis (calcicoptosis) and HCQ-mediated lysosomal cell death (Ghosh et al., 2024)

CONCLUSION AND FUTURE PERSPECTIVES

Nanomaterials serve as effective vehicles for the controlled delivery of therapeutic agents, ensuring optimal accumulation at tumour sites and enabling precise activation within the tumour microenvironment. Innovations such as pH-responsive and redox-sensitive nanoplatforms, photothermal therapies, and multifunctional theranostic systems have demonstrated significant promise in preclinical models, enabling both real-time tumour imaging and synergistic multimodal therapy. The findings discussed in this chapter highlight the potential of nanomedicine-driven metalloptosis, where metal-based nanoparticles initiate programmed cell death pathways that selectively target cancer cells while preserving normal tissues. Significant strides have been made in the development of nanoplatforms engineered to exploit cuproptosis, ferroptosis, and calcicoptosis. Cuproptosis-targeting nanomaterials have shown remarkable potential in disrupting mitochondrial homeostasis and protein aggregation in cancer cells, amplifying cytotoxicity through copper-ion-mediated stress responses. Similarly, ferroptosis-based strategies leverage iron-catalysed lipid peroxidation and reactive oxygen species (ROS) production to induce tumour cell death. Calcicoptosis, characterized by intracellular calcium overload, presents another emerging frontier in metalloptosis, with studies demonstrating its ability to disrupt mitochondrial integrity and metabolic pathways in aggressive cancers.

Despite promising advancements, several challenges remain before metalloptosis-based nanomedicines can be translated into clinical applications. Although metal-based nanomedicines have demonstrated tumour-selective toxicity, concerns regarding their long-term biocompatibility, biodistribution, and potential off-target effects must be addressed. Future research should focus on optimizing biodegradable and excretable nanoplatforms to prevent systemic accumulation and toxicity. Cancer cells exhibit adaptive resistance to programmed cell death pathways, necessitating strategies that combine metalloptosis with immunotherapy, gene therapy, or metabolic reprogramming to enhance efficacy. Understanding tumour heterogeneity at the molecular level will allow for personalized therapeutic interventions. The therapeutic efficacy of metalloptosis hinges on maintaining optimal metal ion concentrations within cancer cells while avoiding cytotoxicity in normal tissues. The development of stimuli-responsive nanocarriers capable of controlled metal-ion release is essential for ensuring precise therapeutic action. The translation of nanomedicines from laboratory research to clinical use is hindered by complex synthesis procedures, batch variability, and regulatory hurdles. Future efforts should prioritize scalable, cost-effective fabrication techniques while adhering to good manufacturing practices (GMP) and regulatory guidelines. While preclinical models have demonstrated the potential of metalloptosis-based therapies, large-scale clinical trials are required to evaluate safety, efficacy, and pharmacokinetics. The integration of patient-derived tumour models and organoid systems will provide a more accurate assessment of therapeutic outcomes in heterogeneous cancer populations.

The intersection of nanomedicine and metalloptosis represents a cutting-edge frontier in cancer research, with multifunctional nanoplatforms offering unprecedented precision in cancer therapy. The ability to selectively target cancer cells through metal-ion-induced cell death pathways, coupled with advanced imaging and drug delivery systems, holds immense potential for overcoming the limitations of traditional therapies. Future research should focus on refining nanoplatform designs, improving biocompatibility, and integrating metalloptosis with diverse therapeutic strategies to develop personalized cancer treatments. The translation of these technologies into clinically viable therapies will require interdisciplinary collaboration between materials scientists, oncologists, and bioengineers to address current challenges and optimize therapeutic outcomes. Ultimately, the continued advancement of metalloptosis-driven nanomedicine will not only enhance cancer treatment but also pave the way for original strategies in precision oncology, offering hope for improved survival and quality of life in cancer patients worldwide.

REFERENCES

Abdolmaleki, A., Ghasemi, F., & Hosseini, M. (2024). Unveiling the promising anticancer effect of copper-based compounds: A comprehensive review. *Journal of Cancer Research and Clinical Oncology*, *150*(5), 1235–1250. DOI: 10.1007/s00432-024-05641-5 PMID: 38662225

Beaudoin, C., & Omran, Z. (2024). Anticancer effects of new disulfiram analogs. *Biological & Pharmaceutical Bulletin*, *47*(11), 1804–1812. DOI: 10.1248/bpb.b24-00538 PMID: 39505546

Berchtold, M. W., Brinkmeier, H., & Muntener, M. (2000). Calcium ion in skeletal muscle: Its crucial role for muscle function, plasticity, and disease. *Physiological Reviews*, *80*(3), 1215–1265. DOI: 10.1152/physrev.2000.80.3.1215 PMID: 10893434

Cheng, Z., Li, M., Dey, R., & Chen, Y. (2021). Nanomaterials for cancer therapy: Current progress and perspectives. *Journal of Hematology & Oncology*, *14*(1), 85. Advance online publication. DOI: 10.1186/s13045-021-01096-0 PMID: 34059100

Cong, Y., Li, N., Zhang, Z., Shang, Y., & Zhao, H. (2025). Cuproptosis: Molecular mechanisms, cancer prognosis, and therapeutic applications. *Journal of Translational Medicine*, *23*(1), 104. DOI: 10.1186/s12967-025-06121-1 PMID: 39844182

Cui, K., Wang, K., & Huang, Z. (2024). Ferroptosis and the tumor microenvironment. *Journal of Experimental & Clinical Cancer Research : CR*, *43*(1), 315. Advance online publication. DOI: 10.1186/s13046-024-03235-0 PMID: 39614322

Dai, Y., Leng, D., Guo, Z., Wang, J., Gu, Y., Peng, Y., Zhu, L., & Zhao, Q. (2023). NIR-II excitation self-assembly nanomedicine for targeted NIR-IIa fluorescence imaging-guided cuproptosis-promoted synergistic therapy against triple-negative breast cancer. *Chemical Engineering Journal*, *479*, 147704. DOI: 10.1016/j.cej.2023.147704

Dixon, S. J., Lemberg, K. M., Lamprecht, M. R., Skouta, R., Zaitsev, E. M., Gleason, C. E., & Stockwell, B. R. (2012). Ferroptosis: an iron-dependent form of nonapoptotic cell death. *cell, 149*(5), 1060-1072.

Feng, L., Zhao, K., Sun, L., Wang, X., Zhang, Y., Yang, G., & Liu, Z. (2021). SLC7A11 regulated by NRF2 modulates esophageal squamous cell carcinoma radiosensitivity by inhibiting ferroptosis. *Journal of Translational Medicine*, *19*(1), 367. Advance online publication. DOI: 10.1186/s12967-021-03042-7 PMID: 34446045

Feng, M., Xiao, S., Liu, Z., Li, M., Zhang, X., Chen, X., Zhang, Y., Chen, B., & Liu, J. (2023). Multifunctional platinum-doped porous FeS2 nanoparticles for photothermal-enhanced photodynamic ferroptosis combination therapy. *Materials Today Nano*, *23*, 100371. DOI: 10.1016/j.mtnano.2023.100371

Ghosh, A. K., Roy, K., & Das, P. K. (2024). Organic Nanoparticle–Carbon dots conjugate for multimodal cancer therapy. *ACS Applied Nano Materials*, *7*(5), 4946–4959. DOI: 10.1021/acsanm.3c05730

Guan, G., Liu, H., Xu, J., Zhang, Q., Dong, Z., Lei, L., Zhang, C., Yue, R., Gao, H., Song, G., & Shen, X. (2023). Ultrasmall PtMn nanoparticles as sensitive manganese release modulator for specificity cancer theranostics. *Journal of Nanobiotechnology*, *21*(1), 434. Advance online publication. DOI: 10.1186/s12951-023-02172-y PMID: 37980476

Hu, J., Yan, L., Cao, Z., Geng, B., Cao, X., Liu, B., Guo, J., & Zhu, J. (2024). Tumor microenvironment activated CU crosslinked Near-Infrared sonosensitizers for visualized Cuproptosis-Enhanced sonodynamic cancer immunotherapy. *Advancement of Science*, *11*(43), 2407196. Advance online publication. DOI: 10.1002/advs.202407196 PMID: 39331855

Hua, Y., Yang, S., Zhang, Y., Li, J., Wang, M., Yeerkenbieke, P., Liao, Q., & Liu, Q. (2024). Modulating ferroptosis sensitivity: Environmental and cellular targets within the tumor microenvironment. *Journal of Experimental & Clinical Cancer Research : CR*, *43*(1), 19. Advance online publication. DOI: 10.1186/s13046-023-02925-5 PMID: 38217037

Huang, H., Guo, H., Liu, J., Ni, C., Xia, L., Cao, X., Xia, J., Shi, X., & Guo, R. (2024). Dendrimer/metal-phenolic nanocomplexes encapsulating CuO2 for targeted magnetic resonance imaging and enhanced ferroptosis/cuproptosis/chemodynamic therapy by regulating the tumor microenvironment. *Acta Biomaterialia*, *183*, 252–263. DOI: 10.1016/j.actbio.2024.05.035 PMID: 38801869

Huang, H., Guo, H., Liu, J., Ni, C., Xia, L., Cao, X., Xia, J., Shi, X., & Guo, R. (2024b). Dendrimer/metal-phenolic nanocomplexes encapsulating CuO2 for targeted magnetic resonance imaging and enhanced ferroptosis/cuproptosis/chemodynamic therapy by regulating the tumor microenvironment. *Acta Biomaterialia*, *183*, 252–263. DOI: 10.1016/j.actbio.2024.05.035 PMID: 38801869

Huang, H., Wu, Y., Sun, X., Zhang, S., Zhang, H., Zhang, M.-R., Wang, R., & Hu, K. (2024). Application potential of 64Cu-elesclomol in theranostics of tumors with high mitochondrial metabolism. *Journal of Nuclear Medicine*, *65*(Supplement 2), 241826. DOI: 10.2967/jnumed.122.265439

Huang, Y., Zhang, Z., & Chen, Y. (2024). Novel insights into cuproptosis inducers and inhibitors. *Frontiers in Molecular Biosciences*, *11*, 1477971. Advance online publication. DOI: 10.3389/fmolb.2024.1477971 PMID: 39659361

Kaouri, K., Bitsouni, V., Buttenschön, A., & Thul, R. (2020). Adhesion-driven patterns in a calcium-dependent model of cancer cell movement. *arXiv preprint* arXiv:2003.00612.

Ko, M. J., Min, S., Hong, H., Yoo, W., Joo, J., Zhang, Y. S., Kang, H., & Kim, D. (2023). Magnetic nanoparticles for ferroptosis cancer therapy with diagnostic imaging. *Bioactive Materials*, *32*, 66–97. DOI: 10.1016/j.bioactmat.2023.09.015 PMID: 37822917

Kumari, N., & Imlay, J. A. (2023). Analysis of copper-induced protein precipitation across the proteome. *Metallomics*, *15*(1), mfac098. Advance online publication. DOI: 10.1093/mtomcs/mfac098 PMID: 36549662

Lei, G., Zhuang, L., & Gan, B. (2022). Targeting ferroptosis as a vulnerability in cancer. *Nature Reviews. Cancer*, *22*(7), 381–396. DOI: 10.1038/s41568-022-00459-0 PMID: 35338310

Li, Q., Han, X., & Lan, X. (2020). Ferroptosis: A novel cell death form will be a promising therapy target for diseases. *Acta Biochimica et Biophysica Sinica*, *47*(10), 857–867. DOI: 10.1093/abbs/gmv073 PMID: 26350095

Li, W., Xiao, Y., Guo, G., Peng, J., Zhu, N., Chen, Z., Peng, B., Jiang, Z., Li, B., Yu, G., Guo, Z., Liang, M., & Guo, W. (2024). Cuprous oxide nanocomposites with photothermal (PTT) and chemical dynamics (CDT) effects induce cuproptosis in breast cancer using the strategy of increasing inflow and reducing outflow. *Nano Today*, *56*, 102223. DOI: 10.1016/j.nantod.2024.102223

Liang, W., Han, C., Zhang, D., Liu, C., Zhu, M., Xu, F., Fang, C., Zhang, S., Liu, C., & Li, Y. (2023). Copper-coordinated nanoassemblies based on photosensitizer-chemo prodrugs and checkpoint inhibitors for enhanced apoptosis-cuproptosis and immunotherapy. *Acta Biomaterialia*, *175*, 341–352. DOI: 10.1016/j.actbio.2023.12.022 PMID: 38122883

Liu, . (2024). Nanobiotechnology boosts ferroptosis: Opportunities and challenges. *Journal of Nanobiotechnology*, *24*(1), 2842. Advance online publication. DOI: 10.1186/s12951-024-02842-5

Liu, Q., Zhao, Y., Zhou, H., & Chen, C. (2023). Ferroptosis: Challenges and opportunities for nanomaterials in cancer therapy. *Regenerative Biomaterials*, *10*, rbad004. Advance online publication. DOI: 10.1093/rb/rbad004 PMID: 36817975

Liu, X., Sun, J., Wang, Z., Chen, R., & Zhou, L. (2024). Engineering a multifunctional copper-based nanoplatform for photoactivated cuproptosis and immunogenic cell death. *Nano Letters*, *24*(3), 1325–1338. DOI: 10.1021/acs.nanolett.3c04789

Lungu, I. I., Grumezescu, A. M., Volceanov, A., & Andronescu, E. (2019). Nanobiomaterials Used in Cancer Therapy: An Up-To-Date Overview. *Molecules (Basel, Switzerland)*, *24*(19), 3547. DOI: 10.3390/molecules24193547 PMID: 31574993

Macomber, L., & Imlay, J. A. (2009). The iron-sulfur clusters of dehydratases are primary intracellular targets of copper toxicity. *Proceedings of the National Academy of Sciences of the United States of America*, *106*(20), 8344–8349. DOI: 10.1073/pnas.0812808106 PMID: 19416816

Nagai, M., Vo, N. H., Shin Ogawa, L., Chimmanamada, D., Inoue, T., Chu, J., Lu, R., Blackman, R. K., & Barsoum, J. (2012). The oncology drug elesclomol selectively transports copper to the mitochondria to induce oxidative stress in cancer cells. *Free Radical Biology & Medicine*, *52*(10), 2142–2150. DOI: 10.1016/j.freeradbiomed.2012.03.017 PMID: 22542443

Nagpal, A., Redvers, R. P., Ling, X., Ayton, S., Fuentes, M., Tavancheh, E., Diala, I., Lalani, A., Loi, S., David, S., Anderson, R. L., Smith, Y., Merino, D., Denoyer, D., & Pouliot, N. (2019). Neoadjuvant neratinib promotes ferroptosis and inhibits brain metastasis in a novel syngeneic model of spontaneous HER2-positive breast cancer metastasis. *Breast Cancer Research : BCR*, *21*(1), 94. Advance online publication. DOI: 10.1186/s13058-019-1177-1 PMID: 31409375

Ni, C., Ouyang, Z., Li, G., Liu, J., Cao, X., Zheng, L., Shi, X., & Guo, R. (2023). A tumor microenvironment-responsive core-shell tecto dendrimer nanoplatform for magnetic resonance imaging-guided and cuproptosis-promoted chemo-chemodynamic therapy. *Acta Biomaterialia*, *164*, 474–486. DOI: 10.1016/j.actbio.2023.04.003 PMID: 37040813

Qin, X., Zhang, J., Lin, Y., Sun, X., Zhang, J., & Cheng, Z. (2020). Identification of MiR-211-5p as a tumor suppressor by targeting ACSL4 in Hepatocellular Carcinoma. *Journal of Translational Medicine*, *18*(1), 316. DOI: 10.1186/s12967-020-02494-7 PMID: 32859232

Rawat, N., Ahmad, N., Raturi, P., Singhvi, N., Sahai, N., & Kothiyal, P. (2023). Nanobiomaterials: Exploring mechanistic roles in combating microbial infections and cancer. *Discover Nano*, *18*(1), 158. DOI: 10.1186/s11671-023-03946-x PMID: 38123864

Razzaque, M. S., & Wimalawansa, S. J. (2025). Minerals and Human Health: From Deficiency to Toxicity. *Nutrients*, *17*(3), 454. DOI: 10.3390/nu17030454 PMID: 39940312

Shapovalov, G., Gordienko, D., & Prevarskaya, N. (2021). Store operated calcium channels in cancer progression. *International Review of Cell and Molecular Biology*, *363*, 123–168. DOI: 10.1016/bs.ircmb.2021.02.016 PMID: 34392928

Shoshan-Barmatz, V., & Nahon-Crystal, E. (2019). Mitochondria as emerging targets for therapies against T cell acute lymphoblastic leukemia. *Journal of Leukocyte Biology*, *105*(5), 935–944. DOI: 10.1002/JLB.5VMR0818-330RR PMID: 30698851

Smith, J., Doe, A., & Brown, L. (2024). Mitochondria and acute leukemia: A clinician's perspective. *International Journal of Molecular Sciences*, *25*(17), 9704. DOI: 10.3390/ijms25179704 PMID: 39273651

Stockwell, B. R., Jiang, X., & Gu, W. (2020). Emerging mechanisms and disease relevance of ferroptosis. *Nature Reviews. Cancer*, *20*(7), 467–484. DOI: 10.1038/s41571-020-00462-0 PMID: 32413317

Sun, B., Gao, W., Yu, X., Zhang, C., Du, H., Luo, Y., Zhu, J., Yang, P., & Zhang, M. (2024). Charge regulated PH/NIR dual responsive nanoplatforms centered on cuproptosis for enhanced cancer theranostics. *Biomaterials*, *122907*. Advance online publication. DOI: 10.1016/j.biomaterials.2024.122907 PMID: 39476451

Tang, D., Chen, X., Kroemer, G., & Klionsky, D. J. (2023). The implications and prospect of cuproptosis-related genes and copper chelators in cancer therapy. *Frontiers in Oncology*, *13*, 1117164. DOI: 10.3389/fonc.2023.1117164 PMID: 36925927

Tang, Z., Chen, X., & Kang, R. (2024). SLC7A11 as a prognostic marker in renal cell carcinoma: Implications for ferroptosis in cancer therapy. *Cancer Research*, *84*(3), 412–425. DOI: 10.1158/0008-5472.CAN-23-0611

Triboulet, S., Aude-Garcia, C., Carrière, M., Diemer, H., Proamer, F., Habert, A., Chevallet, M., Collin-Faure, V., Strub, J.-M., Hanau, D., Van Dorsselaer, A., Herlin-Boime, N., & Rabilloud, T. (2013). Molecular responses of mouse macrophages to copper and copper oxide nanoparticles inferred from proteomic analyses. *arXiv preprint arXiv:1311.0802*. https://arxiv.org/abs/1311.0802

Tsvetkov, P., Coy, S., Petrova, B., Dreishpoon, M., Tong, B., & Yuan, H. (2022). Copper induces cell death by targeting lipoylated TCA cycle proteins. *Science*, *375*(6586), 1254–1261. DOI: 10.1126/science.abf0529 PMID: 35298263

Tsvetkov, P., Coy, S., Petrova, B., Dreishpoon, M., Tong, B., & Yuan, H. (2023). FDX1 regulates cellular protein lipoylation through direct binding to LIAS. *bioRxiv*. https://doi.org/DOI: 10.1101/2023.02.03.526472

Turski, M. L., & Thiele, D. J. (2015). Is copper a new target to counteract the progression of chronic diseases? *Metallomics*, *10*(12), 1712–1729. DOI: 10.1039/c5mt00202h PMID: 30339169

Wan, S. Y., & Stockwell, B. R. (2008). Synthetic lethal screening identifies compounds activating iron-dependent, nonapoptotic cell death in oncogenic-RAS-harboring cancer cells. *Chemistry & Biology*, *15*(3), 234–245. DOI: 10.1016/j.chembiol.2008.02.010 PMID: 18355723

Wang, H., Zhang, Y., Li, X., Zhao, J., & Chen, Q. (2024). Copper-based nanoplatforms for synergistic cuproptosis-immunotherapy: Advances and perspectives. *Advanced Functional Materials*, *34*(5), 2309872. DOI: 10.1002/adfm.202309872

Wang, L., Yu, Y., Zhou, C., Wan, R., & Li, Y. (2022). Anticancer effects of disulfiram: A systematic review of in vitro, animal, and human studies. *Systematic Reviews*, *11*(1), 109. Advance online publication. DOI: 10.1186/s13643-021-01858-4 PMID: 35655266

Wang, S., Ma, R., Mei, Z., & Hou, Y. (2024). Metalloptosis: Metal ions-induced programmed cell death based on nanomaterials for cancer therapy. *MedMat*, *1*(1), 6–26. DOI: 10.1097/mm9.0000000000000004

Wang, Y., Zhang, X., Li, S., Jiang, F., Jiang, P., & Liu, Y. (2023). AuPt-Loaded Cu-Doped Polydopamine Nanocomposites with Multienzyme-Mimic Activities for Dual-Modal Imaging-Guided and Cuproptosis-Enhanced Photothermal/Nanocatalytic Therapy. *Analytical Chemistry*, *95*(37), 14025–14035. DOI: 10.1021/acs.analchem.3c02661 PMID: 37694580

Xiao, C., Wang, X., Li, S., Zhang, Z., Li, J., Deng, Q., Chen, X., Yang, X., & Li, Z. (2024). A cuproptosis-based nanomedicine suppresses triple negative breast cancers by regulating tumor microenvironment and eliminating cancer stem cells. *Biomaterials*, *313*, 122763. DOI: 10.1016/j.biomaterials.2024.122763 PMID: 39180917

Xie, J., Yang, Y., Gao, Y., & He, J. (2023). Cuproptosis: Mechanisms and links with cancers. *Molecular Cancer*, *22*(1), 46. DOI: 10.1186/s12943-023-01732-y PMID: 36882769

Xie, P., Huang, Y., Tang, K., Wu, X., Zeng, C., Yang, S., & Tang, X. (2023). Carbon nanoparticles-Fe(II) complex for efficient theranostics of xenografted colonic tumor. *Cancer Nanotechnology*, *14*(1), 38. Advance online publication. DOI: 10.1186/s12645-023-00196-5

Yang, L., Zhao, Z., Tian, B., Yang, M., Dong, Y., Zhou, B., Gai, S., Xie, Y., & Lin, J. (2024). A singular plasmonic-thermoelectric hollow nanostructure inducing apoptosis and cuproptosis for catalytic cancer therapy. *Nature Communications*, *15*(1), 7499. Advance online publication. DOI: 10.1038/s41467-024-51772-1 PMID: 39209877

Zabala, V., & Suh, N. (2020). Metabolic alterations and vulnerabilities in hepatocellular carcinoma. *Gastroenterology Report*, *9*(1), 1–13. DOI: 10.1093/gastro/goaa057 PMID: 33747521

Zafar, H., Zhang, J., Raza, F., Pan, X., Hu, Z., Feng, H., & Shen, Q. (2024). Biomimetic gold nanocages incorporating copper-human serum albumin for tumor immunotherapy via cuproptosis-lactate regulation. *Journal of Controlled Release*, *372*, 446–466. DOI: 10.1016/j.jconrel.2024.06.059 PMID: 38917953

Zhang, C., Huang, T., & Li, L. (2024). Targeting cuproptosis for cancer therapy: Mechanistic insights and clinical perspectives. *Journal of Hematology & Oncology*, *17*(1), 68. DOI: 10.1186/s13045-024-01589-8 PMID: 39152464

Zhang, H., Li, Y., Wang, X., & Liu, J. (2023). Ferroptosis-related gene expression and breast cancer prognosis. *Journal of Clinical Oncology*, *41*(15, suppl), e12501. DOI: 10.1200/JCO.2023.41.15_suppl.e12501

Zhang, H., Sun, J., & Chen, W. (2024). Calcium peroxide nanoparticles for tumor-targeted therapy: Mechanisms and clinical implications. *Journal of Nanobiotechnology*, *22*, 2873. Advance online publication. DOI: 10.1186/s12951-024-02873-8

Zhang, Y., Li, X., & Wang, Z. (2023). Calcium signaling in cancer: A double-edged sword. *Frontiers in Cell and Developmental Biology*, *11*, 1248763. DOI: 10.3389/fcell.2023.1248763

Zhang, Y., Li, X., & Wang, Z. (2024). The impact of calcium overload on cellular processes: Exploring calcicoptosis as a novel form of regulated cell death. *International Journal of Molecular Sciences*, *25*(24), 13727. DOI: 10.3390/ijms252413727 PMID: 39769488

Zhang, Y., Shi, J., Liu, X., Wang, L., & Chen, Q. (2024). SLC7A11 as a prognostic biomarker for hepatocellular carcinoma. *Journal of Clinical Oncology*, *42*(16, suppl), e16004. DOI: 10.1200/JCO.2024.42.16_suppl.e16004

Zhang, Y., Tan, H., & Tang, Z. (2023). Broadening horizons: Ferroptosis as a new target for traumatic brain injury. *Burns and Trauma, 11*, tkad051. Advance online publication. DOI: 10.1093/burnst/tkad051 PMID: 38250705

Zhang, Y., Tan, H., & Tang, Z. (2023). Proteomic analysis of ferroptosis pathways reveals a role of CEPT1 in regulating ferroptosis sensitivity. *Protein & Cell, 15*(9), 686–704. DOI: 10.1093/procel/pwac080

Zhang, Y., Wang, Y., & Li, X. (2024). The study on cuproptosis in Alzheimer's disease based on the comprehensive analysis of cuproptosis-related genes. *Frontiers in Aging Neuroscience, 16*, 1480332. DOI: 10.3389/fnagi.2024.1480332 PMID: 39759399

Zhao, S., Liu, P., & Li, Y. (2024). Biomineralized apoferritin nanoparticles delivering dihydroartemisinin and calcium for synergistic breast cancer therapy. *Scientific Reports, 14*(1), 29402. Advance online publication. DOI: 10.1038/s41598-024-80735-1 PMID: 39592736

Zhao, Y., Ye, T., & Zhou, X. (2022). Copper-induced tumor cell death mechanisms and antitumor theragnostic applications of copper complexes. *Journal of Inorganic Biochemistry, 226*, 111634. DOI: 10.1016/j.jinorgbio.2021.111634

Zhao, Y., Ye, T., & Zhou, X. (2022). Elesclomol: A copper ionophore targeting mitochondrial metabolism for cancer therapy. *Journal of Experimental & Clinical Cancer Research : CR, 41*(1), 271. Advance online publication. DOI: 10.1186/s13046-022-02485-0 PMID: 36089608

Zhao, Y., Ye, T., & Zhou, X. (2023). Metabolic cell death in cancer: Ferroptosis, necroptosis, and cuproptosis. *Protein & Cell, 15*(9), 642–657. DOI: 10.1093/procel/pwad031

Zhao, Y., Ye, T., & Zhou, X. (2023). Targeting cuproptosis for cancer therapy: Mechanistic insights and clinical potential. *Journal of Hematology & Oncology, 16*, 89. Advance online publication. DOI: 10.1186/s13045-024-01589-8

Zhao, Y., Ye, T., & Zhou, X. (2024). Interplay of ferroptosis and cuproptosis in cancer: Dissecting metal-related cell death pathways for therapeutic insights. *Cancers (Basel), 16*(3), 512. Advance online publication. DOI: 10.3390/cancers16030512 PMID: 38339263

Zhao, Y., Ye, T., & Zhou, X. (2024). Mechanisms of cuproptosis and its relevance to distinct diseases. *Apoptosis, 29*(7-8), 1–13. DOI: 10.1007/s10495-024-01983-0 PMID: 38824478

Zhao, Y., Ye, T., & Zhou, X. (2024). Metal-dependent cell death in renal fibrosis: Now and in the future. *International Journal of Molecular Sciences*, *25*(24), 13279. DOI: 10.3390/ijms252413279 PMID: 39769044

Zhao, Y., Ye, T., & Zhou, X. (2024). Synergistic enhancement of low-dose radiation therapy via cuproptosis induction and mitochondrial damage using a theranostic nanoplatform. *Journal of Nanobiotechnology*, *22*, 3011. Advance online publication. DOI: 10.1186/s12951-024-03011-4

Zhao, Y., Ye, T., & Zhou, X. (2025). Cuproptosis: Molecular mechanisms, cancer prognosis, and therapeutic potential. *Journal of Translational Medicine*, *23*(1), 61. Advance online publication. DOI: 10.1186/s12967-025-06121-1

Zhou, B., Liu, J., Kang, R., & Klionsky, D. J. (2024). FERREG: Ferroptosis-based regulation of disease occurrence, progression, and therapy. *Briefings in Bioinformatics*, *25*(3), bbae223. Advance online publication. DOI: 10.1093/bib/bbae223 PMID: 38742521

Zhou, H., Yang, J., Li, Z., Feng, J., Duan, X., Yan, C., Wen, G., Qiu, X., & Shen, Z. (2024). Hollow mesoporous calcium peroxide nanoparticles for Drug-Free tumor calcicoptosis therapy. *Acta Biomaterialia*, *185*, 456–466. DOI: 10.1016/j.actbio.2024.07.009 PMID: 39004329

Zhou, Y., Luan, S., Jiang, Q., Chen, T., & Tan, J. (2021). KLF2 inhibits cancer cell migration and invasion by regulating ferroptosis through GPX4 in clear cell renal cell carcinoma. *Cancer Letters*, *522*, 1–13. DOI: 10.1016/j.canlet.2021.09.014 PMID: 34520818

Zhu, W., Cheng, X., Xu, P., Gu, Y., Xu, H., Xu, J., Wang, Y., Zhang, L. W., & Wang, Y. (2024). Radiotherapy-Driven nanoprobes targeting for visualizing tumor infiltration dynamics and inducing ferroptosis in Myeloid-Derived suppressor cells. *Journal of the American Chemical Society*, *146*(32), 22455–22468. DOI: 10.1021/jacs.4c05650 PMID: 39094119

Chapter 15
Comparative Insights into Biomaterials from Animal-based and Non-Animal Sources in Biomedical Applications

Imade Armadi
https://orcid.org/0009-0003-3063-5058
Cadi Ayyad University, Marrakech, Morocco

Abdessamad Abana
Cadi Ayyad University, Marrakech, Morocco

Youssef Ait Hamdan
Cadi Ayyad University, Marrakech, Morocco

Souad Loqman
Cadi Ayyad University, Marrakech, Morocco

Anass Belbachir
https://orcid.org/0009-0002-4828-0251
Cadi Ayyad University, Marrakech, Morocco

ABSTRACT

The application of biomaterials in the biomedical field represents a major advancement, offering effective and sustainable alternative solutions. These materials stand out for their unique properties, particularly their biocompatibility and biodegrad-

DOI: 10.4018/979-8-3373-1305-4.ch015

ability. However, the choice between animal or non-animal sources constitutes a primary challenge, directly influencing their use and effectiveness in various contexts. This chapter offers a comparative analysis of biomaterials of animal and non-animal origin, highlighting their distinct properties and adaptability to biomedical applications, while mentioning the limitations of each type of source. This multidimensional analysis thus provides a critical framework for guiding the choice of biomaterials based on the specific needs of biomedical applications and opens up perspectives on the development of hybrid or alternative materials capable of overcoming these limitations.

INTRODUCTION

In 1991, the most widely accepted definition of a biomaterial emerged from the Consensus Conference in Chester, UK, as any substance or combination of substances, other than drugs, of synthetic or natural origin, which can be used for any period of time, which partially or totally augments or replaces a tissue, organ or function of the body, in order to maintain or improve the quality of life of the individual. (Marin et al., 2020). Since then, biomaterials have been widely used in medical treatments such as cancer therapy, ligament and tendon repair, orthopedic applications, drug delivery, wound healing, and many others (Insuasti-Cruz et al., 2022). Biomaterials can be used to improve the function or complete replacement of organs and tissues in damaged or deteriorated parts (Marin et al., 2020). However, their interest lies in their ability to interact with biological systems in a controlled manner, enabling them to be used for therapeutic or diagnostic purposes (Alipour et al., 2020). Moreover, their unique properties, such as biodegradability, biocompatibility and non-toxicity, are highly demanding in the biomedical field (Festas et al., 2020). This makes biomaterials suitable candidates for various medical applications.

Except that, the major challenge remains to choose between biomaterials from animal and/or non-animal sources. Chitosan, collagen and silk are the main animal-sourced biomaterials widely discussed in the literature (Avila Rodríguez et al., 2018; Qi et al., 2017; Tian et al., 2022). Thanks to their qualities, these materials can adopt various forms such as films, hydrogels and sponges to respond to the needs of specific applications. (Fuchs et al., 2020). However, their availability and yields differ from source to source and remain an interesting point of discussion.

On the other hand, non-animal sources are gaining in popularity in the biomedical field due to their biodegradability, biocompatibility, and eco-friendly nature (L. Li et al., 2025). Biomaterials include polysaccharides, proteins and extracellular vesicles and can be adopted into various forms such as nanoparticles, nanofibers and hydrogels for application in wound healing, tissue engineering and drug delivery

(Jovic et al., 2019). This chapter focuses on alginate, cellulose and agarose, three well-known non-animal biomaterials.

In this sense, this chapter presents a comparative vision between biomaterials of animal and non-animal origin, closely analyzing their distinctive properties, their biomedical applications, while concluding with a presentation of hybrid biomaterials as a perspective vision.

I. COMPARATIVE INSIGHTS INTO THE ORIGINS AND PROPERTIES OF BIOMATERIALS

1. Animal Source

- **Collagen:**

Collagen is represented as the most abundant structural protein in the human body, accounting for around 25% to 35% of protein mass. Indeed it has been shown that any protein characterized by a structure based on three helical polypeptide chains (Figure 1) belong to the collagen family (Avila Rodríguez et al., 2018). Collagen is a viscoelastic material with high tensile strength and low extensibility. Collagen sources include chicken skin, bone, duck feet, equine tendons, bird feet, sheep skin, frog skin, and many others (Aleksandra et al., 2020). However, collagen from some sources is misfolded, which can lead to disease (Avila Rodríguez et al., 2018). Its availability in nature makes it of even greater interest, as it is used in various fields including biomedical, particularly in blood coagulation, tissue remodeling and vascular prostheses, generally in the form of microparticles that are easy to inject subcutaneously, or as tissue scaffolding (François Portier, 2017). In the literature we find different types of collagen each with its own sources and properties, which may guide the choice for a specific application, for example, type I collagen is the most widely used in the manufacture of cosmetic products due to its high biocompatibility (Avila Rodríguez et al., 2018). Chemically speaking, collagen has a structure characterized by the presence of particular amino acids such as hydroxyproline (around 14%) and hydroxylysine. These particular amino acids are obtained by hydroxylation of proline and lysine after synthesis of the α chain (Figure 1) (Marin et al., 2020).

Figure 1. Collagen triple-helix structure

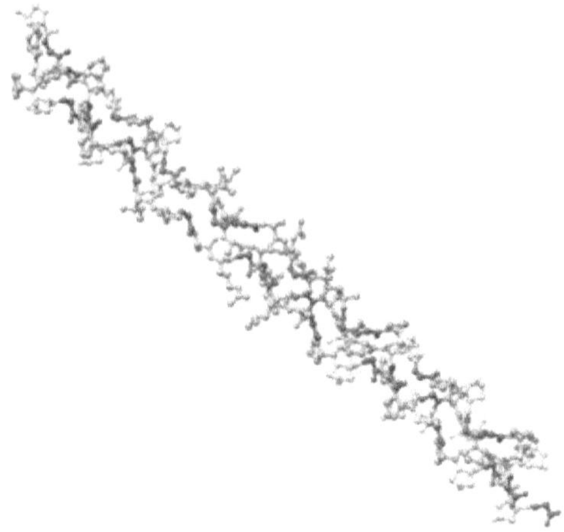

Thanks to its triple helix structure, collagen is characterized by high resistance to stretching and remarkable elasticity (Terzi et al., 2018). This property gives it a generally supportive role to connective tissues in withstanding mechanical stresses, such as shock absorption in articular cartilage (Terzi et al., 2018). In addition, this biomaterial promotes cell proliferation and new tissue formation, making it a key element in wound healing and tissue engineering (Ishigaki & Kubo, 2020). Not to mention its footprint for cell adhesion and migration, playing an important role in the repair of damaged tissue (Ishigaki & Kubo, 2020).

In the same sense, we add that the fibrillar structure of collagen, with its specific topography and sequential exposure of epitopes during tissue remodeling, plays a crucial role in the dynamic binding and controlled release of growth factors (Dong & Lv, 2016). Electrostatic interactions - for example, the heparin-collagen binding of VEGF - promote angiogenesis, while specific binding domains (e.g. CBD-TGFβ) enhance bone healing. In addition, chemotactic gradients generated by constructs such as CBD-SDF-1α stimulate stem cell migration (Baek et al., 2022).

- **Chitosan:**

After cellulose, chitin and chitosan top the list of natural biomaterials found in abundance in nature, usually in a variety of eukaryotic organisms, including crustaceans, insects and fungi (Kou et al., 2021). Recently, the industry has become increasingly interested in these two biomaterials, which are having a very significant and positive impact on research and development in fields as diverse as chemistry, biology, health and environmental preservation. Today, several industrial fields are concerned, from cosmetics to the food industry, via biomedicine (Crini, 2019).

According to the literature, shrimps and crabs are the most common sources for the preparation of chitosan, although other species are also used. In terms of yield, chitin content differs from one species to another, but generally remains between 10 and 75% (Triunfo et al., 2022). Work by (Dima et al., 2017) has shown that around 10-25% chitin (dry weight) is found in crustacean waste. (Tolaimate et al., 2003) states that some lobster species have the highest chitin content of all chitin-containing species, with shells containing 60-75% chitin by weight. Moving on to the chemical structure of chitin, the precursor to chitosan, which is represented by a chain of N-acetyl-β-D-glucosamine monomers linked by a glycosidic (1→4) bond, and nomenclature defines this structure as that of a poly β-(1→4)-2-acetamido-2-deoxy-D-glucopyranose (J. Wang & Zhuang, 2022). Therefore, This biopolymer has a composition close to cellulose with a modification at the C2 position. After deacetylation, we prepare chitosan, whose chemical structure is represented by a chain of ß(1-4)-D-glucosamine monomers. It has three reactive functional groups, amine group at C2 and two hydroxyl groups at C3 and C6 respectively (Younes & Rinaudo, 2015) (Figure 2).

Figure 2. Chemical structure of biomaterials derived from animal sources: A: Collagen, B: Chitosan, C: Silk

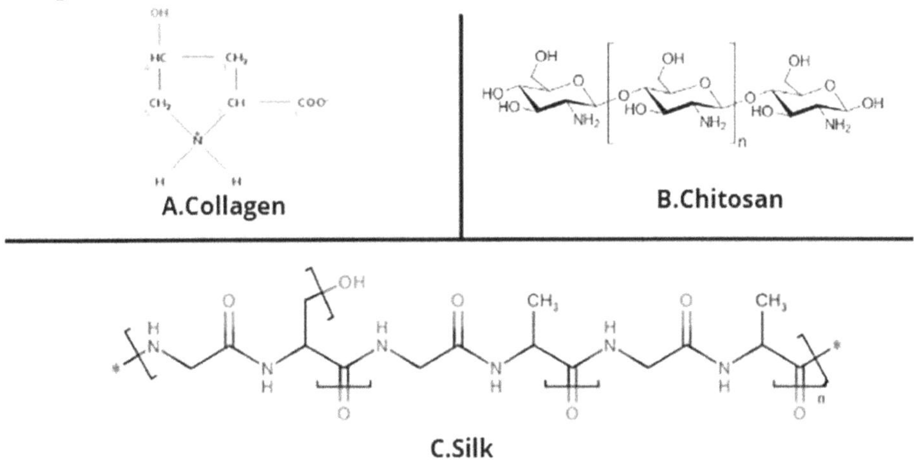

The chemical structure of chitosan, together with its biocompatibility and biodegradability properties, have attracted the interest of scientific researchers. Indeed, these unique properties play different roles in membranes, sponges and scaffolds, in addition to their biological properties, such as biocompatibility and biodegradability (Mohebbi et al., 2019). Thanks also to its non-toxicity to human tissues, while being progressively degraded and eliminated by the body, chitosan reduces the risk of toxic reactions (Azmana et al., 2021). These qualities give it significant potential for the development of drug delivery systems and other biomedical applications (Issahaku et al., 2023; Mohebbi et al., 2019).

- **Silk:**

Silk, another example of a natural biomaterial, is valued in the fields of biomedicine, biotechnology, and materials. The main sources of this natural protein biomaterial are the spider (*Nephila clavipes*) and the silkworm (*B. mori*) (Belda Marín et al., 2020). Despite the remarkable properties of spider silk (*Nephila clavipes*), its large-scale exploitation remains a major challenge, making the silkworm more practical for silk production (F. Wang et al., 2021). Chemically, silk is composed of two proteins: fibroin and sericin. Fibroin (~400 kDa) is the central peptide, and silk fibers are made up of two fibroin filaments linked by sericin, which acts as a glue (Lujerdean et al., 2022). Each fibroin molecule contains two chains, the heavy chain (FibH) and the light chain (FibL), linked by a disulfide bridge (Qi et al., 2017) Figure 2. Fibroin also contains another protein, fibrohexamerin/P25. Thanks to its structure, silk fibroin (SF) has attracted the attention of many scientific researchers in various fields such as chemistry, physics, engineering, biology and biomedicine (Lujerdean et al., 2022). It is considered an outstanding bioactive material for tissue engineering applications due to its biocompatibility, biodegradability and ease of modification. SF can be processed into a variety of formats, including sponges, platelets, gauze, particles, hydrogels, fibers and films, making it suitable for many applications (Lujerdean et al., 2022).

Thanks to its unique properties silk fibroin (SF) remains a biomaterial of choice. It is biocompatible, which has favored its use in sutures and various medical applications (Belda Marín et al., 2020; F. Wang et al., 2021). Studies have demonstrated its safety in contact with several cell types, including hippocampal neurons, skin cells and bone cells (Grabska-Zielińska & Sionkowska, 2021). Biodegradable, SF can be naturally degraded by proteolytic enzymes such as chymotrypsin, carboxylase and actinase, a key asset for biomedical applications requiring gradual resorption of the material (Ranjan et al., 2023). It also boasts excellent mechanical resistance, with high tensile strength, making it ideal for structures requiring strength and stability, such as tissue engineering scaffolds. Finally, its versatility enables it to be processed into a variety of formats, including films, mats, hydrogels and sponges, using techniques such as spin coating, electrospinning, freeze-drying and physical or chemical cross-linking, opening up a wide range of biomedical applications (Lujerdean et al., 2022).

2. Plant Source

- **Alginate:**

Alginates are natural polysaccharides extracted mainly from various species of marine brown algae such as *Padina sp., Dictyota sp., Sargassum polycistum, Turbinaria ornata and Turbinaria murayana.* and from certain bacterial sources such as *Pseudomonas sp. and Azotobacter sp.* The amount of alginate in different species is quite high, and can exceed 18% of dry weight in many brown algae. Alginates are water-soluble, biodegradable, non-toxic and non-irritant by nature. Structurally, and as illustrated in Figure 3 they are linear block copolymers of α-(1→4)-linked l-guluronic acid (G) and β-(1→4)-linked d-mannuronic acid (M) residues with M/G ratios ranging from 1.04 to 4.41 (Belattmania et al., 2020). Alginates are mainly available on the market in the form of calcium alginate and sodium alginate. Sodium alginate turns into an ionic gel in the presence of various divalent metal cations (e.g. Ca2+, Zn2+, Ba2+) and trivalent metal cations (e.g. Fe3+, Al3+) (Nayak et al., 2020). Alginate lyases can degrade alginate polymers into oligosaccharides or monosaccharides, broadening their potential applications (Nayak et al., 2020).

Figure 3. Chemical structure of non-animal-derived sources: A. Alginate, B. Cellulose, C. Agarose

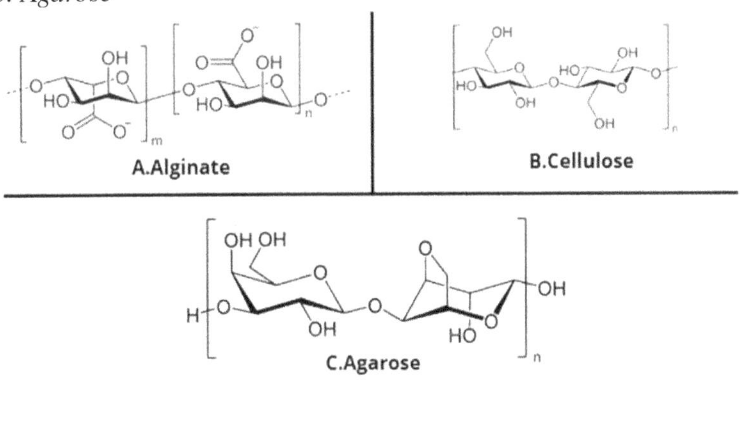

The mechanical properties of alginates are influenced by water content, with soft, extensible behavior at high water contents of 62-93%, but brittle, high-modulus behavior at low water contents of 19-48%. Hydrogels exhibit maximum fracture energy at intermediate water content, which is a measure of toughness; the soft-brittle transition results from aggregation of polymer chains upon dehydration, which activates hydrogen bonding interactions (X. Zhao et al., 2019). Alginate gels alone can have poor mechanical properties and syneresis problems, reducing their effectiveness in encapsulating certain substances such as proteins and bioactive compounds (Ramdhan et al., 2020). Overall, alginate-based materials offer tunable mechanical properties through a variety of methods, including dehydration, functionalization and composite formation, constituting their versatility for applications in tissue engineering and drug delivery.

- **Cellulose:**

Cellulose, the Earth's main organic compound, comes mainly from vascular plants, especially wood and cotton. Other sources of cellulose include jute, hemp, corn, rice, wheat straw, sisal and bacterial sources such as Acetobacter xylinum. Cellulose has many applications ranging from paper products to textiles, and various chemical and pharmaceutical uses (Seddiqi et al., 2021). The molecular structure of cellulose is a recurring unit of β-d-glucopyranose molecules forming a linear chain that can occur in crystallographic or amorphous form Figure 3. Cellulose is insoluble in water, but can dissolve in ionic liquids. Hemicelluloses are the second most abundant polysaccharides in nature, in which xylan is one of the main constituents of this polymer (Seddiqi et al., 2021). Plant cellulose is widely used in industry, while bacterial cellulose, often produced by Acetobacter xylinum, is suitable for non-industrial applications (Amalin Kavitha et al., 2020). Cellulose comes in a variety of forms, including fibers, microfibrils/nanofibrils and micro/nanocrystalline cellulose, each with distinct properties (Seddiqi et al., 2021). Extraction processes vary according to source, with plant and algal cellulose requiring bleaching and purification, while bacterial cellulose can be grown directly (P. K. Gupta et al., 2021; Pesic, 2021).

Cellulose-based materials have tunable mechanical properties; the Young's modulus in compression can be controlled from 30 kPa to 1.3 MPa by adjusting the initial cellulose concentration, with the diameter of the nanofibrous cellulose that forms the hydrogel constant at 15-20 nm, regardless of the initial cellulose concentration. Meanwhile, biocompatible cellulose hydrogel, prepared using a salt leaching process, was able to successfully support cartilage tissue culture (Clare et al., 2019). Cellulose of different molecular weights and concentrations was dissolved in a mixture of ionic liquid and DMSO, coagulated in ethanol which formed highly porous amorphous materials prepared using two drying methods: with scCO2 (aerogels) and freeze-drying (cryogels), cellulose aerogels and cryogels exhibited different mechanical behaviors, with cryogels showing higher compressive modulus and yield strength at the same density (Buchtová et al., 2019). The results of the study exceed those of metals, alloys and glass fibers, enhancing the potential of durable, lightweight and high-performance materials, with stress transfer being efficient and the high degree of alignment in cellulosic fibers enabling them to achieve a Young's modulus of up to 86 GPa and a tensile strength of 1.57 GPa, exceeding the mechanical properties of known natural or synthetic biopolymer materials. The mechanical properties of cellulose-based materials are mainly influenced by factors such as hydrogen bonding, nanofiber size and orientation, and structural interfaces (Ghavimi et al., 2019; Ray et al., 2021).

- **Agarose:**

Agarose is a natural polysaccharide derived from red algae, primarily from species of red algae. The main sources include the genera Gracilaria, Gelidium, Gigartina, and Hydropuntia. Agar, from which agarose is extracted, is composed of agarose and agaropectin (Barbu et al., 2021). It possesses excellent properties such as electrical conductivity, pH reactivity, and the formation of thermally reversible gel. Structurally, agarose is formed from a linear polysaccharide composed of D-galactose and 3,6-anhydro-L-galactose with numerous hydroxyl groups in its structural unit, which on average form hydrogen bonds with the hydrogen atoms of its structure or with those of water (figure 3). Its molecular weight ranged between 80 kDa and 140 kDa. Agarose had the ability to form a controlled hydrogel with stability and hysteresis, making it an ideal adjustable drug delivery system for loading and controlling drug release by stimulating a responsive reaction under different environmental conditions, increasing drug retention time, and thereby reducing the frequency of dosing and the drug's toxic effects. (Irastorza-Lorenzo et al., 2021; Jiang et al., 2023).

The mechanical properties of agarose, particularly the Young's modulus and the shear modulus, are strongly influenced by the concentration. Various methods have been used to characterize these properties, including resonance techniques, tensile and compression tests, rheology, and quantitative T2 MRI (Alam et al., 2020). Agarose spheres showed Young's modulus values ranging from 209 to 646 kPa for concentrations between 2% and 4% (Sacco et al., 2024). The shear modulus and relaxation rate increase exponentially with agarose concentration, with an exponential factor difference observed for concentrations below 2% (Jana et al., 2022). The biomechanical properties of agarose hydrogels were strongly associated with agarose concentration, with highly concentrated hydrogels exhibiting the highest Young's modulus values. Moreover, the type of agarose influenced the biomechanical properties, particularly the strain at break, suggesting that the difference between agarose types could be used to obtain biomaterials with different elastic behaviors. All types and concentrations of agarose exhibited high biocompatibility, with no significant systemic or local adverse effects observed in vivo, and a pro-regenerative immune response (Irastorza-Lorenzo et al., 2021). Although there are many examples of biomaterials from animal and non-animal sources. In this study we have focused more on the biomaterials most discussed in the literature and used in the biomedical field. Table 1, shows a summary of what has been discussed, presenting the main points.

Table 1. Comparative overview of animal- and non-animal-derived biomaterials

Biomaterial	Source	Structure/Composition	Key Properties	Forms	References
Collagen	Animal (e.g., skin, bone, tendons)	Triple helix; rich in hydroxyproline	High tensile strength, elasticity, biocompatibility, supports cell adhesion	Films, hydrogels, scaffolds	(Avila Rodríguez et al., 2018; Marin et al., 2020)
Chitosan	Animal (extracted from crustaceans)	Polymer of ß(1-4)-D-glucosamine (after deacetylation)	Biocompatible, biodegradable, antimicrobial, chemically modifiable	Membranes, sponges, nanofibers	(Crini, 2019; Younes & Rinaudo, 2015)
Silk	Animal (silkworms; also spiders)	Composed of fibroin and sericin	Excellent mechanical strength, biocompatibility, degradable, versatile processing formats	Films, fibers, hydrogels, sutures	(Belda Marín et al., 2020; Qi et al., 2017)
Alginate	Non-animal (brown algae and bacteria)	Linear copolymer of α-L-guluronic acid and β-D-mannuronic acid	Water solubility, biocompatibility, ionic gel formation, tunable properties based on water content	Hydrogels, films, foams	(Belattmania et al., 2020; Nayak et al., 2020)
Cellulose	Non-animal (plant or bacterial)	Linear chain of β-D-glucopyranose	High mechanical strength, tunable by concentration, good biocompatibility	Fibers, aerogels, cryogels	(Buchtová et al., 2019; Seddiqi et al., 2021)
Agarose	Non-animal (red algae)	Linear polysaccharide of D-galactose and 3,6-anhydro-L-galactose	Thermoreversible gel formation, stability, biocompatibility	Hydrogels, spheres, films	(Irastorza-Lorenzo et al., 2021; Sacco et al., 2024)

II. BIOMEDICAL APPLICATIONS OF ANIMAL- AND PLANT-DERIVED BIOMATERIALS

1. Animal Source

- **Chitosan:**

Chitosan, a polysaccharide derived from chitin through deacetylation, as previously described, has garnered considerable interest in the biomedical field due to its unique properties such as biodegradability, biocompatibility, non-toxicity, and antimicrobial activity. It is considered the second largest renewable biomaterial after cellulose. This interest translates into a multitude of potential applications, ranging from antimicrobial wound dressings to drug delivery systems targeting the brain (Crini, 2019).

- **Antimicrobial Dressings:**

Thanks to its properties and antimicrobial activity, chitosan remains the ideal candidate for wound management. It can be used alone or in combination with other polymers, active agents, and metallic nanocomposites to enhance its effectiveness (Kravanja et al., 2019). Studies have shown that chitosan has antibacterial activity against numerous bacteria, yeasts, and fungi, which is very interesting for the biomedical field (Yan et al., 2021). Furthermore, it promotes the regeneration of skin epithelial cells and the production of collagen by fibroblasts, thereby accelerating healing (Confederat et al., 2021). Moreover, studies discuss the possibility of incorporating liposomes containing antimicrobial drugs, such as chlorhexidine (CHX), into chitosan-based hydrogels, which improves the retention of liposomes and the prolonged release of the drug, thus offering enhanced control of skin infections (Yousefian et al., 2023).

- **Wound Healing:**

Chitosan, a biocompatible and bioactive biopolymer, plays a key role in wound healing. Thanks to its hemostatic properties, it promotes the aggregation of erythrocytes and platelets, effectively stopping bleeding. Its antimicrobial activity, due to its interactions with bacterial membranes, helps limit infections while chelating certain metal ions (Cano-Vicent et al., 2023). It also modulates the inflammatory response by acting on the CD14, TLR4, and CR3 receptors of macrophages, thereby contributing to balanced healing. Moreover, its antioxidant effects prevent excessive oxidative stress, thereby protecting the cells involved in tissue regeneration (Pires et al., 2023). Chitosan also stimulates angiogenesis and improves collagen organization, essential for tissue repair. Finally, by promoting the migration of fibroblasts and keratinocytes, it accelerates wound closure and re-epithelialization (L. Zhao et al., 2023).

- **Bone Regeneration:**

Chitosan also has a say in bone tissue engineering (BTE) due to its biocompatibility, biodegradability, and osteoconductivity. Its antimicrobial, bioadhesive, and pro-coagulant properties make it an ideal candidate for bone regeneration, particularly in the design of scaffolds intended to support the adhesion, proliferation, and differentiation of bone cells (Kudiyarasu et al., 2024). However, pure chitosan has limited mechanical strength, which has led to its combination with other biomaterials. Chitosan and ceramic composites such as hydroxyapatite (HA) and calcium phosphate cement (CPC) improve the structural stability and bioactivity of scaffolds, promoting mineralization and osteogenesis (Tao et al., 2020). Moreover, the integration of chitosan with mesenchymal stem cells (MSC) constitutes another promising approach. The CSM-chitosan scaffolds, enriched with growth factors and bioactive molecules, stimulate osteoblastic differentiation and accelerate bone formation. Moreover, chitosan nanofibers improve cell adhesion and activate osteogenic signaling pathways, thereby promoting calcium deposition and tissue mineralization (Guillén-Carvajal et al., 2023).

- **Collagen:**

Collagen is a biomaterial widely used in the biomedical field due to its biocompatibility, biodegradability, and low antigenicity. As a major component of connective tissues, collagen accounts for approximately 20 to 30% of the total proteins in the human body and plays a key role in the mechanical strength of tissues (Aleksandra et al., 2020). It is primarily found in the skin, tendons, and cartilage, where it provides flexibility and strength. This abundance and its structural role make it a material of choice for various biomedical applications (François Portier, 2017).

- **Drug Delivery Systems:**

It plays an essential role in drug delivery systems, particularly in the form of films, membranes, or nanoparticles for the controlled release of therapeutic substances (An et al., 2016). In ophthalmology, collagen shields allow for the direct application of medications to the eye, while collagen sponges are used to promote the healing of burns and chronic wounds. It is also used for gene therapy thanks to nanoparticles loaded with genetic material (Jafernik et al., 2023). Collagen films and membranes are also used as biomedical barriers and controlled drug release devices, allowing them to ensure a gradual release of active ingredients. They can be chemically modified to improve their stability and efficacy (Haider et al., 2024).

- **Tissue Engineering:**

It is used for tissue engineering, particularly in the production of skin substitutes for burn victims and patients with chronic wounds. Its properties also make it a key element in the development of bone matrices, artificial ligaments, and even bioengineered blood vessels (P. Gupta et al., 2024). Thanks to its numerous applications, collagen remains an essential material in modern medicine, paving the way for new advancements in regenerative therapy and bioengineering.

2. Plant Source

- **Agarose:**

Agarose-based hydrogel films exhibit excellent hydration properties, absorbing and retaining large amounts of liquid while maintaining structural integrity for wound healing applications (Autio et al., 2018). Agarose bioplastic films exhibit interesting properties such as transparency, strength, flexibility, and good swelling properties that facilitate drug administration. As shown by cell culture and hemolysis tests, bioplastic films are biocompatible and hemocompatible, as the drugs incorporated into the bioplastic films, including antibiotics and antiseptics, retain their potency (Awadhiya et al., 2017). Overall, agarose-based hydrogel films exhibit numerous properties, such as versatile and biocompatible dressings that provide prolonged hydration and mechanical protection while potentially accelerating the healing process (Irastorza-Lorenzo et al., 2021) . Not to mention the fact, Agaroses used in the fibrin agarose (FA) biomaterials also showed good biocompatibility ex vivo because more than 95% of fibroblasts in the hydrogels were alive, thus the type and concentration of the agarose used in the FA biomaterials had an effect on their biomechanical properties. FA with D1LE agarose had the highest young's modulus and FA with LM agarose had the highest stress and strain at fracture. As such, the FA biomaterials had in vivo biocompatibility with no adverse effects either systemic or local, and the FA biomaterials biodegradation was found to be influenced by the concentration and type of agarose, with the rate of in vivo biodegradation depending on the concentration and type of agarose (Ortiz-Arrabal et al., 2023).

- **Alginate:**

- **Healing Dressings:**

Alginate-based dressings are effective materials for wound healing due to their biocompatibility, non-toxicity, and ability to maintain a moist environment (Aderibigbe & Buyana, 2018). These dressings can absorb excess wound exudate, forming a gel that promotes healing and protects against infection (Mohanto et al., 2021). Alginate-based dressings can be formed into hydrogels, films, pads, and foams, each form offering specific advantages for wound management (M. Zhang & Zhao, 2020). The hydrophilic nature of alginate-based dressings improves in a moist environment, removes wound exudate, and accelerates skin recovery (Varaprasad et al., 2020). Pratically, M. Soleimanpour et al developed a wound dressing using a combination of fibrinogen, nisin, EDTA, and alginate. The hydrogel showed slow leakage of nisin, exhibited antibacterial activity, absorbed water and oxygen, and cell viability tests proved high compatibility, meanwhile blood clotting tests supported the rapid clotting reaction of the hydrogel when in blood. In vivo experiments also resulted in stronger wound healing, re-epithelialization, and collagen deposition (Soleimanpour et al., 2022).

Alginate-based dressings form a gel upon contact with wound exudates, maintaining a moist environment conducive to healing (Mohanto et al., 2021). Alginate dressings have various beneficial properties for wound healing, including antimicrobial, antifungal, antiviral, anti-inflammatory, antioxidant, and hemostatic effects, as well as the ability to promote angiogenesis and tissue regeneration. The formulation of alginate dressings can take various forms, such as hydrogels, nanofiber networks, and 3D scaffolds or sponges, which can trap cells or drugs to enhance wound healing (Barbu et al., 2021). Overall, alginate-based dressings offer numerous advantages over synthetic polymers, making them a valuable option for wound management (Mohanto et al., 2021).

- **Bone Regeneration:**

Alginate-based scaffolds have the ability to promote bone tissue regeneration by enhancing cell proliferation and osteoblast differentiation. Alginate-based scaffolds can be used to deliver drugs and other therapeutic agents for tissue regeneration. These scaffolds provide an environment conducive to the growth and differentiation of osteoblasts (Nayak et al., 2020). Alginate hydrogels have a valuable application in bone tissue engineering due to their excellent biocompatibility, biodegradability, lack of immunogenicity, abundant source, and affordable cost. However, pure alginate hydrogel scaffolds still exhibit drawbacks such as insufficient mechanical properties and low biological activity, which limits their clinical application (Chen et al., 2024).

- **Controlled Drug Delivery Systems:**

Alginate possesses unique properties that make it an excellent support for various therapeutic agents, notably its gel-forming ability and stability (Nayak et al., 2020). Alginate hydrogels possess physicochemical characteristics and a similarity to the native extracellular matrix, both in terms of composition and mechanics, and their high water content contributes to their good biocompatibility, allowing them to be used as a matrix for the encapsulation and distribution of various bioactive compounds, such as drugs, peptides, polysaccharides, antibiotics, antigens, and enzymes(V. Singh & Singh, 2019). The versatility and customization of alginate make it an ideal candidate for future advancements in controlled drug delivery applications (Nayak et al., 2020).

In an animal study conducted to compare the biocompatibility, pharmacokinetics, and bioavailability of a human monoclonal antibody in alginate-based prolonged-release delivery systems after subcutaneous administration in rats. 28 days after injection, the alginate-based hydrogel formed prolonged-release delivery systems, and the in-situ formation system also delayed the time required to reach the maximum serum concentration by 2 to 4 days. The almost complete release of the monoclonal antibody from the alginate matrices occurred during the 28-day study period, without impacting systemic bioavailability (Wani et al., 2023).

- **Cellulose:**

Cellulose nanofibrils (CNF) can form solid 3D porous networks, which can be made bioactive for bone formation through simple and scalable strategies. These scaffolds contribute to the formation of hydroxyapatite, the release of essential ions for bone repair, while enhancing the expression of osteoblastic genes and the production of bone morphogenetic protein 2 (BMP-2) (Ferreira et al., 2019). Moreover, the non-toxicity, biocompatibility, biodegradability, and cost-effectiveness ensure that cellulose-based scaffolds present a promising potential in bone tissue engineering applications, and they can also be used for the localized delivery of growth factors and antibiotics to promote bone tissue repair and regeneration (Janmohammadi et al., 2023). In addition, in terms of wound healing, S. Bhowmik et al. found that gelatin-cellulose nanocrystal (CNC) composite films had significantly better mechanical properties than pure gelatin films. In addition, the incorporation of CNC improved the water absorption and buffering capabilities of gelatin, and gelatin-CNC biocomposite films were biocompatible, non-cytotoxic and proved useful as dressings to absorb wound fluids and maintain moisture for wound healing (Bhowmik et al., 2017).

Cellulose and its derivatives are widely used in bone and cartilage tissue engineering due to their excellent biological properties. However, cellulose-based composites have limitations, such as slow degradation and tight compaction, which can hinder cell penetration into the scaffolds (Tao et al., 2020). Similarly, bacterial cellulose is a promising material for bone tissue engineering, although its lack of bioactivity is a limitation, the use of growth factors can still enhance the bioactivity of materials for bone tissue engineering, improving the properties of cellulose and its derivatives is essential to enhance their application in the treatment of bone diseases (Farnezi Bassi et al., 2020).

III. LIMITATIONS AND CHALLENGES OF BIOMATERIALS BASED ON THEIR ORIGINS

Despite the interesting qualities and the role that biomaterials play in the biomedical field. Limits and challenges are encountered in every study. However, these obstacles in no way represent a negative point for these biomaterials; on the contrary, they represent a motivation to work even harder, advance science, and tackle these challenges. From animal or plant sources, obstacles are present with slight differences, and in this section, we will generally present the obstacles that each source suffers from.

1. For Animal Sources

The use of animal-derived biomaterials in biomedicine presents challenges and limitations related to biocompatibility, regulatory aspects, and the constraints of in vitro and in vivo testing (Amadou Toure, 2018). Ideal biocompatibility is difficult to achieve, requiring a clinically acceptable compromise. It is imperative to maintain the material-tissue relationship over a long duration, which complicates the achievement of perfect biocompatibility. Moreover, the evaluation of biocompatibility itself includes physicochemical studies and cytotoxicity assessments. Short-term and long-term tests are essential to evaluate the potential risks, functionality, and clinical behavior of materials (Cao et al., 2023).

Furthermore, on the testing side, in vitro remains a preliminary step providing quick results and a general idea, making it difficult to generalize and decide to move on to clinical applications. Moreover, animal experimentation, although necessary in some cases for biomedical research, is subject to debates and strict regulations. French law, for example, requires that animal experimentation be necessary, irreplaceable, and conducted while ensuring the health and well-being of the animals (Amadou Toure, 2018).

Finally, natural-origin biomaterials often coincide with raw material obstacles, either in terms of availability or cost, which can sometimes be very high for advanced research. This limits the tests in what is conventional and often hinders the advancement of science in this area (Claudia Spataru et al., 2024).

2. For Non-Animal Sources

Plant-based materials have demonstrated excellent biocompatibility and biodegradability, making them suitable for various biomedical applications, with processing capabilities ranging from nanoparticles and nanofibers to hydrogels. However, the need to develop standardized isolation methods has remained constant for plant-based materials, necessitating continued research to overcome challenges such as variations in material properties depending on the source, microbial contamination, uncontrolled water absorption, low mechanical strength, and unpredictable degradation patterns (J. Li et al., 2025). However, a further transition from preclinical applications to clinical applications is necessary for plant-based materials. Continuous efforts aim to improve the physicochemical properties and expand the applications of these biomaterials in the pharmaceutical and biomedical fields (K. Zhang et al., 2022).

In this sense, we say that biomaterials that are natural-based tend to have numerous functional limitations. They frequently do not possess adequate mechanical strength and stability, possess high degradation rates, and may not offer sufficient signals for cell differentiation and tissue formation (Gomez-Florit et al., 2020). Their use is further complicated by batch-to-batch variations in composition as well as potential immunogenicity issues. Ullah & Chen, (2020) remarked that to solve these issues, researchers are trying blending natural polymers and using classical physical/chemical crosslinking treatments along with cutting edge 3D bioprinting and nanotechnology. However, many natural biomaterials encounter obstacles when optimizing mechanical performance in terms of stiffness and limited extensibility or being 'too compliant' which is defined by increased strain to failure (Miserez et al., 2015).

The chemical modification of plant polysaccharides is a decisive approach to improve their bioactivity and biochemical properties in order to adapt them to biomedical applications. The main modification methods include sulfation, phosphorylation, acetylation, salinization, and carboxymethylation. Chemically modified polysaccharides have improved their biological activities such as antioxidant, antitumor, antiviral, and immunoregulatory effects. On the other hand, the lack of controllability in the chemical modification process, which results in inconsistent substitution degrees and molecular weights from one batch to another, as well as the toxicity and by-products of the catalysts used in chemical modification methods, lead to low yields (Mohammed et al., 2021).

The polysaccharides present in biomaterials are generally used in modified forms, which require effective compatibilization strategies. However, native plant polysaccharides have reduced thermal stability, high moisture absorption, and limited mechanical performance, which hinders their direct use in advanced material systems. The effectiveness of these compatibilization strategies must be critically evaluated based on a detailed analysis of the chemical structures, morphologies, and macroscopic properties of polysaccharide-based materials (Troy et al., 2021).

Furthermore, although cellulose has been used for a long time in pharmaceutical products, nanocellulose is a relatively new biomaterial in this field. Despite the low mechanical strength of non-hydrogel forms of alginate, which limits their potential applications, further functionalization of alginate with a wider range of molecules is necessary to create more interactive forms with tissues (Claudia Spataru et al., 2024). Natural origin polymers offer numerous advantages for tissue engineering due to their similarity to the extracellular matrix and a reduced risk of inflammation or toxicity compared to synthetic polymers. Given that researchers have made efforts to mimic the extracellular matrix using its main constituents, such as collagen, fibronectin, and glycosaminoglycans, in tissue engineering applications, after all, successful tissue engineering requires the development of scaffolds that provide a 3D structure to support cell adhesion, proliferation, and extracellular matrix production (Su et al., 2018). However, the potential for immune response due to impurities and batch-to-batch variability of natural materials needs to be improved in the production, purification, and control of material properties in order to enhance biocompatibility. Despite this, further research and development are still necessary to translate natural origin polymers into successful clinical applications (Imran et al., 2020). Table 2 illustrates the main biomedical applications of the biomaterials discussed, and gives an overview of the major challenges.

3. Regulatory Challenges and Approval Routes for Biomaterials

Developing and authorizing biomaterials for medical devices is governed by intricate processes that follow international standards and policies (Schuh & Funk, 2019). Jurczak et al., (2024) argue that the Medical Device Regulation (MDR) and the In Vitro Diagnostic (IVD) Device Regulation (IVDR) of the European Union (EU) have recently changed to protect patients, but may hinder innovation progression on devices that utilize biomaterials. The Bayon et al., (2024) approach reflects the need for integrating primary regulatory plans to meet specific clinical needs and provides explanation of the apparent "success" in adopting novel biomaterials in clinical products. There is, however, no question that the translation of new biomaterials into clinical practice is complex and current standardization and regulations do not sufficiently address these challenges (Ebrahimi, 2020). The challenges with regulations of using biomaterials in biomedical applications stem from the fact that biomaterials are not a standalone medical product and regulators approve final medical products (Song et al., 2022). There are many issues with the animal studies conducted on biomaterial products, including vague objectives and poorly devised studies which in turn results in failure to translate the studies into regulation (Cheng et al., 2022). Plant-derived materials offer advantages such as lower contamination risk and reduced ethical concerns, but face challenges in standardization and clinical translation (L. Li et al., 2025). To overcome these challenges, cooperation between different stakeholders is necessary, to bridge this gap among researchers, clinicians, industry, and regulatory bodies, with emphasis on early integration of safety considerations and robust research and development phases.

Table 2. Biomedical applications and challenges of biomaterials

Biomaterial	Applications	Main Advantages	Limitations/ Challenges	References
Collagen	Tissue engineering, hemostasis, drug delivery systems	Promotes cell proliferation, excellent tissue integration	Source variability, risk of misfolding	(Avila Rodríguez et al., 2018; François Portier, 2017)
Chitosan	Antimicrobial wound dressings, drug delivery, bone engineering	Antimicrobial activity, accelerates healing, biodegradable	Low mechanical strength when used alone, yield variability	(Crini, 2019; Yousefian et al., 2023)
Silk	Sutures, scaffolds for tissue engineering, implantable devices	High mechanical strength, versatile processing formats	Large-scale production challenges, purity control issues	(Belda Marín et al., 2020; Lujerdean et al., 2022)
Alginate	Wound dressings, bone scaffolds, controlled drug delivery	Ionic gel formation, creates a moist healing environment	Syneresis issues, mechanical weakness under certain conditions	(Aderibigbe & Buyana, 2018; Mohanto et al., 2021)
Cellulose	Bone and cartilage tissue engineering, cell culture scaffolds	High rigidity, mechanical properties can be tuned	Slow degradation, dense structure may hinder cell penetration	(Ferreira et al., 2019; Janmohammadi et al., 2023)
Agarose	Hydrogel films for wound healing, drug delivery platforms	Thermally reversible gel formation, stable gel structure	Sensitive to concentration variations, mechanical limitations	(Irastorza-Lorenzo et al., 2021; Jana et al., 2022)

IV. HYBRIDIZATION AND COMPOSITE BIOMATERIALS

1. Generalities

This term of composite materials has not just come into existence. Indeed, for decades various materials have been combined to produce a new material offering performance and efficiency unattainable by materials taken individually. In reality, many materials can be considered composites (A. Singh et al., 2019). For example, a metal can be seen as a composite made up of various grains. Otherwise, a composite material is a material made up of at least two components with significantly different physical and chemical properties. When combined, they give rise to a material with properties distinct from those of the initial materials (M. Wang, 2016).

They too have their say in this field, offering valuable advantages such as high corrosion resistance, low electrical conductivity, and reduced thermal expansion. Except that the term organic-inorganic hybrid composites has recently emerged in the literature. These hybrid materials are defined by the emergence of new electronic orbitals between two or more materials, thereby generating unprecedented properties (Park et al., 2020).

Let's go back a bit to the 80s-90s, when two researchers significantly developed this term. Niizeki (1986), in his work, defined hybrid materials as two or more types of chemical bonds resulting from the hybridization of monolithic materials. Yamada et al. (1989), on the other hand, showed that hybrid materials are like mixtures of two or more materials, whose new properties emerge thanks to the formation of novel electronic orbitals (A. Singh et al., 2019; M. Wang, 2016).

2. Classifications

We can therefore classify these hybrid composites as follows: Class I hybrids that exhibit weak interactions, such as Van der Waals forces, hydrogen bonds, or weak electrostatic interactions. Or, hybrid composites of class II, which in turn exhibit strong chemical bonds between the two components (Chong et al., 2023).

Another functional classification categorizes hybrid materials into three types: structural hybrid materials (composites), chemically bonded hybrid materials, and functionally hybrid materials. Figure 4 illustrates the relationship between these three categories (Dorozhkin, 2011; A. Singh et al., 2019; L. Zhang et al., 2020).

Figure 4. Classification of hybrid materials

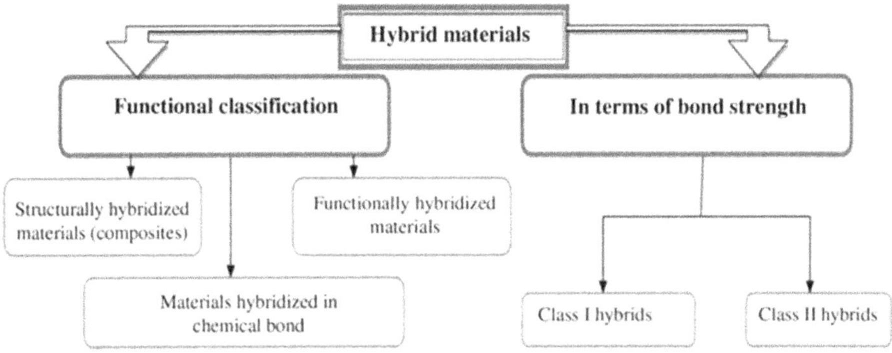

3. Manufacturing and Functionalization Approaches for Hybrid Biomaterials

Hybrid biomaterials often combine a natural polymer, such as chitosan, with inorganic components (hydroxyapatite, calcium carbonate, clays) to enhance their properties (Liu et al., 2021).. Their manufacture is based on several approaches: Mixing of components to optimize their compatibility and functionality. Co-precipitation of the inorganic component in the presence of the polymer, influencing crystal size and organization (Zafeiris et al., 2021). Biomimetic mineralization, mimicking natural processes to control mineral structure. Advanced techniques (freeze-drying, 3D printing, electrospinning) to adjust porosity and three-dimensional structure. Inorganic doping to confer additional properties (antibacterial, osteogenesis). Addition of a third component or cross-linking agents to improve mechanical and biological resistance. Controlled-release methods (layer-by-layer, electrospray) to encapsulate and release drugs in a targeted manner (He et al., 2021).

4. Interest in Biomedical

The primary question in this section remains to determine its relevance in the biomedical field. Indeed, they are generally used in the literature to improve medical treatments through the development of new technologies and advanced devices (Ates et al., 2017).

In this sense, it is noted that hybrid composites in biomedical engineering can be used for the manufacture of medical devices (dental implants, vascular grafts). Moreover, they are involved in drug delivery due to their ability to maintain a stable therapeutic range with minimal variations, reduce side effects, increase the plasma concentration of short half-life drugs, and decrease the number of daily doses (Park et al., 2020; A. Singh et al., 2019). The success of tissue engineering approaches heavily depends on the selection of biomaterials, as they guide the structure and shape of developing tissues, determine mechanical stability, and offer opportunities to administer inductive molecules to transplanted cells (M. Wang, 2016). Hybrid composites, obtained by combining synthetic polymers with other matrices, enhance cell interaction and promote integration into host tissues. These composites also offer tunable material properties to support the formation of bone, vascular, and nerve tissues (Ates et al., 2017; Dorozhkin, 2015).

CONCLUSION

As a conclusion, this comparative study of biomaterials, whether of animal or non-animal origin, highlights the richness and diversity of their biomedical applications.

On the one hand, polysaccharides include types of plant and marine origin, possessing interesting physicochemical, mechanical, and biomedical properties, granting them versatility in various applications (J. Li et al., 2025). Polysaccharide-based materials have proven to be promising in drug delivery, tissue engineering, wound healing, and biosensors due to their structural similarities with the extracellular matrix and their non-toxic degradation behavior (Jin et al., 2021). The versatility and abundance of polysaccharides position them as emerging excipients in pharmaceutical research, with the potential to advance healthcare and improve patient outcomes (Jabeen & Atif, 2024).

On the other hand, animal-derived biomaterials also possess unique properties and are widely discussed in the literature, with well-supported in vitro tests and more advanced preclinical tests, due to their significant availability compared to non-animal sources (Marin et al., 2020). These properties, which manifest in biocompatibility and biodegradability, have been and continue to be the most sought after in urgent clinical applications (Claudia Spataru et al., 2024).

Each biomaterial source has specific advantages and disadvantages, influenced by factors such as cost, extraction methods, and intrinsic material properties. It is therefore very important to recognize that each biomaterial has a unique role to play, depending on the clinical context and specific needs. Hybrid composites, by combining the strengths of different sources, open promising perspectives to overcome these challenges and improve solutions in various biomedical applications (tissue engineering, drug delivery systems, bone regeneration.) (Tsouknidas, 2024). The optimization of these hybrid systems in future research using advanced manufacturing techniques will provide improved scalability and rigorous clinical evaluation, paving the way for customized, multifunctional biomaterials that can meet the evolving needs of modern medicine. Ultimately, there is no universal biomaterial; the choice depends on the specific application, clinical needs, and material performance.

REFERENCES

Aderibigbe, B., & Buyana, B. (2018). Alginate in Wound Dressings. *Pharmaceutics*, *10*(2), 42. DOI: 10.3390/pharmaceutics10020042 PMID: 29614804

Alam, K., Hasan, A., Iqbal, M., Umer, J., & Piya, S. (2020). Experimental study on the mechanical properties of biological hydrogels of different concentrations. *Technology and Health Care*, *28*(6), 685–695. DOI: 10.3233/THC-191984 PMID: 32200364

Aleksandra, O., Robert, K., Karolina, K., Wojciech, R., Agnieszka, S., & Maciążek-Jurczyk, M. (2020). Collagène – structure, propriétés et application. *Ingénierie Des Biomatériaux*, *23*(156), 17–23.

Alipour, M., Baneshi, M., Hosseinkhani, S., Mahmoudi, R., Jabari Arabzadeh, A., Akrami, M., Mehrzad, J., & Bardania, H. (2020). Recent progress in biomedical applications of RGD-based ligand: From precise cancer theranostics to biomaterial engineering: A systematic review. *Journal of Biomedical Materials Research. Part A*, *108*(4), 839–850. DOI: 10.1002/jbm.a.36862 PMID: 31854488

Toure, A. (2018). Contribution au développement de substituts osseux auto-réticulants en ingénierie tissulaire osseuse maxillo-faciale (Doctoral dissertation, Nantes). [Contribution to the development of self-crosslinking bone substitutes in maxillofacial bone tissue engineering].

Amalin Kavitha, A., Thomas Paul, K., & Anilkumar, P. (2020). Cellulose-derived materials for drug delivery applications. In *Sustainable Nanocellulose and Nano-hydrogels from Natural Sources* (pp. 367–390). Elsevier., DOI: 10.1016/B978-0-12-816789-2.00018-3

An, B., Lin, Y.-S., & Brodsky, B. (2016). Collagen interactions: Drug design and delivery. *Advanced Drug Delivery Reviews*, *97*, 69–84. DOI: 10.1016/j.addr.2015.11.013 PMID: 26631222

Ates, B., Koytepe, S., Balcioglu, S., Ulu, A., & Gurses, C. (2017). Biomedical applications of hybrid polymer composite materials. In *Hybrid Polymer Composite Materials* (pp. 343–408). Elsevier., DOI: 10.1016/B978-0-08-100785-3.00012-7

Autio, K. A., Dreicer, R., Anderson, J., Garcia, J. A., Alva, A., Hart, L. L., Milowsky, M. I., Posadas, E. M., Ryan, C. J., Graf, R. P., Dittamore, R., Schreiber, N. A., Summa, J. M., Youssoufian, H., Morris, M. J., & Scher, H. I. (2018). Safety and Efficacy of BIND-014, a Docetaxel Nanoparticle Targeting Prostate-Specific Membrane Antigen for Patients with Metastatic Castration-Resistant Prostate Cancer: A Phase 2 Clinical Trial. *JAMA Oncology*, *4*(10), 1344–1351. DOI: 10.1001/jamaoncol.2018.2168 PMID: 29978216

Avila Rodríguez, M. I., Rodríguez Barroso, L. G., & Sánchez, M. L. (2018). Collagen: A review on its sources and potential cosmetic applications. *Journal of Cosmetic Dermatology*, *17*(1), 20–26. DOI: 10.1111/jocd.12450 PMID: 29144022

Awadhiya, A., Tyeb, S., Rathore, K., & Verma, V. (2017). Agarose bioplastic-based drug delivery system for surgical and wound dressings. *Engineering in Life Sciences*, *17*(2), 204–214. DOI: 10.1002/elsc.201500116 PMID: 32624768

Azmana, M., Mahmood, S., Hilles, A. R., Rahman, A., Arifin, M. A., & Ahmed, S. (2021). A review on chitosan and chitosan-based bionanocomposites: Promising material for combatting global issues and its applications. *International Journal of Biological Macromolecules*, *185*, 832–848. DOI: 10.1016/j.ijbiomac.2021.07.023 PMID: 34237361

Baek, J., Lee, K., Ra, H. J., Lotz, M. K., & D'Lima, D. D. (2022). Collagen Fibrous Scaffolds for Sustained Delivery of Growth Factors for Meniscal Tissue Engineering. *Nanomedicine (London)*, *17*(2), 77–93. DOI: 10.2217/nnm-2021-0313 PMID: 34991339

Barbu, A., Neamtu, B., Zăhan, M., Iancu, G. M., Bacila, C., & Mire an, V. (2021). Current Trends in Advanced Alginate-Based Wound Dressings for Chronic Wounds. *Journal of Personalized Medicine*, *11*(9), 890. DOI: 10.3390/jpm11090890 PMID: 34575668

Belattmania, Z., Kaidi, S., El Atouani, S., Katif, C., Bentiss, F., Jama, C., Reani, A., Sabour, B., & Vasconcelos, V. (2020). Isolation and FTIR-ATR and 1H NMR Characterization of Alginates from the Main Alginophyte Species of the Atlantic Coast of Morocco. *Molecules (Basel, Switzerland)*, *25*(18), 4335. DOI: 10.3390/molecules25184335 PMID: 32971782

Belda Marín, C., Fitzpatrick, V., Kaplan, D. L., Landoulsi, J., Guénin, E., & Egles, C. (2020). Silk Polymers and Nanoparticles: A Powerful Combination for the Design of Versatile Biomaterials. *Frontiers in Chemistry*, *8*, 604398. Advance online publication. DOI: 10.3389/fchem.2020.604398 PMID: 33335889

Bhowmik, S., Islam, J., Debnath, T., Miah, M., Bhattacharjee, S., & Khan, M. (2017). Reinforcement of Gelatin-Based Nanofilled Polymer Biocomposite by Crystalline Cellulose from Cotton for Advanced Wound Dressing Applications. *Polymers*, *9*(6), 222. DOI: 10.3390/polym9060222 PMID: 30970900

Buchtová, N., Pradille, C., Bouvard, J.-L., & Budtova, T. (2019). Mechanical properties of cellulose aerogels and cryogels. *Soft Matter*, *15*(39), 7901–7908. DOI: 10.1039/C9SM01028A PMID: 31535679

Cano-Vicent, A., Tuñón-Molina, A., Martí, M., & Serrano-Aroca, Á. (2023). Biocompatible Chitosan Films Containing Acetic Acid Manifested Potent Antiviral Activity against Enveloped and Non-Enveloped Viruses. *International Journal of Molecular Sciences*, *24*(15), 12028. DOI: 10.3390/ijms241512028 PMID: 37569404

Cao, X., Lin, X., Li, N., Zhao, X., Zhou, M., & Zhao, Y. (2023). Animal tissue-derived biomaterials for promoting wound healing. *Materials Horizons*, *10*(9), 3237–3256. DOI: 10.1039/D3MH00411B PMID: 37278612

Chen, X., Wu, T., Bu, Y., Yan, H., & Lin, Q. (2024). Fabrication and Biomedical Application of Alginate Composite Hydrogels in Bone Tissue Engineering: A Review. *International Journal of Molecular Sciences*, *25*(14), 7810. DOI: 10.3390/ijms25147810 PMID: 39063052

Cheng, M., Liu, W., Zhang, J., Zhang, S., Guo, Z., Liu, L., Tian, J., Zhang, X., Cheng, J., Liu, Y., Deng, G., Gao, G., & Sun, L. (2022). Regulatory considerations for animal studies of biomaterial products. *Bioactive Materials*, *11*, 52–56. DOI: 10.1016/j.bioactmat.2021.09.031 PMID: 34938912

Chong, E. T. J., Ng, J. W., & Lee, P.-C. (2023). Classification and Medical Applications of Biomaterials–A Mini Review. *BIO Integration*, *4*(2). Advance online publication. DOI: 10.15212/bioi-2022-0009

Clare, L., Teale, J. C., Toms, G., Kudlicka, A., Evans, I., Abrahams, S., Goldstein, L. H., Hindle, J. V., Ho, A. K., Jahanshahi, M., Langdon, D., Morris, R., Snowden, J. S., Davies, R., Markova, I., Busse, M., & Thompson-Coon, J. (2019). Cognitive rehabilitation, self-management, psychotherapeutic and caregiver support interventions in progressive neurodegenerative conditions: A scoping review. *NeuroRehabilitation*, *43*(4), 443–471. DOI: 10.3233/NRE-172353 PMID: 30412509

Claudia Spataru, M., Simona Baltatu, M., Victor Sandu, A., & Vizureanu, P. (2024). *General Trends on Biomaterials Applications: Advantages and Limitations*. DOI: 10.5772/intechopen.114838

Confederat, L. G., Tuchilus, C. G., Dragan, M., Sha'at, M., & Dragostin, O. M. (2021). Preparation and Antimicrobial Activity of Chitosan and Its Derivatives: A Concise Review. *Molecules (Basel, Switzerland)*, *26*(12), 3694. DOI: 10.3390/molecules26123694 PMID: 34204251

Crini, G. (2019). Historical review on chitin and chitosan biopolymers. *Environmental Chemistry Letters*, *17*(4), 1623–1643. DOI: 10.1007/s10311-019-00901-0

Dima, J. B., Sequeiros, C., & Zaritzky, N. (2017). Chitosan from Marine Crustaceans: Production, Characterization and Applications. In *Biological Activities and Application of Marine Polysaccharides*. InTech. DOI: 10.5772/65258

Dong, C., & Lv, Y. (2016). Application of Collagen Scaffold in Tissue Engineering: Recent Advances and New Perspectives. *Polymers*, *8*(2), 42. DOI: 10.3390/polym8020042 PMID: 30979136

Dorozhkin, S. (2015). Calcium Orthophosphate-Containing Biocomposites and Hybrid Biomaterials for Biomedical Applications. *Journal of Functional Biomaterials*, *6*(3), 708–832. DOI: 10.3390/jfb6030708 PMID: 26262645

Dorozhkin, S. V. (2011). Biocomposites and hybrid biomaterials based on calcium orthophosphates. *Biomatter*, *1*(1), 3–56. DOI: 10.4161/biom.1.1.16782 PMID: 23507726

Ebrahimi, M. (2020). Standardization and regulation of biomaterials. In *Handbook of Biomaterials Biocompatibility* (pp. 251–265). Elsevier., DOI: 10.1016/B978-0-08-102967-1.00013-X

Farnezi Bassi, A. P., Bizelli, V. F., Brasil, L. F., Pereira, J. C., Al-Sharani, H. M., Momesso, G. A. C., Faverani, L. P., & Lucas, F. A. (2020). Is the Bacterial Cellulose Membrane Feasible for Osteopromotive Property? *Membranes*, *10*(9), 230. DOI: 10.3390/membranes10090230 PMID: 32932731

Ferreira, F. V., Souza, L. P., Martins, T. M. M., Lopes, J. H., Mattos, B. D., Mariano, M., Pinheiro, I. F., Valverde, T. M., Livi, S., Camilli, J. A., Goes, A. M., Gouveia, R. F., Lona, L. M. F., & Rojas, O. J. (2019). Nanocellulose/bioactive glass cryogels as scaffolds for bone regeneration. *Nanoscale*, *11*(42), 19842–19849. DOI: 10.1039/C9NR05383B PMID: 31441919

Festas, A., Ramos, A., & Davim, J. (2020). Medical devices biomaterials <scp>–A</scp> review. *Proceedings of the Institution of Mechanical Engineers, Part L: Journal of Materials: Design and Applications, 234*(1), 218–228. DOI: 10.1177/1464420719882458

Portier, F. (2016). Biomateriaux collagène/gélatine: des phases cristal-liquides aux matériaux hybrides (Doctoral dissertation, Université Pierre et Marie Curie-Paris VI). [Collagen/gelatin biomaterials: from liquid-crystalline phases to hybrid materials].

Fuchs, S., Shariati, K., & Ma, M. (2020). Specialty Tough Hydrogels and Their Biomedical Applications. *Advanced Healthcare Materials*, *9*(2), 1901396. Advance online publication. DOI: 10.1002/adhm.201901396 PMID: 31846228

Ghavimi, S. A. A., Lungren, E. S., Faulkner, T. J., Josselet, M. A., Wu, Y., Sun, Y., Pfeiffer, F. M., Goldstein, C. L., Wan, C., & Ulery, B. D. (2019). Inductive co-crosslinking of cellulose nanocrystal/chitosan hydrogels for the treatment of vertebral compression fractures. *International Journal of Biological Macromolecules*, *130*, 88–98. DOI: 10.1016/j.ijbiomac.2019.02.086 PMID: 30779988

Gomez-Florit, M., Pardo, A., Domingues, R. M. A., Graça, A. L., Babo, P. S., Reis, R. L., & Gomes, M. E. (2020). Natural-Based Hydrogels for Tissue Engineering Applications. *Molecules (Basel, Switzerland)*, *25*(24), 5858. DOI: 10.3390/molecules25245858 PMID: 33322369

Grabska-Zielińska, S., & Sionkowska, A. (2021). How to Improve Physico-Chemical Properties of Silk Fibroin Materials for Biomedical Applications?—Blending and Cross-Linking of Silk Fibroin—A Review. *Materials (Basel)*, *14*(6), 1510. DOI: 10.3390/ma14061510 PMID: 33808809

Guillén-Carvajal, K., Valdez-Salas, B., Beltrán-Partida, E., Salomón-Carlos, J., & Cheng, N. (2023). Chitosan, Gelatin, and Collagen Hydrogels for Bone Regeneration. *Polymers*, *15*(13), 2762. DOI: 10.3390/polym15132762 PMID: 37447408

Gupta, P., Sharma, S., Jabin, S., & Jadoun, S. (2024). Chitosan nanocomposite for tissue engineering and regenerative medicine: A review. *International Journal of Biological Macromolecules*, *254*, 127660. DOI: 10.1016/j.ijbiomac.2023.127660 PMID: 37907176

Gupta, P. K., Keerthi, A. M., Kallapur, S. S., & Choudhary, S. (2021). Overview of Cellulose Types and Applications. In *Comprehensive Glycoscience* (pp. 220–236). Elsevier., DOI: 10.1016/B978-0-12-819475-1.00019-5

Haider, A., Khan, S., Iqbal, D. N., Shrahili, M., Haider, S., Mohammad, K., Mohammad, A., Rizwan, M., Kanwal, Q., & Mustafa, G. (2024). Advances in chitosan-based drug delivery systems: A comprehensive review for therapeutic applications. *European Polymer Journal*, *210*, 112983. DOI: 10.1016/j.eurpolymj.2024.112983

He, J., Hu, X., Cao, J., Zhang, Y., Xiao, J., Peng, J., Chen, D., Xiong, C., & Zhang, L. (2021). Chitosan-coated hydroxyapatite and drug-loaded polytrimethylene carbonate/polylactic acid scaffold for enhancing bone regeneration. *Carbohydrate Polymers*, *253*, 117198. DOI: 10.1016/j.carbpol.2020.117198 PMID: 33278972

Imran, M., Sajwan, M., Alsuwayt, B., & Asif, M. (2020). Synthesis, characterization and anticoagulant activity of chitosan derivatives. *Saudi Pharmaceutical Journal : SPJ : the Official Publication of the Saudi Pharmaceutical Society*, *28*(1), 25–32. DOI: 10.1016/j.jsps.2019.11.003 PMID: 31920430

Insuasti-Cruz, E., Suárez-Jaramillo, V., Mena Urresta, K. A., Pila-Varela, K. O., Fiallos-Ayala, X., Dahoumane, S. A., & Alexis, F. (2022). Natural Biomaterials from Biodiversity for Healthcare Applications. *Advanced Healthcare Materials*, *11*(1), 2101389. Advance online publication. DOI: 10.1002/adhm.202101389 PMID: 34643331

Irastorza-Lorenzo, A., Sánchez-Porras, D., Ortiz-Arrabal, O., de Frutos, M. J., Esteban, E., Fernández, J., Janer, A., Campos, A., Campos, F., & Alaminos, M. (2021). Evaluation of Marine Agarose Biomaterials for Tissue Engineering Applications. *International Journal of Molecular Sciences*, *22*(4), 1923. DOI: 10.3390/ijms22041923 PMID: 33672027

Ishigaki, T., & Kubo, K. (2020). Mechanical properties and collagen fiber orientation of tendon in young and elderly. *Clinical Biomechanics (Bristol, Avon)*, *71*, 5–10. DOI: 10.1016/j.clinbiomech.2019.10.003 PMID: 31675513

Issahaku, I., Tetteh, I. K., & Tetteh, A. Y. (2023). Chitosan and chitosan derivatives: Recent advancements in production and applications in environmental remediation. *Environmental Advances*, *11*, 100351. DOI: 10.1016/j.envadv.2023.100351

Jabeen, N., & Atif, M. (2024). Polysaccharides based biopolymers for biomedical applications: A review. *Polymers for Advanced Technologies*, *35*(1), e6203. Advance online publication. DOI: 10.1002/pat.6203

Jafernik, K., Ładniak, A., Blicharska, E., Czarnek, K., Ekiert, H., Wiącek, A. E., & Szopa, A. (2023). Chitosan-Based Nanoparticles as Effective Drug Delivery Systems—A review. *Molecules (Basel, Switzerland)*, *28*(4), 1963. DOI: 10.3390/molecules28041963 PMID: 36838951

Jana, S., Das, P., Mukherjee, J., Banerjee, D., Ghosh, P. R., Kumar Das, P., Bhattacharya, R. N., & Nandi, S. K. (2022). Waste-derived biomaterials as building blocks in the biomedical field. *Journal of Materials Chemistry. B*, *10*(4), 489–505. DOI: 10.1039/D1TB02125G PMID: 35018942

Janmohammadi, M., Nazemi, Z., Salehi, A. O. M., Seyfoori, A., John, J. V., Nourbakhsh, M. S., & Akbari, M. (2023). Cellulose-based composite scaffolds for bone tissue engineering and localized drug delivery. *Bioactive Materials*, *20*, 137–163. DOI: 10.1016/j.bioactmat.2022.05.018 PMID: 35663339

Jiang, F., Xu, X.-W., Chen, F.-Q., Weng, H.-F., Chen, J., Ru, Y., Xiao, Q., & Xiao, A.-F. (2023). Extraction, Modification and Biomedical Application of Agarose Hydrogels: A Review. *Marine Drugs*, *21*(5), 299. DOI: 10.3390/md21050299 PMID: 37233493

Jin, M., Shi, J., Zhu, W., Yao, H., & Wang, D.-A. (2021). Polysaccharide-Based Biomaterials in Tissue Engineering: A Review. *Tissue Engineering. Part B, Reviews*, *27*(6), 604–626. DOI: 10.1089/ten.teb.2020.0208 PMID: 33267648

Jovic, T. H., Kungwengwe, G., Mills, A. C., & Whitaker, I. S. (2019). Plant-Derived Biomaterials: A Review of 3D Bioprinting and Biomedical Applications. *Frontiers of Mechanical Engineering*, *5*, 19. Advance online publication. DOI: 10.3389/fmech.2019.00019

Kou, S., Peters, L. M., & Mucalo, M. R. (2021). Chitosan: A review of sources and preparation methods. *International Journal of Biological Macromolecules*, *169*, 85–94. DOI: 10.1016/j.ijbiomac.2020.12.005 PMID: 33279563

Kravanja, G., Primožič, M., Knez, Ž., & Leitgeb, M. (2019). Chitosan-Based (Nano) Materials for Novel Biomedical Applications. *Molecules (Basel, Switzerland)*, *24*(10), 1960. DOI: 10.3390/molecules24101960 PMID: 31117310

Kudiyarasu, S., Karuppan Perumal, M. K., Rajan Renuka, R., & Manickam Natrajan, P. (2024). Chitosan composite with mesenchymal stem cells: Properties, mechanism, and its application in bone regeneration. *International Journal of Biological Macromolecules*, *275*, 133502. DOI: 10.1016/j.ijbiomac.2024.133502 PMID: 38960259

Li, J., Ahmed, H. H., Hussein, A. M., Kaur, M., Jameel, M. K., Kaur, H., Tillaeva, U., Al-Hussainy, A. F., Sameer, H. N., Hameed, H. G., Idan, A. H., Alsaikhan, F., Narmani, A., & Farhood, B. (2025). Advances in polysaccharide-based materials for biomedical and pharmaceutical applications: A comprehensive review. *Archiv der Pharmazie*, *358*(1), e2400854. Advance online publication. DOI: 10.1002/ardp.202400854 PMID: 39651831

Li, L., Zhong, D., Wang, S., & Zhou, M. (2025). Plant-derived materials for biomedical applications. *Nanoscale*, *17*(2), 722–739. DOI: 10.1039/D4NR03057E PMID: 39605132

Liu, X., Wu, Y., Zhao, X., & Wang, Z. (2021). Fabrication and applications of bioactive chitosan-based organic-inorganic hybrid materials: A review. *Carbohydrate Polymers*, *267*, 118179. DOI: 10.1016/j.carbpol.2021.118179 PMID: 34119147

Lujerdean, C., Baci, G.-M., Cucu, A.-A., & Dezmirean, D. S. (2022). The Contribution of Silk Fibroin in Biomedical Engineering. *Insects*, *13*(3), 286. DOI: 10.3390/insects13030286 PMID: 35323584

Marin, E., Boschetto, F., & Pezzotti, G. (2020). Biomaterials and biocompatibility: An historical overview. *Journal of Biomedical Materials Research. Part A*, *108*(8), 1617–1633. DOI: 10.1002/jbm.a.36930 PMID: 32196949

Miserez, A., Weaver, J. C., & Chaudhuri, O. (2015). Biological materials and molecular biomimetics – filling up the empty soft materials space for tissue engineering applications. *Journal of Materials Chemistry. B*, *3*(1), 13–24. DOI: 10.1039/C4TB01267D PMID: 32261919

Mohammed, A. S. A., Naveed, M., & Jost, N. (2021). Polysaccharides; Classification, Chemical Properties, and Future Perspective Applications in Fields of Pharmacology and Biological Medicine (A Review of Current Applications and Upcoming Potentialities). *Journal of Polymers and the Environment*, *29*(8), 2359–2371. DOI: 10.1007/s10924-021-02052-2 PMID: 33526994

Mohanto, S., Chakraborty, P., SoundraPandian, C., Manna, S., & Dutta, J. (2021). A Comprehensive Review on Alginate as Wound Dressing Biomaterial. *Current Applied Polymer Science*, *4*(1), 3–14. DOI: 10.2174/2452271604999200518085622

Mohebbi, S., Nezhad, M. N., Zarrintaj, P., Jafari, S. H., Gholizadeh, S. S., Saeb, M. R., & Mozafari, M. (2019). Chitosan in Biomedical Engineering: A Critical Review. *Current Stem Cell Research & Therapy*, *14*(2), 93–116. DOI: 10.2174/1574888X13666180912142028 PMID: 30207244

Nayak, A. K., Mohanta, B. C., Hasnain, M. S., Hoda, M. N., & Tripathi, G. (2020). Alginate-based scaffolds for drug delivery in tissue engineering. In *Alginates in Drug Delivery* (pp. 359–386). Elsevier., DOI: 10.1016/B978-0-12-817640-5.00014-5

Ortiz-Arrabal, O., Irastorza-Lorenzo, A., Campos, F., Martín-Piedra, M. Á., Carriel, V., Garzón, I., Ávila-Fernández, P., de Frutos, M. J., Esteban, E., Fernández, J., Janer, A., Campos, A., Chato-Astrain, J., & Alaminos, M. (2023). Fibrin and Marine-Derived Agaroses for the Generation of Human Bioartificial Tissues: An Ex Vivo and In Vivo Study. *Marine Drugs*, *21*(3), 187. DOI: 10.3390/md21030187 PMID: 36976236

Park, W., Shin, H., Choi, B., Rhim, W.-K., Na, K., & Keun Han, D. (2020). Advanced hybrid nanomaterials for biomedical applications. *Progress in Materials Science, 114*, 100686. DOI: 10.1016/j.pmatsci.2020.100686

Pesic, D. (2021). Cellulose in Nature - Versatile sources for Novel Applications: A Literature Review. *Undergraduate Research in Natural and Clinical Science and Technology (URNCST). Journal, 5*(2), 1–9. DOI: 10.26685/urncst.200

Pires, P. C., Mascarenhas-Melo, F., Pedrosa, K., Lopes, D., Lopes, J., Macário-Soares, A., Peixoto, D., Giram, P. S., Veiga, F., & Paiva-Santos, A. C. (2023). Polymer-based biomaterials for pharmaceutical and biomedical applications: A focus on topical drug administration. *European Polymer Journal, 187*, 111868. DOI: 10.1016/j.eurpolymj.2023.111868

Qi, Y., Wang, H., Wei, K., Yang, Y., Zheng, R.-Y., Kim, I., & Zhang, K.-Q. (2017). A Review of Structure Construction of Silk Fibroin Biomaterials from Single Structures to Multi-Level Structures. *International Journal of Molecular Sciences, 18*(3), 237. DOI: 10.3390/ijms18030237 PMID: 28273799

Ramdhan, T., Ching, S. H., Prakash, S., & Bhandari, B. (2020). Physical and mechanical properties of alginate based composite gels. *Trends in Food Science & Technology, 106*, 150–159. DOI: 10.1016/j.tifs.2020.10.002

Ranjan, C., Sarkhel, G., & Kumar, K. (2023). Investigation of Mechanical, Tribological, and Electrical Properties of Silk Reinforced Polymeric Composite. *Advances in Materials Science and Engineering, 2023*, 1–12. DOI: 10.1155/2023/1507891

Ray, U., Zhu, S., Pang, Z., & Li, T. (2021). Mechanics Design in Cellulose-Enabled High-Performance Functional Materials. *Advanced Materials, 33*(28), 2002504. Advance online publication. DOI: 10.1002/adma.202002504 PMID: 32794349

Sacco, P., Piazza, F., Marsich, E., Abrami, M., Grassi, M., & Donati, I. (2024). Ionic Strength Impacts the Physical Properties of Agarose Hydrogels. *Gels (Basel, Switzerland), 10*(2), 94. DOI: 10.3390/gels10020094 PMID: 38391424

Schuh, J. C. L., & Funk, K. A. (2019). Compilation of International Standards and Regulatory Guidance Documents for Evaluation of Biomaterials, Medical Devices, and 3-D Printed and Regenerative Medicine Products. *Toxicologic Pathology, 47*(3), 344–357. DOI: 10.1177/0192623318804121 PMID: 30392453

Seddiqi, H., Oliaei, E., Honarkar, H., Jin, J., Geonzon, L. C., Bacabac, R. G., & Klein-Nulend, J. (2021). Cellulose and its derivatives: Towards biomedical applications. *Cellulose (London, England), 28*(4), 1893–1931. DOI: 10.1007/s10570-020-03674-w

Singh, A., Verma, N., & Kumar, K. (2019). Hybrid composites: a revolutionary trend in biomedical engineering. In *Materials for Biomedical Engineering* (pp. 33–46). Elsevier., DOI: 10.1016/B978-0-12-818431-8.00002-7

Singh, V., & Singh, A. (2019). Alginate-Based Hydrogels: Synthesis, Characterization, and Biomedical Applications. In *Alginates* (pp. 141–168). Apple Academic Press. DOI: 10.1201/9780429023439-4

Soleimanpour, M., Mirhaji, S. S., Jafari, S., Derakhshankhah, H., Mamashli, F., Nedaei, H., Karimi, M. R., Motasadizadeh, H., Fatahi, Y., Ghasemi, A., Nezamtaheri, M. S., Khajezade, M., Teimouri, M., Goliaei, B., Delattre, C., & Saboury, A. A. (2022). Designing a new alginate-fibrinogen biomaterial composite hydrogel for wound healing. *Scientific Reports*, *12*(1), 7213. DOI: 10.1038/s41598-022-11282-w PMID: 35508533

Song, X., Tang, Z., Liu, W., Chen, K., Liang, J., Yuan, B., Lin, H., Zhu, X., Fan, Y., Shi, X., Zhao, P., Yang, L., Zhang, K., Mikos, A. G., & Zhang, X. (2022). Biomaterials and regulatory science. *Journal of Materials Science and Technology*, *128*, 221–227. DOI: 10.1016/j.jmst.2022.04.018

Su, F., Wang, Y., Liu, X., Shen, X., Zhang, X., Xing, Q., Wang, L., & Chen, Y. (2018). Biocompatibility and *in vivo* degradation of chitosan based hydrogels as potential drug carrier. *Journal of Biomaterials Science. Polymer Edition*, *29*(13), 1515–1528. DOI: 10.1080/09205063.2017.1412244 PMID: 29745306

Tao, F., Cheng, Y., Shi, X., Zheng, H., Du, Y., Xiang, W., & Deng, H. (2020). Applications of chitin and chitosan nanofibers in bone regenerative engineering. *Carbohydrate Polymers*, *230*, 115658. DOI: 10.1016/j.carbpol.2019.115658 PMID: 31887899

Terzi, A., Storelli, E., Bettini, S., Sibillano, T., Altamura, D., Salvatore, L., Madaghiele, M., Romano, A., Siliqi, D., Ladisa, M., De Caro, L., Quattrini, A., Valli, L., Sannino, A., & Giannini, C. (2018). Effects of processing on structural, mechanical and biological properties of collagen-based substrates for regenerative medicine. *Scientific Reports*, *8*(1), 1429. DOI: 10.1038/s41598-018-19786-0 PMID: 29362434

Tian, Y., Wu, D., Wu, D., Cui, Y., Ren, G., Wang, Y., Wang, J., & Peng, C. (2022). Chitosan-Based Biomaterial Scaffolds for the Repair of Infected Bone Defects. In *Frontiers in Bioengineering and Biotechnology* (Vol. 10, p. 899760). Frontiers Media S.A., DOI: 10.3389/fbioe.2022.899760

Tolaimate, A., Desbrieres, J., Rhazi, M., & Alagui, A. (2003). Contribution to the preparation of chitins and chitosans with controlled physico-chemical properties. *Polymer*, *44*(26), 7939–7952. DOI: 10.1016/j.polymer.2003.10.025

Triunfo, M., Tafi, E., Guarnieri, A., Salvia, R., Scieuzo, C., Hahn, T., Zibek, S., Gagliardini, A., Panariello, L., Coltelli, M. B., De Bonis, A., & Falabella, P. (2022). Characterization of chitin and chitosan derived from Hermetia illucens, a further step in a circular economy process. *Scientific Reports*, *12*(1), 6613. DOI: 10.1038/s41598-022-10423-5 PMID: 35459772

Troy, E., Tilbury, M. A., Power, A. M., & Wall, J. G. (2021). Nature-Based Biomaterials and Their Application in Biomedicine. *Polymers*, *13*(19), 3321. DOI: 10.3390/polym13193321 PMID: 34641137

Tsouknidas, A. (2024). Advancements in Biomaterials for Bioengineering and Biotechnology. *International Journal of Molecular Sciences*, *25*(14), 7840. DOI: 10.3390/ijms25147840 PMID: 39063082

Varaprasad, K., Jayaramudu, T., Kanikireddy, V., Toro, C., & Sadiku, E. R. (2020). Alginate-based composite materials for wound dressing application:A mini review. *Carbohydrate Polymers*, *236*, 116025. DOI: 10.1016/j.carbpol.2020.116025 PMID: 32172843

Wang, F., Guo, C., Yang, Q., Li, C., Zhao, P., Xia, Q., & Kaplan, D. L. (2021). Protein composites from silkworm cocoons as versatile biomaterials. *Acta Biomaterialia*, *121*, 180–192. DOI: 10.1016/j.actbio.2020.11.037 PMID: 33249226

Wang, J., & Zhuang, S. (2022). Chitosan-based materials: Preparation, modification and application. *Journal of Cleaner Production*, *355*, 131825. DOI: 10.1016/j.jclepro.2022.131825

Wang, M. (2016). The composite and hybridization approach in developing new biomaterials. *China International Conference on Functional Materials*.

Wani, S. U. D., Ali, M., Mehdi, S., Masoodi, M. H., Zargar, M. I., & Shakeel, F. (2023). A review on chitosan and alginate-based microcapsules: Mechanism and applications in drug delivery systems. *International Journal of Biological Macromolecules*, *248*, 125875. DOI: 10.1016/j.ijbiomac.2023.125875 PMID: 37473899

Yan, D., Li, Y., Liu, Y., Li, N., Zhang, X., & Yan, C. (2021). Antimicrobial Properties of Chitosan and Chitosan Derivatives in the Treatment of Enteric Infections. *Molecules (Basel, Switzerland)*, *26*(23), 7136. DOI: 10.3390/molecules26237136 PMID: 34885715

Younes, I., & Rinaudo, M. (2015). Chitin and Chitosan Preparation from Marine Sources. Structure, Properties and Applications. *Marine Drugs*, *13*(3), 1133–1174. DOI: 10.3390/md13031133 PMID: 25738328

Yousefian, F., Hesari, R., Jensen, T., Obagi, S., Rgeai, A., Damiani, G., Bunick, C. G., & Grada, A. (2023). Antimicrobial Wound Dressings: A Concise Review for Clinicians. *Antibiotics (Basel, Switzerland)*, *12*(9), 1434. DOI: 10.3390/antibiotics12091434 PMID: 37760730

Zafeiris, K., Brasinika, D., Karatza, A., Koumoulos, E., Karoussis, I. K., Kyriakidou, K., & Charitidis, C. A. (2021). Additive manufacturing of hydroxyapatite–chitosan–genipin composite scaffolds for bone tissue engineering applications. *Materials Science and Engineering C*, *119*, 111639. DOI: 10.1016/j.msec.2020.111639 PMID: 33321677

Zhang, K., Ma, B., Hu, K., Yuan, B., Sun, X., Song, X., Tang, Z., Lin, H., Zhu, X., Zheng, Y. J., García, A. G., Mikos, A. M., Anderson, J., & Zhang, X. (2022). Evidence-based biomaterials research. *Bioactive Materials*, *15*, 495–503. DOI: 10.1016/j.bioactmat.2022.04.014 PMID: 35633843

Zhang, L., Liu, T., Xie, Y., Zeng, Z., & Chen, J. (2020). A new classification method of nanotechnology for design integration in biomaterials. *Nanotechnology Reviews*, *9*(1), 820–832. DOI: 10.1515/ntrev-2020-0063

Zhang, M., & Zhao, X. (2020). Alginate hydrogel dressings for advanced wound management. *International Journal of Biological Macromolecules*, *162*, 1414–1428. DOI: 10.1016/j.ijbiomac.2020.07.311 PMID: 32777428

Zhao, L., Zhou, Y., Zhang, J., Liang, H., Chen, X., & Tan, H. (2023). Natural Polymer-Based Hydrogels: From Polymer to Biomedical Applications. *Pharmaceutics*, *15*(10), 2514. DOI: 10.3390/pharmaceutics15102514 PMID: 37896274

Zhao, X., Xia, Y., Zhang, X., Lin, X., & Wang, L. (2019). Design of mechanically strong and tough alginate hydrogels based on a soft-brittle transition. *International Journal of Biological Macromolecules*, *139*, 850–857. DOI: 10.1016/j.ijbiomac.2019.08.057 PMID: 31400427

About the Contributors

Safaa Al-Humairi is a postdoctoral and PhD Mechanical/Biomaterials Engineering graduate from the University of Teknologi Malaysia. His research focuses on the design and development of novel biomaterials and their related applications. He is an associate professor and program coordinator at the Management and Science University, Shah Alam, Malaysia. Dr. Safaa is a registered professional engineer in a number of engineering associations and societies and has more than 15 years of experience in biosensor/materials design and implementation. He is the author of more than 150 research articles published in well-known and highly impacted journals. He has also been awarded a number of special gold, silver, and bronze medals for many innovations and innovative national and international engineering and technology exhibitions. He is also an editor and reviewer for several well-known journals and publishers.

Erkan Koç is an accomplished Associate Professor at Karabuk University, Turkey, specializing in Biomedical Engineering within the Faculty of Engineering. With a robust academic background in metallurgy and materials science, he has dedicated his career to advancing research in biodegradable materials and biomedical applications. Dr. Koç obtained his Ph.D. in 2013, with a thesis focusing on the corrosion-dependent mechanical behaviors of biodegradable magnesium alloys. His earlier Master's thesis (2008) explored the effects of alloying elements on the properties of magnesium castings. His academic journey began as a Research Assistant in 2005, and he has since ascended through the academic ranks, becoming an Associate Professor in 2020. Dr. Koç's leadership roles include serving as the Head of the Biomedical Engineering Department (2021-2024) and co-directing the Materials Research and Development Center. His administrative expertise complements his extensive research contributions. His research interests center on biomaterials, with significant contributions to understanding the mechanical, tribological, and biological properties of novel materials. His works are well-published, featuring articles in high-impact journals such as Journal of Materials Engineering and Performance and Ceramics International. Dr. Koç has also supervised numerous postgraduate theses, including cutting-edge studies on bioactive glass ceramics and magnesium-based biomedical alloys. In addition to his academic endeavors, Dr. Koç has actively participated in and led multiple scientific research projects focused on improving the mechanical properties and biocompatibility of magnesium alloys. His collaborations with international researchers and participation in conferences demonstrate his commitment to global academic exchange. Dr. Koç continues to innovate in the field of biomedical engineering, bridging material science and clinical applications to address critical challenges in medical technology.

Ameer Najah Saud Al-Huamiri is a distinguished academic and researcher in the field of biomedical engineering, currently serving as a Lecturer in the Department of Biomedical Engineering at Al-Mustaqabal University, Iraq. He earned his Ph.D. in Biomedical Engineering from Karabuk University, Turkey, specializing in biomaterials and dental materials engineering. His doctoral research focused on the synthesis and characterization of bioactive glass-ceramic materials for endodontic cements, exploring their properties and biocompatibility. Dr. Al-Huamiri also holds a master's degree in Ceramic Materials Engineering and a bachelor's degree in Materials Engineering from Babylon University, Iraq. His academic journey reflects a strong foundation in materials science, particularly in ceramic processing and characterization techniques. Throughout his career, Dr. Al-Huamiri has contributed extensively to research in porous media, nanomaterials, bioceramics, and corrosion studies. He has expertise in material characterization methods, such as X-ray Diffraction (XRD) and Scanning Electron Microscopy (SEM), as well as in advanced processing techniques like sol-gel synthesis. His work also incorporates modern computational methods, including artificial neural networks for material design and genetic algorithms for optimization. Dr. Al-Huamiri has authored numerous publications in international journals and presented at prestigious conferences, highlighting his innovative approaches to developing biomedical materials for dental and medical applications. His expertise has been recognized through his role as a reviewer for several high-impact journals, including Journal of Materials Engineering and Performance and Advanced Engineering Materials. In addition to his academic accomplishments, Dr. Al-Huamiri has significant experience in engineering simulation and analysis, utilizing software such as SolidWorks, ANSYS Fluent, and MATLAB. His technical knowledge extends to bioceramic material development, thermal analysis, and porosity measurement, which he applies in both academic and industrial contexts. Dr. Al-Huamiri continues to advance the field of biomedical engineering by focusing on interdisciplinary research that bridges material science and clinical applications, with a particular emphasis on sustainable and biocompatible materials.

***

Abdessamad Abana is currently an intern at the Regenerative Medicine Center laboratory, located at the University Hospital Center (CHU) in Marrakech, where he specializes in natural-origin biomaterials. His work mainly focuses on the study and application of biopolymers, such as alginate, for regenerative medicine treatments.

Youssef Ait Hamdan received his PhD in Biology at Cadi Ayyad University.

Imade Armadi is currently pursuing a PhD in Biology and Biomedicine at the Regenerative Medicine Center laboratory at the University Hospital Center (CHU) in Marrakech. His research focuses on the biomedical applications of chitosan, particularly in the context of clinical therapy. His work aims to explore the potential of chitosan in drug delivery systems, tissue engineering, and other therapeutic applications, contributing to advancements in regenerative medicine and clinical treatments.

Ramlath Beegam L. is aPhD Scholar in Biochemistry at MACFAST Tiruvalla (MG University). Their research focuses on Nanoparticles, Green synthesis, and phytopharmacological studies.

Jagadeesh Baskaran is currently working as a Faculty member in the Department of Mechanical Engineering, PSG Institute of Technology and Applied Research. He obtained his B. Tech in Mechanical Engineering and M.Tech in Advanced Manufacturing from SASTRA University. For his performance during the Master's program, he received the best outgoing M. Tech student award recognising his academic record and research publication from his M.Tech thesis. He has two years of work experience in SAP ERP software consulting and one year of teaching experience in Mechanical and Manufacturing Engineering. During his Ph.D. work at NIT Trichy, he got the DORA plus scholarship to undergo research training in the Mechanical and Industrial Engineering department of Tallinn University of Technology, Estonia. His research interests include Metal 3D printing, Design for Additive Manufacturing, Laser Materials Processing, unconventional machining techniques and materials management. He has authored 4 international journal Publications in metal 3D printing in which 3 of them are the outcomes of his PhD thesis. One of the presentations from his PhD work earned a best paper award in the ICPPM conference (March 2023).

Tejasvi Batra is a keen follower of advances in cancer biology and therapeutic applications. He has been involved in various projects in the abovementioned areas and plans to continue pursuing such endeavors.

Anass Belbachir is a Professor of Pathological Anatomy at the Faculty of Medicine and Pharmacy of Marrakech and the Director of the Regenerative Medicine Center. His research focuses on cancer, the use of biomaterials, and stem cells for clinical applications, aiming to advance therapeutic strategies in regenerative medicine and cancer treatment.

Banashree Bandhopadhyay has been working as Assistant Professor-II, at the Centre for Medical Biotechnology, Amity Institute of Biotechnology, Amity University Uttar Pradesh, Noida.Her area of research mainly deals with Cancer Biology, Immunology, Genetics and Theragnostics.

Sunandani Chandel is a Ph.D. Research Scholar in Forest Products & Utilization at Kerala Agricultural University, India. She holds a B.Sc. in Forestry from Dr. Y.S. Parmar University and an M.Sc. in Forestry from Navsari Agricultural University, where she was awarded the Chancellor's Gold Medal. Her research focuses on sustainable forest product utilization, and she has published extensively in peer-reviewed journals. She has received prestigious fellowships, including the SERB International Travel Scheme and the British Ecological Society Travel Grant. She is also a recipient of Best Blog Award at XV World Forestry Congress held at South Korea in 2022. As an active researcher, she is dedicated in advancing sustainable forestry and wood-based innovations.

Chutturi Mahesh, Forestry graduate did his Masters in Forest Products and Utilization from Forest College and Research Institute, Hyderabad. He is ICAR Senior research fellow pursing 3rd year Ph.D in Forestry (Forest Products and Utilization) at Kerala Agricultural University, has qualified UGC NET twice in (Environmental Science), and written peer review articles in various journals, He had rich practical knowledge in Forestry, Had attended various international conference and workshops.

Adil El Housseini is affiliated with Ibn Zohr University. Their research interests include venom of scorpion, Toxicology, animal physiology, neurosciences.

Rajni Gautam received Ph.D., M.Sc. and B. Sc. Degrees in Electronics from University of Delhi, India, in 2014, 2009, and 2007 respectively. She has 16 publications in International Journals of repute and 15 publications in International conferences. Her total citations are 338 with h-index of 10. Her research interests include device modeling and simulation for advanced metal oxide–semiconductor field-effect transistors (MOSFET) structures such as surrounding gate MOSFET with study of Reliability issues and biosensing applications and Synthesis and Characterization of doped metal oxide nanoparticles. She has more than 7 years of teaching experience and currently supervising two PhD scholar. She is supervising two PhD students.

Shreya Gupta is an undergraduate student perusing BSC Biotechnology at Amity University.

Syed Tasawar Hussain is a Biomedical Engineer affiliated with the University of Engineering and Technology, Lahore.

Nida Iqbal is working as chairperson/ associate professor in Biomedical Engineering department, UET, Lahore, New Campus, and Pakistan. She did her PhD in Biomedical Engineering in Faculty of Biosciences and Medical Engineering, Universiti Teknologi Malaysia (UTM), Malaysia. She has 17 years research and academic experience. she have learned and acquired expertise in biomaterials mainly focused on synthesis and characterizations of bioceramics and its composites, tissue engineering scaffolds, bioactive coatings, biodegradable metallic implants, hydrogels, target drug delivery and related fields. She has total 42 Publications in Journals with impact factor 120, h index: 21.

Jenny Jacob is an accomplished researcher and Associate Professor in the Department of Biosciences at Mar Athanasios College for Advanced Studies, Tiruvalla (MACFAST), Kerala. With a robust academic background and over a decade of teaching experience, she is deeply engaged in cutting-edge research in biochemistry, phytochemistry, and bioinformatics. Her research primarily focuses on the therapeutic potential of medicinal plants, with particular interest in anti-inflammatory pathways, dual COX/LOX inhibition, and bioactive compound analysis. Dr. Jacob has contributed significantly to scientific literature through her studies on Tinospora cordifolia and other native medicinal species, highlighting their pharmacological relevance in combating oxidative stress and inflammation. Dr. Jacob has published extensively in peer-reviewed journals, and her work is widely cited in the field of natural product research. Through her research leadership, Dr. Jenny Jacob continues to mentor students and collaborate across disciplines, contributing meaningfully to the scientific community and the development of innovative, plant-based therapeutic strategies.

Rajakumari K. is an Assistant Professor Vels Institute of Science, Technology and Advanced Studies (VISTAS).

Jasmine Kaur is a Master's student currently pursuing her interests at the Amity Institute of Biotechnology with ardor and determination.

Muhammad Zaeem Khalid is a Biomedical Engineer affiliated with the University of Engineering and Technology.

Danie Kinglsey received his PhD from Vellore Institute of Technology and is currently an Associate Professor at VIT University.

Neeraj Kumari did her Ph. D. in analytical chemistry from University of Delhi in 2018 under the supervision of Professor of Ramesh Chandra and co – supervision of Professor Monika Datta. She has presented her work in many international and national conferences where she has awarded two times for giving best oral presentation and for her research work (Dr. Upadhyayula V. Rao Memorial Award, 2017 and Professor V. Panda Rango Rao Award, 2015, in Annual Convention Chemists). She is life member of Indian Science Congress and American Chemical Society. She has guided many B. Sc. students to complete their project work during her Ph. D. work. Dr. Kumari qualified CSIR – UGC NET in June 2011 and CSIR – JRF in December 2011. She has published 25 publications including research articles, books, book chapters, conference proceedings and patents. Dr. Neeraj Kumari has been working as Assistant Professor in K. R. Mangalam University since January 2019. She is teaching inorganic chemistry to B. Sc. and M. Sc. Chemistry students.

Souad Loqman is a Professor of Microbiology at the Faculty of Medicine and Pharmacy at Cadi Ayyad University, Marrakech.

Unnimaya M. is a PhD Scholar in Bioscience at MACFAST, Thiruvalla, M G University, Kottayam. Their research focuses on Nanoparticles, Synthesis, and Phytopharmacological studies

Anusha Mittal is a dedicated Master's student with an avid interest in cancer biology and emerging targets and therapies for various cancers. She is keen to explore the transformative potential of computational simulations and molecular modeling, and looks forward to multi-omics and systems biology integrations to provide new insights. With a focus on leveraging these advanced tools, she aims to advance both basic and clinical cancer research, driving novel treatment pathways and enhancing therapeutic efficacy. Passionate about contributing to groundbreaking solutions, she is committed to advancing the frontier of cancer therapy and improving patient outcomes through technological innovation.

Ruchika Nirala is an undergraduate student pursuing Zoology (H)+ BEd at Amity University.

Dharshika P. is affiliated with the Bio-Engineering department at Vels Institute of Science, Technology and Advanced Studies at Vels University.

Ruqiah Ganda Putri Panjaitan is a lecturer in Biology Education at the Faculty of Teacher Training and Education, Universitas Tanjungpura, Pontianak, Indonesia. She earned her Bachelor's degree (S1) in 1997, her Master's degree (S2) in 2003, and her Doctorate (S3) in 2008, all from the Institut Pertanian Bogor (IPB). With extensive academic experience, Prof. Dr. Panjaitan has contributed significantly to the development of Biology Education. Her expertise and research interests focus on biology teaching methodologies, education, and curriculum development. She is an active researcher and academic, and her contributions are well recognized in the scientific community. Prof. Dr. Panjaitan's scholarly work can be accessed via her ORCID ID: https://orcid.org/0000-0002-2194-8808 and Scopus Author ID: 55656556500. She can be contacted via email at ruqiah.gpp@fkip.untan.ac.id.

Vivek Pazhamalai is working as Associate Professor at Vels Institute of Science, Technology and Advanced Studies, and has teaching experience of 15 years. He has published more than 60 research articles in international and national journals to his credit.

Anita Restu Puji Raharjeng is a Biology lecturer at the Faculty of Science and Technology, Universitas Islam Negeri Raden Fatah Palembang, Indonesia. She holds a Bachelor's degree in Biology from the Faculty of Mathematics and Natural Sciences, Universitas Negeri Malang. Anita pursued her Master's degree in Molecular Biotechnology at the Faculty of Mathematics and Natural Sciences, Universitas Brawijaya, and in Biomedical Science at the Faculty of Veterinary and Biomedical Sciences, James Cook University, Australia. She completed her Ph.D. in Biology at the Faculty of Biology, Universitas Gadjah Mada. Anita is also a contributor to scientific literature, having authored a book chapter titled "Sustainable and Eco-friendly Nanomaterials: Innovation for Eco-Friendly Green Healthcare Solutions", which reflects her commitment to environmentally friendly healthcare solutions through sustainable nanomaterial innovations. Her academic and research interests focus on biology, biotechnology, and biomedical sciences. Anita can be reached via email at anitaraharjeng_uin@radenfatah.ac.id. She is also available on: ORCID: https://orcid.org/0000-0002-8308-4574 Scopus Author ID: 57219323981

Jayasri Rajkumar is a Biotechnology student at Vels University, specializing in microbiology, molecular biology, phytomedicine, and bioinformatics. With a strong interest in advanced molecular biology, Jayasri has also enhanced her understanding of computational tools in biotechnology through bioinformatics studies. Her academic journey is driven by a passion for bridging theoretical knowledge with hands-on experiences, aiming to contribute to the dynamic and growing biotechnology research and industry.

Ivo Romauld S. has a Ph.D in Biotechnology and is an Assistant Professor at Vels University.

Shilpa Rudra received her M.Sc Biotechnology from Pondicherry University, B.Sc from Calcutta University, and is currently pursuing her PhD in the department of Integrative Biology, SBST, VIT Vellore.

Meenamiga S. S. is an experienced Assistant Professor with a demonstrated history of working in the education management industry. Skilled in Lecturing, Protein Structure Prediction, Molecular & Cellular Biology, Cell Culture, and Mycology. Strong engineering professional with a Doctor of Philosophy - PhD focused in Mycology and drug discovery from Vels University.

Evika Sandi Savitri is a Lecturer and the Head of the Study Program at the Faculty of Science and Technology, UIN Maulana Malik Ibrahim Malang. She holds the academic rank of Senior Lecturer. Her research interests focus on plant structure and development, as well as plant biotechnology Evika earned her Bachelor's degree in Biology Department from Universitas Brawijaya (UB) Malang in 1999, followed by a Master's degree from the same university in 2003. She completed her Doctoral degree at Universitas Brawijaya, UB Malang in 2012. With her deep expertise in plant biotechnology, she has contributed significantly to her field of research and education. Evika can be contacted via email for further academic inquiries in evikasandi@bio.uin-malang.ac.id; Evika has been added as an author to this book chapter project due to her expertise in plant biology, particularly in the areas of plant structure and development and plant biotechnology. Her research background and academic leadership as the Head of the Biology Study Program at the Faculty of Science and Technology, UIN Maulana Malik Ibrahim Malang, bring a valuable perspective to the topic. Her inclusion is relevant if the book chapter addresses aspects of plant biology or tissue culture techniques, which are fundamental to advancements in areas such as sustainable agriculture, biotechnology, and eco-friendly solutions. As an experienced researcher and educator, Evika's contributions can help ensure the academic rigor and relevance of the content.

Ashline Shaji is a Ph.D. research scholar at Kerala Agricultural University, Thrissur. She graduated from Rani Lakshmi Bai Central Agricultural University,

Jhansi, Uttar Pradesh, India, and completed her post-graduation at Kerala Agricultural University, Thrissur, India. Her post-graduation research focused on wood anatomy, a core area of wood science, which deepened her passion for the field and shaped her as a dedicated wood anatomist. Her interest in material sciences led her to pursue a Ph.D. in composites. Currently, her research focuses on bio-based wood composites, contributing to the development of sustainable and innovative materials.

Girish Sharma has been a Professor & Dy. Centre Head, Centre for Medical Biotechnology, Amity Institute of Biotechnology; Coordinator – Amity Center for Cancer Epidemiology & Cancer Research. His area of Research Interest includes Cancer Chemoprevention, using both Natural & Synthetic compounds; Epidemiology of various Cancers (Hospital based Cancer Registry) including Breast, Childhood, Prostate, Gall Bladder Cancer etc.; Exploring new drugs and drug combinations, drug resistance mechanisms and targets (for cancer and other related diseases); Uro-oncology patient data compilation and analysis.

Mohsen Sheykhhasan is a Doctor of Philosophy and Assistant Professor at Qom University of Medical Science and Health Services.

Himani Shulka is affiliated with the MCA project at Microsystems Lab.

Adithya Raj U. is a Master's student at College of Forestry, Kerala Agricultural University, specializing in ecology and forest resource management. My research focuses on phytosociology and carbon sequestration in secondary and mature forests, forest fires, flora and faunal diversity in forest ecosystems. I have conducted studies on phytosociology and soil attributes in different forest landscapes. With expertise in remote sensing, GIS and web designing, I integrate technology with ecological research to support conservation efforts.

Muhammad Asad Ullah is a Lecturer in the department of Bio Medical Engineering at University of Engineering and Technology, Lahore, Narrowal Campus.

Tanmay J. Urs is a B.Sc. (Hons/Research) student of Medical Biotechnology at Amity University.

Gowthami V. is an accomplished researcher in nanotechnology, energy storage, and material science. She holds a Ph.D. in Physics from Alagappa University (2016), specializing in thin films and transition metal oxides for supercapacitors, gas sensors, and electrochromic devices. With over a decade of academic and research experience, she has served as an Assistant Professor and Head of Department at multiple institutions. Her extensive publications in high-impact journals focus on sustainable nanomaterials. A passionate educator and scientist, her groundbreaking research in green energy solutions makes her a top contender for the Best Researcher Award.

Thanush V. T. is a faithful BTech biotechnology student specialized in Insilico techniques and clinical pathology expert in docking softwares and have an experience in computer aided studies

Kosireddy Vanitha is a dedicated btech biotechnology student specializing in bioinformatics, clinical pathology, clinical laboratory techniques passionate about unraveling the genomic sequences and docking studies through different softwares, poised to revolutionalize computer studies

Treesa Varghese has a M. Sc. in Biochemistry, PhD. She has 13 years of teaching experience.

Meenupriya V. is a dedicated B. tech. biotechnology student, specialized in microbiological laboratory techniques, docking, molecular biology laboratory techniques and have an experience in computer aided studies.

Index

Symbols

A

B

C

D

O

P

R

S

T

W

www.ingramcontent.com/pod-product-compliance
Lightning Source LLC
LaVergne TN
LVHW080354011026
849161LV00009B/2304